AF770260

FUNCTIONAL ARCHITECTURE OF THE HUMAN MENTAL

A Reference Psychophysics Treatise of Human Mentation and its Disorders

Joseph J. Jean-Claude
Associate Laser Optics Engineer

Caroline Stamu-O'Brien, MD
Assistant Professor of Psychiatry
New York University

Worcester - USA

Publisher's Cataloging-in-Publication Data

Names: Jean-Claude, Joseph J., author. |O'Brien, Caroline Stamu, author.
Title: Functional architecture of the human mental: a reference psychophysics treatise of human mentation and its disorders/ Joseph J. Jean-Claude [and] Caroline Stamu O'Brien.
Description: Worcester, MA: Joseph J. Jean-Claude & Caroline Stamu O'Brien, 2021. | Includes bibliographical references and index.
Identifiers: ISBN 978-0-9647466-8-8
Subjects: LCSH: Psychology, Pathological. | Psychology. | Psychiatry. | Psychophysics. | Physics. | BISAC: PSYCHOLOGY/ Psychopathology / General. | PSYCHOLOGY/ General.| MEDICAL/ Psychiatry / General.
Classification: LCC RC489.P72J43 2021(print) | LCCRC489.P72 (ebook) | DDC 616.89/14--dc23.

©COPYRIGHT 2021

All rights reserved. Printed and bound in the United States of America. No part of this book may be reproduced or utilized in any form or by any means, electronic or mechanical, including photocopying, recording or by any information storage and retrieval system, without permission in writing from the publisher.

International Standard Book Number: 978-0-9647466-8-8

DISCLAIMER

This treatise was designed as a comprehensive source of information for mental health professionals, psychologists, psychiatrists, physicians, counselors, nurses, occupational and rehabilitation therapists, cognitive science researchers, as well as social workers and forensic/legal specialists. It is not intended in any way to provide information of any sort to mental health patients or the public in general. If you think you may be suffering from any medical or psychiatric condition, standard safety should always take precedence by seeking immediate opinion from your physician and/or mental health professionals. You should never delay seeking medical advice, disregard medical advice or discontinue medical treatment because of information in this treatise.

The material in this publication is not intended to prevent, treat, or cure any mental disorder therein discussed. When it comes to diagnosis of mental dysfunctions, interested professionals shall only use the content as an aid in consolidating or ascertaining a particular diagnosis or determination of a specific mental impairment. The authors make no representation of effectiveness and assertiveness of such diagnoses and cannot be held liable of any consequences thereof. This material should not be used in any legal capacity whatsoever, including but not limited to establishing "standard of care" in a legal sense or as a basis for expert witness testimony.

The views and opinions expressed in this book strictly represent the authors' views and opinions, and are not construed in any ways to imply endorsement by institutions the authors may be associated with. The book may only reproduce verbatim such endorsements when they are explicitly and directly expressed or formulated by authorized representatives of said institutions or organizations in their own writing.

In memory of my mother, Anatasie, who knew the deep waters of life and surely lived so much more in spirit than the flesh.

Joseph J. Jean-Claude

To my brother George, an intangible and everlasting bond.
To my parents who inspired me to study the art of medicine, and to reach for the sky.
In memory of Ronald R. Fieve, MD, pioneer of lithium therapy, who took me under his wing, and helped me unravel many mysteries of mind.

Caroline Stamu-O'Brien

PREFACE

The most important trend in the evolution of psychiatric medicine is its struggle to establish diagnostic and therapeutic standards based on the same level of empirical rigor and systematization as biological medicine, let alone the core physical sciences. This long-running quest is responsible for its departure from the organization of the science around and about psychoanalysis, ever since the emergence of the DSM-III in the United States of America, in favor of a preferential arrangement around psychotherapy based on neurochemical agents.

It is not a coincidence that arduous has been the fate of psychiatric medicine as a member of the science of the Mental, given the impenetrability of the Human Mind in the unrelenting quest to see the light inside of this black box. To that extent, the responsibility of psychiatric medicine is unique among the sciences, which the very Human Mind has incidentally developed in fashioning our way of life, our habitat and destiny.

The development of systematic methods inside of the science has faced many insider critics and criticisms since the release of DSM-III, all of which must be understood in terms of own stirs inside of science of the Mental seeking to unleash needed improvements in practice and theoretical representations. Of course, one should also understand the societal pressures of many different orders external to psychiatry onto its proceedings in terms of inevitable currents.

Those criticisms are indeed many. Psychologists, whose primary motivations are the inquest for towering representations that help fully elucidate the transactions of the Mind and gain insight into the bewildering diversity of clinical cases confronting their practice, have grown increasingly dissatisfied with the diagnostic and classificatory solutions proposed by the DSM. The Society for Humanistic Psychology — a division of the American Psychological Association — turned very counter and vocal against DSM-5 in 2015 with the charge of a dangerous broadening of the definition of many mental disorders therein. They believed it could lead to deleterious overtreatment with pharmaceuticals. Further, psychologists want more than a flat recitation of symptoms for every disease. In effect, a disease model that can finally elucidate the root mentation or biological causes of mental dysfunctions, establish clear, unequivocal and objective lines of demarcation between normalcy and abnormality, while remaining consistent with and pegged to a characterological or personality model, has always faltered in psychopathology, despite the DSM many revisions.

Even the then chair of the former DSM-IV, Dr Allan Frances, was among the critics in 2013 at the release of DSM-5, starkly assessing that *"APA's approval of DSM-5 was the "saddest moment" in my lengthy career of studying, practicing, and teaching psychiatry... the revision was "deeply flawed" and contained a number of changes that seemed "clearly unsafe and scientifically unsound."* A former president of the American Psychiatric Association (APA), Dr John Talbott, professor emeritus of psychiatry at the University of Maryland's School of Medicine, was also compelled to join the critics and had this to say to the clinical community: *"If you let the specifics of the DSM tie you down, it prevents you from practicing the art of medicine. So I would hope people would not be bound by it but be flexible and use their clinical judgment instead."*

An institutional reaction took place in the incarnation of the Research Domain Criteria initiative (RDoC) at the **National Institute of Mental Health** (USA) which also sought to lay down an avenue of resolution to the deficiencies historically hampering psychiatric medicine. Effectively, for one, there does not exist any universally accepted prevalence figure for the vast majority of psychiatric disorders, a major deficiency in any science. On another hand, psychiatric diagnoses have not been traditionally based on pure scientific criteria but incorporate factors or preventions of social, legal and historical nature. One could argue that it is not for psychiatry to care for these concerns but for these other venues to take the raw and rigorous determinations from psychiatric science as is and to their own effects. So it runs in the core sciences. Further, the mapping between the functional anatomy of the nervous system and the hierarchy of mental disorders has never been properly addressed, let alone the sought-after relationship between the chromosomal genetic basis and the hierarchy of mental disorders. Effectively, if mental disorders are not normalized etiologically as they naturally occur, it will not be possible to find or delimit their systematic chromosomal genetic basis, since nature is manifestly not disparate, disjoint or chaotic.

Dr. Thomas R. Insel, then director of the National Institute of Mental Health (NIMH), held for a short while the personal critical position that DSM-5 suffered from a *"lack of validity"* and that NIMH should *"stop funding research projects relying exclusively on DSM-5 criteria."* The position was institutionally untenable and NIMH later released a joint statement with the APA pointing out that *"the DSM represents the best information currently available for clinical diagnosis of mental disorders. Patients, families, and insurers can be confident that effective treatments are available and that the DSM is the key resource for delivering the best available care."* Ever since psychiatry turned to neurochemical agents for therapy, the focus in psychiatry, hence the DSM tool, has turned to the prescription of safe drugs, exempt from deleterious side effects, and for good reasons. It is important to recognize that, historically, this tool has come to be developed not to promote scientific research, since it was not based on clinical research, but to respond to pressing clinical demands from the ailing population.

RDoC is probably best tailored, in our view, to support research that can advance the field in its long unsolved quests and feed back onto the DSM tool to improve the taxonomy and etiologies of psychopathology. To that aim, this treatise exposes research that brings the rigor of the core physical sciences incarnated in psychophysics and a constellation of etiological categories, under the umbrella of a new towering architecture of the Human Mental, to the effective elucidation of these long-running pressing challenges in psychiatry. Our ambition with this new reference treatise is to help overcome the current impasse in psychiatric science, and provide the clinical community one more tool for its arsenal in the task of unraveling and probing the depths of the Human Mental. It is our hope that clinicians will make best and copious use of it.

TABLE OF CONTENTS

Chapter 1

PSYCHOPHYSICAL FOUNDATIONS OF THE HUMAN MENTAL

One of the goals of this treatise is to undertake a decisive effort in approaching the Human Mental from a mathematical-physics formalism in order to definitively restrict studies of the Mental in any branch of the field from further unwarranted and unproductive speculations, as well-intentioned as they may be. We develop this psychophysics effort within the theoretical framework offered by the **Quanto-Geometric Theory (QGT)**, an innovative physical science formalism which has successfully addressed developments in both the Quantum realm of matter and the larger-scale universal arena, the latter generally taken to be the object of the Theories of Relativity in physics. In particular, QGT has been able to theoretically compute from first principles a slew of fundamental physical constants, a long-time expected achievement in fundamental physics, but never before delivered by any other theoretical body. We equally hope to successfully put the Quanto-Geometric canon and its numeric prescriptions at work to implant and uphold, once and for all, the formal psychophysics approach to the study of the Human Mental. It is important to recognize that we not only offer formal mathematical description of mental categories but advance an application consistently covering the spectrum of mental analytic exegesis within the theoretical boundaries of QGT.

1.1 Philosophical Views of the Mental Through Consciousness

In philosophy, mind is generally set to equate consciousness, since both Western and Eastern philosophies do not offer a clear distinction between the two notions. René Descartes' ideas about mind had been instrumental in shaping formal visualizations of the entity in particular in the West. He was convinced that the body and conscious mind are two different substances, with the first made of matter and the second being of an immaterial nature. Today's neuroscience, however, has widely adopted the viewpoint that our brains give rise to consciousness.

How the duo mind-matter works together is at the heart of what philosopher David Chalmers at New York University termed the *"hard problem"* of consciousness: how can physical networks of neurons produce experiences that appear to be exogenous to the material world? Despite the evocation of neurons or neural networks in the assertion, this approach to the question remains of a strictly philosophical nature. It is not epistemic either because its ambition is to solve the problem at once, but not to analyze proposed solutions. Many opposing philosophers and neuroscientists counterargue that the hard problem of consciousness as posed by D. Chalmers is simply a faux problem -- *"It's an unsolvable mystery, because the problem is ill posed."* advances neuroscientist Michael Graziano of Princeton University. His argument hinges on the view, as he further argues, that consciousness is nothing but a trick of the mind, with no substance of its own.

Despite a plethora of developments for the last hundred years including the more recent ones, Philosophy has inarguably been unable to resolve the question of the Mental in the least amount and stands far from holding the ultimate word on the representations of mind and consciousness. To say the least, Philosophy of mind has hitherto remained utterly speculative, unable to render a consistent and, most importantly, integral framework for apprehension of the Mind phenomenon.

1.2 Pre-Requisites for a Successful Approach to Consciousness

Everything seems to point in the direction that Mind or Consciousness is real because so much in terms of the manipulation of the natural world can be realized through them. On that account, there should be at least:

1. A successful philosophical approach to it.
2. A successful psychological approach to it.
3. A successful mathematical-physics approach to it.

Even in the surmise that Mind or Consciousness is a trick, one must agree that it is no less phenomenological because we experience it as endowed with structure and systematic operation. For instance, the current writing is a systematic product of mind. The only compelling warrant of adequacy in the proposed 3-tier approach to the question of Mind (meaning that which is true to nature) and promise of falsification or verifiability is for a Theory of Mind to tap into mathematical resources or mathematical logic as a foundation. We have seen that much of the psychological approach, which was always a piggy back on the neurologic approach since J. M. Charcot at La Salpêtrière hospital in the 1800's, has proved unable to eradicate surmises and conjectures in the science of Mind. Neural science itself remains largely speculative in its main propositions which are functional interpretations of behavior.

Furthermore, a consistent and assertive philosophy of Mind must tightly connect to psychology in that it must naturally yield the known forms of mental or personality dysfunctions, as known in psychiatry and neurology, as well as a direct understanding of or model for human characterology. From there, it must come to a rigorous mathematical-physics formulation, final stage of the science of Mind.

It may well be that this 3-tier approach will not be given along a timeline or even in different theoretical bodies, but in a single Theory. So it is because the final Theory must be consistent across the possible different rubriques of elaboration. Next to other possible contributions along that line, this treatise ambitions to precisely offer a single Theory, the Quanto-Geometric Theory of Mind, to deliver this outcome. The philosophical components of the Theory are already exposed elsewhere[1]. This treatise will concentrate on the elements of the 2nd and 3rd tier in the proposed psychophysics approach to Mind.

One may note that in the common discussions taking place in neuroscience and philosophy about Mind, the psychological contributions brought about by Analytic Psychology are rarely examined and properly dimensioned in terms of an overarching architecture of Mind. Perhaps there have not been enough inferences made from Analytic Psychology toward Philosophy of Mind to this day, in order to apportion that towering and thorough comprehension of the mind phenomenon at best insight.

1.3 Human Cognition and Representations

Every science of the mental understandably attempts to construct its own differentiated lexicon. Early neurology and psychology did not dwell on a representation for the notion of cognition, which has come to play an important role in today's cognitive science. This notion is not necessarily equivalent to consciousness in its essence and focuses on the meaning of what a knowable in the mind is. Let's consider for a moment the sentence *"I know that your first name is Peter"*. The most common way for us to know somebody's name first hand is for that person to tell us his/her name in an acquaintance. In a physical encounter, that equates to a single representation or registering in one's mind the image and voice of that person telling us his/her name. Stress the word *representation*. We may define a representation to be the perception, singular or composite, of an object or event, tangible or intangible, which we may otherwise call a *percept*. Once I have registered this percept in my mind, I think I am in full right to say I think *I know that his name is Peter*.

Note that this recognition does not require any pre-registered imagery of event about that person in my mind or anything else - (in which case cognition would be a function of memory) - for me to have gained cognizance of him and his name. From that one single event, I am in full right to say ***"I know him."***

---

[1] Quanto-Geometry, Overture of Cosmic Consciousness and Universal Knowledge for All, Vol I & II.

Perception is not always fully internalized, i.e. when we have our attention focused elsewhere, whatever we perceive with our senses does not fully resonate internally. In that situation, should we happen to have heard spoken words from someone, you might say in that case, as we commonly do, those words have fallen on deaf ears. It is only when attention/volition is focused on perception (or specific perception) that a perception automatically becomes cognition, which then may or may not incite a reaction. There is no intermediacy between perception and cognition in terms of a gradation course, associative or deliberative cogitations, or even memorized patterns, but **only** the intervention of the attention/volition function as a conveyor. A *percept* is thus a *cognos*.

In recalling the notion of consciousness, which is a common concept throughout the sciences of Mind, we must further agree that every conscious being must necessarily *know* or *be cognizant* that he or she is conscious. If being conscious is experiencing at once willpower/attention, motivation and sensations, we are necessarily *aware* of exercising these mental qualities because it is virtually impossible to miss perceiving our own behavior under these faculties. Therefore the state of *awareness* or *cognizance* must be part of being conscious.

1.4 Is the Human Mind Lodged in Neural Structures and Networks?

Many in today's neuroscience may ignore that the decade of the 1990's had been officially declared **Decade of the Brain**, with the hopes that this puzzle would have been then finally unraveled. The decade came and went by, no breakthrough was announced at its term and the puzzle remained as whole as ever. The majority of researchers in neural science have historically posited the putative truism that Consciousness or Mind is or must be a product of the Brain. In that manner, they avail themselves outright for the latter the kind of empirical experimentation traditionally undertaken in science. The view that fuses Mind and Brain has been dubbed *monism* in neural science.

Aside from real-time imaging of blood flow throughout the brain, the investigative methods in use in neural science are generally based on lesions, deficient neuron metabolism, neuron degeneration, all tracked to be associated with observation of particular functional impairments and observable effects in behavior. For instance, the US *National Institute of Health (NIH)* reports the following:

"In patients with neurodegenerative disease, several studies have suggested that impaired self-awareness is ***related to*** *right prefrontal hypometabolism or atrophy, specifically in ventromedial or orbitofrontal regions, though the precise anatomical basis for this phenomenon is* ***still unclear****.*

The suppression of pathways to neural impulses is another method used in neuroscience to investigate behavioral or physiological functions. In that sense, the NIH exposition continues:

"Impaired self-awareness is a common, though not homogenous phenomenon among patients with neurodegenerative diseases. Patients with different diseases ***may exhibit*** *impaired self-awareness at different time points in the disease course, show distinct patterns of preserved and impaired awareness for different deficits, and exhibit divergent degree of impaired self-awareness. Patients with behavioural variant frontotemporal dementia (FTD) characteristically show early, severe lack of awareness of their behavioural and personality decline, and sometimes their cognitive deficits...*

Numerous models have been ***proposed to explain*** *the cognitive processes underlying impaired self-awareness in individuals with neuropsychological deficits. Some have emphasized the involvement of domain-specific processes, such as perception of sensory input, episodic memory, verbal abilities, or executive control mechanisms. Other models suggest the involvement of additional, domain-general mechanisms, such as a conscious-awareness system and comparator mechanisms (McGlynn and Schacter, 1989; Schacter, 1990; Agnew and Morris, 1998). According to these influential models, impaired self-awareness may result from domain-specific dysfunctions of perceptual or episodic memory abilities, preventing 'registration' of one's decreased functioning into one's long-term memory. Additionally, impaired self-awareness may reflect domain-general failures, either due to generally diminished consciousness, or due to failure or disconnection of attentional mechanisms responsible for comparing recently registered self-related information with previous self-knowledge (Agnew and Morris, 1998). Recent models additionally point out the role of motivational and emotional factors (Rosen, 2011)...*

The neuroanatomical basis for self-awareness has been examined by various study paradigms, and direct investigation of ***brain-behaviour correlations*** *sheds some light on the various neuropsychological models. Lesion studies demonstrated that impaired awareness for motor deficits is more related to right hemisphere injuries (Babinski, 1914; Belyi, 1987; Schmitz et al., 2006). Correspondingly, there is more anosognosia for hemiplegia after right Wada test-induced inactivation (Adair et al., 1995). In right lesion patients, anosognosia for hemiplegia and neglect is related to dorsal premotor and primary motor cortices, dorsolateral prefrontal cortex (PFC), and the insula (Berti et al., 2005). Imaging studies involving patients accordingly demonstrated the importance of frontal lobes in self-awareness. Inaccurate self-appraisal in traumatic injury patients is related to reduced medial PFC glucose metabolism (Fontaine et al., 1999), and unawareness of symptoms in schizophrenic patients is related to bilateral dorsolateral PFC atrophy (Flashman et al., 2001). Self-evaluation accuracy is related to anterior dorsolateral PFC activation, particularly on the right, in traumatic injury patients as well as healthy participants (Schmitz et al., 2006). Functional neuroimaging studies with healthy participants correspondingly demonstrate increased right dorsolateral PFC activation during self-referential appraisal tasks (Fossati et al., 2003; Schmitz et al., 2004). Other studies propose that self-referential processing depends on activation of bilateral cortical midline structures (Johnson et al., 2002; Northoff et al., 2006; Schmitz and Johnson, 2007). Neuroimaging studies also emphasize the role of the anterior insula in self-awareness (Berti et al., 2005; Schmitz and Johnson, 2007; Craig, 2009)...*

Neurodegenerative diseases cause progressive, characteristic patterns of decline in various functional domains. The affected domains vary across diseases, and patients may present with a decline in activities of everyday living, motor, cognitive, social-interpersonal or emotional abilities, depending on the regions of atrophy. While many neurological conditions impact some aspects of functioning, patients with different diseases have varying ability to recognize their impairments (Prigatano, 2009; Zamboni and Wilcock, 2011). Lack of self-awareness for neurological impairments such as cortical blindness (Anton, 1898) and hemiplegia has historically been termed 'anosognosia' (Babinski, 1914), a term later used to describe lack of awareness for other more subtle neurological impairments such as cognitive and behavioural deficits (McGlynn and Schacter, 1989). The term 'impaired self-awareness' refers to the inability to accurately estimate one's functional capacity (Prigatano, 2009)."

These are typical analytic examples from the investigative methods in use in neuroscience which tend to blindly credit neural structures and networks with the ownership of human consciousness. Note, however, that no direct cause-effect relationship pertaining to fundamental logic is evoked, but correlations, conditional correlations and hypothetical functional models to that effect. Incidentally, by virtue of that trend, up to the decade of the 1990's, just about almost every structure in the brain gradually became part of the so-called *limbic system!*

It seems that the most sensible and logical interpretation of experimental outcomes in neuroscience to date is that Mind and Brain ***may be two different*** products which nevertheless ***work together***. How they intersect, harmonize and resonate with one another would be a logical consequence, albeit a quite mysterious affair on that account as well.

1.5 Evidence of Dichotomy between Mind and Brain

Against the backdrop of neural science's monist view that the biological Brain lodges the Mind, one important study that has not received the deserved level of attention in the science is the aging relationship between Brain and Mind. Is an aging Brain necessarily associated with an aging Mind, or is an aging Mind a direct function of an aging Brain?

1.5.1 Disparity between Aging Brain and Cognitive Decline of Aging Mind

The monist will thus also have to explain the following paradox: while our brain ages, just as any other histological formation in our human bodies (the strength of homeostasis in our bodies declines as we age), our mental faculties, however, do not exactly follow the same aging process. Why do our minds not appear to age or do not age concomitantly with our aging brains?

Our bodies change in noticeable ways as we age over the life course. Our hair grays out, our skin winkles and, along with our muscles, loses elasticity as joints and muscles stiffen up. Just as those histological changes occur outside of the nervous system altogether, so does the nervous system itself, albeit in more subtle ways. Cognitive decline may begin after age 30 but becomes definitely more and more pronounced starting midlife and into age 70, 80 and 90 successively (Aartsen, et al., 2002). *"... Relatively little decline in cognitive performance occurs until about age 50."* (Albert & Heaton, 1988). While these facts are well known in neural science, the monist perspective generally thwarts the correct interpretation of their peculiarities in persistently conflating Mind with Brain. If we heed the data in terms of highly intelligible functions attributable to the Mental v. more neurologic or nervous aspects of the same, we find a notable distinction between aging of the Brain and that of the Mental. Below is a summary of the facts known about brain aging.

1.5.1.1 Negative Aging Changes

1. *Decline in Declarative Memory (autobiographical memory of life events and accumulated knowledge of learned facts and information) — Registering new information to memory and recalling names and numbers may take longer.*
2. *Decline in Working or Accumulative memory (ability to hold a piece of information in mind, such as a phone number or the location of a parked vehicle).*
3. *Fluid intelligence, such as processing speed and problem-solving, also decrease with age.*
4. *Certain aspects of attention can become more difficult.*
5. *Splitting our focus between two tasks (i.e. holding a conversation while driving) becomes more challenging with age. This type of attention is called divided attention.*
6. *Selective attention diminishes (ability to tune out distractions and focus on a particular stimulus).*
7. *Accentuated synaptic decline along with neuron structural and chemical decline with aging. Also decline in neurogenesis (ability of the Brain to produce more neurons).*

1.5.1.2 Positive Cognitive Changes While Aging

1. *Procedural memories like remembering how to drive, ride a bike, dress up or tie a shoe remain largely intact.*
2. *Better performance on tests of verbal abilities in middle age, per the* Seattle Longitudinal Study, *which tracked the cognitive abilities of thousands of adults over the past 50 years.*
3. *Performed better at spatial reasoning. For instance most known Supreme Court judges, in general having attained their late years in life*

(age 80 is common), are still able to produce brilliant pieces of constitutional logic in jurisprudence.

4. *Performed better at math.*
5. *Performed better at abstract reasoning in middle age than they did when they were young adults.*
6. *Growing evidence that we are perfectly able to learn new things throughout the entire course of life.*
7. *There are always those elders in the population that still qualify as super-achievers in old age (superagers). Late studies indicate that one fifth of septuagenarians perform cognitive tests just as well as their 20-year-old counterparts, and pinpoint the existence of individuals over age 80 with memory as sharp as a 20-30 year old.*

What the above tells us is that the overall histological and physiological capacities of the Brain along with certain mnemonic functions decline with aging of the latter, while the vast majority of cognitive and intellectual functions, including certain aspects of memory, either remain unaltered or improve. In the negative performance rubrique, we must stress the following important adjustments to interpretation:

1. *Memory is a function of sense organs inasmuch as they register afferent information at first instance of treatment. The decline in the strength and vigor of perceptions through the perception channels, caused by their own aging, will necessarily affect their imprint in the mnemonic reservoir, whether it is centralized or distributed.*
2. *The decline in the vigor of anatomic perception channels will also negatively impact attention capacity and thus ability to execute tasks.*
3. *Intellectual capacity tends to remain with those who used to exercise it throughout their life course, just as muscles' elasticity is a function of their continued use (use it or lose it). Therefore an elderly person who uses to be much more manually handy than intellectual in his/her lifetime occupation should not be expected to demonstrate intellectual agility.*

The minimal logical conclusions admissible from the above considerations altogether are the following:

1. *A function of a mathematical nature must be found to support the truism claim that aging of the Brain in histological and physiological terms*

causes aging of the Mind in terms of decline in cognitive capacity, such that:

$B = f(M) = k \cdot M$, *where* B *is Brain age,* M *is cognitive ability and* k *a proportionality constant as a real number different than 0 or positive definite (* $k \in R^+$ *).*

2. *The known facts do not support a direct linear proportionate relation between aging of the Brain and aging of the Mind, since late Brain age may correspond to high cognitive capacity.*
3. *If the function is non-linear, as it ought to be in this case according to the diverse facts, then there are other intervening factors that create the non-linearity such as a square, a root, etc., possibly in provenance of other variables or phenomal dimensions different than the time variable inherent to aging.*

We must forcibly conclude that there is indeed a large disparity between aging brain and cognitive decline of an aging mind. Despite the use of the term aging, what we have just studied is indeed not an evolution in time on both sides of the equation but a physical (or psychopshysical) phase correlation between the two tenets.

1.5.2 Phylogenetic Perspective of Biological Evolution Invalidates Monism

Whilst the notions of Mind, Consciousness and Cognition do not appear to have yet received in current literature a *physical* definition that confers them a particular ontological connotation, they have more or less been hitherto interchangeable terms for the same experience of mindfulness in phenomenology, notwithstanding our preliminary discussion attempting to frame Cognition. Much of what the Mind "box" or Mental Body creates is inarguably observable in behavior or phenomenology, in particular its sensation and motivation products, through specialized anatomic effectors and receptors. It is fair to say that this descriptor takes the like of a framework for the living at large as represented in the concept of model organism adopted in experimental Biology.

1.5.3 Many Protists Show Animal-like Intelligent Behavior in Phenomenology

A model organism in Biology is a non-human species destined to extensive dedicated studies in order to explain particular biological phenomena, with the expectation that it will help gain further insight in ontology and phenomenology of more complex organisms, notably humans. Many model organisms have been adopted, among them the protist ***Euglena***, which is a monocellular eukaryote. Its cellular configuration and bio-chemical processes are expected to provide more insight into the same in higher organisms such as plants and humans.

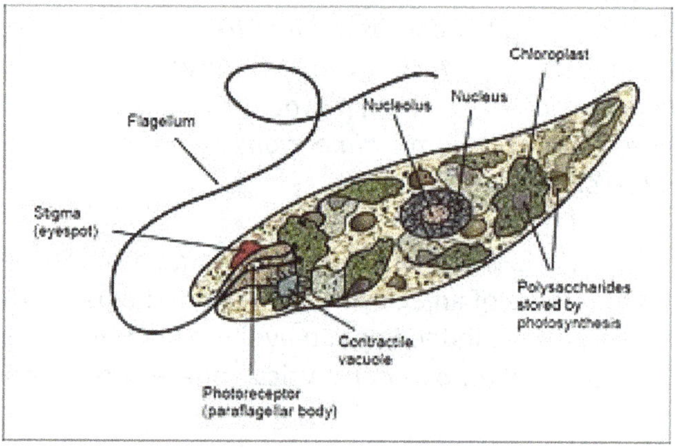

Fig. 1.1 Transverse cut of a Euglena protist

Euglena individuals have two flagella rooted in basal bodies located in a small reservoir at the front of the cell. Typically, one flagellum is very short and does not protrude from the cell, while the other is long enough to be seen under a light microscope and may be even longer than the cell body. The surface of the long emergent flagellum bears a coating of roughly 30,000 extremely fine filaments (Fig. 1.1). These organisms use the long flagella to swim through the liquid medium where they live in colonies.

The variant ***Euglena gracilis*** has secondary chloroplasts, thrives as a so-called mixotroph since it is able to feed both by photosynthesis and phagocytosis. In phagocytosis, a portion of the very flexible cell membrane invaginates like a mouth and locks the prey to form a food bowl that detaches from the membrane and travels into the cytoplasm. In addition, all *Euglenae* possess a red eyespot organelle composed of carotenoid pigment granules. While the red eyespot is not photosensitive, it filters sunlight that comes to fall on a light-detecting structure (paraflagellar body) at the base of the flagellum, allowing only particular wavelengths of light to pass through. As the cell rotates with respect to the light source, the eyespot partially blocks the source, so permitting the *Euglena* to detect the direction of the light source toward which it moves for more bathing (phototaxis). When the living medium is full of nutrients and light is plentiful, *Euglena* kicks off its reproduction mechanisms to deliver more of its kindred to the world in best living conditions. Whereas in low moisture conditions, or when food is scarce, *Euglena* forms a protective wall around itself and honkers down to lie dormant as a resting cyst until living conditions improve again.

Therefore, the least that the research analyst is able to conclude from this phenomenological framework is that *Euglena* displays a broad and precise level of ***understanding*** in how to interact with its living medium from the point of view of developing adequate metabolic and reproductive activity for successful living, metabolism and reproduction being the two fundamental components of Life. In addition, many of the biological phenoma that this organism implements, such as feeding through a mouth or invagination, using a flagellum for displacement or swimming, vision through eyespots for spatial orientation, are precursors in geometry of comparable ontological elements in display in the higher multicellular organisms we call animals[2].

Consequently, it is incumbent on the monist neuroscientist to present evidence that Euglena **does not experience the mindfulness** of comprehension, self-interest and integrated cognition, despite the many ontological and phenomenological traits it presents in common with higher forms of the living endowed with a central nervous system. So the monist ought to explain, on the basis of what we can see of Euglena in terms of duly witnessed behavior:

1. Why it would be that she does not feel?
2. Why it would be that she does not want?

---

[2] In Volume III of the series **Quanto-Geometry**, author Jean-Claude J. exposes an extensive development concerning the biogeometric foundations of Phylogenetic evolution.

3. Why she does not feel happy when she finds that which she wants or desires?
4. Why she would not feel unhappy when she cannot find what she wants or desires?

Answers to these questions are necessary not because we arbitrarily pose or impose them but because in fundamental logic if you cannot directly prove a predicament, you ought to at least prove it through the method of *reductio ad absurdum*, which is what these interrogations represent as formulated. Yet it remains utterly difficult to construe the set of facts known about this ***living*** model organism as simple mechanical responses of a machine to the conditions of the environment. We are keenly confronted with that predicament, should we consent to the clear similarities between the ontological definitions borne out of Euglena's body with observable phenomenological responses and those developed in animals like humans. In any case, the differences do not seem to pertain to the order of quality but quantity as relates to the number of effectors and receptors involved. Everything considered, the final question the monists ought to unequivocally answer is: why even in the absence of a biochemical structure surrogating animals' nervous system this ***living*** monocellular model organism displays evidence of mindfulness in terms comprehension, self-interest and integrated cognition?

1.5.4 Cognition without a Nervous System Exists Among the Living

The challenge of finding among the living a conscious or mindful entity which does not rely even remotely on something akin to an incipient brain or a rudimentary nervous system of sorts for cognition seems to be a good one to take on, in order to irrevocably depose the monist case or attitude.

A fact that has been very much long under-appreciated or muted among neuroscientists is the implication of the existence and anatomy of these animals called sponges belonging to the genus *Spongia*. They live under the ocean waters in about 6000 different species pertaining to the genus. Paradoxically, these animals are brainless and present no nervous system whatsoever, not even individual nerve cells; yes, zilch!

However, sponges do exhibit physiognomic **sensori-motor reactions**! Now, if a minimal sensori-motor reaction is not the beginning of consciousness or cognition, we will have to redefine cognition in neuroscience and throw away everything we learned since Cajal and Charcot about the nervous system and its functional anatomy.

A brief review of the anatomy and physiology of sponges throughout their life cycle is pertinent and immediately follows. They are multicellular organisms in their own right. However, they lack organs and histological organization akin to those of most other animals. Nevertheless, they present specialized groups of cells which perform the necessary vital functions. Some of these cells are in charge of digestion, some others are responsible for reproduction, yet others are in charge of circulation bringing water into the system so the organism can innerly feed through filtering. Other groups of cells specialize in getting rid of wastes resulting from digestion.

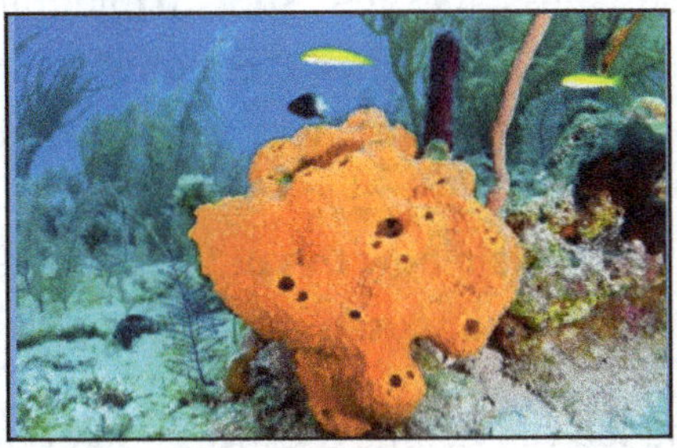

Fig. 1.2 A sponge in its underwater habitat.

Sponges present a wide variety of shapes or physiognomy, some featuring a cluster of tubules that may reach a dozen meters in height (Fig. 1.2). Part of their diet are bacteria and organic matter which they seize by actively drawing water in through pores denoted ostia. Along the channels in these pores lie collar cells, with their collars surrounding a hair-like structure designated a flagellum. The flagella beat to create water currents. Most sponges are carnivorous and also feed on many small organisms just brought in by the water. A few other species very actively engage in carnivorous behavior by using their spicules to capture prey such as small crustaceans.

Sponges feature prolific methods of reproduction, in both the sexual and asexual capacities. Sexual reproduction occurs through the production of eggs and sperm. In some species, these gametes are from the same individual making them hermaphrodites. In other species, heterosexuality assigns certain individuals with the production of eggs and others the production of spermatozoids in sperm. Water currents mediate fertilization by bringing the male and female gametes into the inner body of the organism for reunion. A larva is then formed, which in this phase will maintain a life of swimming around the water all by itself. At the end of this life cycle phase, the larva settles on a substrate to which it becomes attached for the remainder of its lifetime for growth and development.

Is it not quite remarkable that the above-depicted entire sum of ontology and phenomenology as developed by this organism can be thoroughly accomplished without a single nerve cell, let alone the layout of a nervous system, central or autonomous? If purposefulness may at all sum up mindfulness or simply cognition as captured in the notion of function, the monist neuroscientist must explain why this particular form of mindfulness is patently not based on the functional distribution inherent to the histology of the common animal nervous system. The monist must also explain how this peculiar implementation of mind and matter is realized, with matter putatively creating Mind.

This implementation indeed represents the inception of the animal form of the living. Could one of the deepest and most important secrets of life unsuspectingly lie therein? While it is incontrovertibly accepted that the genus *spongia* represents the first sprout of the living in the animal form, we do not know of any individual of the genus to have received the stature of a model organism in neuroscience. So it must have been, if a model must contain the very primeval baselines that profile posterior developments to be of express interest for scrutiny. In fact, beyond the question of the nervous system, the foundational precursors of histological organization of the living in its animal form are cast therein. It is regrettable that this vector has never been perceived and granted due attention in Biology.

1.6 The Mental as a Physical Entity in Itself

Once we are able to firmly visualize a decoupling of the Mental from the nervous system as discussed above, we free ourselves up for a more genuine examination of the Mental in its composition and operation.

Effectively, the question of whether or not the brain can define Mind or consciousness is well warranted. The search to define consciousness as a product of the brain almost amounts in a way to the brain taking on itself to define consciousness. Do we really want our brain to define consciousness for us or do we want to define it out of our own abstract Sense of Conscious Self? It is paramount to realize the de facto difference between these two propositions.

Should we want the brain to define human consciousness, we find ourselves in the predicament of having to uncover in the brain something like a *Rosetta stone* that extols the defining clues to consciousness, since it probably could not develop mentation as a whole without a program. We have not found this program after over two centuries of investigation and over two millenia of pondering. Nor do we have experience of our brains telling us (Conscious Self) anything in any form of communication, *whereas we do have experience of our Abstract Selves examining the brain itself and acting on it through intelligence*. The brain cannot objectivize the Mind, whereas the Mind is fully able to objectivize the brain. The Mind is capable of objectivizing not only the brain but uncannily itself as well, as we all know, through introspection.

Therefore all explicit definitions of Mind or Consciousness must come from the Abstract Sense of Conscious Self regarding itself (or itself as the object of the definition) and it will automatically be a working definition in the act, whether it is optimal or not. In that way, the question of whether Consciousness originates from the brain or not is immaterial to the investigation and does not require any cooperation from the brain for such, not even recourse to the act of examining the structures of the Brain!

We do not bother to wonder why such magic is even possible, we pragmatically realize that it is, because the Conscious self is aware of itself, fully endowed as it is with the magic of introspection and, in the social context, intelligentsia (social or collective insight). The Abstract Self can assuredly acquire knowledge of itself, of its own abstraction, that is. In the abstraction of Consciousness, there is Anatomy, Structure and Dynamics, per our own copious experience. No one should ever claim that these specific definitions of the properties of Consciousness do not exist towards an overall definition and study of consciousness, and pretend that Consciousness is a nebular, amorphous phenoma. No less than the monist proposition, such a claim is vacuous because, for one, on account of that nebula their proponents might as well claim that they don't have any consistent Conscious Self themselves, and for the other, it is indeed out of the exercise of a structured and dynamic Consciousness that they can even make the strange claim that they think they lack one or a formed one.

The quest by the Mind to understand the Mind represents the very human cognos attempting to profile the definitions subtending its own proceedings. In the undertaking, the inquisitive cognos automatically gains the distance normally required between object and subject to make this analytic feat possible. This represents an undeniable objective dimension of Mind which makes the proceedings of Mind underlying awareness permeable to individual insight and intelligentsia. The Mind or Mental Body is flexible enough to allow for self-reflection (reflection taken as both mirror duplication and ponderation), which is achieved in a form of detachment from own awareness, emotions and motivations. Introspection or the knowledge of self entirely develops through that analytic capacity whereas, through direct observation of the kindred, one can find an objective path to the broad study of Mind generically in its human dimension, conformally to how one experiences one's own. This is how all Theories of Mind have emerged for the most part. Consequently, it is clear that as the Mind breaks itself into subject and object, it is poised to acquire legitimate knowledge of itself.

All in all, the very minimal definition of Mind or Consciousness is the notion of *Me* or *I*. And anytime we step outside of the Conscious Self to say or think *You, He, She, We* or *They,* we make a recognition that that which is in us by which we say *I* or *Me* is also within our kindred, as an extension of the representation of Self. These are implicit workings of Consciousness or Mind because it enjoys its own degree of freedom in autonomy and absence of immanent physical dependency. This absence of inner physical dependency is very clear in such properties as imagination or logical analysis. In all, the human Mind does behave as an independent body, consistent with the traditional representation of the Mental Body in psychology and psychiatry. Its intangibility does not make it completely unphysical. We will later discuss what that exactly means from a psychophysics approach.

1.7 Psychology as a Disincarnate Cognitive Science

It is by virtue of the veracity of the above views that S. Freud was able to depart from his tutor, Jean-Martin Charcot, influential founder of worldwide notoriety of the science of neurology, to cast the revolutionary bases of the new science of Analytic Psychology (Fig. 1.3). S. Freud created the science of Psychology by visualizing the functional categories that must be proper to the Mental on its own, having witnessed the behavioral manifestations of the Mental in deep dysfunction at La Salpêtrière under Charcot.

Many important contributions were brought about since inception of the science by other influential thinkers such as Carl G. Jung, Alfred Adler, John B. Watson, Pierre Janet, Jean Piaget, etc., who continued to visualize a disincarnate Mental Body of its own and a broad spectrum of its transactions. Of course such developments never had the favor of the larger public because, for one, they uncovered the deep motivations of human behavior, both in the mundane and moral order, and, for the other, such heed is hopeless until the citizenry falls prey to mental dysfunctions of more or less severe morbidity. The schism inside the science over time between the analytic stream of Freudian origin and the behavioral stream of Pavlovian inspiration, must remain segregated from the larger monism problem of neural dependency or origin of Mind.

The relationship between neural anatomy and the Mental Body with its own transactions is of course a very narrow one and remains the foundation and justification of Psychiatry as a branch of medicine that unites neurology to psychology. However, it has not been able to date to spell out the seminal nature of this important relationship. Furthermore, it is on account of the monist problem that Psychiatry today is still based on empirical pharmacotherapy with psychopharmacological agents discovered by serendipity for the most part as well as significant problems in disease classification and etiology, despite the enormous services it has rendered to public health worldwide since its inception.[3]

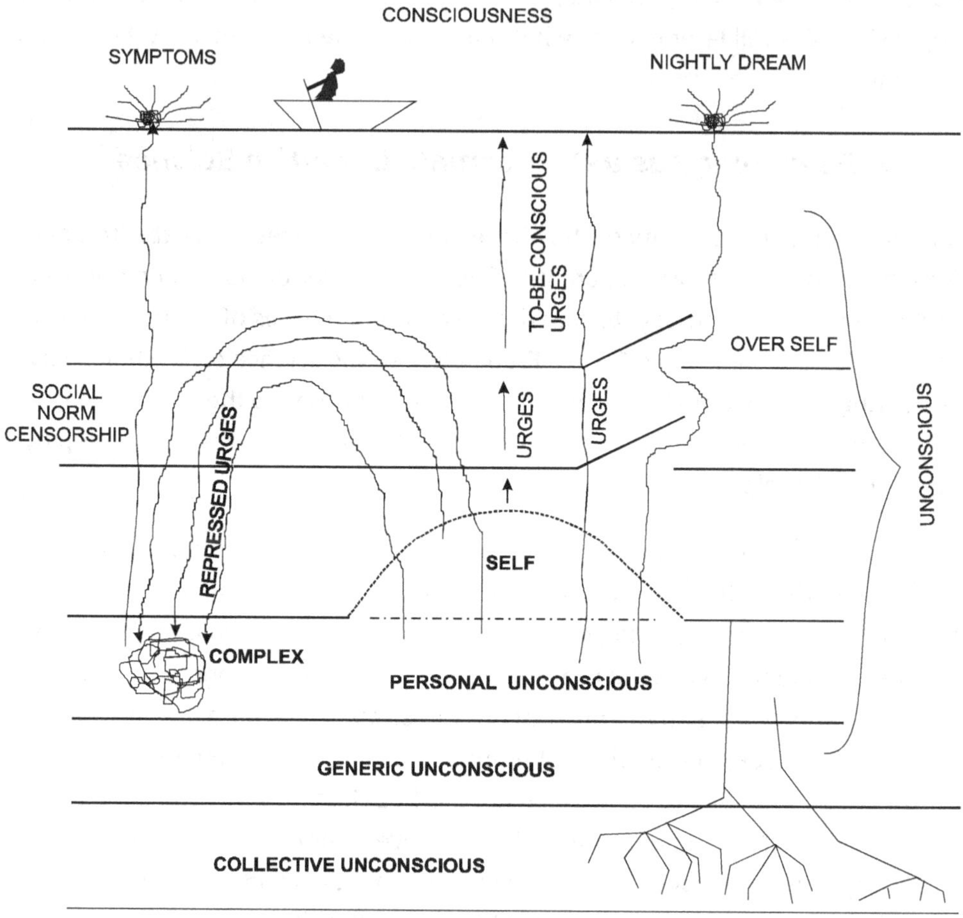

Fig. 1.3 The psychoanalytic model of Mind organization

It may well be that the medical science of Psychiatry to date is just not equipped with the tools for such an endeavor, given the psychophysics implications of the latter. We make it our objective in this treatise to fill this void.

---

[3] **Is Psychiatry Scientific? A Letter to a 21st Century Psychiatry Resident**, Jose de Leon, Print ISSN 1738-3684 / On-line ISSN 1976-3026 - http://dx.doi.org/10.4306/pi.2013.10.3.205

1.8 Visualizing the Mental Under Linear Algebra Categories

Many different mental categories had been studied in detail by S. Freud, from which he proposed early on a Mental Architecture that remained unchanged in Analytic Psychology in almost two centuries. It is based on what Freud had witnessed at La Salpêtrière under Charcot, with additions by Carl G. Jung, which resulted in a layered spectrum of the Mental. It equally involves dynamics based on impulses traveling across layers with or without filtering or blockage. This architecture also proposes a disease model based on conflicts between personalities (or complexes) incarnated within the layers and their interactions in terms of drives or impulses.

This construction is an approach to the configuration of the Mental Body and, despite being largely grounded on empirical facts, it lacks the formalism that would be required in the core sciences such as the physical sciences in order to further solidify the proposed knowledge. Except perhaps for Piaget's incipient exercises in using the mathematical categories in **Representation Theory of Groups** to express certain psychological objects and processes, there have been no attempts that we know of in using mathematical formalism to formulate a stringent and coherent architecture of Mind. Without being a prisoner of mathematical logic, one ought to acknowledge that it is at least a good warrant of consistency and accuracy. Its inherent logical methodology will not only help us stay clear of unproductive speculations but also constrain and discipline our attempt to comprehend the Mental beyond the old diagrammatic models. One of the reasons why this is even possible is because the Mental very largely expresses itself through the very mathematical language. We are going to show next how the codification encapsulated in Linear Algebra is inherent to the dynamic transactions of the Mental with a simple example.

Say that somebody named Peter burned George's home to ground with everything in it. Ever since that day George developed the greatest hatred for that individual. On a scale of 1 to 10, George's hatred is rated at 10. Peter was indicted, convicted and went to prison for a number of years and George never heard of him since then. But in later years, George fell sick and was in need of a kidney transplant. George received that transplant at some point, although the identity of the donor was kept incognito per clinical policy. So now George is in joy that someone donated a kidney to him and feeling gratitude in his heart for the unknown donor. He later made a request to the clinical personnel to meet with the donor, and at some point they granted his wish and arranged a meeting between the two. When Peter crossed the door to meet with him, George was in shock and could hardly believe that Peter's kidney was the one that saved his life. Feelings of gratitude now invaded him. On the scale of 1 to 10 George's feeling of joy at that meeting could be rated at 10.

Let's analyze this situation numerically. George's hatred for Peter and his eventual gratitude towards Peter are antithetic quantities to one another. They both cannot be graded in the domain of positive Real Numbers R^+, as mentioned. They have to be graded in the entire Domain R of both positive and negative real numbers, which now makes them algebraic quantities. We would have to assign -1 to George's feeling of hatred instead of -10 because in the hierarchy inherent to the Domain of negative real numbers, -1 is greater than -10. So we have the following numeric outcomes to the situation:

The end result feeling that George is going to have for Peter may be projected to be neutral or 0 because of the algebraic sum:

$H+J=-10+10=0$, where *H* stands for Hate and *J* for Joy.

When George fell seriously ill, his daily sentimental state was likely to be around the sadness of grievance, probably to be graded at around -3 or:

$\frac{S_1+S_2+S_3+...+S_i}{i}=-3$, where S_i is the level of sadness mind states he experiences throughout the day, a negative real number.

When he received the news of a donor willing to give him a kidney, his daily feelings must have flipped to joy and hope, perhaps to be graded daily average of +8, given that this is going to save his life, such that:

$\frac{J_1+J_2+J_3+...+J_i}{i}=+8$, where J_i is the level of joyful mind states he experiences throughout the day, a positive real number.

When, in the meeting with Peter, he was in shock realizing unexpectedly that Peter was the donor that saved his life, his hatred for Peter may have at one brief moment altogether changed to total empathy making true the projection at the first item: $H + J = -10 + 10 = 0$. That would have left him thereafter with no particular feeling for Peter, which is indifference towards him.

However, if after the fact, George comes to believe that his life was worth more than all the possessions that Peter formerly deprived him of, so that Peter's donated kidney is worth even more to him, then we have to reshape the grading or the etalon and say that the hatred is rated at -9 and the joy graded at +10 so that:

$H + J = -9 + 10 = +1$, which is the amount of gratitude that is left for George to feel for Peter.

In fact, that value is a variable which depends on the amount of valuation that George places in the donation of the kidney with respect to the value of his own life.

Furthermore, as we said at the outset, those sentiments (hatred and joy/gratitude) are antithetic to one another, which means that they are suitable to an even higher categorization that is vector representation (or trigonometric symmetry).

One does not witfully effect all these computations in one's mind, since we only experience direct feelings and personal cogitations. However, the exercise portrays underlying algebraic mathematics through which our mind constructs them in its operation. It is thus entirely possible to apply linear algebra to human mentation by assigning an algebraic number to states of mind and applying algebraic computational rules to follow or describe their evolution.

1.9 Stochasticity and Determinism in the Dynamics of the Mental Body

Qualia is one of these modern terms frequently used in Mind literature with apparently rather vague connotations. Likewise, the term sentience, which was originally used to mean the ability to think as opposed to feel, has over time come to mean feelings, just as qualia. For the purpose of this text, let's broadly define sentience or qualia as the diverse possible *states of mind*. We must keep to the understanding that, although sensations bear a physiological undertone, they are fully experienced in thoughts. In that context, a rather strange paradox about human consciousness in this stage of Human culture is how the common person can foul himself or herself into believing that thoughts in qualia or sentience develop in a deterministic fashion, against the background of Time. Meanwhile, the Mind itself, in terms of flow of thoughts, is in actuality framed to project itself as distributed stochastic bundles of thoughts.

Nobody can tell what their exact thoughts from one moment to the next, or throughout successive moments will be as the day unfolds, in an unequivocal show that Mind develops in stochastic jets, even though inside each jet there may be a relatively short span of continuum or predictability. It seems as though there is only a certain likelihood that we may know or define at one moment the content of our next span of thoughts. This is not about futuristic projections. Although we may decide to think about something in particular, how we come to decide those particular pensive moments is mostly a random event, while the very specific content of those pensive moments may or may not be randomized. When we decide on something of any nature, the decision with the implicated desire and motivations are formed as projections or representational projections, which may or may not be deterministic through volition, however the next decision along our pensive thread is never entirely predetermined, if for no other reason because *"we can change our minds"* unexpectedly from very own volition in course. The evolution of our pensive thread is thus heavily mutational, the only true constant about it being its continual unfolding.

Even considering larger spans of time or circumstances, we would be drawn to the same conclusion. I can plan to do something sometime later in the day, the week, the month or the year and effectively execute on it in due course, but the overall representational course (or thread of specific volitional events) that takes me to that moment of completion is completely random. And it may well be that the specifically planned action in original representation never materializes per my given pensive flow.

Hence, if Mentation always concerns feelings, rationales and desires or motivations (willingness), the train of thoughts that vehicle this qualia overwhelmingly obeys stochasticity in the majority of its expression. If we develop the living experience of our lives entirely through the process of Mentation as what chiefly orchestrates actions and transformations making up the *fabric of our days*, the above also incontrovertibly means that the teleological thread of our lives is globally and predominantly stochastic, notwithstanding its continuous substrate. And that time, as a well-behaved deterministic variable, was **never** a bona fide descriptor of the Human teleological mentation experience in its continuity.

I shall briefly mention that it is possible, on one's own accord, to break the mentation substrate as well and so interrupt its continuum. However, because most people are unfamiliar with that personal mentation experience, we will discard it from the analysis.

If this all means that Mentation is fully accessible to a mathematical formulation of stochastic or statistical category, it also means that notwithstanding the omnipresence of Time in our Minds, it was never an effectual determinant in our Mentation processes in terms of directing and mediating our continual flow of thoughts with qualia. A mathematical function to describe the evolution of human thoughts is therefore best chosen as a probability or statistical representation than a well-behaved functional expression or functional[4].

1.10 Self-Awareness and Consciousness Modeled as a Differential Geometry Symmetry

We are now going to introduce technical distinctions between the terms awareness, self-awareness, consciousness and Mind by incipiently extolling the Anatomy of the mentation body in pursuing with the formal mathematical-physics vantage formerly initiated. A few common dictionaries define awareness as the *state of knowing something*. Awareness must further imply some sort of distinction between two or more entities, the knowing and the knowable, with the knowing tenet subject to information gathering from the knowable. The state of

---

[4] A functional in Mathematics is a function of a function.

awareness implies as well the act of filtering such information in terms of that which the knowing agent is concerned about, and might subsequently act upon.

In one of its acceptions, the term *consciousness* intently qualifies the process of being *aware* of a knowable or an observable by capturing some of its specific characters or attributes. We are going to encapsulate this fact under the term *awareness*. When the knowable is the very cognos of the inquesting individual, it becomes *self-awareness*. We are further going to relate self-awareness to the *Sense of Self*, in the understanding that a sensory-like intake is necessary to orchestrate the cognition in awareness or a cognos, whatever the nature of the knowable. Furthermore, there is clearly an effector component in the notion of self-awareness, evidenced in the fact that the self tends to act in certain particular ways. That is what we mean when we say i.e. *"I do not see myself doing this."* or *"That kind of thing, that's not me."* or *"This is my thing."* in the sense that this is the kind of thing I like or tend to do. So there surely exists a *Self-effector* component to *self-awareness* as well.

We thus arrive at the following important definition:

Self-awareness is a cognitive bundle encapsulating a Sense of Self and a Self-Effector in the form of a monolith.

The most important property of self-awareness is its constancy over the entire course of an individual's life cycle. For certain, we all know at every minute of life that **we** are **ourselves** and **not** somebody else. Furthermore, we know ourselves to be the **same** inner person all the time, from infancy to teenage to adulthood to elderly, despite the many different transformations that our body experiences throughout. Even when we experience important psychological changes, as relate to our emotional and intellectual states and remain fully cognizant of these changes or alterations, we still believe that we are the same Self and not another Self or somebody else. In a word, our sense of personal identity or cognition thereof remains always unchanged. Therefore our Self-Awareness is fundamentally an **invariant**. It is important to recognize that said invariant remains preserved under all the developmental **transformations** that we go through in our life cycle, and while we are, by mental instigation, in perpetual action **transforming** the environment or habitat. This makes Self-Awareness within the Mental Body altogether a definite mathematical-physics Symmetry in its own right.

Let us now briefly examine what a Symmetry is in Geometry. A Symmetry in Geometry is defined to be an **invariant** that is preserved under **transformations** of some kind, most of the time rotational or translational. For example, the homes and streets and cities we live in remain completely unaltered as the earth's globe continually spins around its polar axis. The symmetry here is formed by humans and their artificial habitat with the spinning globe altogether as a system. Mathematician Emmy Noether had axiomatized this concept in the formulation of the following Theorem:

> *"Every differentiable symmetry of the action of a physical system has a corresponding conservation law."*

Translation for the non-experts: there is a conservation constraint or invariance associated with every continuous action or transformation of a physical system. The theorem had been numerically expressed in the category of the integral of an action in time, the latter being translated in a Lagrangian representation *(I)*, such that:

$$I = \int L(q,\overline{q},t) \cdot dt,$$

where q is the coordinate set, $\overline{q} = \dfrac{dq}{dt}$ and L the Lagrangian notation.

A Lagrangian may otherwise be simply viewed as the sum of all energies making up a dynamic system. In catering to this definition of a Symmetry, we realize that it perfectly applies to Self-awareness, leading us to propose the following definition of Self-awareness:

Self-Awareness is the invariant discrete bundle of sense of self and adjunct self-effector which remain preserved under emotional alterations, exercise of reason and purposeful activity as well as across changing developmental stages during the lifecycle. It is expressed both during the mental states of arousal and during the phases of nocturnal sleep eliciting dreaming activity.

Once it is formed, arguably at age 3, the self-awareness monolith remains inalterably the same in relation to the rest of the Mental Body until the end of an individual's lifecycle, since there will never be an instance of life where the individual will normally think that he/she is no longer himself or herself but someone else. Inasmuch as the Mental Body will orchestrate the medium of inhabitation which includes both the natural world and kindred, as well as all the other sentient activities performed by the Mental, one may consider the *system* covered by the symmetry to be Self-Awareness and the Mental Body. Noether's Symmetry concept is expressed in time, which is, however, a moot variable in the Quanto-Geometric framework. We will later show that the Self-Awareness symmetry is a psychological incarnation of what we dub in this framework Quintessence, along with its due numeric expression.

1.11 Primitives of Human Memory

In analyzing the structure of Human Memory, *retention* appears to be the most fundamental property of the phenomenon of Memory which of course has a number of different dimensions. Psychological Memory is the collection of registered events that chiefly involve the Self. All collected information must have a "Self" index in one way or another. Even in the possibility of the existence of a Collective Memory as known in collections of Collective symbols or archetypes, either the stack or elements of the stack must have a "Self" index to relate the stack to the particular person who is the beholder. In addition, the act of memorization requires the catalytic intervention of the faculties of attention and volition, two sentient elements that appear to hold their own segregated life from the essential elements proper to Memory.

1.11.1 Mnemonic Retention or Collection

The first manner of expression of the Retention attribute is indelibility. This function must be soundly given in the artifact of individual Memory. Without it, the edifice or container cannot be built. If it is not given, the container is comparable to a reed basket, which evidently cannot retain liquid content. When it is given, the container is by comparison as solid and waterproof as a clay jar. Everything that makes it into the container will forever perdure as content. ***Nothing can vanish from the stack, it is indelible, except for catastrophic structural ac-***

cidents such as degeneration or lesions of any nature. While a loss in memory may be a result of a loss or structural impairment in the mnemonic stack or container, forgetfulness is not to be considered a result of destruction of a part of the stack or the container, but strictly a miss or dysfunction in the Recollection function, which we will shortly review.

The Collection function is an absolute that is invariable from one individual to the next. We all have in our Mental a stack of all events that ever occurred to us and as we registered them. We may have totally forgotten some of them, nevertheless they are still there all intact. That is the reason why we can recollect those forgotten ones at the favor of a particular situation, or by following clues to their recollection, or even as content of nightly dreams. We could not remember them if they were not part of the basis indelible stack.

1.11.2 Recent Memory v. Remote Memory

It is easy to represent that the retention stack must be in some way layered in terms of recent memory and remote memory, since we know we can forget something that occurred yesterday or the day before, while we still have vivid memory of an event from remote past. There must therefore be a differential by which we can distinguish between retention of fresh events and that of remote past events. One may argue that the differential may reside at the Recollection level and not the Retention level. One may counterargue, however, that a dynamic model that envisions the transitioning of events from one layer of the stack to another or the continual formation of stack layers gives a more sensible account of recent events versus remote events than misses or gaps in a recollection index.

Furthermore, one of the most important aspects of Freudian Architecture of the Mental involves two important provinces of Mind, namely the Generic Unconscious and the Collective Unconscious, which are to be visualized as genuine mnemonic containers in and of themselves. Consistent with the Freudian mental model, one may also justifiably consider the Personal Unconscious layer to be the principal siege of individual psychological Memory as discussed above. Very specifically, the Personal Unconscious layer appears poised to play the pivotal role of remote-event container and the more superficial layers including the Conscious layer the role of recent-event container. This hypothesis concords with the fact that the latter are in charge of dealing with the day-to-day interfacing with the living medium which provides immediate treatment of the information coming in through the external or sensory perceptive channels. Considered in that manner, the Freudian model ends up proposing psychological Mnemonic organization on the basis of both a cumulative and a distributed arrangement. It also proceeds from here that one same packet of representations may be duplicated throughout the entire set of layers in accordance with the distributed type of arrangement. Such a model appears to be consistent with:

1) The functional neuro-anatomy of Memory which encompasses a plethora of structures and pathways precursed from all three primeval prosencephalic, mesencephalic and robencephalic formations in the ontogenetic development of the human Brain.
2) And the somatotopic arrangement alike in the afferent wing of the entire nervous system.

These remarks do not constitute a validation of Monism as we remind the reader to never lose sight of the distinction between correlation and causal factor. In addition, the known cases of individuals starting inexplicably to speak a different language after a coma and what is known as the *Foreign Language Syndrome* have not yet received sufficient sensible neurofunctional analysis on the part of Monists to solidly credit their claim in the Memory chapter.

1.11.3 Mnemonic Registration

Before events and objects can be collected into the container, they must be registered or brought in through a perception channel. Therefore the registration function is primeval in Memory. It is important to realize that the registration function apportions to mnemonic content, or the memory payload, the beholder's individual mark. One same event will not be perceived in the same way by all individual observers, in light of their varied idiosyncracies. The reality before us all is always the same. It exists in an immanent manner, in and of itself. Nevertheless, the way that we perceive an event or object of reality is observer-dependent. Through a feedback loop, our Mind reshapes perception to some extent in quality and amplitude according to the individual observer's own temper or character.

The above may be put in evidence by having different observers render their perception of the image of an object intently made to be ambiguous in representing two different things. Likewise, on that same account, a scene is likely to be reported in different ways by their observers in good faith. For instance, certain sounds may have a greater effect on some characters than others: not everyone perceives musical notes the same way or with the same intensity, certain characters may be indifferent to music altogether, or a certain style of music, whereas in some others it may reverberate profoundly in their psyche and get them humming. From there, one can see how they may report in different ways scenarios involving sounds or tunes. Likewise certain colors have more effect on some people than others, some people are very sensitive to the play of colors and how they harmonize, while that association will leave others indifferent. So two people may in very good faith perceive or report a scene in slightly or vastly different ways in its attributes and qualifiers, with no negative implication in the integrity of the inalterable reality that has been there all the time as an object or circumstance of its own. Hence the registration function is very significantly a dependency of an individual's character in general.

It is important to keep in mind that perceptions are not always internalized in thorough percepts or payloads since they are dependent on the attention/volition faculties. There may even be times when perceptions do not result in internalized percepts at all. If during the act of registration of a perception we have our attention momentarily deviated elsewhere, whether partially or fully, whatever we perceive with our senses in the act in regards to the primary observable of interest will not fully resonate internally or will be doomed to falter altogether, respectively. Retrieval of this information in the exercise of Recollection will consequently suffer a more or less important recall deficit.

1.11.4 Mnemonic Recollection

Recollection of events and objects sitting in memory as memory content is another separate function of Memory. Some have a prodigious memory or power of recollection while others may have poor recall capability or recollection ability. When the recollection capacity is vigorous and effective, we say that we have good memory. Good memory or poor memory is not a result of mnemonic container capacity in terms of limits or even defects in cumulation or retention. The common notion of good or poor memory largely relates to the Recollection function. We call a deficient recall forgetfulness. A forgetful act may also result from deficient registration of the payload as mentioned before or interlayer dynamics that result in blocking or trapping the targeted payload for recollection.

A notable example of a deficient registration of the payload is whenever we accomplish an act exclusively with the hand or foot that is not the one pertaining to our skillfull anatomic side, left side for right-handed individuals, right side for left-handed individuals. Chances are that in those instances we were not "minding" what we were doing. Therefore the payload or perception did not get a chance to be properly registered and did not quite make it to retention or storage. The only way to retrieve that information, for instance where we placed that hammer or that book, is by recollecting prior and/or posterior events to the act, and executing on what that information leads you to. There is no recollecting the payload at its face value in that instance because it did not make it to retention due to very deficient registration.

Analytically, the pathway for registration appears to be different than the pathway for recollection. Recollection operates in terms of pulling information from the container, while registration inputs information into the container. Furthermore, recollection seems to operate in terms of applying a pass-through filter for a particular kind of information. What there is in our minds when we try to recollect an object, person or event, is an image that vectorizes the disbursement of a discrete part of the container content through duplication of a model image. We are not aware of any index table, so to speak, or numerically stacked bank of information in our minds, which we taxonomically refer to whenever we attempt to retrieve information from our Memory. While the latter represents the approach that we had chosen for all of our common computing devices in modern technology, it is not necessarily the method mother Nature has followed in organizing human Memory. The act of recollection is incipiently shaped as a projection of a mental model image or an image sketch destined to select from the container a bundle of representations that best mimics or relates to the sketch. Therefore, if registration is essentially a sensory-like act that funnels information into the container, recollection is an effector-like act that outputs information from it.

One can also see that the artifact of the model image can influence through its quality the outcome of the act of recollection. The greater its duplication value the more efficient the recollection effort.

In addition, we shall mention that the recollection function may also develop through association. For instance, you may recollect someone's forgotten name, by implicit association with other persons in his/her occupation or dwelling, or by common endeavors, until the name of that particular person extemporaneously pops in the conscious mind. The exercise of one or the other method of recollection may be singular or plural, and, in their action, concomitant or successive, as one attempts to overcome forgetfulness.

Moreover, there exists delayed recollection or scheduled recall among the many variants of the recollection function. For instance, when going back home at the end of the workday, it came back to mind that I needed to pick up the clothing from the Cleaning service, not far from my residence. But it was only when I was parking the car in my garage when I got home that I realized I had forgotten to stop at the Cleaning service. In that case, the recall did not occur, although it is clear that it was duly issued or pre-scheduled. The miss may have been due to overriding preoccupations of the moment which filled up the conscious mind and interfered with the recall or perhaps an interim event of significance that impacted the conscious mind in the meantime. Therefore, the recollection function is subject to interference in its scheduled mode.

Lastly, spontaneous recall is another recollection artifact worth mentioning here in this review. It concerns a recall event or action spontaneously arising from the unconscious layers, without a conscious trigger, that is. The mnemonic payload simply pops up to the conscious mind (cursor). This occurs notably in the recollection of nightly dreams during daytime, away from the awake moment. Sceneries or dream scenarios will at times spontaneously surface up with no consciously recognizable reasons or no attempt of recollection. This is not to be confused with the semi-deliberate attempt to let the dreams of the night flow in replay as we remain in the gray zone (semiconscious) following sleep before transitioning to fully awake. This exercise is virtuous in pulling the dreams out of unconscious incognito into conscious awareness for posterior at-will recollection.

1.11.5 Sameness and Repeatability in Memory

While retention stands for one major attribute of memory organization, the second major operator in that mentation Function is Sameness or Repeat. The criterion of sameness or association based on sameness in kind seems to overwhelm intralayer organization of the container's content. For memory to be effective as a function, the payloads must not only be indelible, but they must also remain the same throughout the many strings of recalls that they may be submitted to and at every recall they must be externally expended in their exact original form. Repeat becomes an important element that the entire mnemonic architecture must provide for. Therefore, the beat of a clock is an ineluctable requirement to furnish the foundational basis for continual endless repeat as much as count. It may be visualized as the trunk of the tree of Memory.

One of the things that we are fully aware of by introspection is that we are more or less able to remember every aspect of our lives ever since perhaps age 3. Although many details will escape the recollection function, we remain cognizant that the uninterrupted suite of events in our lives is retained in our individual Memory. The view of an album photo when we were a toddler or perhaps age 5 or 7 may bring back to mind events such as when the infant that we were was attending kindergarten. Therefore autobiographical memory is undoubtedly a given.

In addition, many anecdotal NDE reports[5] exist where the subjects reveal having had an experience of a flash review of his entire life span akin to a motion picture film scrolling in the mind. Were human Memory a tree, the continual count provided by the human heart would be somewhat comparable to the layer count of new wood added to the cambium block every year (Fig. 1.4). One can see how the successively grown branches around the trunk partake of the cam-

[5] NDE stands for Near Death Experience.

bium ring cycles in continual development by the plant. Every branch bears the mark of its own age. Evidently this is not about the age in time of the element but its age in terms of its evolution in space, since there is only herein an account of the dynamic space spread of one earth orbital (not about how long the planet takes to orbit around the sun but strictly the orbital space spread itself as perceived by the plant, independent of a fictitious set duration).

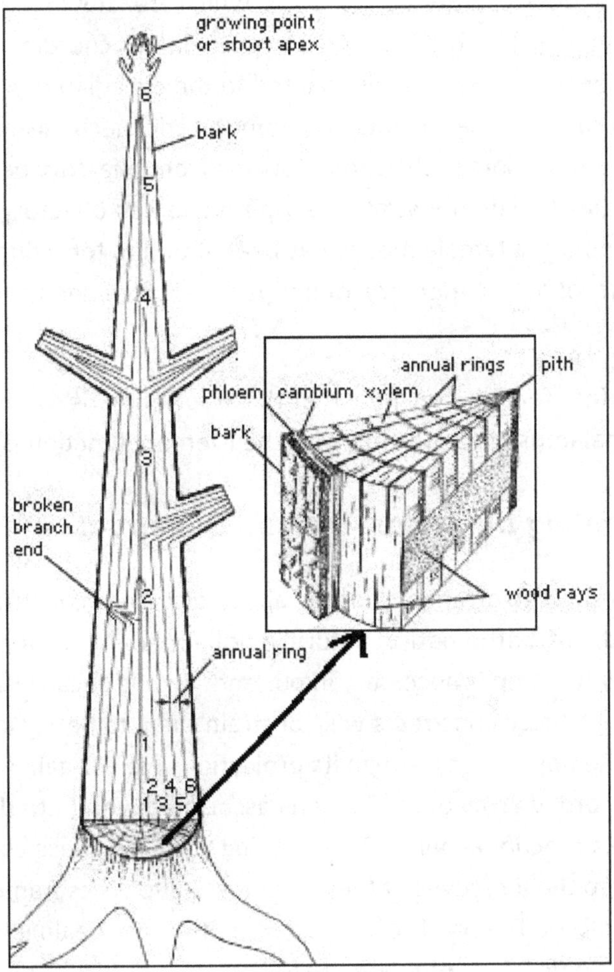

Fig. 1.4 How a tree implements memory in the cambium of its trunk section and branches

The biological heart represents the one single clock that can provide the repeat in cyclicity and endless count that the mnemonic function fundamentally requires for its development. Effectively, the association between the heart and the hypothalamus in the development of Memory is well known in neural science. It has been unequivocally proven that the heart communicates with the brain, in particular the hypothalamus, in various pathways: via direct neural transmission, neurotransmitters and endocrine connections. Posterior Mammillary in its medial and lateral layout shows two nuclei, namely the mammillary nucleus and the tuberomammillary nucleus, which are known to play a role in the Memory functions. Furthermore, the hypothalamus coordinates a number of hormonal reactions and behaviors related to the circadian rhythm, complex patterns of neuroendocrine outputs and homeostatic mechanisms, as well as other important behaviors such as those arising from olfactory perception. The hypothalamus has well demonstrated responsiveness to olfactory stimuli, including pheromones: a female mouse has been found to form during intercourse a precise 'olfactory **memory**' of her partner which persisted for several days thereafter.

We must therefore forcibly conclude that the association between the heart and the hypothalamus in connection with the Memory function is undeniable.

1.12 Integrating the Major Analytic Constructs of the Mental

Our challenge now is to arrange all of the above discussed constructs in a single integrated model of mathematical nature, if not a mathematical-physics nature. The reason why this step is necessary in our endeavor is because a mathematical formulation of these constructs will constrain them to better intellectual discipline and in the hopes that through its projections we will gain working insight into a desirably broad array of phenomena associated with both the normal mind and the dysfunctional mind. We are going to model these constructs by mapping them to the directives of the mathematical-physics framework at work in Quanto-Geometric Theory. The constructs that we are dealing with which need formal numeric integration are the following:

1. Mind or Mental Body
2. Consciousness
3. Cognition
4. Awareness
5. Representations
6. Conscious and Unconscious
7. Qualia and Sentience
8. Willingness and Attention
9. Motivations
10. Memory

We are going to imbue all these qualities in an Analytic Geometry function of two variables based on a particular orthonormed coordinate system which will also share three of the aforementioned mentation qualities. This function has the likes of or may be incipiently assimilated to the Normal Density Function to which a number of canonical dimensions in the Quanto-Geometric mathematical-physics framework have been added.

1.12.1 Axial Descriptors for Volition, Motivation and Sentiments

The 3-space Quanto-Geometric coordinate system directly models the three major components of the act of Mentation. We discuss below how each of these components maps to a specific axis.

1.12.2 The vertical q-axis as a descriptor of Volition

The vertical axis *(q-axis)* of the coordinate system incarnates the mental quality of willingness or volition. Volition is a measure of the level of concentration or focus of our thoughts. It is the reciprocal of attention, because to more volition less attention. This is reflected in the alert condition, which constrains the mind to narrowly and intently focus on a percept or an observable by minimizing or atomizing the scope of attention. Therefore:

$V = \frac{1}{A}$, where *V* stands for Volition and *A* for Attention.

Thus we need not include Attention *(A)* in the Cartesian model, since the above formula allows us to compute *A* separately whenever Volition *(V)* is known. Therefore the vertical *q-axis* tallies the actual values of the Function itself. The reason why we have chosen the *q-axis* to model the level of mental concentration is because in the original Quanto-Geometric framework that axis represents *density*, a parallel to concentration. The selection is therefore not arbitrary.

1.12.3 The horizontal t-axis as a descriptor of Motivation

The horizontal motile axis *(t-axis)* models the phenomenon of motivation. We make a clear distinction between volition and motivation. In motivation, there is only a certain disposition toward action. So one may experience negative motivation, which is what we feel when we experience such sensations as terror which predisposes us to paralysis; or we may experience positive motivation, which is what we feel when we experience such sensations as fury which predisposes us to motion. In positive motivation, we thus experience a propositional or motional potentiality.

In the Quanto-Geometric framework, physical space is *innerly* motional as the very origin of motion, giving rise to the concept of *space momentum*. Such a quality is modeled in the Theory with the *t-axis*, reason why we hereby surrogate this attribution by assigning the artifact of motivation, with its motional quality, to this axis.

1.12.4 The horizontal m-axis as a descriptor of Sentiment

In Quanto-Geometric Theory, the horizontal *m-axis* is a morphic axis grading forms. In this application of the framework to mentation, it will be used to give the measure of morphogenic amplitude or *re-presentational multiplicity* in a thought. This is an ability to foment or handle *presentation,* which may be likened to the common notion of *sentiment* or the aforementioned notion of qualia. It is very difficult to conceptualize a thought without a level of representation, minute though it might be. If we think hate, for instance, as a singlemost form of thought, we can see that therein lies something more than a propositional or motional potentiality, what we termed motivation, that is. It takes representation to comprehend the meaning of that other "thing" in the notion, without representation you cannot access that meaning. Note that it does not take behavior per se to access that meaning, in fact it is this pensive "echo" imbued in the notion that informs subsequent behavior. This echo or inner evocation in the thought is *representation* or *presentation*, if you will.

Just like the other two components of mind currently in discussion, representation as a component of thought exists before any language is learned and before the Mind is delivered in the natural world for the living experience. If you slap the buttock of a new born, like nurses or midwives commonly do while holding him or her upside down, a cry ensues in signal of a profound "dislike" or hate. If the new born could speak, the midwife would hear from him or her "I hate being slapped." Or perhaps "I hate you or whoever/whatever is slapping me."

In summary, we have posed that the three most generic components that make up the sentience inherent to the Mental Body are volition, motivation and representation (sentiment). This is to mean that every thought or thought unit will have a gradient of volition, a gradient of motivation and a gradient of representation (sentiment). Further, the function representing the Mental Body is expressed in terms of volition playing the role of dependent variable (or the function itself) and the other two components, motivation and representation, playing the role of independent variables.

1.13 Expression of the Mathematical-Physics Function Encapsulating the Mental Body

We first offer a complete view of the expression and graph of the Quanto-Geometric Function of two variables (Fig. 1.5).

$$Q(t,m) = \pm\left|\frac{(m+t)^0}{\sigma\sqrt{2\pi}} \bullet e^{\left(\frac{-(m+t)^2}{2\sigma^2}\right)}\right|, \text{ for } (m,t) \neq (0,0), [(m,t) \in R^+)] and [-(m,t) \in R^-]$$

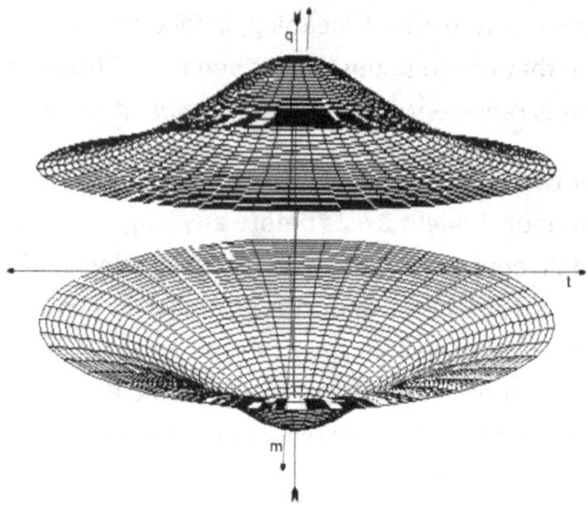

Fig. 1.5 A complete view of the graph of the Quanto-Geometric function of two variables *(m,t)*

To remain compliant to the constructs discussed above, we apply a restriction to the domain and range of the function. We do so because on the Cartesian plane of representation there is no negative value of the *presentation (sentiment)* variable *(t)*, nor is there any negative value at all for the volition variable *(q)*, the very function itself. So it turns out because, for one, within our sense of self, we feel endowed with only one Mental Body altogether, not two or three. Hence the function cannot be defined on the negative *q-axis*. Likewise we do not know of antithetic forms of sentiments, i.e. two forms of hate, therefore the function is not defined on the negative *t-axis*. These restrictions we introduce in the expression and graph of the function as displayed below (Fig. 1.4).

$$Q(m,t) = \left| \frac{(m+t)^0}{\sigma\sqrt{2\pi}} \bullet e^{\left(\frac{-(m+t)^2}{2\sigma^2}\right)} \right|,$$

for $(m,t) \neq (0,0), (t \in R^+) and (-t \in R^-) and (m \in R^+)$

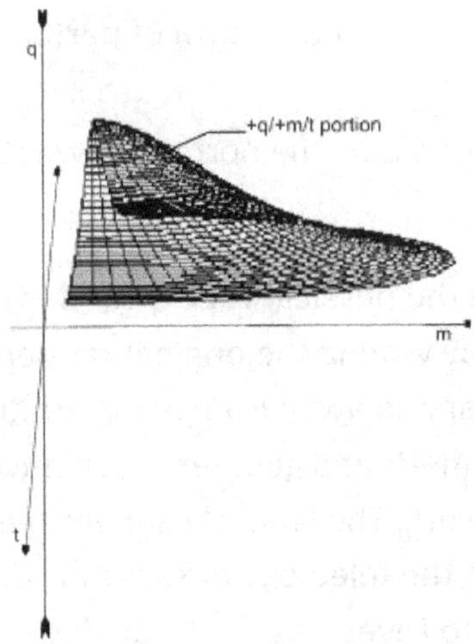

Fig. 1.6 A view of the graph of the Mental Body Function of two variables *(m,t)*

Further developments in the physical Theory have considered the implications of curvature evolution of the Function through differentiation. The outcome of this analysis has highlighted a form of normalization of the Function in accordance with the sectionals of the graph, casting a spectrum of 9 horizontal normal layers (Fig. 1.7 & 1.8). This form of normalization runs contrary to the vertical percentage account of Gaussian normalization that is generally done to the parallel Normal Distribution Function. At that point, the function is best considered a Differential Geometry foliate divided in 9 sectional manifolds or curved layers of the graphical layout.

In the physical Theory, each of these layers is identified with an ontological definition or norm as follows:

- Layer 1 is underscored by the norm of **monolithisation.**
- Layer 2 is underscored by the norm of **ambivalence.**
- Layer 3 is underscored by the norm of **association.**
- Layer 4 is underscored by the norm of **manicheism.**
- Layer 5 is underscored by the norm of **metamorphogenesis.**
- Layer 6 is underscored by the norm of **harmony.**
- Layer 7 is underscored by the norm of **paradox.**

- Layer 8 is underscored by the norm of **perfection (equanimity** or **self-detachment).**
- Layer 9 is underscored by the norm of **asymptotic expansiveness** or **serialization.**

There are good reasons in the physical Theory for this characterization, which the reader may prospect by visiting the original referenced publication. The specificity of these norms is far and away from being arbitrary as they arise from the very philosophical, numeric and geometric primitives that subtend the canon at work in the framework. The label chosen for the layer is of little import but the ontological type in the teleology or semantic of the descriptor. For instance, whether we refer to Layer 1 as the Unary layer or the Monolithic layer does not matter, what is essential is the focus on the central idea of *one in compactification*.

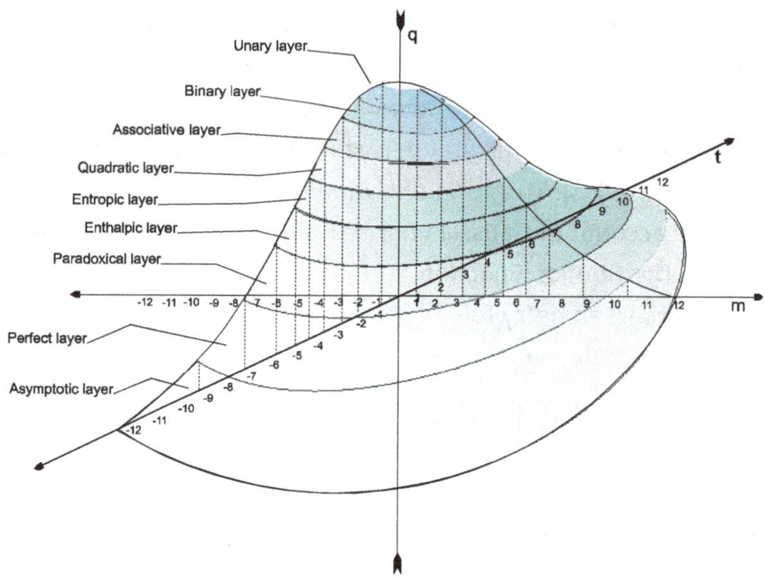

Fig. 1.7 The quanto-geometric coordinate system as a direct descriptor of volition, motivation and thoughts multiplicity with a spectrum of 9 horizontal normal layers.

When it comes to the application of these fundamental Quanto-Geometric norms in universal ontology to the Human Mental in particular, they become emulated in the following manner:

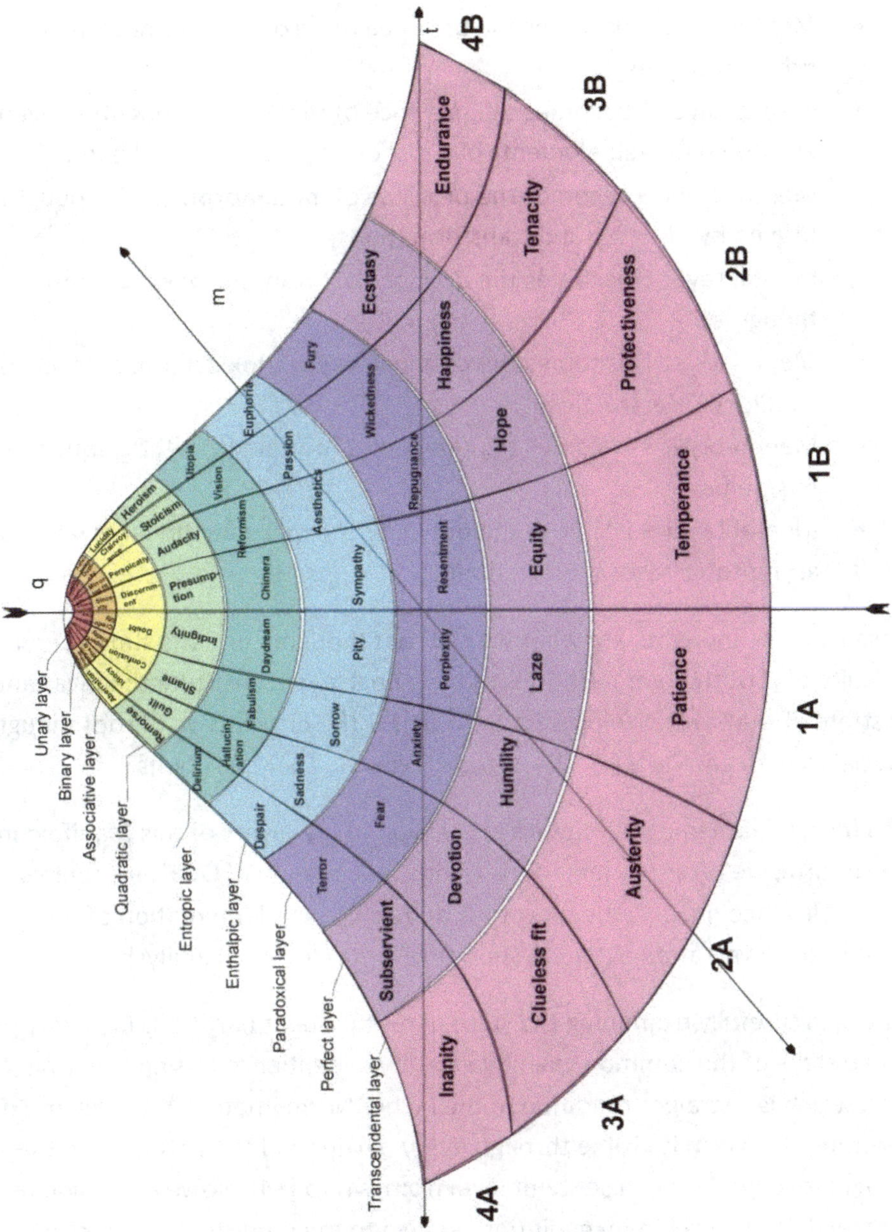

Fig. 1.8. The Human Mentation Manifold displaying its complete distribution of pensive partitions and pensive layers.

- Mental Layer 1 becomes the province of **egocentric** thoughts.
- Mental Layer 2 becomes the province of **ambivalent** thoughts.

- Mental Layer 3 becomes the province of **associative** or **analytically-driven** thoughts.
- Mental Layer 4 becomes the province of **manicheic** thoughts (driven by election between elements of a dichotomy, i.e. good and bad).
- Mental Layer 5 becomes the province of **metamorphogenic** thoughts (driven by disorder and transformations).
- Mental Layer 6 becomes the province of **harmonic** or **empathetic** thoughts.
- Mental Layer 7 becomes the province of **paradoxical** thoughts (chaotic, conflictive, destructive).
- Mental Layer 8 becomes the province of **perfect** thoughts (equanimous, selfless).
- Mental Layer 9 becomes the province of **expansive** thoughts (endless, asymptotic, resistive, deferment).

These forms of thoughts are what we call root thoughts or basis states of mind. The suite of root thought partitions making up a layer constitute the invariant substrate of the Layer. We present in Table 1.1 the distribution of root thoughts associated with each layer of the Mental Foliate in their partitions.

For a formal mathematical-physics expression of the layers of this Manifold in Tensor form, we refer readers to the orginal publication of QGT[6]. It acquires particular relevance mostly when it comes to machine implementation of this Theory, conceived as an eventual supporting tool to clinical analysis.

It is worth carefully examining the suite of root thought partitions in each layer to take stock of the common cognitive quality or sentience arising from the layer, which is a straight rendition of the higher Norm imbued in the layer. So therefore, the Norm is visible through every partition of the Layer, while there is a progressive gradation in sentient level from [-4] to [+4]. However, inside of that trend, there is a binary evolution relative to the intensity in expression of the morphogenic descriptor which progresses from Thread [1] to [4] and from Thread [-1] to [-4]. The group labeled A with the negative numbers represents

---

[6] Quanto-Geometry, Overture of Cosmic Consciousness and Universal Knowledge for All, Vol I

the left chiral side of the distribution (Table 1.2), whereas the group labeled with the positive numbers represents the right chiral side of the distribution, the entire distribution being of a binary nature and originally symmetric around horizontal *m-axis* of the graph, the morphic axis.

	PASSIVE LATENCY - ANIMA					ACTIVE LATENCY - ANIMUS			
	-4	-3	-2	-1		1	2	3	4
	Dramatism	Pessimism	Negativity	Disapproval	Hybrid	Assent	Assurance	Optimism	Excitement
1	Timidity	Introversion	Solitude	Indifference	←→	Conservativenes	Possessiveness	Competitivenes	Cupidity
2	Inquisitiveness	Curiosity	Superficiality (In	Credulity	←→	Sincerity	Mirroring	Duplicity	Authoritarianism
3	Aberration	Idiocy	Disorientation	Doubt (Perple:	←→	Discernment	Perspicacity	Clairvoyance	Lucidity
4	Remorse	Guilt	Shame	Regretfulness	←→	Presumption	Audacity	Stoicism	Heroism
5	Delirium	Dystopia	Fabulousness	Daydream	←→	Chimera	Reformism	Visionary	Utopia
6	Despair	Sadness (Disapp	Sorrow	Pity	←→	Sympathy	Admiration	Euphoria	Passion
7	Terror	Fear (Anguish)	Angst	Anxiety	←→	Resentment	Repugnance	Wickedness	Fury
8	Subservience	Devotion	Humility	Laziness	←→	Equity	Hope	Happiness	Ecstasy
9	Inanity	Cluelessness	Austerity	Patience	←→	Temperance	Endurance	Resilience	Tenacity

Table 1.1 Map of the Human Mentation Manifold with its distribution of pensive Layers and partitions in a tabular view.

There is symmetry of the antisymmetric class between the partitions in both Groups beholding the same number identifier, in a one-to-one fashion. Therefore the progression that we observe across a layer is expressible in terms of an angle-related parameter, i.e. the cosine of an angle to typify the presentation capacity of the varied partitions, such that:

$P = cos(1/\Theta)$, P being the *presentation capacity* of the mentation partition or its *morphic multiplicity*, and Θ being its trigonometric angle (angle formed with the *m-axis* and taking the same as the cosine axis), per the Manifold in Fig. 1.8.

A top down projection of the Quanto-Geometric function (as well as its Mental Body surrogate) immediately gives us on the *m-t* plane a trigonometric layout where all the normal layers are represented as semi-circular bands (Fig. 1.9). Each quadrant in the illustration is partitioned in 4 slices, thus yielding 4 partitions per layer and a representative angle for each partition. Which lateral side of the partition we choose to measure the *morphic* angle is inconsequential as we might choose the median segment through the partition instead for that measure.

Table 1.3 shows an example of the antisymmetric character as realized between elements pertaining to Threads [-4] and [+4] across the entire spectrum.

	◄ [-4] Dramatism	◄ [-3] Pessimism	◄ [-2] Negativity	◄ [-1] Disapproval
1	Timidity	Introversion	Solitude	Indifference
2	Inquisitiveness	Curiosity	Superficiality (In	Credulity
3	Aberration	Idiocy	Disorientation	Doubt (Perplexit
4	Remorse	Guilt	Shame	Regretfulness
5	Delirium	Hallucination	Fabulousness	Daydream
6	Despair	Sadness (Disap	Sorrow	Pity
7	Terror	Fear (Anguish)	Angst	Anxiety
8	Subservience	Devotion	Humility	Laziness
9	Inanity	Cluelessness	Austerity	Patience

Table 1.2 The left hemi-chiral grouping of the Human Mentation Manifold with its distribution of pensive Layers and partitions in a tabular view.

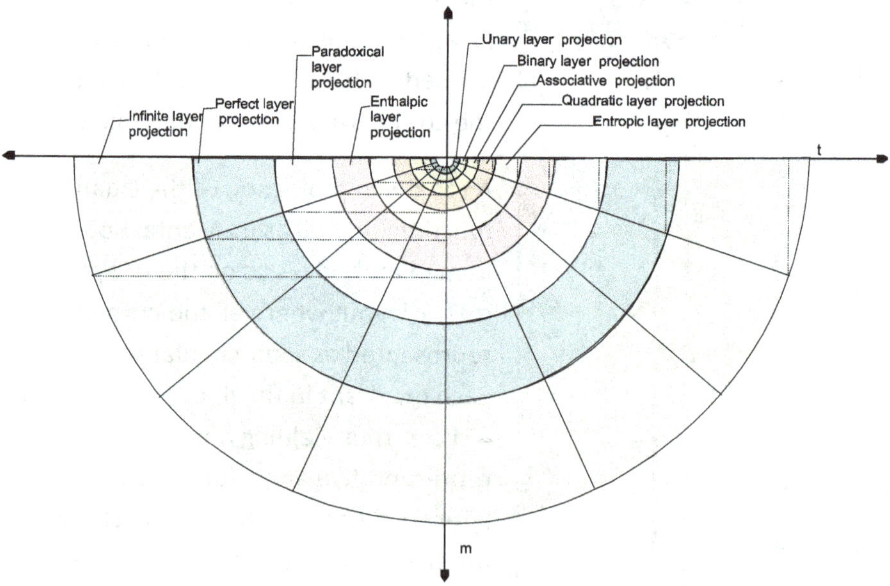

Fig. 1.9 Progression of multiplicity and motivational index of thought partitions across a thread as evidenced by their projections on the *t*-axis and the *m*-axis.

Layer	[-4] Thread	[+4] Thread
1	Timidity	Cupidity
2	Inquisitiveness	Authoritarianism
3	Aberration	Lucidity
4	Remorse	Heroism
5	Delirium	Utopia
6	Despair	Passion
7	Terror	Fury
8	Subservience	Ecstasy
9	Inanity	Resilience

Table 1.3 The antisymmetric character of the Human Mentation Manifold exemplified in the [-4] and [+4] threads

We have labeled the elements at the left chiral side (Table. 1.2) with a negative number due to the passive quality there is to these mental fits, whereas the elements at the right chiral side have been labeled with a positive number due to the active quality to their mental fits. Everyone can easily understand the antisymmetric behavior between somebody torn in *remorse* and someone else boasting *heroism*, or between someone paralyzed and *terrified* by an object or circumstance and someone in a *fury* or rampage of destruction. Furthermore, the level of presentation capacity (morphic multiplicity) in each antisymmetric state has the same value. According to trigonometric rules, whether an angle *Θ* is positive or negative, its cosine is the same positive value. Accordingly, it is easy to concur that the level of presentation (issuing or supporting the amount of *representations*) in *terror* must be rated at the same exact value as the level of presentation in *fury*, both being experientially two paroxysmal mind states. Same would hold true for the presentation level or morphic multiplicity by someone in the profound *despair* of Grief Reaction compared to the emotion she experienced at the height of *passion* in that relationship. Keep in mind that the presentation capacity property we otherwise call morphic multiplicity supports and controls the amount of representations, as percepts or incepts, the discrete pensive partition is able to handle. As we can see, in the above Presentation relation, as the angle *Θ* becomes larger, the quantity *1/Θ* becomes smaller, accordingly the quantity *cos(1/Θ)* becomes larger, which is the Presentation value. Concordantly, the extreme mind states in Groups -4A and +4B show the highest morphic multiplicity and the most central ones in Groups -1A and +1B show the lowest value for this variable.

Should the reader wonder why the entire partitioning is based on a division of 4, we have found that the entire spectrum of human root thoughts available in language and literature yields both in nomenclature and ensuing dynamics to this set division. In the pure mathematical-physics Quanto-Geometric Theory, this partitioning is controlled through a formula denoted *azimuthal genic relation*[7], which we spare the reader of this publication, in the desire to conveniently keep everything mathematical as simple as possible. At the end, the partitioning in 4 is not a critical aspect of the psychophysics application of the Model, the binary aspect of the distribution holding prepronderance over the partitioning. Should one decide to include, say one more partition in one layer, same must be done to the opposite side of the layer at the antisymmetric location, which in turn mandates that two inclusions of the kind must be done to every other layer, so that the integrity of the entire distribution is preserved.

1.14 Ultra-Structure and Dynamics of Pensive Normal Layers

The Normal Layer of the Mental Foliate must be visualized with at very least two major strata longitudinally, which are relatively independent from one another (Fig. 1.10). One embodies the root thoughts as inventoried in the Foliate Map and the other the actual representations brought in by the living experience or from intralayer genesis as a result of inter-partition interaction. The representational stratum is implanted within the root layer and stands for a specialization of the latter at early stages of the lifecycle as they were being permeated by living experience perceptions and slated to issue responses through effectors. The representation sublayer(s) are thus superimposed on the root thought's principal substratum.

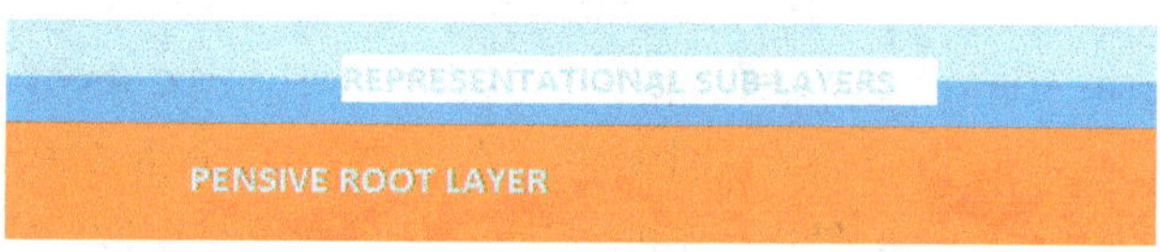

Fig. 1.10 Structure of a normal Mental Layer on the Mentation Manifold

[7] Quanto-Geometry, Overture of Cosmic Consciousness and Universal Knowled for All, Vol II.

The deep portion of the root layer remains more or less immutable after its initial period of consolidation, whereas the representational strata are subject to changes or content additions in the lifecycle. Nonetheless, as we previously mentioned, the autobiographical formation in this layer remains forever unchanged in its condition of indelible basis memory. It is likely that the autobiographical mnemonic information resides in the representational sub-stratum contiguous to the root layer. As previously mentioned, a representational packet incrusted in the representation layer may be repeated indefinitely on any number of partitions cross layer and along the same layer.

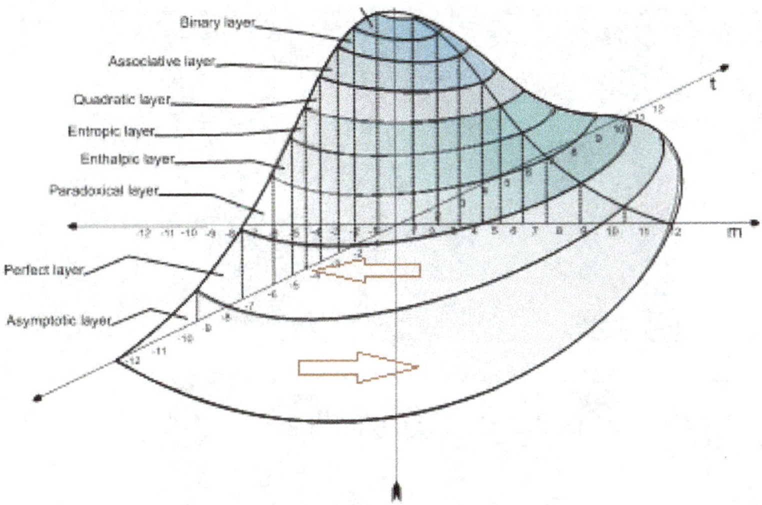

Fig. 111 Two arrows showing the two possible directions of transflow impulses as they travel longitudinally across the Perfect Layer and the Asymptotic Layer of the Manifold.

The pensive impulse of its own, which is not to be confused with the nervous impulse per the monist perspective, bears similarities with the latter, however. The Mental Foliate Manifold showcases vertical pathways along which the pensive impulse travels from one partition to the next one up across the layer stack, in an either up or down direction. We call these impulses *orthoflows*. Across a layer, the impulse travels longitudinally from one partition to the next lateral one, in an either left or right direction. We call these impulses *transflows* (Fig 1.11). We visualize a pensive impulse as an all-or-none signal output by a partition altogether, akin to the nervous impulse. It is best represented as the domino drop model, where an impulse is borne out in the form of numeric binary logic as a result of a full throw/no-throw event. The impulse travels across the partitions akin to a domino swing scrolling along the chain of prearranged domino keys (Fig 1.12). Perhaps the spiral spring in experimental physics is an even better illustration for the transitioning of the mental impulse, since after the strike of one turn of the spiral onto the next, the former returns to the stand-by position ready to transmit the next impulse. There is here similarity with the nerve cell of the nervous system, since after discharge the nerve cell quickly restores the bio-chemical potential for the next electric strike.

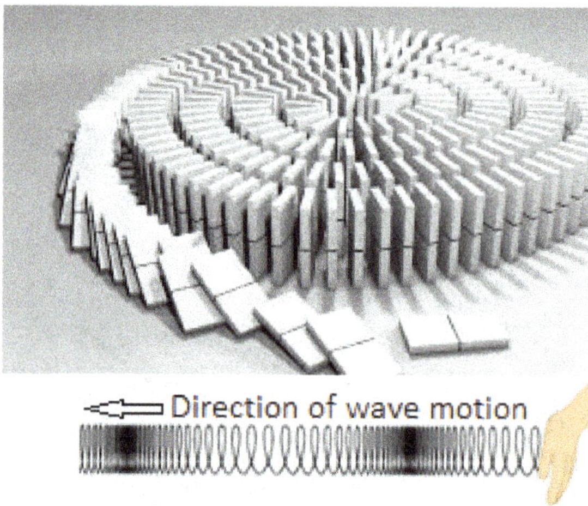

Fig. 1.12 An emulation of travel mental pulses

This impulse would be unsuitable as an alternative signal similar to alternative electric current in a wire, due to the topological arrangement based on broad discrete partitions stacked against one another. At the macroscopic level, the impulse is not based on particulate quantum units of matter transitioning between energy density states. It is seemingly unnecessary to delve any further into the physics of this artifact, since it is an experimental endeavour which requires many fundamental questions of the metric order in the physics of matter to be satisfactorily resolved, as a theoretical precondition. For further analytic details on the pensive impulse model, we refer the reader to the publication of reference[8] by one of the authors.

1.15 The Conscious v. the Unconscious

One unmistakable characterization of human mentation that every human individual is fully aware of is the division between the realm of conscious thoughts, which is the matter of conscious experience, and that of unconscious mental activity, which we experience in regular nightly dreams or occasional daytime dreams. We are quite cognizant that our conscious thoughts are cogent and rational while our unconscious cognitive universe seems to be utterly irrational and emotional. We are well aware that in consciousness we exert our highest level of volition which is the driver allowing us to mobilize the world around us at every moment, whereas in unconscious state volition is at a low gradient, given that when the unconscious takes over in normal conditions we are motionless for the most part with very minimal interaction with the environment. The level of irrationality and the strength of emotions that our unconscious minds are able to reach are such that we wittingly avoid bringing them back for examination once back to conscious, remaining in so much awe of this potential.

We surmise that everyone is well aware that a clear-cut line between our conscious universe and the unconscious falters because of this gray zone of semiconscious and semiunconscious that we are well aware we go through when we are about to fall asleep, as much as we are aware of going through this transition zone when we awake from sleep before turning fully conscious.

We make this triplet stage of conscious – semiconscious/semiunconscious – unconscious a direct match to the three Quintessential phases of the Quanto-Geometric Function in our mathematical-physics analysis. A brief explanation of what Quintessence in Quanto-Geometric Theory is follows. It is a construct that arises from redimensioning what a derivative is in Analytic Geometry and what it says of the curvature evolution of a function. Trivalent Quintessence results from differentiation of the Quanto-Geometric Function.

---

[8] **The Human Mind Inside**, A Novel Interpretation of the Structure and Operation of the Human Mind, Jean-Claude, Joseph J.

$$\frac{dQ(m,t)}{ds} = \frac{-(m+t)}{\sigma^3\sqrt{2\pi}} \cdot e^{\frac{-(m+t)^2}{2\sigma^2}}$$

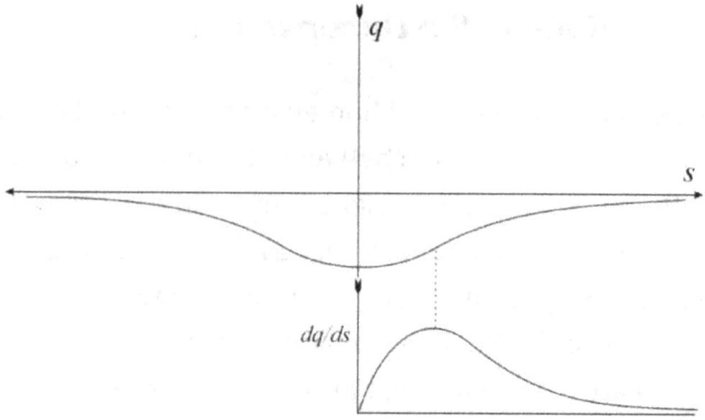

Fig. 1.13 First-order Derivative of the Quanto-Geometric function of one variable *(s)*

In effect, the first-order derivative of the Function has the virtue of extolling the three grand moments or phases enclosed in the first-order correlation between the independent and dependent variables. We remind the reader that a Function is essentially a specific form of correlation between a set of two variables, the independent and the dependent variable(s). The independent variables are always understood to be the due instantiators of change or variation, and the Function as the dependent variable responds to those forerunner changes. Alternatively, if we extemporaneously assign a value to the function, then we may deduce the corresponding value of the independent variable(s). The first-order derivative discloses the first-order correlation between the independent and the dependent variables. At higher canonical level of the Quanto-Geometric framework, the Function *Q(s)* or *q* stands for a *scalar* tenet (or mass physically) and the variables *m* and *t* the *space* tenet, which begets motion and geometry. The numeric expression of the first-order derivative is expressed Fig. 1.13 and a transversal cut of the 3-dimensional manifold represented in the graph. An analysis of the graphic evolution of the partial derivatives casts the following observations.

In one phase or Phase 1 → partial derivatives $\left.\frac{\partial q}{\partial t}\right|_{m} > 1$ and $\left.\frac{\partial q}{\partial m}\right|_{t} > 1$, which translates into the scalar tenet dominating or eclipsing the space tenet in the correlation (second graph in Fig. 1.13).

In the second phase or Phase 2 → $\left.\frac{\partial q}{\partial t}\right|_{m} < 1$ and $\left.\frac{\partial q}{\partial m}\right|_{t} < 1$, which translates into the space tenet dominating or eclipsing the scalar tenet in the correlation.

In the third or Mid-Phase → $\left.\frac{\partial q}{\partial t}\right|_{m} = 1$ and $\left.\frac{\partial q}{\partial m}\right|_{t} = 1$, which means equated co-variant influence between the scalar tenet and the space tenet. The first-order derivative monotonically increases in Phase 1, monotonically decreases in Phase 2 and remains invariant in the Mid-phase. Phase 2 has a broad spread trending to infinity, Phase 1 has a limited and finite spread and the Mid-Phase has an extremely limited spread.

When it comes to applying this characterization to the analysis of the Conscious and Unconscious domains of the Mental Body, we see that this triplet categorization perfectly applies to the three grand mentation domains, well characterized in Freudian Analytic Psychology. We remind the reader that *q* is emulated here by the volition faculty; *m* and *t,* originally space variables, are hereby emulated by the motivation and presentation faculties. Even individual experience brings us the introspective awareness that the universe of our conscious rational thoughts has a much smaller spread than the vast amplitude, range and depth of emotional mind fits accessible in the sleep cycle. If there is a gray zone between the two universes, we have the sense that it must be topologically singular, with much less amplitude than the other two universes, because we essentially transition through it and in rather short order. The Mentation Manifold clearly displays a demarcation consistent with these boundaries, where layers 5 to 9 stand from the Unconscious realm, Layers 1 to 3 the Conscious realm and Layer 4 the Semi-Conscious realm. So therefore:

$\left.\frac{\partial q}{\partial t}\right|_{m} > 1$ and $\left.\frac{\partial q}{\partial m}\right|_{t} > 1$ → Conscious Realm

$$\left.\frac{\partial q}{\partial t}\right|_m < 1 \quad \text{and} \quad \left.\frac{\partial q}{\partial m}\right|_t < 1 \quad \rightarrow \text{Unconscious Realm}$$

$$\left.\frac{\partial q}{\partial t}\right|_m = 1 \quad \text{and} \quad \left.\frac{\partial q}{\partial m}\right|_t = 1 \quad \rightarrow \text{Semi-Conscious/Semi-Unconscious}$$

Upon first-sight examination, it would seem that our conscious thoughts are strictly volitive, rational or realistic and our unconscious thoughts strictly emotional and dispersive, as perceived from our dreams. Viewed from the covariant vantage between two orthogonal variables, however, it is because our conscious thoughts feature dominance of volition over presentation/motivation that they acquire the constricted quality which characterizes them. They are sober and constrained thoughts, so to speak, with a realistic quality to them. On the other hand, it is only because our unconscious thoughts feature dominance of presentation/motivation over volition that they acquire the emotional and dispersive quality normally attributed to them. That also explains at once why the language of the Conscious (common human languages) is logical, straightforward and one-dimensional, while the language of the Unconscious is a symbolic and multidimensional language in the terms perceived and instructed by S. Freud for the interpretation of nightly dreams. The conscious language only bears one dimension in that every term means one thing, synonyms and homonyms being a few exceptions to the rule. The unconscious language is multi-dimensional in that a word is an imagery that represents something else in the sense of holding for a symbol, and that image set may be meaningful only to a particular person, while other image sets are common in meaning to a collective or mankind altogether, such as an archetype. It is the afore-discussed covariance between the variables, in their dependency relation, that is responsible for the difference in the form of expression inherent to each domain of the Mental. One can forthrightly see that when the motivation/morphic factor is dominant the language is symbolic, and when the volition factor is dominant, the language is on point and constrained.

1.15.1 Configuration of the Mental Cursor

The last mental descriptor to introduce in this study is what we have dubbed the Mental Cursor. This characterization provides a material quality to Self-

Awareness in the Symmetry terms that we have defined it, as much as it extols the connection of Self-Awareness with the delimitation of Conscious and Unconscious in the Mental Body. Effectively Self-Awareness is not only a conscious artifact, it spreads the Unconscious alike. Everybody has an experience of Self in their nightly dreams. Our dreams are comparable to a movie with the principal protagonist being the Self entity. We are however aware that there is a different quality to this unconscious Self than there is to the conscious Self. First of all, the unconscious Self does a lot of irrational or unrealistic things. Note that the possibility well exists that it could instead behave in a realistic fashion, despite its intangible character. For instance, it could engage in realistic stories, like the protagonist of our movies, unreal but reality-driven. It materially does not implement reality-driven sceneries, however. It could speak like the conscious Self does. It does not, either. But it will do such things as flying, unlike the Conscious Self. It is further engaged in a symbolic expression of behavior, unlike the Conscious Self.

At times, when the heuristic behavior becomes so stressful, in order to escape the distress of such nightmares, it can say to itself, *"I am not experiencing this for real, this is a dream, an unreal dream*" and subsequently wakes up from it, in order to put an end to the distress. These are formally denoted *lucid* dreams. Therefore the Unconscious Self is self-aware. It too is invariant. By virtue of this invariance we do not find ourselves a different personage every time we go to bed and sleep, we invariably remain the same personage therein. In fact, a significant number of dreams are recurrent throughout a lifecycle, just as the thread of life of the Conscious Self is largely repetitive, on a day-to-day and weekly basis as we well know. Furthermore, the thread of life of the Unconscious Self is episodic as well, in the sense that it takes off every night from where it left it the night before. This is evidenced in artificial or provoked somnambulism by an operator across sessions. We will not pursue that line of analysis however, since it lies beyond the original motivation for this treatise.

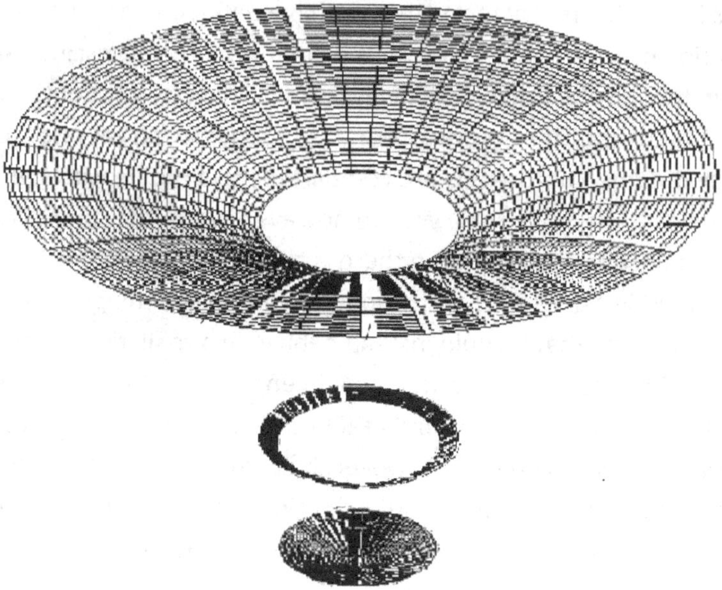

Fig. 1.14 Origin of Quanto-Geometric Tri-Valent Quintessence

Hence our previous definition for the Conscious Self-Awareness fully holds for the Unconscious Self-Awareness as well. Be that as it may, one should not mistake this characterization for two independent Mental entities that concomitantly exist in the Mental Body. Self-Awareness incarnates one single entity of a monolithic nature that takes different faculties or properties depending on its location within the three realms of the Mental. We duly call this entity the Mental Cursor. When it is located in the Conscious realm, we call it the *Hypocursor*; when located in the Unconscious realm, we call it the *Hypercursor* and when located in the quadratic realm we call it the Quadratic Cursor or *Quadracursor*. We have a clear sense of this continuity in the Awareness monolith when we examine the transitioning that occurs between wake and sleep, in both directions. When we are head butting again and again as we are falling asleep, we do not experience a gap or jump between the two states, but a smooth transition in awareness. Likewise, if we direct ourselves to experience a slow transition from sleep to wake, we will acquire the clear sense that the transition between one state and the other is a conversion in the sense of Self. The sense of Self or the Self-Awareness monolith simply takes the attributes of the Mental domain to which it migrates.

In the physical Theory, we invoke the first derivative of the Quanto-Geometric Function to explain the meaning and implications of covariance between the variables and have denoted that categorization Trivalent Quintessence (Fig. 1.14). In the psychophysics application, first-order Quintessence perfectly describes the high-level tripartite partition of the Mental Body as previously exposed. Second-order Quintessence, incarnated in the second derivative of the Quanto-Geometric Function, stands for appropriate and complete formal description of the Mental Cursor here in discussion. The calculus rule has it that when the second derivative of a function is equal to 0, there is an inflexion point at that location on the graph. In the 3-dimensional or Manifold representation of the graph, the inflexion is given by a whole set of points instead of one point. Second-order Quintessence has the virtue of describing at once all 3 phases of the Mental Cursor. When

$$\frac{d^2Q(m+t)}{d(m+t)^2}=0 \text{ for } (t=\pm\sigma) and (m=+\sigma)$$

then the set of standard deviation points delimit and show the inflexion region in the curvature development of the graph. This sector of the Manifold represents the domain of the Quadracursor. The sector that lies at the left side of the inflexion point represents a region of the Mental manifold where the curvature is closed, formally expressible as follows from the second derivative:

$$\frac{d^2Q(m+t)}{d(m+t)^2}>0 \ ,$$

for $(+\sigma<t<+\infty) and (-\infty<t<-\sigma) and (+\sigma<m<+\infty)$, province of the Hypocursor.

The sector lying at the right side of the inflexion points represents a region of the Mental manifold where the curvature is open, formally expressible as follows:

$$\frac{d^2Q(m+t)}{d(m+t)^2}<0 \ ,$$

for $(+\sigma < t < +\infty) and (-\infty < t < -\sigma) and (+\sigma < m < +\infty)$, province of the Hypercursor.

The cursor moves from partition to partition and may be represented as a mini manifold sectional of its own inside the main Mental Manifold, somewhat akin to the needle of a scale or the sweeping lit span of a radar monitor or the spotlight on a theater stage. It entertains its own dynamics, although it does not know of or adjust to any interstitial location between partitions of the main Manifold or Foliate: it sweeps discretely from one partition to the next. Furthermore, it represents a major focus or destination for the flows taking place in the subdomain of its presence, whether the Conscious, the Unconscious or the SemiConscious. For instance, the stealthy hunter, in deep concentration awaiting to shoot a deer, will have the Hypocursor momentarily posted on the Cupidity or Competitive partition. Everything else going on in the mind remains under conscious control of the Hypocursor instance, which will refrain every subjacent pulse or urge coming in from other regions of the positive side of the Foliate, or every other feeling or sensation coming in from the negative side of the Foliate that do not play outright into the situation.

1.16 Conclusion

It is our hope that the above study has set a new paradigm in the thorough visualization of the architecture of the Human Mental. We also hope to have set the definitive basis for a mathematical-physics formalism able to insightfully embrace the entire phenomenon of the Human Mental. One of the virtues of such an effort has been to capably integrate a large number of the constructs in use in the diverse fields of mental science. It has notably uncovered the root levels of the anatomy and the dynamics of the Human Mental. The effort to constrain these constructs with mathematical logic further promises to show fruits when we next address the question of human Characterology and human Mental dysfunctions.

Chapter 2

REDIMENSIONING HUMAN SEXUALITY FROM A PSYCHOPHYSICS PERSPECTIVE

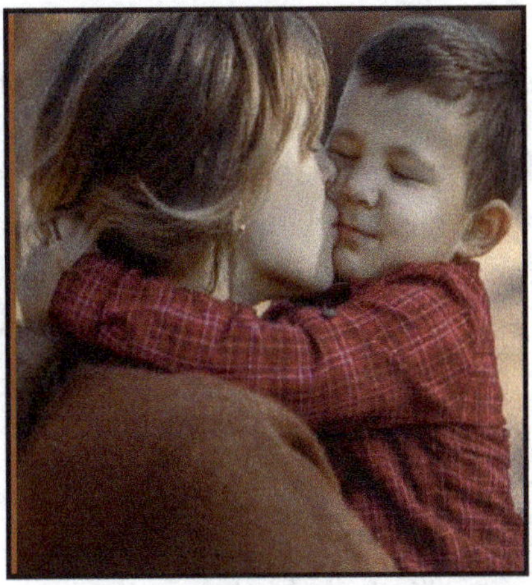

Human sexuality has always been a delicate, uncomfortable and controversial subject in all-time human culture and under all latitudes. Yet it remains one of the most central aspects, if not the most significant aspect, of human ontology. It is manifest not only at the individual level in the act of intercourse between male and female (or their surrogates), but also at the social level both in the societal adoption of a form of gender primacy in social organization as portrayed in patriarchal v. matriarchal organization and in the overt censorship of the female gender and its attributes in certain patriarchal cultures.

The study of human sexuality in the West has been exclusively based on the history of sexuality as it has been experienced in Europe and North America. Inasmuch as the results of such studies are aimed at consolidating a science to be applied in the Western World, in therapeutic settings involving dysfunctions experienced by people in the West, this limitation in scope is quite understandable from a practical point of view. However, the conclusions of such studies should not be considered universally applicable or imposed to practice under other latitudes where social elements of the sexual phenomenon significantly differ from the experience of the West, and even in the West amongst indigenous cultures.

It is also clear that most practitioners in those other countries or regions of the world do apply the corresponding restrictions demanded by culture in their clinical practice.

That said, one must understand that there are observable facts common to the experience under all latitudes and which should inform theory in the quest for a universal science of Mind. Incompatible with science in its quest for objective and unbiased understanding of observable reality is the game of group influence attempting to impose their views and own way of life within the social corpus. The demarcation line here is certainly not easier to delineate than it is when attempting to evaluate whether sexual taboos of a different nature are justified or unjustified.

2.1 Psychoanalytic Perspective of Human Sexuality

It is understandable that Dr. Sigmund Freud had sought in Greco-Latin mythology the necessary metaphors to assist him in a detached exposition and dispassionate interpretation of sexual behavior of the puritan European culture of his time. He built his theory as he discovered more and more sexual motives in human behavior and strived to find the necessary language to explain it, without incurring untimely rejection from the public at large and academics alike. One of the sustained criticisms long levied against Freudian psychoanalysis is *pansexuality*, despite the fact that sexuality is irrefutably and irrevocably present in human life from birth, one being born out of it, to early phase of development when gender intermingling is socially inevitable, to the ubiquitous presence of mature love in society (workplaces, churches, sporting venues, etc.), to the momentous and sumptuous marriage ceremonies, to the pursuance and experience of life in couple for the long haul, and to the elderly still actively looking for love in their late lives. On that account alone, one should be ready to flatly consider the existential interpretation of an individual human life essentially along the sexuality storyline, due to its undeniable extensive life-long footprint. It may well be that other longitudes exist in a human life, but it is also possible for that one particular longitude to be the most central in the span of a human life. That assessment, under the weight of several millennia of Puritanism in the West, does not come as a matter of course.

Dr. Sigmund Freud's psychoanalysis, along with its Jungian variant and others, had also been criticized of lacking experimental basis, a criticism most often levied in modern times as scientism is taking stronger and stronger hold in Western Culture. The idea that in the intricate and complex matter of Mind, the inquesting subject must turn the Mind into a material object for observation, as if no form of introspection was possible or that the Mind cannot reasonably reflect onto itself, is as preposterous and unsound as pretending that nobody else around us has consciousness or has nightly dreams because we cannot directly put them under observation. This criticism generally comes from social science intellectuals who ignore the fundamental role played by thought experiments in the experimental science of theoretical physics, an example of which is the prominent role played by such systematic thought projections in the development of Einstein's Theory of General Relativity or the EPR paradox in Quantum Physics.

Furthermore, the criticism that Freudian analysis lacks experimental basis comes from total ignorance or inconsideration of the fact that before the advent of Freudian psychoanalysis, Dr. Jean Martin Charcot, father of the science of Neurology, had put the unconscious on firm empirical grounds in the 1800's at *La Salpetrière Hospital - Paris*, where he treated hundreds of highly psychotic patients, induced in the very stylized forms of unconscious sleep. It was there that neurologist Sigmund Freud had witnessed the profound sentient states of the human unconscious right before his eyes, which gave him the basis for sketching the overall structure of the Unconscious. The influence of Jean Martin Charcot's empiricism on Sigmund Freud was instrumental in the development of his vision of a Mental Architecture and the psychoanalytic technique. The knowledge of these historical facts seems to have insufficiently transpired in the teachings of Anglo-American psychology and psychiatry; even in Europe they seem to have been forgotten, and that is indeed a problem.

2.2 Sexual Undercurrents in Family Units of More Than Two

The fundamentals in the behavior exposed under the *Oedipus complex* in psychoanalytic theory are this: the young child finds himself or herself in a shelter dominated by two figures, namely the mother and the father; and the question for the child is how do I interrelate with the two? The child has behind himself or herself a short life as a baby where he/she is intimately or bodily related to the mother figure, as an extension of her experience of carriage. Our responsibility as academics, researchers and practitioners is to gather the full extent of facts involved in that phase of human development, under all latitudes, in order to best comprehend the interactions taking place within the experience and best project from there the lines of development of a young human life. This requires from the analyst's mind an explosion of all taboos and freedom from all types of social and cultural pressure or impositions, and the courage to put the finger on the wound alike. In the following, we will attempt to do just that.

We all recognize that what makes the situation in the Oedipus complex so controversial is the sexual undertone possibly involved in the relationship between the child and one of the two parenting figures. We are going to anchor our analysis on this central aspect of the controversial experience. We unreservedly believe that if the situation captured under the Freudian term of Oedipus complex was to be put under the spotlight, as a first, by a female analyst in a matriarchal society, it would have been treated in a much different manner than it was and still is today in the male-dominated Western culture.

2.3 Pivotal Role of the Mother Figure

One of the questions seldom prospected in the concerning situation is how the mother figure feels and orchestrates it. Notice that she is in fact the most pivotal figure in the tripartite relationship. Best understanding of the Oedipian situation can be derived from the viewpoint of the mother being at its center stage. The child, whether male or female, entertains a bodily relationship with her as a baby and a toddler. Save the cases of C-section operations, she had both a conception and vaginal experience with the infant which, as a female undertaking, was an aspect of her sexual experience. In popular culture in the West, one of the things that young men hold as a taboo, albeit one apparently in decline, is to avoid looking at a partum to witness how the baby is coming out of the dilated vagina, in order to avoid disturbing or damaging the young husband's libido in post-partum life. This is, however, only the beginning of the mother's sexual experience with the newborn baby. In general, the partum sexual experience is

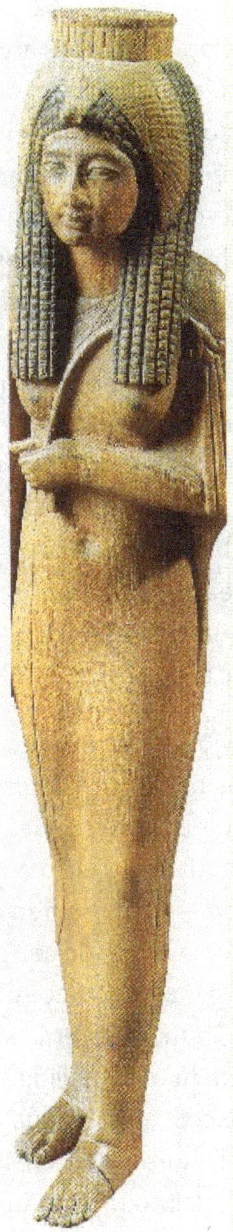

a painful one as we know, but one mixed with the joy of giving life to a man, and to give the world something out of herself.

2.4 Breast Feeding as the Beginning of Sexual Experience

For sure, one of the most important mutual sexual artifacts between mother and baby is breast feeding. While for the baby it will be a pleasurable lingual, labial, gustative and visual experience, for the mother it is a pleasurable sensual experience, which is outright a sexual experience. And so it is under all latitudes.

It is well known that nipple stimulation releases oxytocin which leads to milk secretion and in some instances uterine contractions. In addition, prolactin release equally occurs. Sexual arousal of the mother is clinically known to occur during breastfeeding. Quite tellingly, breastfeeding may result in euphoria, in which case it is coined “milk drunkenness”.

In the more equalitarian societies such as the ancient Pharonic culture of the Saharan Kemets, women used to expose on their naked tops the physical attribute of their globular breasts as a way to manifest their personal feminine presence. In matriarchal or matriarchal-leaning societies, such as the Fon-Yoruba culture of Western Africa, a close parent to the Kemetic culture, women used to remain topless, even to this day, as a way to impose their personal feminine presence. In that cultural area of the world, where the habit of wearing western-style clothing covering the entire body has somewhat solidified, a woman experiencing anger out of personal matters would take to the street completely naked, top, bottom and butts, to explode and, in that manner, impose her feminine presence.

It is safe to say that in general women's breasts, which develop as a secondary sexual characteristic at puberty under hormonal stimulation, are indeed for them a sexual attribute, beyond their phylogenetic function of feeding the young for survival. It is likely for the same reason that nature has turned the act of feeding with the breast or breastfeeding an enjoyable exercise for those entrusted to carry on the continuation of the human race. In the northern Puritan cultures, the very fact by women of protecting their breasts with a piece of clothing is yet another pointer to the sexuality it arouses in them: at the beach, they bear nothing on their bodies except for squint clothing on their bottom and their breasts. There are thus good reasons to believe that all women everywhere enjoy giving their breasts to the men they love, not as a result of learned developmental behavior, but as a sexual phylogenetic trait. By the same token, it is fully justified to say that adult men who love to suckle their fiancés and wives, and take sexual enjoyment in contemplating their breasts and watching breastfeeding, do so as a result of learned behavior in their early relationship with their nurturing mothers, but not as a sexual phenotypic dictate.

Furthermore, the male co-author of this study was able to witness the experience of a mother who had no issue breast feeding her male baby, but felt uncomfortable enough in regards to breast feeding her daughter child to refuse doing it at all. Save the case when a lack of bond between mother and child or an impending depression is to blame, it may well be that women in Puritan societies, who altogether refuse to breast feed their children at any rate, do so due to the very sexual sensations that the exercise arouses in them. In that assessment, we set aside the push by today's farming industry in the Western world to move women away from breastfeeding for own benefit of supplying vast amounts of baby milk formulae. At the other side of the coin, one is equally in good right to speculate that the stories known in popular culture in the West about some modern-day women breast feeding their child well into their toddler years tell us of some examples of women willing indeed to go these extra lengths for personal sexual enjoyment for whatever reason, without us casting any judgement whatsoever on them. We duly acknowledge the exception in yesteryears when late breastfeeding might have been done under the intent purpose of contraception, since breastfeeding outright inhibits ovulation.

2.5 Preserving Pleasure with Wet-Nurses

There is every reason to believe that the practice of employing wet-nurses by aristocrat women throughout the history of Europe and in colonial America goes principally on account of this feeling of discomfort aroused in them by breast-feeding due to its sexual connotation. The practice reached summit in 19th Century Europe and colonial America. Philip Vickers Fithian wrote as a tutor in Robert Carter's household in the state of Virginia at the time: *"I find it common here for people of fortune to have their young children suckled by the Negroes!"* A newspaper advertisement in Jornal do Comercio in Brazil, dated Dec 10, 1827 publishes: *"For rent, a wet nurse with very good milk, from her first pregnancy, gave birth six days ago, in Rua de Pescadores, N° 64. Be it advised that she does not have a child."* Anyone is free to guess what was the fortune or misfortune of the child born in bondage so that his mother could be rented as a wet nurse. Further, many may allege that the refusal by women to breastfeed a child is due to the physical pain that continued breast feeding sessions may cause to the mother. That can only be part of the truth, since some young modern women, who are more open on these subjects than any previous generation, will confess that they find it, in their own words, *"divine, as it is meant to be"*.

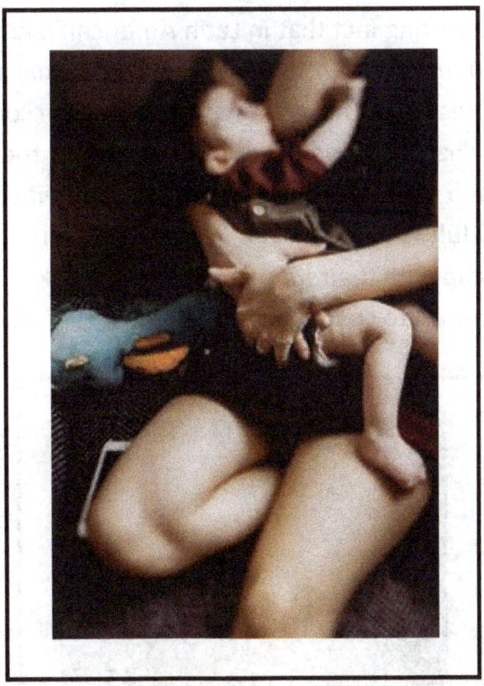

2.6 Deary Names Betraying Breast-Feeding Sexual Undercurrents

To this record, we have to add the fact that sweetie names socially in use in many countries around the world, in particular in Latin American countries, give clues to the sexual character of the relationship between young male progeny and their mothers. As Freud did write in an 1897 letter, *"I found in myself a constant love for my mother, and jealousy of my father. I now consider this to be a universal event in early childhood."* The earliest known stage in human history that the word *"mama"* was used by young children to refer to their mother was the Saharan Kemetic culture where the word *"mammisi"* was used to indicate the houses where pregnant women in labor were taken to for care. In the 10 most common human languages, the word in use is specifically: *māma, mama, mamá, ma, mama, mamã, maa, maman, haha and mamī.* To state that it is a long-known and long-in-use universal word is a fair assessment. Is it not an interesting fact that in Latin American countries men commonly use the word *mami (sweet little mama)* during sexual intercourse in the sweetie language addressed to their female mate which accompanies arousal and orgasm? They only have one *mami* and the uttering of the word during adult sexual intercourse, and even at other times during their life in couple, is a clear indication that their adult sexual behavior has been fully informed by their infant sensual relationship with their *mami*. By the same token, it is quite relevant to mention, when it comes to characterize their early day relationship with their fathers, that Latino women do the same by calling their male partner *"papi"* in those intimate moments or to otherwise be affectionate with their husbands.

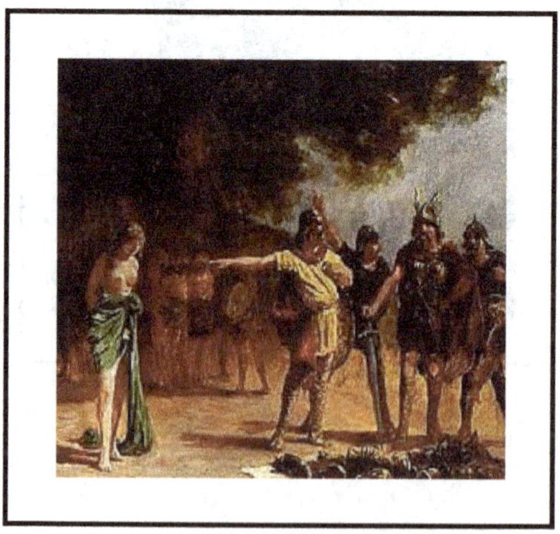

2.7 Topless Women as Booty of War

Another practice of old, as depicted by some, to cast to this record is the one known in Vikings tradition that has a girl excite and lead warriors to the battleground by riding topless on a horse before them. Being in a state of uncontrollable sexual arousal, they would expectedly charge against the enemy with absolutely everything they got. They later expose the captured enemies' women in topless appearance as part of booty for their victor soldiers to choose from.

2.8 Breastfeeding in Public

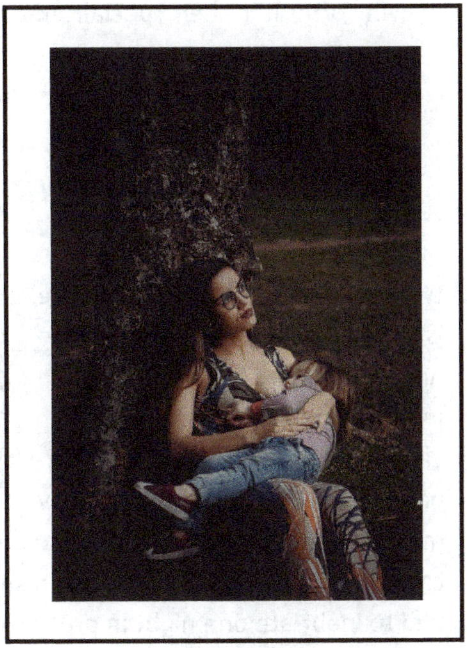

Another interesting situation is that of women who take to public places such as malls, street curbs, pool sides, churches, etc., to breastfeed their child, exposing their breasts in the making. Some women critiques argue that those do not do it in response to urgent need of feeding their babies but for exhibitionism poses. Needless to say that, in most countries, breastfeeding in public is considered *indecent exposure*, notwithstanding the global feminine initiative dubbed *World Breastfeeding Week*, where women rally in open venues to overtly breastfeed their babies. Whether considered exhibitionism or indecent exposure, the rather disapproving reaction to breastfeeding in public in Northern cultures puts before us the clear sexual undertone that women's breasts connote to men. It is not about whether the act is justified or not - i.e. the baby needs feeding in the moment - but the sensitive disapproval or discomfort that the act causes to the rest of the citizenry due to its sexual undertone (or overtone).

2.9 Breast Surgery for Enhanced Sexual Attraction

To this dossier, we have to likewise add the sexual motives behind the individual resolution by modern-day women to effect breast surgery to the aims of giving their breasts a more attractive and provocative appearance. Of course, some respond to their partner's desire of more bountiful breasts. However, recognition of these connotations comes from medical science itself, with all its male and female physicians, who have strived to make the procedure possible and actively offer it in their specialized practices.

2.10 A Rational Basis for the Incest Taboo

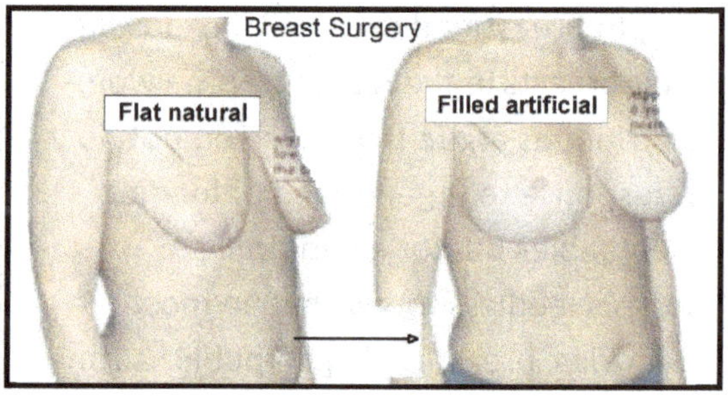

In virtually all human cultures, sexual relationship between mothers and their sons, and between fathers and daughters alike, is under strict incest taboo, a prohibition that we can ultimately justify from a genomic point of view. In the Bible story of Lot, her daughters, who could not find any man around for sexual intercourse and marrying owing to their apparent physical isolation, resorted to engage in such relations with their father, who they had to inebriate one night in order to have sex with him. The Bible relates this story as a forfeit. We know the human genome is looking for diversity in the name of survival, and from that point of view, in the family unit, sexual relations between its inner members, which knowingly produce defective human specimens, is justifiably universally prohibited by social taboos. These taboos however shall not foul the analyst into dismissing the motives of sexual nature that naturally arise within intrafamily relations on account of the simple fact that human beings are indefectibly sexuate.

Some, in the post-modern era of psychoanalysis, have attempted to explain the incest taboo by disqualifying the unconscious motives as genuine *instinctual sexual desire*, and qualifying them instead as *instinctual sexual aversion* against these relations (Westermarck effect). Steven Pinker wrote that "*The idea that boys want to sleep with their mothers strikes most men as the silliest thing they have ever heard.*" That may be true, just because they never get to be aware of these impulses, let alone to remember them once they had become adults, even less to admit that they ever had them. The aforementioned assessment from Steven Pinker is a statement of how well the incest social taboo had worked across generations. Since every time a baby boy has been lying in bed with his mother, with his frail body against her chest and suckling her breasts, he has been materially sexually in bed with her. But as far as sexual intercourse, note that: 1) the incest social taboo has already well solidified in the mother's mind to guard against it at the first place, 2) the situation is not given or cannot materialize with an impuber boy, and 3) by the time of puberty around age 16 the social taboo has already taken firm hold as well in his mind. So therefore the question of sexual intercourse between mother and son is moot and would qualify as a straw man argument. Be all that as it may, the case exists in the world psychiatric record of an 18-month old boy who was unusually rubbing his genitals on his mother's body during breastfeeding and later at age 6 on his caring grandmother's buttocks (See Frotteurism in the *Commented Bibliography* section).

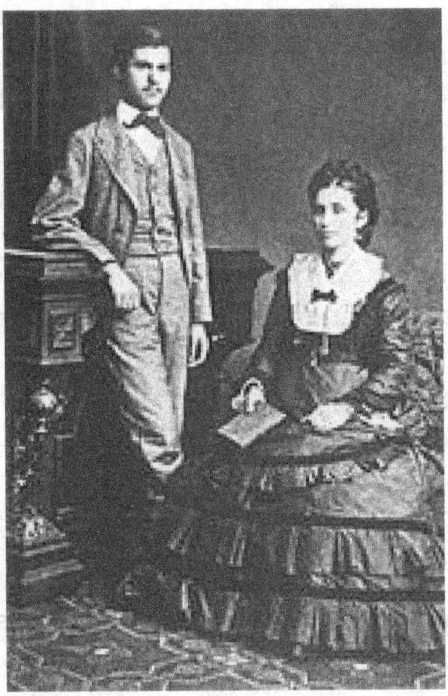

On the account that Freud as a boy once had an erotic reaction to watching his mother dressing, per his own admission, a psychologist explains that "*Freud's mother Amalia Nathansohn Freud was relatively young and of reproductive age during his childhood and since he had a wet-nurse, he may not have experienced the early intimacy with his mother that would have tipped off*

his perceptual system that the woman on his watch was his mother!" This is a funny explanation postulating an instinct of no reaction to a particular percept! Further, in many if not most countries around the world beyond the West, most people marry and have children at very young age, that is to say in their twenties.

2.11 Unavoidable Oedipian Situation

The idea that, in modern-day societies where same-sex unions have become lawful, a young infant in that environment does not experience the conflicts arising from the Oedipus complex is a dead idea on arrival, for the simple reason that in the parental couple one has to play the role of mother and the other the role of father, lest they should be considered a dysfunctional couple. When society puts in the hands of the psychoanalyst cases of that nature, it has not given him or her simpler cases to resolve but otherwise difficult or complicated cases to resolve, for the simple reason that the analyst has now to decipher how the child had resolved the gender identity scheme upon which to map the traditional sexuality motives of the subject in development. Nonsexuate human beings do not exist and intergender relations constitute an inevitable outcome in a family unit. The problem here is this: one cannot assume that same gender parent-child relation, in this case mother-daughter relation, does not entail sexual undertone. It matter-of-factly does, and it is the very reason why mothers in the West have historically chosen to not breast feed at all for the most part. What the daughter child learns in that early experience is *gender empathy*, which characterizes women as a social group. There lies the very important asymmetry that has not been captured by either Freudian, or Jungian psychoanalytic theory in its revisionist approach. Breast feeding informs the early sexual experience of babies in differing phenotypical ways, depending on whether the baby is a male or a female. It is worth underscoring the fact that, at the physiological level, boys and girls get different breast milk as well from their mothers. Mother's milk as the first food for infants is *not created equal*. Research in biology has found that, in humans and other mammals, milk composition changes depending on the infant's gender and on whether conditions are good or unfavorable. Studies have also shown that boys drink more milk on average than girls do.

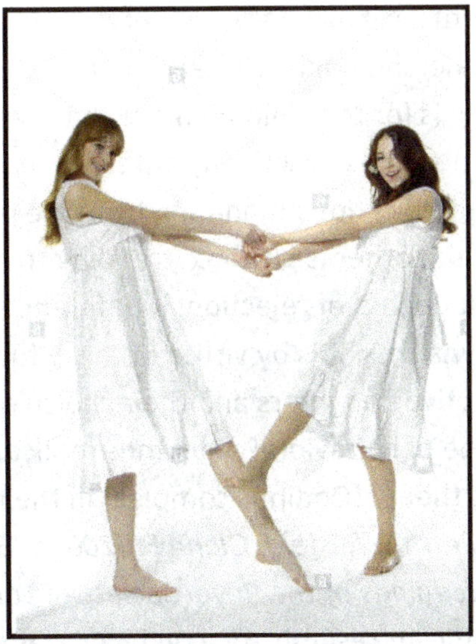

Should we boldly make a projection from this physiological asymmetry, we would state that the empathetic tender that an adult woman feels towards other women, manifest when we see them kindly hold each other's hands for instance in one situation or another, is the same kind as the empathetic tender that she experiences when breastfeeding a baby girl. And quite possibly, it is because the experience of breast feeding baby girls is first, that culturally it continues in adult life in the form of empathy towards other women, manifest behaviorally in the holding of each other's hands as an admitted and accepted form of relational closeness. The contention that women tend in general to be as solidary with each other in patriarchal societies as they do in matriarchal societies, much more so than men who always seem be competitive with one another everywhere, seems to be a valid one. If true, this observation means to bring more support to our hypothesis of a phenotypical origin of the gender empathy behavior in the context being discussed. We conclude by stating that Freud and Jung, in our appreciation, have been too quick to transfer the sexual motives underlying the Oedipian complex to genitalia.

The physical closeness or attachment of the child to the parents is inevitable and potentially results in more attachment of the child to one of the parents specifically. Inequality in that attachment shall reasonably be expected due to the potential that the child will logically tend to attach a good deal more to the more caring or nurturing parent than the other. The power relation between the child and the two parents is another ineluctable since the child will and must perceive that, in the tripartite relation, the parents have the upper hand on him or her, which will effect the child's preferential attachment relation he/she holds with one of the parents – except perhaps in some cultures which attribute special faculties and capacities to twins in particular. Furthermore, the closeness, affectionate and visible commitment of the relationship between the two parents will inevitably be perceived by the child as a competing relation with the one he/she holds with each parent individually. Additionally, it is also clear that there is for the child no more than two elections naturally given in the form of relationship he/she may entertain with the parents: one is *empathy* resulting in exemplification emanating from the parent or identification with the parent, and the other is *distance* trending to antipathy, resulting in a more or less significant degree of rejection; indifference not being an option within these relational dynamics. It is by virtue of these fundamentals that studies conducted on adoptive daughters and their choice of husbands have shown conclusive evidence of behavioral outcomes replicating those posed in orthodox psychoanalytic theory (Oedipus complex) in their basics. A study by *Bereczkei, Tamas; Gyuris, Petra; Weisfeld, Glenn E. (2004). "Sexual imprinting in human mate choice". Proceedings of the Royal Society of London. Series B: Biological Sciences* found significant resemblance on facial traits between daughters' husband and their adoptive father. The study also found that this effect may be modified by the quality of the father–daughter relationship during childhood. Daughters who grew up with more emotional support from their adoptive father were more likely to choose mates with the same characteristics as their adoptive father than those whose adoptive father provided a less positive emotional atmosphere.

2.12 Sexuality is Central to Evolution of Men

There is no evolution of Men without evolution of his sexuality, for it is only through sexuality that Man exists. If sexuality continues to be this uncomfortable thing in human beings' minds, it is thus a significant problem waiting to be solved. If sexuality continues to be this filth in the minds of Men, it is then a very serious problem to resolve. If Men continue to suffocate their sexuality, that equates to a diminishment and a loss of self. It is through sexuality that Man comes to life, and it is his sexuality that opens the gateway to the world, the Cosmos and the Universe for him to prosper therein. If there is something about our sexuality that makes us feel uncomfortable, shameful about ourselves, or outright distraught, whatever its nature, even if it were to be of phylogenetic and ontological nature, it is our responsibility to find out the reasons behind the predicament and to endeavor finding the means to solve it. Because Nature is perennially moving and everything in it is in evolution. It will be Renaissance in Mankind's history the day that Man is born through and to celebration and not through a mother's horrific hollers of pain and the herald of trauma in the lacerate slap on an innocent new butt.

S. Freud had sought support in Greco-Latin mythology for the formulation of his Oedipian psychosexual theory. Likewise, this attempt at redimensioning the essence of the theory finds firm support in the Judeo-Christian sacred texts, notably the Book entitled Song of Songs, attributed to King Solomon. Exegetically, this Book relates King Solomon's very luscious sacred sexuality with the Black Mother. It is within the perspective that we have sketched here that many passages of the aforementioned book as well as some other passages of the Bible (Old Testament) must be read and understood.

That the sons of God saw the daughters of men
that they were fair; and they took them wives
of all which they chose.
Genesis 6:2

Your breasts are like two fawns,
like twin fawns of a gazelle
that browse among the lilies.
Song of Songs 4:5

If only you were to me like a brother,
who was nursed at my mother's breasts!
Then, if I found you outside,
I would kiss you,
and no one would despise me.
2 I would lead you
and bring you to my mother's house—
she who has taught me.
Song of Songs 8:1-2

We have a little sister,
and her breasts are not yet grown.
What shall we do for our sister
on the day she is spoken for?
9 If she is a wall,
we will build towers of silver on her.
If she is a door,
we will enclose her with panels of cedar.

10 I am a wall,
and my breasts are like towers.
Thus I have become in his eyes
like one bringing contentment.
Song of Songs 8:8-10

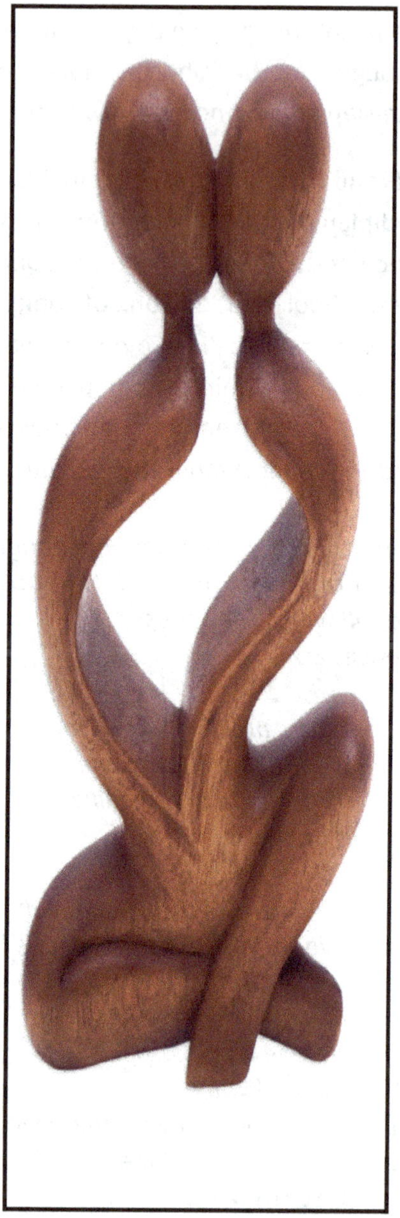

How beautiful are your feet in sandals,
O noble daughter!
Your curving thighs like jewels,
the product of skilled hands.
[3]*Your valley, a round bowl*
that should never lack mixed wine.
Your belly, a mound of wheat,
encircled with lilies.
[4] *Your breasts are like two fawns,*
twins of a gazelle.
Song of Songs 7:1-4

How beautiful you are, how fair,
my love, daughter of delights!
[8]*Your very form resembles a date-palm,*[*]
and your breasts, clusters.

[9]*I thought, "Let me climb the date-palm!*
Let me take hold of its branches!
Let your breasts be like clusters of the vine
and the fragrance of your breath like apples,

[10]*And your mouth like the best wine—*
What flows down smoothly for my lover,

gliding over my lips and teeth.
11 *I belong to my lover,*
his yearning is for me.
12 *Come, my lover! Let us go out to the fields,*
let us pass the night among the henna.
Song of Songs 7:7-12

King Solomon's wisdom has said it all, whether directly or through interpreter: there is only one love. And it never dies. Note well that the inspiration in these verses, in testifying that there is only one love, becomes so elevated in its artistry that, for the most part, it echoes as a single voice speaking for two, or coming from two, as though reflecting their intertwining with one another: expression of the most perfect union between the lover and the loved one.

It is a grave error to discredit, detract or reject human sexuality in any way in the name of the Holy Testaments because it amounts to an abject misinterpretation of Holy Scripture of whatever religion or denomination the claim seeks to lean on, since 1) there is no religion that promotes unisex of the human kind, 2) the Mother figure is capital in all religious testaments, and 3) there are good 'circumstantial' reasons of historic nature for sublimation of sexuality when it exists in a particular culture. It is not our intention to discuss in greater depth this perspective here, since it was not part of the original motivation for this publication. However, there are very good rational arguments that would assist us in making those claims. It remains that in the Christian Church of the West, scriptures hold, against the wish of many priests, that human sexuality of the very carnal luscious nature is Holy!

2.13 Revisit of Freudian Psychosexual Phases

Psychoanalytic theory presents the following psychosexual stages of development per Table 2.1.

Many today contest this breakdown and even the individual content of such phases. Though they may hold good supporting reasons, it may be sad to note that what had been retained of the Oedipian complex, as exposed in 21st Century literature of Anglo-American psychology, does not quite reflect what the original theory had proposed in first half 20th Century. One may read such common interpretations as reported below in as textually faithful a reproduction as possible.

Organ	Age	Activity	Mental Entity
Oral	*up to 1 year old*	*Mouth sucking, swallowing*	*EGO*
Anal	*1-3 year old*	*Anus, withholding and expelling feces*	
Phallic	*3-6 year old*	*Penis or clitoris, masturbation*	*SUPEREGO*
Latent	*6-13 year old*	*Little or no sexual motivation*	*PUBERTY*
Genital	*13-*	*Penis or vagina activity, intercourse*	

Table 2.1 Freudian Psychosexual Phases

The little boy wants to unite with his mother and wants to get rid of the obstacle represented in his father. The boy irrationally thinks that, if his father becomes aware of the forfeit, he would take away his most precious possession, his penis. Hence he develops castration anxiety. He then sets out to resolve the problem by imitating, copying and adopting masculine or dad-like behaviors by identification.

The girl desires her father and realizes that she does not have a penis, which leads her to develop a penis envy and the wish to be a boy. The girl resolves this conflict by repressing the desire for her father and substituting the wish for a penis with the wish for a baby. The girl blames her mother for her "castrated state", which creates great tension. She then represses her feelings to appease the tension and identifies with the mother to take on the female gender role.

Original theory did not quite teach that boys become fearful of their fathers taking away their penis, nor that girls experience a substitution of their wish for a penis by a wish for having a baby! Since it is not our intention in this study to be indiscriminately apologetic for the Oedipian complex as presented in Psychoanalytic Theory, we are not going to debate what appears to be its oversimplification or misinterpretation in its modern version in Anglo-American psychology. The latter overall apparently tends to dismiss it anyway, per the many late studies in the field. Our intention is instead to evolve psychosexual psychoanalytic theory in catering to certain elements of the Oedipian complex characterization that are factually observable and, most notably, by showing the connection or the continuum between overall physiological development of the human body and psychosexual development.

2.14 Psychoanalytic Motives to the Oedipian and Electra Complexes are Far-Fetched

The most significant criticism that the Oedipus complex characterization rightfully deserves in our sense is over-analysis and calling upon forms of interpretation that seem to be far-fetched. That there is a sexual attraction, because it is gender-based, between boy and mother, on one hand, and girl and father on the other hand, can be cast to be factual. However, the underlying motives and behavioral effects advanced in the theory seem to be purely hypothetical. One may reasonably wonder:

1. When or why does a girl's love for her father become admiration and/or a desire to equate him in achievements or out-compete him?
2. Why does a girl have to resort to outlandish femininity in order to obtain her father's presumed absolute protection?
3. To obtain her mother's empathy and forgiveness for her attraction to her father, why does she presumably have to resort to become again a very "small little girl", as contended in orthodoxy?
4. Else she becomes "masculine" by placing herself "under" her mother, so avoiding the woman-to-woman opposition... why?

These are hypotheticals that are posed but not substantiated in the Theory. It is not enough for them to simply *seem* logical.

2.15 Broadening the View of Psychosexual Development

When it comes to the psychosexual stages of development, it is possible that Freud had developed this scheme retroactively in an effort to decipher the origin of unconscious motives he saw at work in the mechanism which he ended up denoting *regression*. Postmodern research in the field has knowingly not borne out factual existence of these stages. The identification of the erogenous zones themselves, on which each is based for the most part, is however an undeniable. It is relevant to note that the wake of any one of the noted erogenous zones does not eclipse any other, and the question then becomes whether or not there is one that is slated to become prevalent.

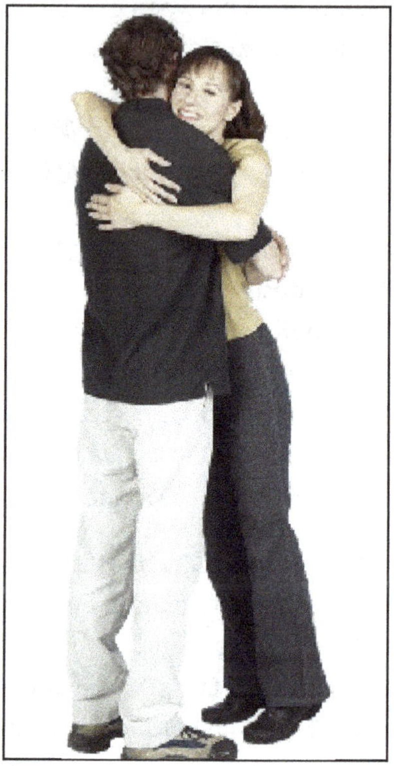

The analysis that we have conducted above has shown that breast-centric libido, although its actual libidinal level had been underestimated, runs throughout the entire course of human life. It is originally placed at the center stream of the metabolic function of the human body, whereby a female is set to *give* and the male is set for *intake*. On the parallel side, genitalia, once awaken, is placed at the center stream of the reproductive function of the human body, whereby a male is set to *give* and the female set for *intake*. This complementarism is what is in display out of the two engaged loving bodies of a male and a female.

The entire development of male and female bodies concurs to a summum phase where the potential for this complementarism reaches its peak. This generally occurs between age 20 and 25. Maximal rate in the flow of estrogen in the female body induces maximum growth of the uterus, proliferation of the endometrium, and regularity in menstruation, with, in particular, maximization of the female secondary sexual characters, namely:

- Enlargement of breasts and erection of nipples.
- Widening of hips and butts with lower waist-to-hip ratio than in adult males.
- Growth of body hair, most prominently in armpits and over pubis.
- Labia minora, the inner lips of the vagina's vulva, prominently grown and exhibiting changes in color.

- Multiplication of the erogenous zones, which include the cervix, neck (back and taper), inner ear, butts, etc.

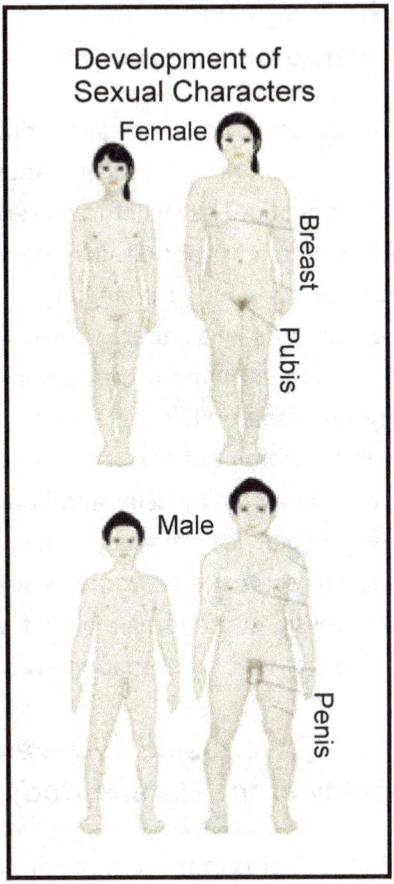

As to the male body, in the referred phase, it notably becomes more muscular and physically stronger. And if sporting is a practice by the individual, his body reaches the maximum muscular development it is naturally able to. More broadly and comprehensively, at its top flow rate, secretion of testosterone from the testes causes the male secondary sexual characters to be manifest in increased size and mass of muscles and bones, in taller stature making adult males taller than their female counterparts, increased mass and size of vocal cords causing a deepening of the voice, and the consummate change in shape of the face and skeleton. Other male secondary sexual characters include:

- Increased muscle strength.
- Heavier skull and bone structure.
- Broadening of shoulders and chest with the shoulders grown wider than hips.
- Increased secretions of glandular oil and sweat.
- Growth of facial and body hair, chest and pubic hair, including in underarm and on abdomen.
- Growth of penis length.
- Enlargement of larynx (Adam's apple).

2.16 Psychosexual Development Emerges from Tripartite Development of the Human Body

It is difficult to draw a clear dividing line between what has been called secondary sexual characters as listed above and physiological extensions of the metabolic function. The structural strength acquired by the male body through bones and muscle mass definitely enhances the projective capacity required for foraging or in more modern language to put food on the table from manipulation of the elements, in a general sense; whereas the normal enlargement of breasts through their mammary glands in the female body definitely pertains to an extension of the body's metabolic activity equally. Said enlargement becomes particularly prominent and quite notable at every pregnancy. Notice the lack of strengthening of muscles and bones in the female body in favor of greater softness and plastic or malleable mass of the body. We shall also note that pregnancies, a direct result of women's sexual activity, put a huge burden on the overall metabolism of the female body for the duration, whose level considerably increases for the 9-month long event.

2.17 Psychosexual Development is Spurred by Physiological Vitality of the Human Body

What is clear is that, from the broadest perspective, there is a phase of accelerated development in anatomic and physiological terms which peaks in the early 20's and from there a long slow phase of decline in vitality. Vitality is to be defined as the combination of metabolic capacity, regenerative capacity and reproductive capacity of the human body. The psychosexual ability or what we have come to call sexuality is not limited to the reproductive capacity and related activities, but remains at the heart of all three of these fundamental functions, which altogether produce the vitality of the human body. From that vantage point, sexuality starts with birth and only disappears at the last breath of the human body. It is important to recognize that its psychological expression maintains a tight connection with the physiological streams subtending the vitality of the human body. This proposition will not be difficult to accept when one remembers the amount of work that a male, for his own, has to develop, labially, with abundance of manual caresses and forceful penetration, in order to contribute to the paroxysm of orgasm in the act of copulation, all of which leaves him completely vacated of his vital forces immediately thereafter! Perhaps with good reason, nature has also granted men the very real capacity for pleasure of giving pleasure.

2.18 Tight Connection between Metabolism and Sexuality

In this context, it is very relevant to point out the notable connection that exists between sexual arousal and metabolic activity resulting in perspiration or sweats. We must remember, at this effect, that sweating is a result of muscular activity, which accordingly increases the metabolic rate of the entire human organism. Effectively, the release of pheromones in animal sweat, particularly the scent of sweat emanating from the armpits in humans, appears to act as a potent aphrodisiac. Some early studies had suggested that both women's hypothalami are activated when they smell the pheromone chemical similar to testosterone but not the estrogen-like substance, whereas men's hypothalami have the opposite response of only turning them on by the estrogen-like pheromone chemical. There also appears to be sexual disparity between the specific subregions of hypothalamus that are activated. Because in this way we chemically perceive the opposite sex in a very different manner than the way we perceive members of the same sex, some early researchers have suggested that pheromones could explain why some of our behaviors are gender-specific. The consensus today has settled around the fact that, notwithstanding the dysfunctionality of the human vomeronasal organ, whose par in animals incontrovertibly processes pheromone signals, we humans are able to detect pheromones through the rest of the olfactory system.

2.19 Pheromonal Expression of Metabolism in Psychosexual Behavior

While pheromones may be present in all bodily secretions, including saliva, research has focused on axillary sweat which contains the very odorous 16-androstenes. Very importantly, one of these steroidal compounds, androstadienone, exists at much higher concentrations in male sweat than female sweat and can be detected by women at different levels of sensitivity. Upper lip application of a pharmacological dose of androstadienone to women has demonstrably resulted in improved mood and heightened focus, particularly in capturing emotional information, as well as urges for attractiveness to potential male mates. Generally, positive mood knowingly facilitate women's sexual response while increased focus improves sexual satisfaction. Quite conclusively, further studies have shown a beneficial effect of androstadienone on sexual desire and arousal in women. In summary, evidence thus exists that 16-androstene pheromones, in particular androstadienone, play a beneficial role in women's mood, focus and sexual response, and quite possibly in mate selection as well.

The female pheromone, estratetraenol (estra-1, 3, 5(10), 16-tetraen-3-ol) was first isolated from the urine of pregnant women (Thysen et al., 1968) and is likely to be secreted in women's armpit sweating equally. Although the evidence is less compelling, pheromones in female axilliary sweat, which also has a very characteristic odor, does trigger the same pattern of behavior with regards to males as does men's androstadienone to females; it has also been found that estratetraenol additionally has what appears to be a contagious effect on other women knowingly heterosexual in triggering sexual arousal. The consensus seems to be around the fact that behavior induced by androstadienone is much stronger and characterizable than that induced by estratetraenol. Be that as it may, the keynote here is how psychosexual behavior arises from metabolic physiological functions beyond the known physiological reproductive ones.

2.20 Energy Boosting Herbs Also Effect Libido

One of the most popular herbs in traditional folk medicine, in particular Traditional Chinese Medicine, is ginseng. The herbs consist of a light-colored, forked-shaped root, a relatively long stalk, and green leaves with an oval shape. Both American ginseng (*Panaxquinquefolius, L.*) and Asian ginseng (*P. Ginseng*) are credited to boost energy, lower blood sugar and cholesterol levels, reduce stress, promote relaxation, treat diabetes, and, very significantly, manage sexual dysfunction in men. Ginseng contains two significant compounds: ginsenosides and gintonin, which complement one another in providing health benefits. A study by the *Journal of Korean Medical Science,* republished by the USA's NIH explains: *"As for physical fatigue and physical performance, ergogenic aids are believed to increase performance by some of the following mechanisms: renewing or increasing energy stored in the body, facilitating the biochemical reactions that yield energy, reducing or neutralizing performance-inhibiting metabolic by products, and facilitating recovery."*

Anecdotal evidence exists that a concoction of ginseng used to treat nervous fatigue can induce unexpected potent erections. The libidinal effects of the herb are not limited to men but extend to women as well.

2.21 Stages of Development from the Quanto-Geometric Vantage

There have been many attempts to define universal human development stages by world health organizations, national governments' health organizations and the academic life and social sciences alike. There is to this day no consensus on that subject, while the related nomenclature is extremely flourished, not to say confusing. If we agree with the vitality parameter as defined above, and that its course in a human life is the 3-step tempo that we mentioned, then we shall consequently agree that the Quanto-Geometric Grand Eigenfunction may perfectly encapsulate the course of human development. The rest would only be a matter of defining the subpartitions that identify the different phases. The Quanto-Geometric Grand Eigenfunction readily provides the basis for that distribution. We have posed elsewhere that developmental evolution of all Karyots, including human beings, obeys the differential distribution deriving from the Quanto-Geometric Grand Eigenfunction (Fig. 2.1).

The *v* coordinate in the graph stands for biological vitality as defined, and the *r* coordinate the age in terms of relative astrophysical cycles (not time duration through Ephemeris time flow). The curve describes ascending vitality from birth through infancy, to childhood, to adolescence, reaching a peak in the middle of youth. From that point on, the trend is to descent, going from early adulthood, to maturity, to seniority to elderly and finally to complete senility in the asymptotic neighborhood. In that demarcation, we have attempted to make the stages as granular as might be.

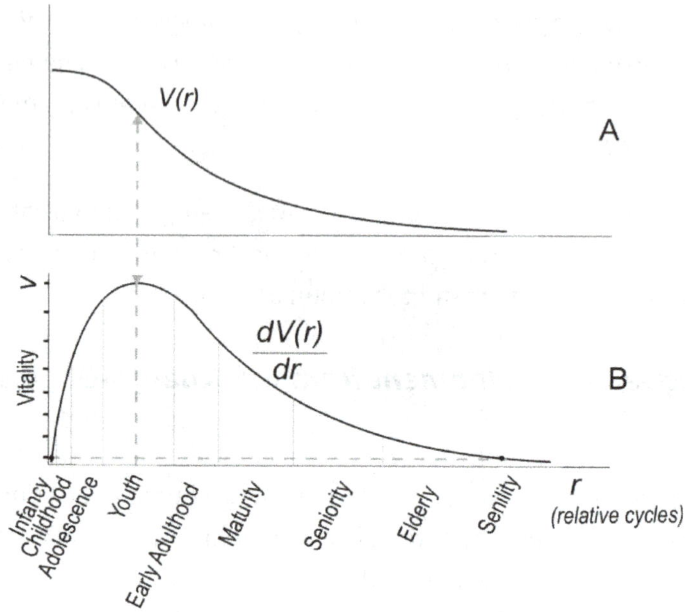

Fig. 2.1 Developmental phases through the life of a Karyot as a function of correlational astrophysical cyclicity

In Table 2.2, we include the age span as commonly understood for each of the first 4 phases exhibiting an increasing slope of vitality, which is one area where the analytic disparities generally abound.

The breakdown is shown in Table 2.2.

Phase Identity	Duration	Activity	Freudian Phase
Infancy	*up to 3 years old*	*Mouth sucking, swallowing Anus, withholding and expelling feces*	*Oral - Anal*
Childhood	*4-12 years old*	*Socialization and cognition*	*Phallic-Latent*
Adolescence	*13/15 -19 years old*	*Puberty and rationalization*	*Puberty*
Youth	*20-25 years old*	*Autonomy and ontological maturation*	

Table 2.2 Freudian Psychosexual Phases with age span

The interpretation is as follows:

1 The Infancy phase spans the first 3 years of life, where the infant is generally confined at the parental shelter, and under intensive care and attention by the parents. His/her life of an infant is heavily based on *instinctual imperatives and their satisfaction*. This phase would encompass the Freudian oral and anal phases.

2 In the Childhood phase, spanning 4 to 12 years old, the young life essentially develops *socialization and cognition* by leaving the household for the wider world beyond, notably schooling, and learning the world as it is. This phase would encompass the Freudian phallic and latent phases.

3 In the Adolescence phase, extending from 13 years of age for girls and 15 for boys and up to 19 years of age, the teenager experiences momentous changes with the body, which take place very fast. This is puberty, as universally acknowledged. The young life specifically gets acquainted with *change and transformations, learns to rationalize the world and to visualize their personal role therein.*

4 In the Youth stage, spanning 20 to 25 years of age, humans become their full man and their full woman as they make the *experience of freedom and autonomy, in maximal possession of their ontological capacities:* metabolic, regenerative and reproductive.

2.22 Biophysical Foundations of Human Sexuality

In the puberty phase of life is where the final elements of sexuality are put in place in both the biological body and the Mental body, and at the same time the human being starts experiencing sexual life. We are next going to explore this edifice from the QGT psychophysics perspective, in the hopes that it brings new light to the so crucial phenomenon of sexuality in human life.

2.22.1 Sexuation or Gender Determination Under the Mentation Foliate

The mental cartography reflecting the Mentation Foliate gives a very clear view of what constitutes sexuation on the mental plane from the QGT biosphysics perspective. We have discussed above many aspects of sexuation on the biological plane. One of the most important elements of that characterization is the biochemistry that supports the production of primary and secondary sexual characteristics in the development of the human body. The hormonal production that subtends this development represents the deepest marker of sexuation which proposes a configuration based on two principal hormones, testosterone and estrogen, in each of the two polar forms of sexuation, the masculine and the feminine gender, that is. It can never be overstressed that sexuation does not rely on the presence of one and only one of these two hormones in the sexuate individual. Both hormones are always present; however they entertain a major-minor relationship which is the sole determinant of gender.

	PASSIVE LATENCY - ANIMA					ACTIVE LATENCY - ANIMUS			
	-4	-3	-2	-1		1	2	3	4
	Dramatism	Pessimism	Negativity	Disapproval	Hybrid	Assent	Optimism	Assurance	Excitement
1	Timidity	Introversion	Solitude	Indifference	↑ ↓	Conservatives	Possessiveness	Competitivenes	Cupidity
2	Inquisitiveness	Curiosity	Superficiality (In	Credulity	↑ ↓	Sincerity	Mirroring	Duplicity	Authoritarianism
3	Aberration	Idiocy	Disorientation	Doubt (Perple:	↑ ↓	Discernment	Perspicacity	Clairvoyance	Lucidity
4	Remorse	Guilt	Shame	Regretfulness	↑ ↓	Presumption	Audacity	Stoicism	Heroism
5	Delirium	Hallucination	Fabulousness	Daydream	↑ ↓	Chimera	Reformism	Visionary	Utopia
6	Despair	Sadness (Disapp	Sorrow	Pity	↑ ↓	Sympathy	Admiration	Euphoria	Passion
7	Terror	Fear (Anguish)	Angst	Anxiety	↑ ↓	Resentment	Repugnance	Wickedness	Fury
8	Subservience	Devotion	Humility	Laziness	↑ ↓	Equity	Hope	Happiness	Ecstasy
9	Inanity	Cluelessness	Austerity	Patience	↑ ↓	Temperance	Protectiveness	Tenacity	Resilience

Fig. 2.3 Male Mentation Map with color highlight at Right-Chiral side

The hormonal dualism is duly reflected on the mental or psychological plane in the binary distribution that belies the Mentation Body in both males and females. As previously mentioned, the distribution is binary in that one side reflects states of mind that denote a passive-latent character, thereby supporting feminity, and the other side denotes an active-latent character, supporting thereby masculinity (Fig 2.3). Thus our psychophysics gives total support to the Jungian view of sexuality and gender definition, as well as the known hormonal distinction that defines gender in the science of Biology. C. G. Jung had correctly viewed that a state of mind he dubbed Anima is responsible for psychological female characteristics in women, whereas a state of mind he dubbed Animus is responsible for the male characteristics in men. He further had the insight that there is a bit of Animus in women and a bit of Anima in man equally. Under our psychophysical umbrella, the passive-latent side of the Mental Foliate or Manifold translates the Anima and the active-latent side the Animus (Fig. 2.3).

At the top of the Distribution displayed in the Foliate map, we noted Anima and Animus, to mean that the entire left chiral side of the distribution composes feminine mentation, whereas the entire right chiral side of the distribution composes masculine mentation. The biological determinant marked by dual hormonal biochemistry with a major-minor relationship supports the Jungian view of sexuation by upholding the pair Anima-Animus. Likewise the QGT Foliate map orchestrates the proposition, through its dual chiral distribution with, very importantly, a major-minor in the *accrual level* of mind states and inner dynamics of each chiral set. The map in the illustration effectively shows the right chiral side with color tones that are stronger than their counterparts at the left chiral side. The illustrative map in Fig. 2.3 thus shows a male Mental Body.

The map in Fig. 2.4 represents a female Mental Body, where the left chiral groups show a more intense tone than the right chiral ones. Hence, what makes the difference between a male and a female individual is the accrual level in the intensity of one or the other chiral group of the entire distribution in the Mental Foliate Map. This concept of *accrual level* is a prominent trait in the configuration of the Mental and remains the defining quality subjacent to many conditions of the Mental as we shall study later.

PASSIVE LATENCY - ANIMA					ACTIVE LATENCY - ANIMUS			
-4	-3	-2	-1		1	2	3	4
Dramatism	Pessismism	Negativity	Disapproval	Hybrid	Assent	Optimism	Assurance	Excitement
Timidity	Introversion	Solitude	Indifference	↑ ↓	Conservativenes:	Possessiveness	Competitivenes	Cupidity
Inquisitiveness	Curiosity	Superficiality (In	Credulity	↑ ↓	Sincerity	Mirroring	Duplicity	Authoritarianism
Aberration	Idiocy	Disorientation	Doubt (Perple:	↑ ↓	Discernment	Perspicacity	Clairvoyance	Lucidity
Remorse	Guilt	Shame	Regretfulness	↑ ↓	Presumption	Audacity	Stoicism	Heroism
Delirium	Hallucination	Fabulousness	Daydream	↑ ↓	Chimera	Reformism	Visionary	Utopia
Despair	Sadness (Disapp	Sorrow	Pity	↑ ↓	Sympathy	Admiration	Euphoria	Passion
Terror	Fear (Anguish)	Angst	Anxiety	↑ ↓	Resentment	Repugnance	Wickedness	Fury
Subservience	Devotion	Humility	Laziness	↑ ↓	Equity	Hope	Happiness	Ecstasy
Inanity	Cluelessness	Austerity	Patience	↑ ↓	Temperance	Protectiveness	Tenacity	Resilience

Fig. 2.4 Female Mentation Map with color highlight at Left-Chiral side

Hence the following principle:

1 **Ground State 1** of a human Mental Foliate is one where there is a natural enhancement in intensity (accrual) of one or the other side of the entire distribution. This natural level of accrual is what determines psychological gender in a human being. A person is psychologically a male because of this natural accrual of the right-chiral side of the Foliate distribution. A person is psychologically a female because of the natural accrual in the left-chiral side of the Foliate distribution.

2 It follows that every person is hybrid on the psychological plane and that only the prevalence in the particular accrual set of chirality gives the person his or her specific psychological gender, whether male or female gender.

2.22.2 Dynamics of Love and Sexuality Deriving from the Mentation Foliate

Once we understand the mentation basis for psychological gender, we are in a position to have a better grasp of gender in action or interaction, aka sexuality or love. While gender pertains to ontology, sexuality is not ontology but phenomenology because it duly involves interaction between gendered individuals. Sexuality is the pairing between masculinity and feminity on both the intellectual-psychic plane and the physical-biological plane. One must be sure to visualize the full Foliate in pairing or match with another, resulting in a left-side-prevalent Foliate in a match with a right-side prevalent Foliate, for the exercise of sexuality or love to be given. The match is essentially a coupling in space between the two prevalent sides of the two pairing Foliates, Layer to Layer. One half Layer in one Foliate pairs with the other half Layer in the other Foliate, across the entire 9-stratum spectrum of the mental Manifold.

2.22.3 Each Layer of the Mental Foliate Influences Sexual Behavior

Every layer of the Foliate brings its own "color" to sexuality. The Unary Layer elicits sexuality or mutual attraction based on the value of possession or material assets. In North America, popular culture has it that all marriage means is that *"they [the spouses or partners] are going to be spending money together"*. Making money and spending money creates the node of attraction between the two partners. In general, people at the top of the socio-economic ladder everywhere tend to develop their sexuality along that line predominantly. Stress *predominantly*, since this trend does not mean at all that there will be no other intervention by the other Layers in their love relationship.

A pairing Ambivalent Layer will elicit sexuality or mutual attraction based on the value of perceptiveness of the elements of reality. A couple moved by the imperatives of that Layer may find themselves very actively engaged in Tourism endeavors, sharing occupations and interests involving frequent travels. For instance, they may find themselves sharing the occupation of transporters, travelling cross-country together in their transportation truck and loving this way of life together.

The Associative Layer in pairing elicits sexuality or mutual attraction based on the value of intellectualism. The couple will tend to have an admiration for each other based on the brilliance of their minds as high intellectual achievers. Liberal arts professions will tend to cement their attraction for each other.

The color that the Quadratic Layer brings to mutual attraction or sexuality is the element of Heroism or grandiosity. Sharing interest in the public good, the law as well as social welfare and order will tend to provide the elements for their bond as a couple. In other words, discovering in each other these sorts of feelings and interests will drive them all the more tightly close to one another.

The Metamorphogenic Layer brings to mutual attraction elements of concern for disorder, for newness and social change. Sharing those concerns brings their spirits together in mutual attraction.

The Harmonic Layer makes sexuality or mutual attraction a harmonic "concave-convex" experience through coupling (copulation). In pairing, it is the Layer of love par excellence because the artifact of matching is an essential part of its typology. It will make the couple experience deep passion.

In pairing, the Paradoxical Layer makes mutual attraction an instigative and distressing experience through pain (or hurt). The couple is united in sharing hurt and pain as they tend to experience on that mode coitus and intimacy.

The Perfect Layer makes mutual attraction or sexuality an experience of share in universalism (pairing with Universe) through Ecstasy (Bliss), etc. These couples are united in their selflessness and religious sense, which may bring them to pastoral life together.

The Asymptotic Layer brings to sexual pairing a sense of Platonism, remote mutual devotion, disincarnate expression and even long-stretched patience to sexuality, its best love expression being what has been termed platonic love.

2.22.4 Complementarisms in Love

The above narrative spells out how the prime typological norms influence match in sexuality and love and what the couple's behavior tends to show when a particular layer has its way in the interaction. There is obviously a gender *complementarism* that plays out in the interaction, since a major subset of negative chirality in one gender couples with a major subset of positive chirality in the other gender. So therefore, popular wisdom is justified in the view that, in general, the husband goes out there and makes the money, while the wife controls the spending of the money, as would totally be the case in a traditional couple.

Nonetheless, we shall keep in mind that the coupling involves not only the two major sets but the two minor sets as well, wherein the roles are inverted, albeit remaining complementary to one another. There is thus passive-latency in the minor set for the husband and active-latency in the minor set for the wife. On that very account, popular insight, since the mid-1940's, has it well spotted when stating that *"behind every successful man is a great wife."* Translate busy and discriminate wife. A fitting example is how First Lady Eleanor Roosevelt supported her ailing husband and US President, Franklin D. Roosevelt, by doing herself most of his public appearances and developing herself many of the popular political positions upheld by the federal government during Roosevelt's presidency. Modern world history has also shown in repeated instances how the spouses of incapacitated or repressed political candidates took to replace them on the political stage, for one reason or another, in campaigns and elections where their husband's sympathizers still gave those leaders' acting wifes their votes. At the other side of the scale, every man that can be attentive to and heartily have ears for his wife will contribute to her greatest happiness and greatest amount of love in the couple. Because these qualities are here intervening as minors, we can understand why they represent ideals that are not always cast in a relationship at their best.

2.22.5 Disparity between Psychological Gender and Biological Gender

Our study thus far has put in evidence two distinct types of determinants for gender, one that is based on biological ontogenesis in the determination of genitalia in the human body and the hormonal system in the determination of secondary sexual characteristics, and one other that is based on chirality in the distribution of basis mentation states in the human Mental Foliate. When everything goes well, nature correspondingly and harmoniously maps the biological sexuation formations to the Mental Foliate's sexuation or gender formations. Accordingly, our psychophysics vision of the Mental Body duly predicts that there may be accidental instances where biologically produced gender characteristics do not match gender characteristics produced by the Mental Foliate. One ought to outright abandon the monist perspective in order to comprehend this outcome. In the hypothesis that the Mental Body is a product of the biological brain and its neural networks, we are in good stead to reason that the Mental Body must mandatorily replicate gender characteristics determined from biological ontogenesis along with the brain's electric and biochemical activity, in particular the neural endocrine system, later on. There is for sure a monist problem to solve when there is a de facto or highly plausible disparity between the two.

2.22.6 What Feeling Trapped in One's Own Body Means

Contrary to the above, the distinct possibility of a significant disparity between the two developments in gender determination, which is so central to human ontology, strongly advocates for a notable level of independence between the biological brain or central nervous system and the Mental Foliate as studied thus far. This possibility had materialized since mankind's history of old and in modern times alike. Reported in the 4000-year old Christian Bible or Judaic texts, it has been described in various ancient sacred texts of different civilizations such as Greece, Egypt, Rome, and China in one form or another. The German author Magnus Hirschfeld coined for it the term *transvestite* in 1910 to specifically describe individuals who customarily and voluntarily wore clothes of the opposite sex. Hirschfeld's group of transvestites consisted of both males and females, with sexual habits verging in the heterosexual, homosexual and bisexual. Quite aside from their sexual orientation, what is interesting with this group of individuals is their desire to cross-dress and to effectively wear clothing of the opposite sex, either circumstantially or permanently in their lives, demonstrating thereby self-conscious psychological gender contrary to their biological gender. It is not uncommon to hear these individuals say that *"they feel trapped in their body"*. This gender determination disparity between the biological body and the Mental body or Foliate, in the terms posed in our psychophysical framework, represents the very first dimension of all direct cisgender issues and cisgender-related issues in individual behavior or sexuality.

Our attempt here is to make clear the psychophysics basis for transgender consciousness and deriving sexual behavior, **at first order**. It does not pretend to substitute the tendencies for transgender identification and same-gender sexuality that may arise from psychosocial development in traditional theory. The latter represents **second-order** transgender orientation.

2.22.7 Imperative of Gender Duality Even in Transgender Relations

The second dimension of this question relates to the unique binary choice represented in gender orientation as displayed in same-gender sexuality in general. We well understand the reason for binary biological sexuation, or two sexuate choices, since we know it is based on two chief hormones, the estrogen and the testosterone hormones which determine one or the other sexual characteristics (male or female). At the psychological level, the question as to why all homosexual or lesbian individuals must either play a male behavioral role or a female behavioral role in a relationship is a legitimate one, though not always posed or answered. Our framework gives straightforward answer to this non-trivial question. The Mental Foliate knows of only two binary chiral sides of the distribution of mentation states informing behavior and which at the same time constitutes gender and gives way to sexuality. There exists in human groups no sexual relationship between two people behaving the both, or self-identified, as either males or females. That is because the distribution is such that it naturally and unequivocally results in a necessary matching between two chiral complementary sets of basis states. That is what is given in the so-called same sex relationships or unions. In their Mental Bodies or Mentation Foliates, these individuals are slated to be indeed the gender that they claim for themselves.

2.22.8 Asexuality under the Vantage of the Mentation Foliate

Another interesting fact to put under scrutiny is the uncommon existence of psychologically asexual individuals, characterized by the lack of sexual attraction to others, or low or absent interest in or desire for sexual activity. While some asexual individuals may practice solitary masturbation or have sex to procure enjoyment to a romantic partner, others strictly do not. Although in principle in our framework one side of the distribution bears prevalence in *ground state 1* of the Mental Foliate, one can visualize an accidental *ground 0 state* whereby there is no emphasis whatsoever of any chiral side of the distribution, making it a flat equated distribution throughout. In that event, gender distinction based on accrual levels disappear and we have a psychologically asexual individual with nevertheless a sexuate biologically-determined body.

Last but not least, of note is the distinct real possibility that while the body of an asexual person may be experiencing sexual arousal, he experiences no such feeling or emotion at all mentally or psychologically. Author Fischer et al. reported that "*scholars who study the physiology around asexuality suggest that people who are asexual are capable of genital arousal but may experience difficulty with so-called subjective arousal.*" By subjective arousal he meant arousal sentimentally felt or experienced in Mind. This is another clear and compelling evidence of the disparity between biological sexuality supported by the nervous system and psychological sexuality supported by the Mentation Foliate, an independent body of its own. Clearly in this case, the Mental Foliate is at an accidental *ground 0 state*, as far as chiral emphasis or lack thereof, which is thus notably unable to manifest gender-oriented sentience or to elicit gender-oriented behavior.

2.23 Conclusion

It is important for the sciences of Psychology and Psychiatry to remain dispassionate in their understanding of behavior in order to provide the best humanism possible in the service to human health and mental equilibrium. Without proper comprehension of the breadth and depth of the Human Mental and its structures, it will be difficult to exercise the equanimity required in provisioning solace to those who fall prey to distress in a condition and are desperately looking for help and those others who are desperate for social acceptance. We believe that what is of import is the endeavor to reach the deepest and finest level of comprehension in structures and transactions of the Mental and to remain uncompromisingly non-judgemental in order to help human individuals fully conquer their destiny. We recognize the difficulty there is in acknowledging the freedom of personal expressions that every individual is entitled to for their own personal emancipation, while upholding norms and standards for normalcy from a health provider perspective. Medical science, however, shall not renounce to the search for insights in the deepest principles that compose the canon of life and uphold these principles and norms in the very exercise and advocacy of humanism and ethics that the science has forever claimed. We believe that the advent of biophysics and psychophysics represent both a sine qua non requisite and a warrant for those ontogenetical and phenomal norms to be formulated in the most objective and assertive manner possible in Psychological and Psychiatric sciences.

Chapter 3

HUMAN CHARACTEROLOGY THROUGH QGT PSYCHOPHYSICS VANTAGE

The science of psychology generally understands human behavior to be the way that a person acts or conducts himself/herself, particularly in relation to other people. It thus involves actions and mannerisms undertaken or expressed by individuals in their interaction with others and the living environment. Therefore the semantics of the term generally implies someone *in action in a certain way* based on personal attributes. It is however difficult to reduce behavior strictly to action, regardless of the particular way the action develops. For instance, in the physical action of applying a Force to a wall with one's fist or fingers, it is clear that a perceptual sense of pressure must intervene in order to give one a sense of the resistance of the wall to the applied force, so that we do not destroy our arm and fingers in the act. So therefore the action of applying a force cannot be completely reduced to that of a pure *effector* in human physiology and psychology.

Consequently, the notion of acting within the semantics of the term human behavior must include a certain level of sensing or responsiveness in its physiological and psychological application. By contrast, if the behavior were to be more passively emotional than active – i.e. someone restrained in tears because he is feeling physical pain or in response to inflicted humiliation – it remains equally clear that in that case, there is less action than there is an emotional response. Of course, this behavior is majorly a sensation or sentimental response, otherwise called an *affect*, physiologically and psychologically. The ocular glands in the tear shedding intervene as effectors, albeit in the condition of a minor component of the behavior overall.

In this text, especially this Chapter and the next two, we are going to apply to the notion of human behavior the broad physical sense of an *observable*, as understood in physical science. It assumes that both efferent and afferent elements participate in the behavior. When the efferent element is the major we will speak of *active-reactive* behavior as opposed to *passive-responsive* behavior whenever the afferent element is the major.

3.1 Parents' Role in Child Development and Character Formation

The influence of parental behavior on the development of a young life in formation along with psychological character has been amply studied, notably in analytic orthodoxy. Setting aside the objections that we have raised in Chapter 2, our psychophysics largely conforms to those views in terms of parental influence on their children's broad psychological development. There is ample consensus at this point on the psychodynamics playing out between the two parents and the child in development. Psychological parental influence, however, is not an irrevocable direct causal factor in the formation of the child's personal character. We view parents' role as phylogenetic actors in prolonging life in a lineage according to specific directives proper to the lineage. Therefore, on the phylogenetic plane, they are entrusted to image the new life to their own self in a very large measure[9] and, on the psychological plane, to adapt that new life to the physical and human environment which is to be the theater of existence for the new person. They will transmit to the same their own value system and later on induce their own life experience in the choices the young adult will face. With good reason, popular wisdom has it that "Like father, like son."

Parents' value system is based on their role in society, the society's traditions, and their personal worldview which will include both positive emancipating mental attitudes and taboos, negative stereotypes and biases in personal and social terms. Come the phase of development when the new adult faces important life choices, parents will attempt to intervene in order to ensure that what they understand to have been their own mistakes the child will not repeat, they

---

[9] It is understood in this case that the self includes inherited traits, tendencies and potentialities arising from the history of the lineage.

will particularly intervene in career and love partner choices to ensure best outcome in their judgment. They will further ensure the child obtains best educational benefits than they personally could for themselves as well as better standard of living or higher level of wealth than was accessible to them.

All of this background comes to play on the new person's psychological landscape or a Mental Foliate which is not necessarily permeable to it all. It will meet predispositions that dictate the ensuing level of receptivity to its prescriptions. If that were not to be the case, then all of the progenitors to a couple would have to relatively present the same personal characteristics, setting aside gender differences. We know that is not at all the case, while it well seems to be the case for homozygotic twins raised by the same parents. Early childhood, when self-identify had been defined, appears to be the phase of life where personal characteristics or psychological character are born. It must be equally concomitant to the phase of life when the child is able to decisively show preferences in taste, i.e. the ability to say "I like this but not that".

3.2 Gender-Based Behavior: First Causal Factor of Character

In this study, we make no difference between temperament, character, temper or personality; we view them all from the same psychological vantage and the same psychophysics standpoint. The very first level of characterization for human temperament is undoubtedly marked gender tendencies, decried in modern days under the impulse of a negative reaction to so-called gender stereotypes. Yet the secondary sexual characters and the ontogenic chromosomal sex determinants are unbeatable reminders of nature's viewpoint to anyone desiring to obliterate those differences. That being said, it is justice to acknowledge social disfavor imposed on the weaker sex in all human societies, whether male- or female-dominated.

We have spoken in the previous Chapter of the innate hybrid character of the human Mentation Foliate, which is a normal distribution body that presents both chiralities in every human being. On that account, the difference between a male and a female is not one of quality but one of quantity or intensity specifically.

Where these differences show in the most incontestable manner probably resides in the love-passion and sports chapters of life. Women do show a tendency to experience love in a more contemplative, attraction-driven or expectant, not to say heart-felt manner than men do. These qualities arise from the left-chiral side of mentation Layer 6, and what makes them more accentuated in women than men is the much higher intensity of the referred sub-group of pensive partitions with their super-imposed representations in the female Foliate. Contrastingly, men tend to express sexuality in a more instigative and proactive manner, with freedom above deep heart attachment, a sort of more detached passion. These qualities pertain to the right-chiral side of Layer 6's root partitions. Their much higher intensity in males along with the associated representational processes is responsible for the well-known distinctive behavior. It must be said however that, if passion is more broadly the force of love in pairing, it is not quite true that female are more passionate than male, but instead that the former tend to predominantly live their love-passion specifically on the side of the left-chiral pensive roots of Layer 6. This undergirding makes women appear more steady, attached and heart-felt in their love sentiments. When men take pleasure in giving greatest pleasure to their adored princess, and go to the stretches of building castles for them, figuratively or not, this love is not little and bears the true likes of great passion.

As to the matter of sports, women are knowingly more prone to bone fracture than men and tend to be much less projective than men due in no small part to their anatomic sexual characters.

Lastly, women's natural voice pitch turns out to be a very reliable distinctive trait to gender differentiation that should not be underestimated. Men's voice pitch tend to be characteristically grave in contrast to women's.

	PASSIVE LATENCY - ANIMA					ACTIVE LATENCY - ANIMUS				
	-4	-3	-2	-1		1	2	3	4	
	Dramatism	Pessimism	Negativity	Disapproval	Hybrid	Assent	Assurance	Optimism	Excitement	QG CHARACTER
1	Timidity	Introversion	Solitude	Indifference	← →	Conservativenes	Possessiveness	Competitivenes	Cupidity	*EGOCENTRIC*
2	Inquisitiveness	Curiosity	Superficiality	(In Credulity	← →	Sincerity	Mirroring	Duplicity	Authoritarianism	*REALISTIC*
3	Aberration	Idiocy	Disorientation	Doubt (Perple:	← →	Discernment	Perspicacity	Clairvoyance	Lucidity	*INTELLECTUAL*
4	Remorse	Guilt	Shame	Regretfulness	← →	Presumption	Audacity	Stoicism	Heroism	*HYPERBOLIC*
5	Delirium	Dystopia	Fabulousness	Daydream	← →	Chimera	Reformism	Visionary	Utopia	*UTOPIAN*
6	Despair	Sadness (Disapp	Sorrow	Pity	← →	Sympathy	Admiration	Euphoria	Passion	*MATRIXIAL*
7	Terror	Fear (Anguish)	Angst	Anxiety	← →	Resentment	Repugnance	Wickedness	Fury	*PARADOXICAL*
8	Subservience	Devotion	Humility	Laziness	← →	Equity	Hope	Happiness	Ecstasy	*PERFECT*
9	Inanity	Cluelessness	Austerity	Patience	← →	Temperance	Endurance	Resilience	Tenacity	*ASYMPTOTIC*

Fig. 3.1 Example of a Mental Foliate accusing the Intellection temper based on Layer 3 paroxysm.

3.3 QG Psychophysics Model of Human Characterology

QGT psychophysics erects the principle that human character is a product of a specific accrual level in the intensity of root thought partitions with their super-imposed representations in primarily one mental layer (Fig. 3.1). In Chapter 4, we will show how to determine the intensity gradient of this accrual in numeric terms. We nominally grade the accrual level for human character as accrual level 2, in consideration to the fact that accrual level 1 is given in gender ontology. We shall thus keep in mind that accrual level 1 is only applied to either the left-chiral pensive group of partitions on a Layer or the group of partitions composing its right-chiral side. Accrual level 2 equally applies to the entire set of partitions forming the Layer. *We further set all first-order intensity accruals for a Foliate to have the same incremental value or Δ throughout the entire Foliate,* whenever they occur, exception being made for developmental and menstrual accruals which are second-order, and of a periodic nature in the case of the catamenial ones.

Hence what we have so far in the accrual scale is Ground State 0, where there is no accrual at all but simply a basis level. Let's arbitrarily set 1 to the numeric figure for this state, so that:

$I_0 = 1$, where I_0 is the intensity level at Ground State 0.

The accrual level is a Δ or an increment, so that:

$\Delta_{A1} = 3$, where Δ_{A1} is accrual level 1 for gender identity and 3 is an arbitrarily set incremental number.

Hence, $I_1 = I_0 + \Delta_{A1} = 1 + 3 = 4$, where I_1 is the intensity level at Ground State 1.

Again, I_1 accrual figure only applies to one chiral side of a Layer. We will differentially label it I_{1L} for the left-chiral side and I_{1R} for the right-chiral side. In continuing with the formalization, for character definition we have accrual level Δ_{A2} such that:

$\Delta_{A2} = 3$, where Δ_{A2} is accrual level 2 for character and 3 is the set incremental number for all accruals.

Hence we would have: $I_2 = I_1 + \Delta_{A2} = 4 + 3 = 7$ *(2)*, where I_2 would be the intensity level for Character setting.

However, because I_1 does not apply to the entire layer from gender characterization, equation *(2)* must be broken in two equations, one for I_{2L} or the intensity on the left-chiral side for Character setting and I_{2R} or the intensity on the right-chiral side for Character setting. We thus obtain the following set:

For Females: $I_{2L} = I_{1L} + \Delta_{A2} = 4 + 3 = 7$ and $I_{2R} = I_{1R} + I_0 = 4 + 1 = 5$

For Males: $I_{2L} = I_{1L} + I_0 = 4 + 1 = 5$ and $I_{2R} = I_{1R} + \Delta_{A2} = 4 + 3 = 7$

Therefore, despite the fact that the accrual incremental develops homogenously across the Layer, there is an asymmetry in the intensity of the pensive partitions across the Layer due to the one-sided accrual arising from gender ontology.

Thus, human character consists in a passive-responsive and active-reactive mode, the integration of which we call behavior and the type of which corresponds to one quanto-geometric ontogenetic type or normal. It is only when a quanto-geometric mental normal expresses an overrate within the framework of the mental spectrum that the characterological orientation of a subject expresses its specificity and becomes distinguishable. Put simply, a character is:

1. a particular way to perceive the world around us
2. a particular way to respond in affects to stimuli and observations
3. a particular way to manipulate the world and interrelate due to:
4. an inner and natural overrate of one mental normal with respect to all others including its superimposed representational processes.

We have shown above how this overrate pans out in term of intensity of the pensive partitions and operations belonging to a Layer of the Foliate.

3.4 The Egocentric Character

Below a display of the partitions the Monolithic Layer consists of.

1	Timidity	Introversion	Solitude	Indifference	↑	↓	Conservativenes	Possessiveness	Competitivenes	Cupidity

We expect these root partitions of the Mental Foliate to model the Egocentric Character type when stamped with an accrual level 2.

3.4.1 Personal Identity and Attributes

In general, force, obstinacy, reservation, conservativeness, aspiration to domination and power are the great highlights of the Egocentric character. He usually thinks highly of himself and may display arrogance.

He is also a great introvert who strongly resists expressing his emotions. Despite his strong character, there is a shyness side to him. He will scarcely talk about himself, however. Very much a stay-at-home person, he is particularly attached to his home. One of his strongest dislikes is extravagant life.

This character type is loath to getting rid of anything and thus tends to accumulate even that which is out of use or of no usefulness to him any longer. Change, travels and communication are not very much among his likes. He will even forego due leisure as he tends to keep constantly busy.

3.4.2 Love and Interpersonal Relations

Prone to many reservations about other people's capability for achievements. He shows no propensity to congratulating anyone but remains sensible to flattering remarks to his ego. He scarcely considers giveaways or giving gifts and maintains a stingy attitude.

Though not a violent subject by definition, this type of individual is able to react with extreme violence to protect his belongings, to vindicate what he believes to be entitled to. However, these violent reactions quickly leave the way to his usual composure.

In the love chapter, he will mainly practice love materialist or love partnership. This means not at all, however, that he is a stranger to love passion. He keeps his home as a stronghold where he likes to remain in peace and surrounded by his family's best belongings.

3.4.3 Education/Profession/Occupation

His creativity and ability to develop sustained effort are unparalleled. He frequently develops into an autodidact or self-trained individual in the skills he finds interest in. Frequently, he will show a workaholic attachment to his occupation. He will be amongst the first or the most competitive achievers in the fields of activity of his interest. He also invariably shows sound views, for he holds a very practical and materialistic sense of existence.

Since he is strongly realistic, common sense generally assists him. His personal, professional or occupational considerations almost never lack cogency.

Loath to disclose or talk about his assets and his financial resources, he keeps them under the stamp of high discretion and even secrecy.

3.4.4 Language

The egocentric character tends to be direct, concise and very economic in speech. Many are even blunt. His writing is compact, dense or forceful.

3.5 The Realistic Character

Below a display of the partitions the Binary Layer consists of.

2	Inquisitiveness	Curiosity	Superficiality (In	Credulity	↑ ↓	Sincerity	Mirroring	Duplicity	Authoritarianism

We expect these root partitions of the Mental Foliate, when stamped with accrual level 2, to model the Realistic Character type.

3.5.1 Personal identity and attributes

This character type frankly displays a nervous temper. One of their main traits is mobility, verging on agitation. They are constantly on the move and have great difficulty remaining quiet.

A notable propensity to open themselves up to others makes them prone to indiscriminate and ingenuous confidences. One might say they easily deliver their soul to others, as a consequence of an extremely limited sense of intimacy. They do not seem to care enough about the possible damage that such unrestrained sincerity and confidences might cause them.

Frequently, their opinions are quite superficial. Furthermore, those often show an angle of duplicity which materializes as keenness hidden under kindness or statements that are intentionally partly true, partly untrue. This ambivalent slant seems to be what they mostly care about when expressing opinion.

3.5.2 Love and Interpersonal Relations

Due to their unrestrained openness, more than any other character, this type is very much vulnerable to libel and all forms of aggression. At the same time, the realistic character types may actively engage in many forms of imposture, imbroglio and dupery.

Constantly moving from one place to another makes them fond of traveling. To those who are led to go as far as imbroglios, traveling may even become part of the imposture schemes.

They will seek or share the love of travel with their partners, which may stir them to form couples sharing the occupation of transporters, travelling cross-country together in their transportation truck and loving this way of life together. It is also possible that they consciously react compensatively to their tendency to constant commotion by choosing a partner who is calm, stable and even sedentary. It is their very sense of ambiguity that brings them to such considerations of compensation.

3.5.3 Education/Profession/Occupation

These tempers are occupationally very dynamic and full of initiatives. Pushed by an unrivaled curiosity, they are continuously in search of new fields of activity. Informed about everything, they never stop enlarging their scope of knowledge. Their ineradicable inconstancy, however, prevents them from completing their many enterprises. Tourism may be one of these activities with much appeal to them.

3.5.4 Language

The language is given to puns and deliberately ambiguous statements. They tend to make their language pretty colorful along that line.

3.6 The Intellectual Character

Below a display of the partitions the Associative Layer consists of.

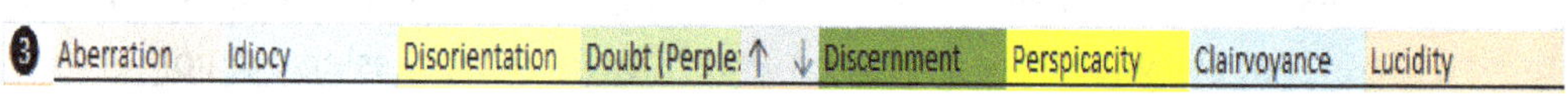

We expect these root partitions of the Mental Foliate, when accusing accrual level 2, to model the Intellectual Character type, which is thereby given to the exercise of associativeness.

3.6.1 Personal Identity and Attributes

Individuals with this temperament want to appear smart and intellectually achieved. They will often go to lengths to become indeed high intellectual achievers. They are convinced of their intelligence and superiority, let alone their infallibility.

Their sense of personal publicity is very developed. They thus live in the expectation of acknowledgement and recognition from others. Their acute sense of association confers them the capability to quickly adapt to new and adverse circumstances or living conditions. However, the tendency to associate trumps constancy and stability. That is why they will frequently display inconstancy of mood as well as inconstancy of opinion. They may instantly change an opinion that they had just firmly contended, because a new window of association just popped in their minds.

These characters may readily submit to other people's influence, although for the most clever ones, it will be necessary to judiciously penetrate their sensibility and their fit of mind in order to create a favorable framework for a new opinion or disposition.

The Associative character holds a defective practical sense. Even when they have accumulated sufficient resources to secure their material existence, they will still feel insecure about their condition and possibilities. The decisions they ought to make generally cost them lots of stress, because it is oftentimes difficult for them to choose one avenue among the many that their higher intelligence opens up to them.

3.6.2 Love and Interpersonal Relations

These characters love to make others feel good by congratulating them. They are always looking for ways to bond with or relate to others. They are kings and queens of networking and prone to help others out. Despite their personal vanity, they tend to display the most contagious sociability, which goes along with unequaled courtesy and kindness. At times however, in particular when faced with troublesome obstacles, they may show outright bad mood and verbal harshness, which equally materialize their sense of relatedness. Not at all here the indifference of the Egocentric temper, for instance.

These characters are given to love-courtesy and love-enlightenment. They commune in the admiration of the artful and luxury. They tend to be quite mundane in sentimental relations.

3.6.3 Education/Profession/Occupation

These characters are often high intellectual achievers and endeavor to be as thorough and perfect as possible in their occupations. Their peers, however, will often see them in doubt and insecurity in situations that would seem to call for straightforward responses, frequently out of an urge for perfection for the high achievers. The others are held back by their natural tendencies to doubtfulness and confusion, with which they have to struggle in order to attain higher levels of achievement.

3.6.4 Language

The Associative temper type is the most talkative of all temperaments. They experience enormous difficulties with silence, and when in company they virtually speak nonstop.

3.7 The Hyperbolic Character

Below a display of the partitions the Quadratic Layer consists of.

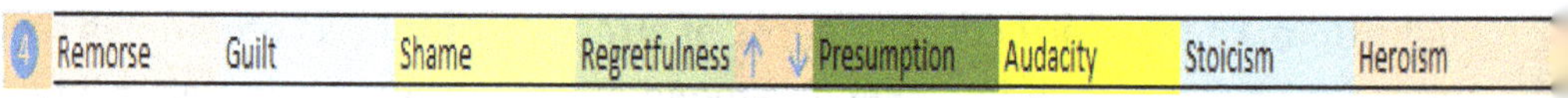

We expect these Layer 4 root partitions of the Mental Foliate, when stamped with accrual level 2, to model the Hyperbolic Character type. It will be thereby given to the display of grandiloquence and pomposity as its prime mark.

3.7.1 Personal Identity and Attributes

The Hyperbolic character type cultivates and aspires to highness, grandeur and majesty. He or she wants to be seen as sublime, magnanimous and supreme. Among their aspirations is to become a guide to others, a ruler or agent of social norms.

They are much given to fanfaronades, they speak aloud with great enthusiasm, whether men or women, also with a condescending and rhetorical tone of voice. You might say they have the tendency to be theatrical. Any trifle may spark a burst of enthusiasm with them. Many such characters lean toward displaying extravagance and extravagant luxury.

3.7.2 Love and Interpersonal Relations

They love to display their strength and resources in an attempt to intimidate others. They drive their peers to believe they nourish grandiloquent ambitions, which turn out to be sometimes futile aspirations. Nevertheless, their enthusiasm is so overwhelming that if it should fail to become contagious, at least it will earn then their peers' favorable disposition. So much so that peers will be willing to help and assist them in their tasks or endeavors or join in their groups.

These characters do not know of greediness. Their contagious optimism will erase any greedy attitude from peers, and they are never resentful. However, they will find it difficult to forgive or tolerate any offense to what they hold for sacred. And so they will unforgivably pursue whoever has offended what they hold for untouchable or sacred.

Condescending by nature, these characters consider themselves the owner of virtue, rules and laws, and thus best placed to tell everyone how to organize their existence!

3.7.3 Education/Profession/Occupation

The Hyperbolic temperament is sensible to the call of duty, with an unmatched sense of honor. For that matter, he will be quick to enroll in the defense of causes generally considered noble. When engaged in such struggles, he will show great capacity for sacrifices and heroism if need be. Hence, these characters lean toward enrolling in the army where uniforms, decorations, patriotic exhortation to defend the mother country strongly appeal to their sense of greatness.

Their great energy and huge pride grant them the assurance that they will eventually overcome any obstacle confronting them in life.

3.7.4 Language

This character type has speech and body language virtually evocative of a theatrical play. Verbal language tends to extrapolation or exaggeration in the form of hyperbolic expressions, i.e.: *"My hand hurts so much it's going to drop off."*

3.8 The Utopian Character

Following is a display of the partitions the Entropic Layer consists of.

5 Delirium	Hallucination	Fabulousness	Daydream	↑ ↓	Chimera	Reformism	Visionary	Utopia

We expect these root partitions, as they reach accrual level 2, of the Mental Foliate to model the Utopian or Metamorphogenic Character type.

3.8.1 Personal Identity and Attributes

Individuals with the Utopian or Metamorphogenic character type are generally quite healthy, yet they worry excessively about their body and their state of health. Few human beings are as meticulous about their diet as the Metamorphogenic characters are. Some would even commonly wear gloves to protect themselves from germs, while they carry on their cottage pharmacy everywhere they travel to. Their concern with disorder and aspiration to purity remain the highlights of these characters' lives.

The Metamorphogenic character pays close attention to the world around. Nature exerts on them an almost mystical appeal as they will spend long hours observing a sunset, the remote horizon, a moonlit night... they are fascinated dreamers. What they are looking for in these sunsets and these moonlit skies is the feel of how things change in nature, second after second, minute after minute. Their interest for natural life and a great dedication to learn nature will turn them into learned individuals, well-informed minds about any subject. Intellectually speaking, a Utopian temperament is an eclectic. The extent of their scientific and philosophical erudition is vast. As a living encyclopedia, they will frequently behave pedantically, however.

3.8.2 Love and Interpersonal Relations

On the sentimental plane, these individuals, men or women, tend to consider marriage very late in their lives. They so tend to remain celibate. They are generally lonely and go across affectively cold lives: they are apparently reluctant to undo their virginity!

This loneliness is, however, not similar to that of the Egocenric character, which the egocentric mind directly elicits. The loneliness of the Utopian temper comes from their inclination to contemplation of nature and daydreaming. With few friends generally, they may not be very sociable.

They also tend to be given to sexual eccentricities driven by a rejection of natural sexual intimacy. It is their sense of newness and novelty which most likely leads them to the rejection of sexual intimacy. Determined to keep themselves always fresh and new, they come to execrate sexual or affective experience which they feel is a violation of their physical integrity. This form of behavior in intimacy is opposite to the Matrixial temper's, a character that is forthright in looking for love match, as we will shortly see.

3.8.3 Education/Profession/Occupation

The Metamorphogenic character tends to become extremely and amply knowledgeable as a result of narrow attention to new objects, new facts, new situations which they never stop scrutinizing and compiling. Their outstanding critical and discriminating abilities are a product of their entropic predisposition to fragment and dis-order or dis-organize constitutive elements of an ensemble. This approach elucidates at a stroke relationships that were originally hidden. However, their ability to synthesize is poor because synthesis is typically an associative skill. They ought to overcome the pitfall of getting lost in too much analysis without ever settling to synthesize and integrate their novel knowledge to their intellectual background. Their thirst for new knowledge never abates, making them recycle constantly that which they have already acquired.

3.8.4 Language

Their language may be quite formal and sophisticated. In that, they rejoin the Intellectual character type. However, their language effervescence is measured, not at all the verbosity characterizing the Intellectual type.

3.9 The Matrixial Character

Below a display of the partitions the Entropic Layer consists of.

6	Despair	Sadness (Disapp	Sorrow	Pity	↑ ↓	Sympathy	Admiration	Euphoria	Passion

We expect these root partitions of the Mental Foliate, when stamped with accrual level 2, to model the Utopian or Metamorphogenic Character type.

3.9.1 Personal Identity and Attributes

Individuals with this character type believe they are physically "handsome" or "attractive", much more so than any other character type. They maintain an unending care about their physical appearance, while they invariably nurture a profound artistic sense. Few human beings use the mirror as much. Fair to say that their appearance is of paramount importance to them. Women usually arrange themselves to be the cutest in vestimenta, hairdresses and facial expression.

These individuals are frequently gifted with prodigious memory. Their penchant for the past and history will make them convinced patriots. At times they find it a challenge to adapt to new life circumstances. Their success in adopting a new living condition, which is more often imposed to them than willfully desired, is contingent upon the possibility of adapting easily to the new situation. They experience great difficulty in modifying life circumstances to best advantage or to overcome them. These characters sleep very little, and generally wake up early in the morning.

3.9.2 Love and Interpersonal Relations

They are very insistent characters, not to say repetitive. The pressing insistence and repetition that characterize them might be mistaken for an imposing personality. In fact, it is a mild prelude to obsession, the individual not being able to control it at all.

They expect from everybody a disposition of collaboration and assistance towards them. You will always see them demand others to behave at the fit of their own expectation and exhaust their relatives in recommendations as to how to organize their own existence.

Sometimes they fall into sudden crises of pessimism and depression, particularly after a peer might have caused them serious grief and mistreated them or even after unexpected misfortunes. They are however very compassionate individuals that are quick to empathize with others and sincerely share their grievances and sufferings. They always generously assist whoever approaches them in need of help. Their identification to and empathy with others may reach such depth that their peers may come to the point of considering them their alter ego.

Love-passion is the sentimental province of these characters. Women of this temperament are very maternal and often seek to shape up a family early in their lives. In general, these characters' ability for tight matches in love, to charm and cherish their pair, as well as taking care of their children, is unrivaled among all character types. At the same time sentimental disappointments will have on them the greatest impact. Love relation breakups will leave them in profound despair and grief from which they have utter difficulties to come back from.

Suicide is a serious problem with these characters. Not because of being prone to annihilation, but as a consequence of their tendency to experience the depth of despair from aggravating life circumstances.

3.9.3 Education/Profession/Occupation

They report that these natives always entertain, in one way or another, some sort of involvement with the arts.

Whenever they become able to sustain systematic effort in developing and promoting their art, oftentimes in the field of music, they would rise up to the apex of artistic creation. Women of this temperament will go through entire days cleaning up, ordering and decorating their homes. Even exhaust will not keep them from proceeding late into the night if necessary.

3.9.4 Language

Matrixial characters are very talkative, akin to the Associative type, but more often than not incur verbal lapses, slips of tongue, and incorrect grammar. They are tireless in repeating themselves, the same views, the same recommendations...

3.10 The Antagonistic Character

The partitions making up Layer 7 are displayed below.

7	Terror	Fear (Anguish)	Angst	Anxiety	↑ ↓	Resentment	Repugnance	Wickedness	Fury

We expect these root partitions of the Mental Foliate to mold the Paradoxical or Antagonistic Character type, when they have been stamped with accrual level 2.

3.10.1 Personal Identity and Attributes

The main trait of the Paradoxical character is conflict and contradiction. They also invariably fall prey to conscientious conflicts, temptations, chronic torments of their inner self. They tend to hatch burning secrets they cannot confide to anyone else.

Their behavior overall materializes chaos, conflicts, aggressions and violence, in greater or lesser measure. We must not conclude, however, that all Antagonistic tempers must be either potential or declared criminals. Many are quite sociable and peaceful characters. Nevertheless, no matter how sociable they might appear, one significant conscientious conflict of whatever nature, a temptation or a secret torment will be with them through the course of their lives.

They maintain a keen awareness of danger and what evil may be around them.

3.10.2 Love and Interpersonal Relations

They are naturally predisposed to betrayals, morbid jealousy, and even incommensurate vindictive acts in response to possible offenses to their personal pride. For all that matter, it will not be rare to see them frequently involved in legal matters. Often they are foiled in a sort of mystery to those around them. They may appear to others under the light of impenetrable individuals.

The exercise of bigotry is not stranger to them either. In attempting to assert the exact contrary of what they know to be true, they will engage in decisive attempts to fool others or to "backstab" them as popular culture has it.

The Antagonist character assumes sexuality in its clearest and most genuine paradoxical expression, sadism and masochism, that is. The practice of sexuality tends to make up an essential thread in their lives. Eroticism on the aggression or victimization slant, almost always imbued in their thoughts, generally constitute the deepest motive of their acts. Well aware of the social unfitness of these types of sexual urges, these characters find themselves more often than not unable to overcome them, which creates a constant internal discomfort or tension. In some extreme cases, as they succumb to these stingy urges, they slip into passionate crimes, rapes, rape-murders, dismemberments, etc.

3.10.3 Education/Profession/Occupation

Quite unintuitively, it is not rare to find these character types in liberal professions, in particular those which give them the opportunity to flush the urge of dealing with evil, such as combating diseases or crime, to rupture and bust an enemy, figuratively or realistically. They will rank in all ladders of social occupations, but it will be no surprise to find many on the conflictive or delinquency side of these activities. One can also see from our premises the enormous appeal that the military will have on most of them.

Further, the Antagonist characters are prone to penetrate human nature, in an attempt to acquire deepest knowledge about individuals and human affairs, which may turn many into true erudites. No surprise that they also are notably in search of vulnerabilities. Their keen sense of good and evil, comparable to that of the Quadratic or Hyperbolic temper, is nevertheless distinguishable from the latter in that it is not primarily driven by personal pride but by a motivation for disruption.

3.10.4 Language

For those with lesser education, language may employ either frequent or sporadic curse words. In others, it may be violent and quite obscene.

3.11 The Perfect Character

The partitions making up Layer 8 are displayed below.

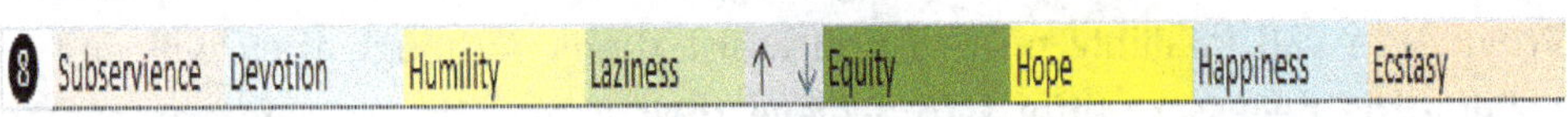

As these root partitions of the Mental Foliate accuse accrual level 2, we expect them to ground the Perfect Character type.

3.11.1 Personal Identity and Attributes

The perfect character features a peculiar religious sense and a tendency to spirituality in views and beliefs. They will be among the faithful for whom regular participation in religious ceremonies is very serious matter. Not all of them necessarily hold a vocation for sacerdotal office, though many do. In any case, their altruistic sense and social sensibility are unpaired. Parental bonds bear a sacred character to them as well.

The Perfect character is full of goodwill and above all an ineradicable optimism. Their behavior is fueled by an aspiration to elevation. They consider that luck is with them to stay. No one will remove from them the belief that they are "elected sons of Providence" to benefit from its justice and mercy.

Quite frequently, their nightly dreams are stylistically symbolic and achetypical.

3.11.2 Love and Interpersonal Relations

They like to imagine enterprises that make them the great protectors of others, akin to philanthropists. The exercise of philanthropy tends to be widespread among them. So pronounced is their sense of solidarity that they will sacrifice themselves to lend help to others.

In the love chapter, they seem to be more in search of a detached happiness such as bliss than love-passion. Consequently, they tend to remain celibate, akin to the Utopian character types. Among those who accede to marriage, divorces, separations and new marriages appear to be quite frequent, more so with them than any other character type. Further, the passion in marriage will not do away with their desire for celestial bliss.

3.11.3 Education/Profession/Occupation

These individuals are convinced that any enterprise of their undertaking will succeed, less because they are going to input a lot of work into it than because Providence will infallibly protect and assist them. Although they will end up making the necessary efforts to achieve their goals, they remain partisans of lesser efforts. Their tendency to laze, pleasure and adventures remain latent and will spring up at times. Others plainly devote their lives to them. Speed, sports cars, airplanes, the rolling tracks... enthrall them all.

3.11.4 Language

Their language typically invokes providence, deference to providence, or wishes for good luck from above.

3.12 The Asymptotic Character

The partitions making up Layer 9 are displayed below.

9	Inanity	Cluelessness	Austerity	Patience	↑ ↓	Temperance	Endurance	Resilience	Tenacity

As these root partitions of the Mental Foliate accuse accrual level 2, we expect them to ground the Asymptotic Character type.

3.12.1 Personal Identity and Attributes

Resistance, endurance and tenacity are very ostensible traits of the Asymptotic temperament. These characters' impassivity and patience endure it all. Indeed it takes a lot for them to display bad mood and impatience, except in front of what qualifies as pettiness in their judgment. Short-tempered behavior or meanness are almost stranger to these characters who are capable of enduring profound suffering for an extensive number of years.

The moderate and sober nature of the typical element under this character type together with an ample supply of endurance endows them with such a potential for survival that they tend to preserve in their entirety the vitality and freshness of their mental faculties very late in their elder years of life. They seem to be defying old age decline.

The Asymptotic character type shares with the Perfect character a profound spiritual sense, leaning toward self-sacrifice. In addition, the asymptotic character seemingly takes it to the specific direction of ascetism.

3.12.2 Love and Interpersonal Relations

These character types particularly show the most inflexible serenity in front of affective and moral suffering from interpersonal relations, and all manners of misfortune or adversity alike. Mothers of this character type may completely forget about their persona during the years devoted to raise their children and indulge very lately in the endeavors they had envisioned for themselves in their younger years.

In love, physical separation does not pose a problem to faithfulness and persistence in their feelings for the cherished person. They are able to maintain durable relations in the distance, should life circumstances forcibly keep them away from their partners. However, in love relationship they are not particularly passionate and may drive the relationship to boredom.

3.12.3 Education/Profession/Occupation

The Asymptotic character never seeks positions of command. These types maneuver in the background, behind the scene, to the aims of fortifying and judiciously tailoring the enterprises in which they get involved. They are the backup resource the outsider will not see, although their unnoticed presence remains strongly active. As entrepreneurs, they are tireless and almost never advertise their persona. No one (except perhaps the Hyper type) has a deeper sense of self-sacrifice and austerity. An Asymptotic temper is able to renounce for long to greatest personal satisfactions if he or she perceives this renouncement as a condition to pursue an essential goal in life.

3.12.4 Language

Silence appears to be their preferred form of communication. Those who become spiritual agents find in prayer, whether mentalized or spoken, the best and most elevated exercise of language or communication.

3.13 The Hyper-Characters or Quintessential Temperaments

As explained earlier in this study, in the physical QGT, Trivalent Quintessence delineates three hyperoperators, namely the Hyper-Quantum operator, the Hyper-Space operator and the Hyper-Quadratic operator. The first maps back to Unary norm, the second to the Asymptotic norm and the third to the Quadratic norm. In their application to the configuration of the human Mental, the Hyper-Quantum operator, as a descriptor of utmost quantum ontology, multiplies by many folds the monocentrism of the unary or egocentric character type. The Hyper-Space operator, as a descriptor of utmost expansive ontology, multiplies by many folds the expansiveness of the asymptotic character type. Lastly, the Hyper-Quadratic operator, in its condition of a descriptor for utmost quadratic ontology, multiplies by many folds the ambivalence of the quadratic character type.

Below a description of these three additional character types deriving from Trivalent Quintessence.

3.14 The Hyper-Egocentric Character

The partitions making up Layer 1 are displayed below.

1	Timidity	Introversion	Solitude	Indifference	↑ ↓	Conservativenes	Possessiveness	Competitivenes	Cupidity

As the Norm of conservation or monocentrism subtending these root partitions of the Mental Foliate accuses an overrate, we expect a form of exaggeration in their expression to ground the Hyper-Ego character type.

3.14.1 Personal Identity and Attributes

This character type presents with an overwhelming enthusiasm, capable of suddenly turning crazy about something that will nevertheless fall completely off his radar very shortly thereafter. He turns out to be a tactless temper with a sheer aspiration to domination. If the aspiration to dominate is common in the Egocentric character, here it is overamplified and you no longer see the quiet strength of the Egocentric temper but storms. The fight for self-ascendancy and domination makes for the bedrock of the hyper type's existence.

The Hyper-Egocentric character tends to behave as if always mad at everything in order to avail himself an opportunity to impose on and subdue everyone. He is tirelessly fighting against the world and, like a true despot, everything must start and end with him.

3.14.2 Love and Interpersonal Relations

He tends to be an impetuous and quite irascible person in interrelating with others. Nevertheless you will see him feeling sincerely regretful when, after an access of anger and regaining his senses, he becomes aware that he has just emotionally hurt someone or upset everyone. Discomforting everyone and unhappy with everybody around him, one might think that solitude would make him happy. Wrong, he needs others around him for the chance to exert tyranny. Sometimes these characters feel completely disarmed in front of other people's silence and complete submission to their wants. No fight no winner. They then feel deprived of the pleasure of acting like the great conqueror or despot they purport to be, since they had not the chance to deliver a fight. One might say that they are truly and deeply alone, in their egocentric bid to single themselves out, without realizing it.

Constancy in relationships may be a problem with this type. Because of the superficiality resulting from their overall behavior, they may not entertain durable relationships. Women of this character type frequently show virile tendencies: they actively seek independence and, when engaged in a couple relation, they will tend to dominate their mate or husband and assume the direction of the family.

These characters will not find faithfulness a great quality for themselves in sentimental relations due to their commitment to sheer domination.

3.14.3 Education/Profession/Occupation

The Hyper-Egocentric character may find it quite difficult to function in a team, especially when the team leader does not possess specialized or higher level professional skills and qualifications that set him or her apart. In the latter case, the Hyper-Ego character will find it strenuous to work under the team leader whom he will attempt to undermine or compete with for superiority and dominance of the group. His bullish attitude with other members of the team with lesser skills will also cause constant friction, unless they resort to either avoid him altogether or be completely submissive to him.

In general, these characters tend to muster the courage and obstinacy that it takes for their enterprises to culminate. Stubbornness and inflexibility will be at the rendezvous as well whenever unexpected obstacles occur. They will be relentless in pursuing that which will give them that aura of super achiever.

The Hyper-Ego character may run the risk of associating with people he had not correctly or sufficiently assessed due to his overboard enthusiasm and irascibility which all hinder judicious critical thinking.

3.14.4 Language

May be clearly bullish in permissive environments.

3.15 The Hyper-Hyperbolic Character

The partitions making up Layer 4 are displayed below.

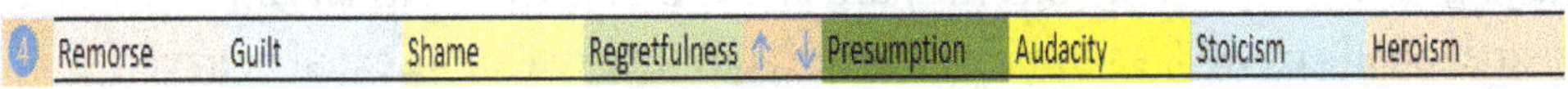

As the Norm of ambivalence subtending these root partitions of the Mental Foliate accuses an overrate, we expect a form of exaggeration in their expression to ground the Hyper-Hyper character type.

3.15.1 Personal Identity and Attributes

The Hyper-Hyperbolic character presents with a frankly illusive temper with a tendency to exercise loose logic or rationalization. This type may indulge in presumption and vanity, believing that humanity or superiors must accept his ideas for sake of evolution or progress, respectively. They may, however, come to harbor rather genuine social and humanitarian preoccupations.

Determined to be seen as ingenious, original and exceptional, they are given to play tricks or games and fanfaronades. Notwithstanding these excesses, they remain sociable characters, displaying ample courtesy to everyone. Being unusual and refined in their tastes, this quality tends to very much transpire in their clothing and the decoration of their home. Note that they may indeed become pretty ingenious and especially talented individuals.

The Hyper-Hyper temper is not exactly concerned with the higher norms of ethics and equity per se, such as the Golden rule, despite the likes and appearance. Indeed the nature of their normative aspirations relate to morale principles or Manichaean morale principles, to be exact. So much so that the social and humanitarian preoccupations these tempers tend to cater coexists with an enormous vanity.

3.15.2 Love and Interpersonal Relations

The Hyper-Hyper characters want to improve and perfect everything for greater societal benefit. Their great personal aspiration is to become role models to others.

In the sentimental aspect, these characters tend to bear on the pros and cons of relationships, virtues and defects they find in prospective partners, before engaging for good in a relation. They are likely to take their extravaganza slant into sexual habits as well, as some may even show asexual or bisexual behavior.

3.15.3 Education/Profession/Occupation

This category of tempers shows many thinkers with ideas that might qualify as original or eccentric, all eager to be part of the social vanguard. They generally seek to belong in select circles of society.

3.15.4 Language

Their language may be super-hyperbolic: *"I'm so hungry I could swallow a horse."*

3.16 The Hyper-Asymptotic Character

The partitions making up Layer 9 are displayed below.

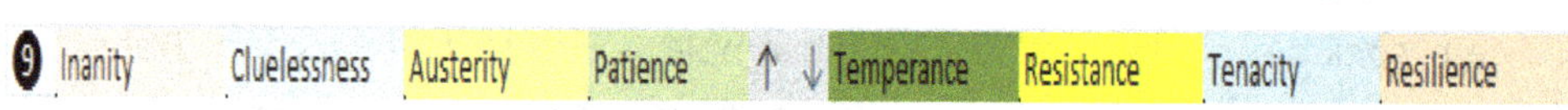

As the Norm of expansiveness subtending these root partitions of the Mental Foliate accuses an extrapolation, we expect a form of exaggeration in their expression to ground the Hyper-Asymptotic character type.

3.16.1 Personal Identity and Attributes

The Hyper-Asymptotic temper presents an extrapolation of the psychic traits emanating from the asymptotic mental layer. In effect, the mind of the Hyper-Expansive character tends to embrace and pursue in perception vast swaths of reality at a time, which gives them the like of escaping the discreteness of the real world. In that manner, their minds are uncharacteristically open to the void of space, conferring them an aura of proneness to fancy and realistically-detached imageries and desires. An absence or withdrawal fit stamps their mind set.

The above causes them to oftentimes show a rather deficient practical sense. However, they are at the same time the most resilient and enduring characters among the twelve.

The Hyper-Asymptotic personality is also marked by an extreme sensitivity which may tend to make these tempers highly impressionable. In that event, they may find it quite challenging to handle or control their intimate feelings. By the same token, they are extremely intuitive individuals, with an extremely high level of perceptiveness.

These individuals thus reveal a gentle and easy-flowing fit of character which may take the likes of weakness when compared to most others. As adults, they tend to show what would qualify as childish or immature behavior.

The asymptotic temper's tendency to ascetic renouncement proceeds here: the idea of owning and accumulating material belongings is unusual to the Hyper-Asymptotic type. Nevertheless, her sense of personal responsibility is well developed. This sense of solidarity and collectiveness joined to the very high level of perceptiveness may grow in these tempers into very elevated forms of spiritualism.

3.16.2 Education/Profession/Occupation

The pursuit of spatialization (or expansiveness) stirs these individuals to expand in their physical space of occupation. Therefore, they tend to spread out, which makes them prone to compulsively multitask in their occupations. They are prone to accuse a significant lack of the ability to focus.

Embracing too much at a time, and with a strong tendency to deferment, they will find it quite challenging to finalize their enterprises.

3.16.3 Love and Interpersonal Relations

Asymptotic characters tend to repress their desires and impulses, to be exact they tend to sublimate them. No one is more selfless than these tempers. They develop long-lasting relationships with distant others and are so given to lasting platonic loves. This is their way of *not* living something that must be part of their lives: they "virtualize" it by turning it into void. In other words, they partially renounce to it or experience it through the void of spatial distance. In addition, this kind of platonic relationship fully satisfies their spirits.

3.16.4 Language

Highlight tends to be evocations of morrows, extrapolations and resignation: "What will be will be".

3.17 A Corroboration of QG Characterology with Public Figures

It is important to realize that the above discussed character types are pure types or characterological primitives. They define the directives along which human lives are profiled from pure psychological determinants at the individual level. There are no other *ways* for human beings to ontologically personify their mental body. In practice, these types are subject to intercomposition or intermingling due to external influences exerted on every individual's Mentation Foliate originating from parents, educators, society and the culture in which they have been evolving. These influences have no other descriptors however than the same evoked types or qualities when they come to orchestration inside of the individual's Mentation Foliate.

As mentioned previously, external influences are internalized within the representational sublayers and modulate the expression of the root partition impulses, namely the *transflows* and in particular *orthoflows*. The 12 types that we have delineated do not always each realize in their pure and exclusive traits. If we consider each primitive in their operator quality, it is mainly when an operator *overloading* occurs as a result of intermingling between differing factors that the pure type will realize and become observable. Understand operator overloading as a repetition or multiplication of the same operator, keeping in mind that they do not necessarily have the same weight within the expression or string, i.e. $\left[\vec{2}\right]\left[\vec{2}\right]\left[\vec{2}\right]$. Operator composition is discussed in Volume II of the QGT publication[10]. By properly taking into account parents' interaction as a major, it is possible to identify and predict a much closer biographical portrait of any individual. However, it remains beyond the scope of this treatise to discuss the numeric systematic within the QGT framework that produces such results.

On another hand, it is of high import to reiterate that, circumstantially, the dynamics proper to a mental layer other than the characterologically determinant one may slightly rise above ground level or Ground 1. Women regularly experience such an increase at the level of the Paradoxical Layer and/or the Matrixial Layer of their mental Foliate throughout the span of their menstruation cycle. Usually, they will then become aggressive and conflictive, or perhaps anxious, distressed, with the kind of common cravings in pregnancy, etc.

The development stage that corresponds to adolescence propends a slight increase in the dynamics of Mental Layer 5 (through operator composition $\left[\vec{3}\right]\left[\vec{5}\right]$ in this case). Such an increase is responsible for the "weird" behavior characteristic of teenagers, their typical motivation to change the world, and their vision of anarchy and a new world. This slight increase above ground level the elderly generally develop in the asymptotic layer of their mental Foliate. It is responsible for their characteristic patience, austerity, temperance, and, if you will, wisdom. Not because they have lived it all and seen it all they ought to become wiser. They become wiser due in essence to this condition of the asymptotic stratum of their mental Foliate, just as teenagers, who have not seen much of the world, are already willing to change it under the instigation of their metamorphogenic mental stratum. The slight increase above ground state in question infants will develop at the level of their Unary or Binary mental Layer. Such an increase accounts for their characteristic tyranny, their stubbornness as well as their unparalleled curiosity and inquisitiveness (they never stop asking questions).

When it comes to a possible increase above ground state due to ingestion of chemical substances, we must point out that alcohol and drugs will definitely

10 Quanto Geometry, Overture of Cosmic Cosnciousness and Universal Knowledge for All, Vol II

produce such effects. Alcohol will specifically cause an over-excitation of the Paradoxical Layer. Each type of drug affects one specific mental layer. Narcotics are devastating to the mental Foliate in two ways. For one, they may increment the accrual level of a normally accrued mental layer far beyond level 3 threshold, else they may disburse the constitutional accrual level of one layer into a distinct layer if not simply provoke a second accrued layer beyond the first and the second threshold. In all three cases constitutional damage result which qualifies not just as dysfunctions but severe or catastrophic trauma.

The majority of these cases may be analytically interpreted in terms of operator composition as explained above. Phases of development throughout the lifecycle are all Quanto-Geometrically typed and stamped with the fundamental norms, per Fig. 2.1 and the details below:

$\left[\vec{1}\right] \rightarrow$	Infancy
$\left[\vec{2}\right] \rightarrow$	Childhood
$\left[\vec{3}\right] \rightarrow$	Adolescence
$\left[\vec{4}\right] \rightarrow$	Youth
$\left[\vec{5}\right] \rightarrow$	Early Adulthood
$\left[\vec{6}\right] \rightarrow$	Maturity
$\left[\vec{7}\right] \rightarrow$	Seniority
$\left[\vec{8}\right] \rightarrow$	Elderly
$\left[\vec{9}\right] \rightarrow$	Senility

Therefore, each developmental phase of the lifecycle, from birth to expiration, takes the weight of one of the 9 primary operators. To project very specifically pensive habits or observable behavior for an individual conjuncturally requires factoring in the individual's actual phase of life, resulting in operator composition with his character-defining operator. Be all that as it may, what will always be there as a major in the biographical narrative is the thread profiled by character definition. This thread is an irreducible constant.

We next showcase examples of application of the QG characterological types with well known public figures, both contemporaneous and from past epochs. For unquestionable credibility, these biographical reports are complete excerpts from their original narrative sources in which we do no more than highlight the traits that exemplify in earnest the descriptors we have profiled from the primitives. They each represent a compelling case of the QG-defined character type, as relates to the principal thread representing the center axis of those lives.

Pope John Paul II

Monolithic Character

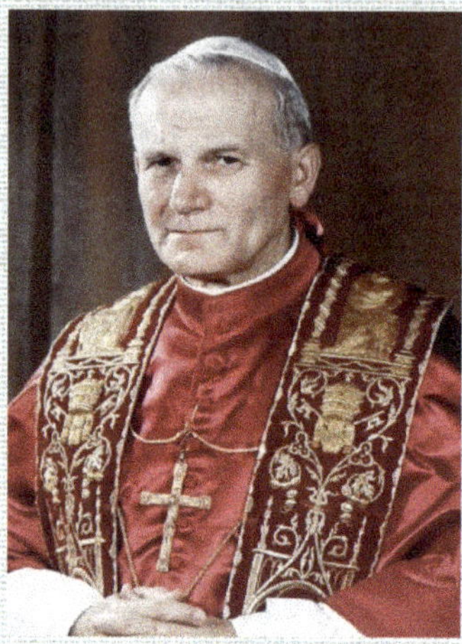

***Biography.com** – Born Karol Józef Wojtyla on May 18, 1920, in Wadowice, Poland, Pope John Paul II's early life was marked by great loss. His mother died when he was 9 years old, and his older brother Edmund died when he was 12.*

Growing up, John Paul was athletic and enjoyed skiing and swimming. He went to Krakow's Jagiellonian University in 1938 where he showed an interest in theater and poetry. The school was closed the next year by Nazi troops during the German occupation of Poland. Wanting to become a priest, John Paul began studying at a secret seminary run by the archbishop of Krakow. After World War II ended, he finished his religious studies at a Krakow seminary and was ordained in 1946. Pope John Paul II became the bishop of Ombi in 1958, and became the archbishop of Krakow in 1964. He was made a cardinal by Pope Paul VI in 1967.

***Crisis Magazine** - (https://www.crisismagazine.com/2020/how-great-was-john-paul-ii) "Pope John Paul II was unquestionably the most dominant figure in Catholicism in the last quarter of the twentieth century. He loomed large over every aspect of Catholic life, directing the Church through one of her most troubling times. And his influence transcended the confines of the Church; at the height of his popularity in the 1990s, he was arguably the most dominant figure on the world stage. He helped bring down the Soviet Union, one of the most terrifying forces of the twentieth century, and he likewise stood up to the Culture of Death that was infecting the West. He was a globetrotting rock star of a pontiff, commanding huge crowds and earning the respect and even adulation of millions of people worldwide."*

Canada One –
(https://www.canadaone.com/ezine/may05/pope_john_paul_leader.html)

Introspection and Solitude

*While Wojtyla had two doctorates in his field, he also studied philosophy and literature and was also a playwright and a poet... he took the time to gain knowledge of the world, himself, and beyond. As a chaplain for university students in Krakow, he used to go on frequent camping and kayaking trips and offered counseling and mentorship to the students. On these excursions, he would usually take an hour or more to be alone by himself to reflect, read, and pray. These **moments of solitude** gave him a strong internal compass and **knowledge of self** required of all great leaders.*

Humility

1978: Elected Pope John Paul II becoming the 264th pope and first non-Italian pope in 456 years; refuses formal papal coronation in favor of a simple inauguration ceremony and chooses not to use the royal plural "We" referring to himself plainly as "I". Wojtyla was not impressed by the trappings of power and its symbols and made that clear from the day he was elected Pope. He had a very simple, plain, and honest way of communicating that endeared people to him. He exemplified the servant-leader role by embodying one of the titles of the Pope: Servus Servorum Dei (Servant of the Servants of God).

Responsibility

2000: Offers a day of apology for sins committed by members of the Catholic Church over the centuries; visits Israel and pays homage to the victims of the Holocaust. Wojtyla was the first pope to visit the Auschwitz concentration camp in Poland in 1979, and later in 2000, he visited Jerusalem's YadVashem in remembrance of the six million Jews who died in the Holocaust, praying for reconciliation between Christians and Jews and apologizing for the sin of anti-Semitism by Christians. The day that former U.S. President, John F. Kennedy, took full responsibility for the Bay of Pigs fiasco, was the day he became a leader. The day that Wojtyla apologized and took responsibility for the sins of anti-Semitism committed by Christians, was the day he became a truly respected global leader.

Uncommon Leadership

1982 – 2003: Receives PLO leader Arafat; Meets Gorbachev as first pope to meet with a Kremlin Chief; visits Cuba and meets with Castro; becomes first pope in history to enter a mosque. Despite criticism from many corners on the controversial issues he supported, Wojtyla was not one to ever back down. He stood for what he believed in and had the courage of convictions. As a leader, he was tough but flexible. His flexibility allowed him to meet famous, and infamous, world leaders and address difficult issues that made him unpopular in certain circles. But he also had the inner toughness and steely resolve to break down walls and foster reconciliation. As Pope and head of the Roman Catholic Church he knew his role was to unify the Church while serving as an apostle of justice and peace. He stood his ground and never wavered, even if it meant alienation.

These (above) are a few of the "firsts" ever: the first pope to visit Auschwitz and the YadVashem's Center in Jerusalem who reconciled Christianity and Judaism for anti-semitism; the first pope to enter a mosque, bringing reconciliation between Christianity and Islam. Meets with his assassin in prison, forgives and asks for clemency for him.

Taavana **-** https://tavaana.org/en/en/content/solidarity-pope-john-paul-ii-and-orange-alternative-bringing-down-communism-poland-0 *"- In Poland, the Communist leadership arrested, executed, and exiled Polish anti-Soviet political dissidents in order to consolidate political power. By the time Poland instated its new Soviet-inspired constitution in 1952, Poles had witnessed the abolition of their Senate, rigged elections, Communist land reforms, and their country's social and political introduction into the sphere of influence of the Soviet Union.*

The opposition movement was comprised of a diverse group of political activists including Pope John Paul II and the Catholic Church, Lech Walesa's Solidarity movement, and the Orange Alternative Movement. While some of their goals varied, they shared a vision of a free, democratic Poland.

In 1978, the movement for a free Poland gained early traction with the election of Karol JózefWojtyła, better known as Pope John Paul II, to the Papacy. The Pope was motivated by a belief that Catholicism and the individual conscience stood diametrically opposed to Communism's suppression of religious, economic and political freedoms, which established the state as an alternative to a higher being. He saw Christianity as an inseparable part of Poland's rich cultural histo-

ry, and sought to re-establish a society where Poles could freely embrace their national and religious identity.

Fourteen months later the Solidarity movement would emerge, uniting many workers and intellectuals in pursuit of the aspirations articulated by the Pope. The Solidarity movement spawned from a labor strike in August 1980, when workers shut down the Gdansk shipyard over new limits on wages. After successful negotiations with the government, the strike leaders formed Solidarity on September 17, 1980, making it the first independent labor union behind the Iron Curtain. Yet Solidarity was not simply a trade union; it was a social and political movement that strove for human dignity and full citizenship, rights and freedoms for all Poles.

...Though mass citizen participation was vital to the success of the anti-Communist movement in Poland, a democratic transition could not have happened without the leadership of people like Lech Walesa, founder of Solidarity; Pope John Paul II, head of the Catholic Church; and the founder of the Orange Alternative, Colonel Waldemar Fydrych, who was generally known by his satiric nickname "Major." While each person had his own life history and style of leadership, they shared a deeply personal commitment to the cause: an open Polish society."

Leading the World Youth

***Diocese of Phoenix** – (https://dphx.org/tob-tuesdays-18/)- Lasting Legacy #3: The Globetrotting Pope.- During his papacy, Pope John Paul II logged more foreign trips than all previous Popes combined. He visited 129 countries, traveling more than 725,000 miles, and was seen in person by more than 150 million people.*

As part of his globetrotting adventures, Pope John Paul II initiated World Youth Day beginning in 1986. At the time, some of the Pope's advisors and admirers thought he was crazy. Why would young adults, increasingly disenchanted with the Church and pursuing a path of secularization, travel significant distances to spend a few days with the Pope? The answer: Because the Pope wanted to spend time with them!

The success of the first World Youth Day in Rome (1986) surprised Church authorities and launched a pattern of global gathering every two years: Buenos

Aires, Argentina (1987), Santiago de Compostela, Spain (1989), Czestochowa, Poland (1991), Denver, Colorado (1993), Manila, Philippines (1995 – where upwards of five million people attended the papal mass and Pope John Paul II had to use a helicopter to get to the stage), Paris, France (1997), Rome for the Great Jubilee (2000), Toronto, Canada (2002), and Cologne, Germany (2005, with Pope Benedict XVI).

World Youth Day was Pope John Paul II's attempt to personally reach the next generation of Catholics, to speak to them from his heart, to sing and laugh with them, and always, always to invite them to follow Christ, who alone is the fullness of life and happiness. Through his magnanimous and playful interactions with youth and young adults, Pope John Paul II changed the way young people viewed the papacy and inspired numerous vocations to the priesthood and religious life. As a result, reaching out to youth and crisscrossing the globe has become standard for the Vicar of Christ.

Moral and Spiritual Authority

***Legacy: Rebel with a Cause** -1920 – 2005: A legacy of leadership. Pope John Paul II was a rebel with a cause. A champion of human worth and dignity, a freedom fighter, a torchbearer for social justice, he left a lasting legacy of leadership and moral example that the world can follow. Asked once, if he feared retaliation from government officials, he replied (according to biographer George Weigel), "I'm not afraid of them. They are afraid of me." Indeed, he relayed a message to the world that will echo through eternity: "Be not afraid!"*

***Forgiveness -** 1983: Meets with assassin Ali Agca in prison. Just two years after the assassination attempt on his life by gunman, Mehmet Ali Agca, and several months of painful recovery, the Pope visited Agca in prison and offered forgiveness. (Much later, in 2000, the Italian government granted clemency to Agca, on the Pope's request).*

***The Catholic Thing** -*
https://www.thecatholicthing.org/2015/02/05/understanding-jpii-oscar-romero/ *- These are just several examples of the enduring myth that John Paul II mistreated Romero. What really happened?*

In Romero's diary, we read about the two audiences John Paul II granted him, in 1979 and 1980. During the first meeting, Romero spoke of the difficulties of his ministry in a country lacerated by political violence. John Paul listened attentively, and compared these experiences with his own in Poland, yet encouraged "prudence." Romero's impressions were that the pope listened to him, but did express worry that John Paul II's aides had told the pontiff critical things about him: "Although my first impression was not altogether satisfactory, I believe it was a most useful visit and talk, since he was very frank."

Before the second meeting, however, John Paul's collaborator, Argentinean Cardinal Eduardo Pironio, gave the pope a glowing report of Romero. The Holy Father encouraged the archbishop to fight courageously, hugged him and told him he prayed for El Salvador daily.

The future martyr was joyous. In his diary, he writes that he felt full approval from the pope and "God's confirmation and his force for [his] poor ministry" and that the day was "filled with great satisfaction and much pastoral accomplishment." Shortly afterwards, Romero quoted John Paul II in his Lenten homilies.

After Romero's death, John Paul II defied prelates who painted him as a crypto-communist. After Romero's assassination in 1980, he sent a telegram condemning the killing and sent his personal delegate, Mexican Cardinal Ernesto Carripio, to preside over the funeral Mass.

In 1983, he visited El Salvador. Latin American prelates begged the pope to not visit Romero's tomb, yet during the motorcade he unexpectedly turned his popemobile towards the cathedral. It was closed, but John Paul II stubbornly waited until someone got the key. He then prayed at Romero's tomb, praising him as a "zealous pastor who tried to stop violence."

John Paul II prays at the tomb of Archbishop Oscar Romero in 1983. He prayed there again in 1996. During a 2000 ceremony in Rome's Coliseum, some Latin American cardinals begged John Paul II not to invoke Romero as an American martyr. Wojtyła did so anyways.

***About Spiritual work and Exorcism** -(https://ucatholic.com/blog/little-known-exorcisms-performed-at-the-vatican-by-pope-john-paul-ii-and-benedict-xvi/)- According to the late Father Gabriele Amorth, who was the exorcist for the Diocese of Rome, Pope Saint John Paul II performed his first exorcism as Pope in the Vatican on March 27, 1982. Bishop Ottorino Alberti of the town of Spoleto, Italy brought a young woman by the name of Francesca Fabrizi to the pope asking for his aid. Immediately after he met the young woman, she starting writhing un-*

controllably on the ground, sobbing, despite John Paul II's interventions. She only calmed when he said "Tomorrow I will say mass for you."

A few years later after the successful exorcism, a happy and peaceful Francesca Fabrizi visited with her husband and children to meet once again with the pope. In the private memoirs of Jacques-Paul Martin, the Prefect of the Papal Household during John Paul II's papacy, he wrote that the pope said that "I've never seen anything like this before. It was a biblical scene."

Pope John Paul II performed another exorcism in Saint Peter's Square during a weekly audience in 2000. A woman by the name of Sabrina was brought to the Vatican, and as soon as she entered the square she immediately began to yell and tried to lunge at the pope, requiring ten people to hold her down. She started drooling and yelling blasphemies. After finishing his weekly address, John Paul II asked to meet with Sabrina. According to Father Amorth, as soon as she got close to the pope her eyes glazed over and her head was thrown back and she yelled "No, leave me alone!" John Paul II performed an exorcism on the spot, blessing her several times. The initial attempt, however, failed to completely exorcise her and Father Amorth was required to perform several more exorcisms with Sabrina to completely rid her of demons.

Love Life and Marian Devotion

The Guardian – *(https://www.theguardian.com/world/2016/feb/15/pope-john-paul-ii-letters-reveal-32-year-relationship-with-woman) - "Pope John Paul II had an intimate 32-year relationship with a Polish philosopher who is believed to have once declared her love to him while he was still a cardinal, according to letters discovered by the BBC.*

There is no indication that the former pope, who died in 2005 and was made a saint by Pope Francis, had a sexual relationship with Anna-Teresa Tymieniecka or ever broke his vow of celibacy, but the correspondence sheds light on the depth of the relationship Pope John Paul II had with Tymieniecka when he was archbishop of Kraków, including the possibility that he struggled to come to terms with his feelings for her."

The BBC contends that Tymieniecka may have confronted the future pope about her feelings for him in Vermont, because he later wrote a letter to her confessing that he was struggling with their relationship. After telling her he believed she was a gift from God, he wrote: "If I did not have this conviction, some moral certainty of Grace, and of acting in obedience to it, I would not dare act like this."

In one letter after that period, he wrote: "My dear Teresa, I have received all three letters. You write about being torn apart, but I could find no answer to these words."

... Reflecting on the importance of priestly celibacy, Pope John Paul II once wrote that it expressed "the church's will" that "the church, as the spouse of Jesus Christ, wishes to be loved by the priest in the total and exclusive manner in which Jesus Christ ... loved her".

The Vatican said in response to the BBC programme that it was already known that Pope John Paul II "was friendly" with Tymieniecka.

University of Dayton – *(https://udayton.edu/imri/mary/p/pope-john-paul-ii-and-consecration-to-mary.php) - In his last apostolic letter,* Rosarium Mariae Virginis, *the Pope cited a statement he had made in 1990 in which Scheffzcyk sees a summary of the Pope's Marian thought: "Our entire perfection consists in being conformed, united and consecrated to Jesus Christ. Hence the most perfect of all devotions is undoubtedly that which conforms, unites and consecrates us most perfectly to Jesus Christ. Now, since Mary is of all creatures the one most conformed to Jesus Christ, it follows that among all devotions that which most consecrates and conforms a soul to our Lord is devotion to Mary, his Holy Mother, and that the more a soul is consecrated to her the more it will be consecrated to Jesus Christ. Never as in the Rosary do the life of Jesus and that of Mary appear so deeply joined. Mary lives only in Christ and for Christ!"... John Paul II's notion of Mary's spiritual maternity includes a "Marian dimension in the life of Christ's disciples."(RM 45) In comparison to the consecration to Christ at baptism, Marian consecration is a freely willed expression of a special spirituality which however is indispensable to the Church.*

"Love that leads to marriage is a gift from God and a great act of faith toward other human beings."

QG Psychophysics Interpretation

The Catholic Church is in and of itself bastion of Tradition, Conservatism, Authority, and, if one remembers the Crusades that took place over 500 years,

Competitiveness as well. On that account the infrastructure of the Church rests on a psychosocial emporium whose signature is predominantly the set of qualifiers laying at the right-chiral side of Layer 1 of the QG Mentation Manifold. Joining the church is squarely joining this psychosocial emporium, want it or not. However, the authentic mission of the Church is of a transcendental order in fashioning a path for spiritual elevation of mankind and consecrating of the spirit. Descriptors of those qualities predominantly lay along both Layer 8 and Layer 9 of the QG Mentation Manifold. Consequently, joining the church is also expressly joining this creed, in this case by voluntary and unbreakable vows. The Church is thus primarily a spiritual family, towered and regimented by immaterial divine entities, and very secondarily a human family.

It is probable that the Polish boy Karol Józef Wojtyla who lost his mother at the very young age of 9, in full peg to her maternity, and his older brother at age 12, a painful loss of kindred and companionship, felt the appeal of the church as that of joining a family in the fullness that life had denied him. He therefore went on to attend the seminary even in secrecy during the WWII and pressed on to succeed in being ordained in 1946 after the war ended. These impacting life events are likely to have preshapped him to become the profound humanist that he was. He sought not one but two doctorates in the theological field, studied philosophy and literature and was also a playwright and a poet…

His role of chaplain for university students in Krakow also provided occasions for the introverted and solitary side of his personality as a Layer-1 prevalent character to be at play. The biographer notes that during the frequent camping and kayaking excursions with students, he would usually take an hour or more to be in solitude and to reflect, read, and pray, adding that *"these moments of solitude gave him a strong internal compass and knowledge of self required of all great leaders."*

As a character loath to any form of extravagance and prone to self-restrain, it is not surprising that when elected pope he declined a formal papal coronation in favor of a simple inauguration ceremony and chose not to use the royal plural "We", referring to himself plainly as "I". The biographer further notes that *"Wojtyla was not impressed by the trappings of power and its symbols and made that clear from the day he was elected Pope. He had a very simple, plain, and honest way of communicating that endeared people to him."* All of which is perfectly predictable from a Layer-1 prevalent character stirred by the specific partitions lying at the left-chiral side of the Layer.

When it came to matters of faith, Pope John Paul II was brought to conflate his personal peg to Tradition and Conservatism to that of the Church in the conduct of Church affairs, while intending to fully play his role of Church topmost authority. Therefore his papal tenure has been first and foremost expression of the Theology of Traditional Canon and its enforcement. It is well known that this paramount concern is what guided his choice of the very orthodox cardinal Ratzinger for prefect of the Congregation for the Doctrine of the Faith in 1991. In 1998, Ratzinger became vice dean of the College of Cardinals and was elected dean in 2002. Ratzinger firmly defended and reaffirmed Catholic doctrine, including traditional teachings on topics such as birth control, homosexuality and interreligious dialogue.

John Paul's stance for enforcement of Catholic Tradition is clearly what guided his early interactions with Salvadoran archbishop Monsenior Romero, whom he publicly confronted in rebuttal of Theology of Liberation which Archbishop Orcar Romero had espoused. This confrontation almost created a rift within the Church in Latin America and a widespread negative reaction to the Vatican among Latin intellectuals. It appeared to many that the pope prioritized matters of faith over the cause of the poor in that region of the world and misunderstood that anti-communism resonated therein in a different manner and had a different context than it did in the Eastern Europe soviet block. It was only after the brutal killing of Monsenor Romero at the paramilitary hand of the political extreme right, turning him into a martyr, that the Pope changed gear and appeared to reconnect to the profound human dimension of the problem of poverty in that region of the world. This issue remained so extremely sensitive to the end of his Papacy that Latin clergy always exhorted him to avoid bringing it to surface during his visits. To no avail however, since he was determined to mend what he was likely to have perceived as an error or a shortcoming.

In that and many other ways reported by the biographers quoted in this review, John Paul II showed the world his immense qualities as a spiritual leader and his enormous capital of moral authority. In particular, he maintained his pro-life stance against contraception to the very end, consistent with the Marian doctrine which otherwise foots the Church and its intangibles on a material tangible anchor, and is further deeply teleogical to the Church in so many regards. In that he showed the world that the task of a leader is to uphold Truth and Rightfulness as it is respectively described and prescribed in the fundamental societal charters, and not to please popular tastes and demands of the moment for self-serving purposes.

There is a long string of firsts in the religious, political, and social order accomplished by Pope John Paul II, per the aforelisted biographers' reports and quotes, which underscore his authoritative leadership of very high caliber. They shall be put on the account of his personal character which is again prevalently anchored on the pensive partitions at the right-chiral side of Layer 1 of his Mental Foliate. Many of them must also be credited to the profound humanistic dimension expected from papacy and which he was able to deliver given the early psychosocial contributions to the formation of his personal character as discussed.

Of course, he was not the perfect Pope. His peg to Tradition and Institution is for certain responsible for the catastrophic failure of spotting and curing sexual abuse perpetrated by clergy against women and children, for decades and decades, worldwide. This problem did not obviously start with him but continued to fester on his watch, hit, and hurt the Church at its very core. This rather dark stain cannot be discarded from his legacy.

Jacques-Yves Cousteau

Realistic/Ambivalent Character

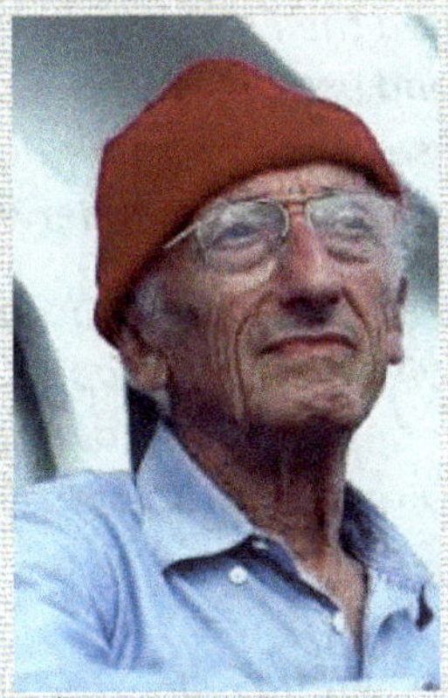

Biography.com *- "Explorer Jacques Cousteau co-invented the Aqua-Lung, a breathing device for scuba-diving, in 1943. In 1945, he started the French Navy's undersea research group. In 1951, he began going on yearly trips to explore the ocean on the Calypso. Cousteau recorded his trips on the TV series The Undersea World of Jacques Cousteau. In 1996, the Calypso sunk.*

Notable Biographies – *(https://www.notablebiographies.com/Co-Da/Cousteau-Jacques.html) - Jacques Cousteau was an undersea explorer, a photographer, an inventor of diving devices, and a writer. Most important was his work that he produced and wrote for television, which enlightened audiences around the world on the subjects of the ocean's natural treasures and the effects of pollution.*

Early Life and Inspiration

Jacques-Yves Cousteau was born June 11, 1910, in Saint-André-de-Cubzac, France, to Daniel and Elizabeth Cousteau. After their son's birth, the Cousteaus returned to Paris, France, where Daniel worked as a lawyer. Although Cousteau was a sickly child, who the doctors told not to participate in any strenuous activity, he learned to swim and soon developed ***a passionate love for the sea****. He combined this love with an early interest in invention and built a* ***model of a marine crane*** *when he was eleven years old.*

[It is] at age 4 [that] Cousteau learned how to swim, [which] started a lifelong fascination with water. As he entered adolescence, he showed a strong curiosity for mechanical objects and upon purchasing a movie camera, he took it apart to understand how it operated.

Cousteau's curiosity notwithstanding, he did not do well in school. At 13, He was sent to boarding school in Alsace, France. After he completed his preparatory studies, he attended Collège Stanislas...

In school Cousteau was bored and often misbehaved. He was even expelled at one time. In 1930 Cousteau entered France's naval academy, the Ecole Navale, in Brest. He graduated three years later and then entered the French navy. In 1936 he was given a pair of underwater goggles, the kind used by divers. Cousteau was so impressed with what ***he saw beneath the sea that he immediately set about designing a device that would allow humans to breathe underwater****.*

This project was put on hold during World War II (1939–45; a war in which England, the Soviet Union, and the United States clashed with Germany, Japan, and Italy). Cousteau became a gunnery (heavy guns) officer and was later awarded the prestigious Legion d'Honneur for his work with the French resistance, a military group fighting against the occupying German army.

Even during the war Cousteau turned his attention to the world below the sea. In 1942 he designed the Aqua-Lung, an early ***underwater breathing device****. Cousteau then helped remove mines from French seas left over from the war. One of these minesweepers (boats used to remove mines from the bottom of the ocean) would become Cousteau's research ship, the Calypso.*

On the Calypso 's first research voyage to the Red Sea, the maritime (having to do with sea travel) and diving expertise of her crew was combined with the scientific expertise of academic scientists who came aboard. These expeditions advanced knowledge of the deep by gathering underwater flora (plants) and fauna (animals) and by ***extensively photographing the underwater world,*** *which is more vast than the surface above water.*

When the French Ministry of Education finally provided grants to cover two-thirds of the expenses, Cousteau resigned from the navy in 1957, with the rank of lieutenant commander, to become director of the Oceanographic Museum in Monaco.

The National Wild Life Federation –
(https://www.nwf.org/Magazines/National-Wildlife/2001/Conservation-Hall-of-Fame-Jacques-Cousteau) "Until Jacques Cousteau came along in his trademark black-and-yellow wet suit with camera in tote, most people thought of the ocean as little more than a giant pool of lapping waves. But when the Frenchman dove deep

beneath the sea's surface, ***he emerged with films depicting an entirely new dimension****: unforgettable landscapes of coral reefs and brilliantly colored fish swirling through endless miles of blue. And by revealing that, Cousteau almost single-handedly moved the public both to marvel at and care deeply about the Earth's oceans.*

Before Cousteau, only a handful of explorers--burdened by heavy tanks strapped to cumbersome, helmeted diving suits--had ventured to the ocean's depths. But with an engineer's help in 1943, he adapted a valve pipe (designed to feed French cars cooking gas during gas shortages) to make a lightweight breathing apparatus that enabled users to inhale one breath at a time. Dubbed the Aqualung, the device gave Cousteau and other scientists a new opportunity to stay submerged long enough to study--and capture on film--underwater life.

Both the Aqualung and Cousteau's famous films inspired a generation of future oceanographers. *"We grew up watching Jacques Cousteau," says Larry Madin, senior scientist at the Woods Hole Oceanographic Institution. "We feel a certain allegiance, a certain connection to him."*

But Cousteau may have had a more powerful impact on the general public. The Aqualung, later known as SCUBA gear, eventually ***allowed people from all walks of life--explorers, scientists, treasure hunters and sightseers--to interact with marine life****, providing them personal experiences that spawned countless new advocates of marine conservation.*

His films--aired mainly on a 1960s-70s television show, The Undersea World of Jacques Cousteau--reached even farther. ***Zooming in on the gigantic eyes of whales and the slinky tentacles of octopuses, he brought such exotic sea creatures into the homes of millions of viewers.*** *"Because of the voice for the ocean that Cousteau provided--and for a while he was pretty much alone in this--people have been drawn to the sea to see for themselves," says oceanographer Sylvia Earle, an explorer-in-residence for the National Geographic Society. "That is really the key," she adds. "If you don't know, you can't care."*

Many of Cousteau's films took a bold conservationist stand. "I credit him with some of those first startling images of animals trapped in nets and of turtles strangled by plastic bags," says Bruce Robison, senior scientist at the Monterey Bay Aquarium Research Institute. "The stunning imagery had a real impact." Indeed, through film, Cousteau unveiled destructive practices that most people knew nothing about--the use of dynamite by fishing fleets to stun and kill hundreds of fish, for example. He also exposed the devastating impact of lost fishing gear, which traps or entangles sea lions, dolphins and other marine life.

Cousteau coupled his activist cinematography with public speeches and lobbying. In 1960, for example, he challenged France's plan to dump radioactive waste into the Mediterranean Sea, and policymakers subsequently canceled the proposal. In the 1970s, he convinced the Italian government to remove some 500 drums of toxic chemicals dropped into the Mediterranean by a sunken freighter. Before Cousteau's efforts, the deadly cargo had been tossing about the sea for three years."

Discovery of Underwater Treasure

The Famous People *(famouspeople.com) - The next mission to Toulon (1952) brought fame to Cousteau, as they found a wrecked Roman ship, 'Mahdia,' filled with treasure, near the South Coast of Grand-Congloué. This was the first underwater archaeology operation. The publication of his book, 'The Silent World,' immensely added to his increasing eminence.*

Raising [marine ecology] awareness

In 1960 Cousteau was an important part of the movement to prevent the dumping of French atomic waste into the Mediterranean Sea. This movement ended in success. ***Throughout his life Cousteau enjoyed much recognition for his tireless support of ocean ecology (the relationship between organisms and their environment).*** *In 1959 he addressed the first World Oceanic Congress, an event that received widespread coverage and led to his appearance on the cover of Time magazine on March 28, 1960.*

In April of 1961 Cousteau was awarded the National Geographic 's Gold Medal at a White House ceremony hosted by President John F. Kennedy (1917–1963). It was through Cousteau's television programs, however, that his work captured the imagination of a worldwide audience. In 1966 Cousteau's first hour-long television special, "The World of Jacques-Yves Cousteau," was broadcast. It was well received by critics. The program's high ratings were important in landing Cousteau a contract with the American Broadcasting Company (ABC), which resulted in the series "The Undersea World of Jacques Cousteau" in 1968. The program ran for eight seasons and starred Cousteau, his sons, Philippe and Jean-Michel, and sea creatures from around the globe. In order to raise public opinion against pollution, in 1975 he founded the Cousteau Society, an international organization with branches in several countries (including the United States at Norfolk, Virginia).

In honor of his achievements, Cousteau received the U.S. Presidential Medal of Freedom in 1985. In 1987 he was inducted into the Television Academy's Hall of Fame, and later received the founder's award from the International Council of the National Academy of Television Arts and Sciences. In 1988 the National Geographic Society honored him with its Centennial Award, and in 1989 France admitted him membership in its prestigious Academy.

Cousteau died in Paris, France, on June 25, 1997, at the age of eighty-seven. While some critics have challenged his scientific credentials, Cousteau never claimed "expert status" in any discipline. But perhaps to a greater degree than any of his fellow scientists, Cousteau enlightened the public by exposing the irreversible effects of environmental destruction.

Marital Life

Fampeople.com – Simone Melchior Biography *- Simone was born on 19 January 1919 in Toulon, France. Her father Henri Melchior and both grandfathers Jules Melchior (paternal) and Jean Baehme (maternal) were admirals in the French Navy. Simone's mother was Marguerite Melchior, affectionately called Guitte. She had two brothers: Maurice, and Simone's twin, Michel... Simone met her future husband, Jacques, at a cocktail party in 1937. He was a naval officer of 27 and she was 18. They were married at Saint-Louis-des-Invalides, in Paris, on July 12, 1937.*

After a honeymoon in Switzerland and Italy, the Cousteaus settled in Le Mourillon, a district of Toulon. Jean-Michel was born May 6, 1938 and Philippe Pierre December 30, 1940. Both sons were born on the family's kitchen table... In 1942, Simone's father provided financing and the manufacturing expertise of Emile Gagnan at Air Liquide to build Jacques Cousteau's aqua lung. Simone was indirectly to hold the key to this significant step in diving history.

Describing his wife, Jacques Cousteau said, "She was the happiest out of camera range, in the crow's nest of Calypso, for example, scanning the sea for whales. Nothing would get by her." He continued, "She lives to spend hour after hour in the wind and the sun, watching, thinking, trying to unravel the mystery of the sea." Simone died in 1990 of cancer.

Undercurrent.org - The Bitter Legacy of Jacques Cousteau September 2001 - Jacques had lived a lie for more than a decade, fathering two children with his long-term mistress. When he died, aged 87, in 1997, he left control of the Cousteau empire, the rights to his name and his huge archive of television footage to Francine, who also runs the Cousteau Society.

Says [granddaughter] Alexandra "Dad [Pierre Philippe] was the one Jacques had groomed to take over everything. They were like two peas in a pod. My grandmother Simone ... was an unsung hero, who never sought any glory or attention, but she kept the Calypso running smoothly and she helped make my grandfather the man he was. He would never have been the Captain Cousteau everyone knows and loves without her."

Weeks after [Simone] died, Jacques moved in with, and then quietly married, his secret mistress Francine Triplet. Then came another rift. Relations between Jacques and his other son, architect Jean-Michel, had never been good and in 1993 they hit rock bottom when Jacques sued to prevent Jean-Michel from using the Cousteau name to plug a resort he owned in Fiji. They eventually settled their dispute.

...

***The Baltimore Sun – October 12, 1997**- In 1990, Simone Cousteau, Jacques' wife and Jean-Michel's mother, died. The next year Jacques married his longtime mistress, Francine Triplet. When the Cousteau Society and Equippe Cousteau encountered financial troubles in 1992, Francine ordered the closing of the California offices where Jean-Michel was based.*

That year, the younger Cousteau left to produce documentaries about marine life and design excursions for environmentally minded travelers. His father apparently wasn't sorry to see him leave the Cousteau Society.

Jacques later told Figaro magazine: "My succession is a perpetual tragedy. The one I had chosen was my son, Philippe." -Jacques expanded on that for Nouvel Economiste magazine: "My son Jean-Michel is charming, but not capable."

In 1995, Jacques filed a lawsuit against his son's use of the Cousteau name in promoting a marine sanctuary resort. Father claimed son was tarnishing his reputation, while son claimed a right to his own surname.- When the dust settled, the resort was called Jean-Michel Cousteau Fiji Islands Resort, and father and son were not speaking....

Jean-Michel says the media attention was generally beneficial -- "wonderful publicity." But others admit the public feuding clouded the younger Cousteau's reputation -- among them Henry, who invited Jean-Michel to the National Aquarium.

"Yes, I was concerned," Henry said, " But when I met him, I was immediately impressed by his commitment to the environment."

As for the future, Jean-Michel plans to keep the Cousteau name in the spotlight. "My best skill is expressing complex environmental issues in language that the person in the street can understand, I want to do that as much as possible," he said.

Henry echoed that Jean-Michel is a valuable spokesman, as much for his speaking abilities as for another attribute:

"It's still the best-known name the environmental community has."

QG Psychophysics Interpretation

Inhabited by a marked sense of curiosity and ambivalence, Cousteau pushed his own limits and the limits of human nature. He was for certain not satisfied with what was observable in the natural world of lands and was intractably attracted to the underwater natural world guarded beneath the oceans of the World. The conjugate formed by the undersea world and the surface world of human inhabitation became the axis that guided his deep and insatiable sense of observation.

He employed his inventive abilities to fashion innovative devices from elements of the surface world into underwater exploratory aids to humans in order to facilitate and promote oceanographic exploration, hitherto largely unfeasible. At the same time, he brought back to the airborne surface world a string of captivating testimonies of underwater life, in films and photography, to be credited for an unprecedented impulse to the science of oceanography. Perhaps what our modern world has learned from Cousteau's underwater journeys is only comparable to what we have learned from Darwin's journey of exploration of the natural world one and a half century before.

While one may believe that his joining and graduating the Ecole Navale, and his subsequent enrolling with the French Navy constitute a definite stepping stone to his underwater exploration career, in fact at age 4 the young Cousteau was already swimming and his lifelong fascination with water and the undersea universe had already kicked in. In his teenage he further bought a movie camera and took it apart in order to “see” with his own eyes how this “viewing box” worked. The ontological directive of natural world observation through ambivalent lens set by the Binary Norm inherent to QG Layer 2 had constructed the axis of life that later took him to Ecole Navale and the French Navy under apparent personal choices.

We all recall his trips on his research ship “Calypso” aired on TV series. Interestingly, the momentum Cousteau’s exploration had reached in bringing to the young and old of the world the underwater marvels of the ocean was realized through this **viewing** box that we call “television”, then still at its debut. Overall Cousteau produced about 115 outstanding TV films and 50 illustrated books about underwater life.

His fund of knowledge from observation was utterly broad and captivating at the same time. Travels and exploratory expeditions made up the bulk of his adult life. His spirit of adventure and on the move dispose, which were prime products of his ‘realistic’ interest in real-world observation, manifested in his personal relationships as well. He shared his love of travel with his first wife, Simone Melchior and their two sons. After the death of Simone, he married Francine Triplet, with whom he had two daughters that he for sure initiated to exploratory travel as they came to share with him the same passion for the ocean.

He won a long string of highly prestigious awards for his oceanographic realizations and coinvented a large number of artifacts for oceanographic exploration. *“While some critics have challenged his scientific credentials, Cousteau never claimed "expert status" in any discipline. But perhaps to a greater degree than any of his fellow scientists, Cousteau enlightened the public by exposing the irreversible effects of environmental destruction. Cousteau died in Paris, France, on June 25, 1997, at the age of eighty-seven.”*

His being undeterred by critics of his scientific credentials is another testimony of a realistic mind that was irreversibly and exclusively stirred by appeal of the natural world, as well as the weight of observation in the buildup of knowledge and stewardship of this planet, our so-called habitat.

Of note is the important fact that Cousteau's ambivalent character has been in full display in the marital chapter of his life as well. That he chose for wife a twin female in the persona of Simone Melchior is not to be underestimated from the viewpoint of a character undergirded by ambivalence. So meaningful was Simone's twin status in their couple that they gave the name of Michel to their first son as Jean-Michel, Michel being the name of Simone's twin brother. Furthermore there was an important 10-year age difference between the two, since he was 27 years old when he married her at age 17, still in her teens. Just at the edge of what can be considered same generation.

Furthermore, beyond the quasi age disparity that seems to suggest that their marriage was both a love affair and a convenience decision on his part, the crucial help that Cousteau received from Simone's father early on to kick off his nascent career firmly authorizes that conjecture, no matter how unflattering for the man and non-judgemental this review portends to be. Cousteau himself acknowledges the tremendous material help that his wife Simone turns out to represent for their enterprise. Grand daughter Alexandra, and many biographers alike, acknowledged that *"she helped make [him] the man he was. He would never have been the Captain Cousteau everyone knows and loves without her."*

What's more, Cousteau entertained for a long while the ambivalent life of a married man with a secret mistress, Francine Triplet. We do not however share the characterization by the biographer that *"Jacques had lived a lie for more than a decade, fathering two children with his long-term mistress."* It is not clear whether his wife Simone was aware of the relationship or not and we know nothing of the possible climate that existed between the two due to this relationship. We do not know for certain either if the relationship with Francine might have predated his marriage with Simone. Therefore the qualifier of a "lie" may be as hasty as inappropriate. What this circumstance duly stands for at face value is ambivalence. At the very least, he had his heart divided between two women. And it is also clear that he had two households at the same time, since he had two "legitimate" children with Simone within their marriage and two other so-called "illegitimate" ones with Francine.

The very fact that he had two children in each of the two households is not to be underestimated either since it may reveal ambivalence in taste and an innate peg to parity. Along that line, how interesting is it that even his descendants embodied his ontological ambivalence in that he had two *sons* with Simone and two *daughters* with Francine. His heart was clearly divided between his two sons, Jean-Michel and Pierre Philippe, from Simone. He favored the younger one over the elder, for reasons that appear to be totally germane to Cousteau's own psychology. We learn from grand daughter Alexandra that Pierre Philippe and father Jacques *"were like* ***two peas*** *in a pod"* whereas he openly considered Jean-Michel *"an incapable"*. What we can see from the reports is that Jean-Michel had a personal take on environmental issues and a different view of social enterprising because he did not see it as antagonistic to personal benefits. Father Jacques made it an imbroglio in which he saw Jean-Michel taking advantage of his name branding, perhaps forgetting that it is also the son's name to freely use. At the same time, one can also understand Cousteau's frustration, disappointment and pain at the untimely death of his son Pierre Philippe, whom he hoped would become his material heir in the direction of the Cousteau world.

Jacques Cousteau wasted no time to marry Francine at the untimely death of Simone from cancer. In those circumstances, a storm between the Francine side of Jacques Cousteau's descent and the Simone side of his descent was all too predictable. However, it is very important to understand that, more than the other involved protagonists, the animosity stems from deep-seated ambivalence in the central figure of the saga, Jacques Cousteau himself.

We strongly hope that the analyst will see in the above not liberty to pass judgement on human lives but an effort to unravel the ways in which a characterological norm may tightly stamp a particular human life.

Nikola Tesla

Intellectual Character

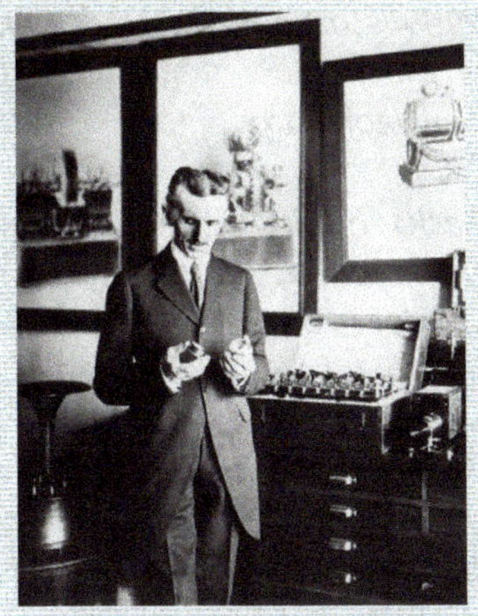

History.com *- Nikola Tesla was born in 1856 in Smiljan, Croatia, then part of the Austro-Hungarian Empire. His father was a priest in the Serbian Orthodox church and his mother managed the family's farm. In 1863 Tesla's brother Daniel was killed in a riding accident. The shock of the loss unsettled the 7-year-old Tesla, who reported seeing visions—the first signs of his lifelong mental illnesses.*

History.com *– (https://www.history.com/topics/inventions/nikola-tesla) - Serbian-American engineer and physicist Nikola Tesla (1856-1943) made dozens of breakthroughs in the production, transmission and application of electric power. He invented the first alternating current (AC) motor and developed AC generation and transmission technology. Though he was famous and respected, he was never able to translate his copious inventions into long-term financial success—unlike his early employer and chief rival, Thomas Edison.*

Thoughtco.com *– (https://www.thoughtco.com/nikola-tesla-1779840) - Nikola Tesla (July 10, 1856–January 7, 1943) was a Serbian-American inventor, electrical engineer, and futurist. As the holder of nearly 300 patents, Tesla is best known for his role in developing the modern three-phase alternating current (AC) electric power supply system and for his invention of the Tesla coil, an early advancement in the field of radio transmission.*

Early Life and Education

Nikola Tesla was born on July 10, 1856, in the village of Smiljan in the Austrian Empire (now Croatia) to his Serbian father Milutin Tesla, an Eastern Ortho-

dox priest, and his mother Duka Tesla, who invented small household appliances and had the ability to memorize lengthy Serbian epic poems. Tesla credited his mother for his own interest in inventing and photographic memory. He had four siblings, a brother Dane, and sisters Angelina, Milka, and Marica.

In 1870, Tesla started high school at the Higher Real Gymnasium in Karlovac, Austria. He recalled that his physics teacher's demonstrations of electricity made him want "to know more of this wonderful force." Able to do integral calculus in his head, Tesla completed high school in just three years, graduating in 1873.

Determined to pursue a career in engineering, Tesla enrolled at the Austrian Polytechnic Institute in Graz, Austria, in 1875. It was here that Tesla studied a Gramme dynamo, an electrical generator that produces direct current. Observing that the dynamo functioned like an electric motor when the direction of its current was reversed, Tesla began thinking of ways this alternating current could be used in industrial applications. Though he never graduated—as was not uncommon then—Tesla posted excellent grades and was even given a letter from the dean of the technical faculty addressed to his father stating, "Your son is a star of first rank."

***Thoughtco.com** - During the 1880s, Tesla and Thomas Edison, inventor and champion of direct electrical current (DC), would become embattled in the "War of the Currents" over whether Tesla's AC or Edison's DC would become the standard current used in long-distance transmission of electrical power.*

***History.com - Did you know?** During the 1890s Mark Twain struck up a friendship with inventor Nikola Tesla. Twain often visited him in his lab, where in 1894 Tesla photographed the great American writer in one of the first pictures ever lit by phosphorescent light. Tesla studied math and physics at the Technical University of Graz and philosophy at the University of Prague. In 1882, while on a walk, he came up with the idea for a brushless AC motor, making the first sketches of its rotating electromagnets in the sand of the path. Later that year he moved to Paris and got a job repairing direct current (DC) power plants with the Continental Edison Company. Two years later he immigrated to the United States.*

Nikola Tesla and Thomas Edison

Tesla arrived in New York in 1884 and was hired as an engineer at Thomas Edison's Manhattan headquarters. He worked there for a year, impressing Edison *with his diligence and ingenuity. At one point Edison told Tesla he would pay $50,000 for an improved design for his DC dynamos. After months of experimentation, Tesla presented a solution and asked for the money. Edison demurred, saying, "Tesla, you don't understand our American humor." Tesla quit soon after.*

Nikola Tesla and Westinghouse

After an unsuccessful attempt to start his own Tesla Electric Light Company and a stint digging ditches for $2 a day, Tesla found backers to support his research into alternating current. In 1887 and 1888 he was granted more than 30 patents for his inventions and invited to address the American Institute of Electrical Engineers on his work. His lecture caught the attention of George Westinghouse, the inventor who had launched the first AC power system near Boston and was Edison's major competitor in the "Battle of the Currents."

Westinghouse hired Tesla, licensed the patents for his AC motor and gave him his own lab. In 1890 Edison arranged for a convicted New York murderer to be put to death in an AC-powered electric chair—a stunt designed to show how dangerous the Westinghouse standard could be.

Buoyed by Westinghouse's royalties, Tesla struck out on his own again. But Westinghouse was soon forced by his backers to renegotiate their contract, with Tesla relinquishing his royalty rights.

In the 1890s Tesla invented electric oscillators, meters, improved lights and the high-voltage transformer known as the Tesla coil. He also experimented with X-rays, gave short-range demonstrations of radio communication two years before Guglielmo Marconi and piloted a radio-controlled boat around a pool in Madison Square Garden. Together, Tesla and Westinghouse lit the 1891 World's Columbian Exposition in Chicago and partnered with General Electric to install AC generators at Niagara Falls, creating the first modern power station.

In 1895 Tesla's New York lab burned, destroying years' worth of notes and equipment. Tesla relocated to Colorado Springs for two years, returning to New York in 1900. He secured backing from financier J.P. Morgan and began building a global communications network centered on a giant tower at Wardenclyffe, on Long Island. But funds ran out and Morgan balked at Tesla's grandiose schemes.

Tesla lived his last decades in a New York hotel, working on new inventions even as his energy and mental health faded. His obsession with the ***number three*** *and fastidious washing were dismissed as the eccentricities of genius. He spent his final years feeding—and, he claimed, communicating with—the city's pigeons.*

Tesla died in his room on January 7, 1943. Later that year the U.S. Supreme Court voided four of Marconi's key patents, belatedly acknowledging Tesla's innovations in radio. The AC system he championed and improved remains the global standard for power transmission.

Absent Love Life

Thoughtco.om - *Feeling that chastity would help him focus on his career, Tesla never married or had any known romantic relationships. In her 2001 book,* ***"Tesla: Man Out of Time,"*** *biographer Margaret Cheney writes that Tesla felt himself to be unworthy of women, considering them to be superior to him in every way. Later in life, however, he publicly expressed strong dislike for what he called the "new woman," women he felt were abandoning their femininity in an attempt to dominate men.*

Medium.com – *(https://medium.com/belover/the-queer-life-of-nicola-tesla-2809416d79c9) He would say he "never touched a woman."He needed to be single, he said. "I do not think you can name many great inventions that have been made by married men."*

He was just too busy being a genius to be married? His friends seemed not to understand. In a 1981 biography, ***Tesla: Man Out of Time****, Margaret Cheney notes "the pressures upon him to marry were unrelenting." There were "whispers that he was a homosexual."*

There's evidence for it. In a 1956 interview, Richard C. Sogge, a longtime member of the American Institute of Electric Engineers (AIEE), is recalling from the late 1880s that Tesla had a "reputation for voyeurism which was embarrassing to the older members." He continues:

"The stories of Tesla's sexual episodes were at one time the talk of the Institute, and we didn't know how to deal with it if the matter should somehow become publicized. You must be aware, of course, that he never went out with women."

In his mid-30s, he was close with Richard Hobson, a Navy hero of famous good looks.Though fourteen years younger, a friend introduces them as they "of course have much in common." They would prove to have a long-lived relationship. Richard Munson writes in Tesla: Inventor of the Modern:

"The famous and muscular officer — striking in his uniform and possessing deep-set eyes, prominent chin, thick beard, and handlebar mustache — often shared dinner with Tesla at the Johnsons', and the two exchanged regular notes, with Hobson in one suggesting: 'Now, my dear fellow, if you are doing nothing over the next ¾ of an hour come over for a short tête-à-tête — I feel I have not seen half enough of you on this visit and I have so much to talk with you about.'"

QG Psychophysics Interpretation

No other word qualifies more appropriately Nikola Tesla's psychological qualities than the word *genius*. He was an uncommon prodigy at the pinnacle of stardom already in his teens when he could successfully perform mathematical integral calculus in his head. His college dean later acknowledged his prodigious mind in a letter to his father. The qualification of "life-long mental illnesses" by one or other biographer, while catering to the mental shock caused by the early death of his brother, his possible voyeurism in adult life and his claim of being able to talk to the pigeons he was feeding at New York's Bryant park toward end of his life, is probably an exaggeration. These impairments never precluded him from properly functioning in important areas of life, such as profession, education, social settings, etc. as psychiatry of this day would have concluded. For certain, his voluntary sublimation of love and interaction with women into professional inventive work are frankly simply comparable to celibacy vow by the religious, which no one in psychiatry would qualify as a dysfunction.

Nobody has done more to impulse the technological grounds of today's human civilization than Nikola Tesla did, inasmuch as his prodigious electromagnetic inventions have come to fahion our way of life, from street lights to in-home electric appliances to power plants, to airborne radio transmission, to the universal and ubiquitous role of AC electricity in industrial production settings. As a man who at times appeared to have the 'magical' power of producing fluorescent fireballs in his hands from electricity, Tesla's genius, was simply outworldly.

It is fair to recognize that Teslas' genius was caught between the greed that plagued the industrial revolution era and formalist practice in academic physics at the time in relenting turmoil between classical physics and the new revolutionary theories of relativity. Tesla was in our judgement castigated by the academic physics establishment ultimately for not holding or pursuing one of these flamboyant formal titles that it sanctimoniously bestows. Instead of his prodigy in fundamental physics and experimental physics, what was praised north and south in academic physics were and still are the perennial Maxwell equations and his theoretical work in unifying magnetism and electricity into what became known as *electromagnetism*. Even Albert Einstein sought to model Maxwell's development with his set of relativistic tensor equations in describing the inner geometry of 'spacetime'. In fact, Maxwell equations are inarguably at the heart of the tremendous blockage physics has experienced for the last century or so. Yet without a Tesla coil and Tesla's alternating current, there is not much "electromagnetism" to have. Today Tesla's name is virtually nowhere to be found in academic records. All one can find for a reference to Tesla in a 1000-page undergraduate physics textbook[11] among many is the following:

"The SI unit for B (magnetic field) that follows from Eqs. 29-2 and 29-3 is the newton per coulomb-meter per second. For convenience, this is called the telsa (T):

1 tesla = 1T = 1 newton/[(coulomb)(meter/second)]

Recalling that a coulomb per second is an ampere, we have:

1T = 1 N/(A x m)

An earlier (non-SI) unit for B, still in common use, is the gauss (G), and :

1 tesla = 10^4 *gauss"*

---

[11] **Fundamentals of Physics,** 5th edition, Halliday, Resnick, Walker

The tesla unit appears out of nowhere in the textbook at that point, completely contextless, and just for 'convenience'! And that's the only place where the word or name tesla appears in the more than 1000 pages of physics!

The industrial 'war of currents' ended up falsely setting Marconi to be the inventor of radio transmission. Matter-of-factly, with the invention of alternating current and the induction coil, Tesla not only discovered the means for putting together the electric generators that went on to illuminate important sections of American cities like New York and Chicago, he also discovered that by feeding high frequency alternating currents to the coil the energy detached from the coil and propagated. Radio communication was no doubt in use when Tesla demonstrated for the U.S. military the operation of remote-controlled watercrafts, a historic and undeniable fact, which occurred much before Guglielmo Marconi appeared on the scene. Many suspect that Guglielmo Marconi was in fact a British spy of sorts, despite his enterprising and scientific tenure, otherwise hired by the then JP Morgan banking group to exact vengeance against Tesla who repeatedly refused to give in to his financier pressures. This was around the time that Tesla's lab caught fire without a forensic explanation. A biographer, Gary Lite, wrote the following in that regard:

369news.com - *(https://369news.net/2018/04/01/what-caused-nikola-teslas-1895-lab-fire/) -"J.P. Morgan was an American financier, banker, and art collector who dominated corporate finance and industrial consolidation. At the height of Morgan's career during the early 1900s, he and his partners had financial investments in many large corporations and had significant influence over the nation's high finance and Congress members. Morgan's total wealth was about $41.5 billion at that time. That is about $2.6 trillion as per today's standards. This was the clout J.P. Morgan had and hence everyone feared him; everyone but Nikola Tesla.*

J.P. Morgan wanted Tesla to sell all his patents to him and his businesses so that he could maximize his gains further.

He was willing to pay Tesla rich returns for the same. Tesla realized that consolidation of the patents in the hand of such a wealthy tycoon would mean that its benefits would never reach the common man and hence Nikola Tesla re-

fused. Morgan was not a man to let go of an insult. With his refusal to sell his patents Tesla had now snubbed Morgan thrice.

Tesla was habituated to working late in his lab. Once immersed in work he used to forget time and even skipped his food. One night he was similarly busy working in his lab when an impulse made him leave the lab for dinner. As he dined, there came a knock on the door. A messenger had arrived with the news that there had been an explosion in the building housing Tesla's laboratory and everything had been destroyed. Tesla ran through the street to where all his dreams, his visions, his work, his patents, his memories were housed but in vain.

The fire brigade was dousing the flames and nothing remained. The greatest monument to the technological advancement of mankind had been wiped off within no time. The totality of his technological achievements was burned into vapor. All that remained was Nikola Tesla himself.

Was it Tesla's refusal to grant his patents to Morgan that resulted in the blaze? Was this the fallout of War of Currents that Edison had badly lost to Tesla? Was it any other adversary of Tesla who did it? Or was it just another accident? No conclusive evidence to the end exists and time will keep its secrets.

Tesla was totally distraught by this loss mentally as well as financially. The fire destroyed all his research papers, notes, patents which awaited filing, books, and journals and also all of his apparatus. It left Tesla penniless. It would have been Tesla who would have been burned and buried in his own lab. But with good grace, Nikola Tesla was still alive...

Tesla told The New York Times *"I am in too much grief to talk. What can I say?" After the fire Tesla moved to 46 & 48 East Houston Street and rebuilt his lab on the 6th and 7th floor."*

Tesla went on with his inventiveness and dedicated his high intellection and energy to the creation of radio transmission hardware. ... "By July 1901, Tesla had expanded his plans to build a more powerful transmitter to leap ahead of Marconi's radio based system, **which Tesla thought was a copy of his own system**... Investors on Wall Street were putting their money into Marconi's system, and some in the press began turning against Tesla's project, claiming it was a hoax." There are clear signs however that the JP Morgan group, the project financier, was engaged in a double game of exhausting and killing it, since they arrested the project near its culminating point without any financially justifiable reason.

"Over the next five years, Tesla wrote more than 50 letters to Morgan, pleading for and demanding additional funding to complete the construction of Wardenclyffe. Tesla continued the project for another nine months into 1902. The tower was erected to its full 187 feet (57 m)... The project came to a halt in 1905, and in 1906, the financial problems and other events may have led to what Tesla biographer Marc J. Seifer suspects was a nervous breakdown on Tesla's part."

The late 1800 was a very tumultuous period in industry, engineering and physics. Suffice it to conclude, as previously reported, that the U.S. Supreme court, shortly after Tesla's death, officially and posthumously granted him priority in the invention of radio transmission in an attempt to restore impartial justice.

The inner workings of Layer 3 of the Foliate are patently all accountable for the psychological charater stamp that accompanied the course of Nikola Tesla's life. The partitions of *Discernment, Perspicacity, Lucidy and Clairvoyance* functioned for him at a very high level as an inventiveness engine. At the same time the naivete and defective practical sense proper to the left-chiral partitions of the same Layer were also responsible for his inability to turn his inventions into solid and durable financial gains for his own benefit in the long run. It was for sure naivete on his part at the beginning of his career to put stock in Thomas Edison's word that if he could fix his DC machines, he would reward him with $50,000, which Edison wisely dismissed when it came time to make good on the promise. Tesla's grand plans that were too often incommensurate with means and left his financial partners with lingering doubts about project completion also significantly mired his commercial enterprises. It is not clear either that he ever visualized the possibility that his own partner could be the force that for own reason and purposes undermined his late enterprises as well as his reputation.

Our last remark will go to his eponymous obsession with number 3 in his late life. Understanding the number as a true operator, most likely not just a conscious infatuation but an ontological adscription transpiring in his personal taste or personal turmoil. If Nikola Tesla was ever mentally unstable in the last phase of his life, one can see the contributing psychosocial circumstances that he had been up against in the course of a life which had been marked by not only prodigious inventiveness but also unrelenting jitters of wars. He died in his apartment in 1943 at the age of 86.

Elizabeth A. M. Bowes-Lyon

Hyperbolic Character

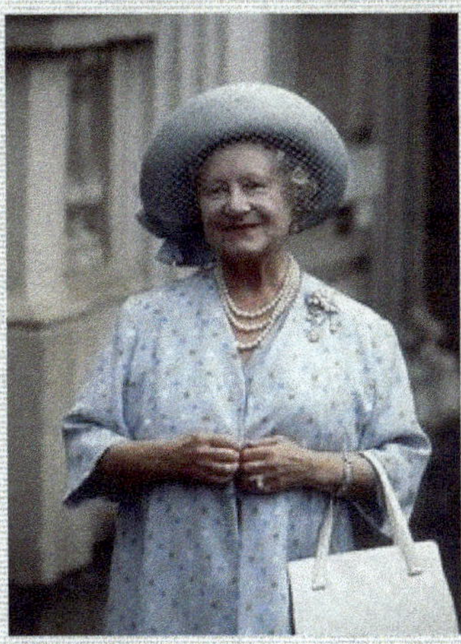

Britainexpress.com *(https://www.britainexpress.com/royals/queen-mother.htm)- Born on August 4, 1900, Elizabeth Angela Marguerite Bowes-Lyon began life as a commoner... Four years after her birth, her parents [Claude Bowes-Lyon and Cecilia Cavendish-Bentinck] became Lord and Lady Strathmore. They remained somewhat impoverished for much of their lives.*

Personal Life

... From an early age, Elizabeth and her younger brother David – referred to affectionately by their mother as the "two Benjamins" – exhibited a great sense of fun and mischief, a quality that she is still known to possess in abundance. On one occasion, after a frantic search around the grounds of St Paul's, the pair were discovered in the "flea house" ***sharing a cigarette****. The family spent much of its time at Glamis Castle, in Scotland ... Elizabeth and David would amuse themselves thereby pouring "boiling oil" (in fact, nothing more harmful than water) on their mother's guests from the castle turrets, and take the grounds people hostage, tying them up until* ***a "ransom" was paid for their release****.*

... [World War I broke out] when she was just 14 years old. Soon after her [14th] birthday, she returned to Glamis, which was now being used as a military hospital for wounded soldiers. With her mother and her elder sister Rosie, Elizabeth cared for soldiers, writing letters for them to their loved ones and running errands to buy their tobacco. She also enjoyed many a high-spirited game of cards with them. It was this experience which enabled the future Queen of England to relate to people of all backgrounds and social classes – a quality which continues to make her one of the most popular Royals.

... Despite the attentions of her Royal inamorato [Prince Albert Stuart], Elizabeth maintained a shrewd distance. She was reluctant to enter into Royal life and to take on all the accompanying trappings, and was cautious of such a match after her father's determination that none of his children should ever "have any post about the Court". From an early age, ***Lord Strathmore had warned Elizabeth that she should avoid Royal entanglements at all costs****. On such advice, and no doubt for her own personal reasons, Elizabeth twice rejected Bertie's proposals [Prince Albert's], much to the shock of his mother, Queen Mary. Finally, on January 13, 1923, as they walked in the woods at St Paul's Walden Bury, Elizabeth accepted his proposal of marriage.*

... In 1937, Bertie's brother King Edward VIII, abdicated in order to be with Wallis Simpson. Bertie, although reluctant to undertake the responsibility of public office, felt he had little choice but to succeed Edward as his natural heir. He was crowned George VI in Westminster Abbey on May 12, 1937, [she became Queen Elizabeth, Queen consort], and the family moved into Buckingham Palace.

Life as a Monarch

The Queen Mother never forgave her brother-in-law nor Mrs Simpson, and was ***instrumental in securing their "exile" from Britain****... The new pressures throughst upon the couple were only exacerbated by the outbreak of World War II. Despite strong advice that the Queen and the two princesses should leave London for Canada,* ***the Queen refused to go****.*

... After air raids, the King and Queen – she dressed in the finest satin and furs – would visit the scene of devastation and offer consolation to those who had lost their homes. It was only after Buckingham Palace was bombed, however, that the Queen felt she could really relate to the people of London. "I'm glad we've been bombed. It makes me feel I can look the East End in the face," she famously said.

... With the outbreak of war in 1939, there was some suggestion that the Queen and her daughters should evacuate to North America or Canada. To this the Queen made her famous reply: 'The children won't go without me. I won't leave the King. And the King will never leave.' ***Thus throughout the Second World War the Queen and her children shared the dangers and difficulties of the rest of the nation.*** *She was in Buckingham Palace when it was bombed in September*

1940. She and the King visited badly damaged areas throughout the country after the air-raids, and toured Britain visiting hospitals, factories and troops.

... After the King's death, The Queen Mother continued her public duties in the UK and overseas... Her Majesty was Patron or President of some 350 organisations. She was Commandant-in-Chief of the Army and Air Force Women's Services, and for Women in the Royal Navy, and held other Service appointments. For many years she was President of the British Red Cross Society, and she was Commandant-in-Chief of the Nursing Division of the St John Ambulance Brigade. She was also Colonel-in-Chief or Honorary Colonel of many UK and overseas regiments, and Commandant-in-Chief of the Royal Air Force Central Flying School.

Biography.com - *She was popular with the public, earning the nickname "Smiling Duchess" because of her consistent indomitable spirit. She was of great moral support to the British public during WWII.*

... After the war, Britain's economy was all but bankrupt. Many of its former colonies were striking out for independence. Great Britain went through several years of harsh austerity, rebuilding its economy and shedding its colonies to form the British Commonwealth.

The royal couple also faced personal challenges: In 1949, a blood clot was removed from the king's right leg. From then on, Queen Elizabeth and her daughters fulfilled many of the king's public engagements.

... Queen Elizabeth deeply loved her late husband, and for a time after his death, it looked as though she would become a recluse. ***But remembering her duty, she accepted the tragic loss with stoic courage and soon resumed her public duties.*** *She would go on to become a wise and respected leader. After her daughter's coronation as Queen Elizabeth II, she took on the name "Queen Mother" so as not to be confused with the new queen. Following her service as queen, the Queen Mother said, "My only wish is that I may be allowed to continue the work that [George VI and I] sought to do together."*

Over the next three decades, the Queen Mother became the royal family's matriarch, but was always careful not to overshadow her daughter's reign as queen.

...In her later years, the Queen Mother Elizabeth became known for her longevity... [she] continued to stay active with appearances at official celebrations. She

also successfully underwent surgeries for a cataract, hip replacements and a broken collarbone. In December 2001, at age 101, the Queen Mother had a fall and fractured her pelvis. She recuperated well enough to attend a memorial service for her late husband in February of the following year. On February 9, 2002, her youngest daughter, Princess Margaret, died at the age of 71. Despite falling and injuring her arm a few days after Margaret's death, the Queen Mother managed to attend her daughter's funeral.

On March 30, 2002, the Queen Mother died in her sleep at her home, the Royal Lodge at Windsor Great Park

QG Psychophysics Interpretation

The hyperbolic quality of Layer 4 of the Mental Foliate was ostensibly manifest early on in Elizabeth Bowes-Lyon's life course when as a child she used to hide out in the flea house to puff cigarette smoke with her younger brother, as well as mischievously playing ransom demands on visitors at Glamis castle. It is clear that Royalty always had a great appeal to her since she managed to be among royalty and participate in royal ceremononials during her upbringing. As a character under the Hyperbolic stamp, it is predictable that law and order, duty and honor would be at the forefront of her personal pursuits in the many endeavors of her life.

On the matter of Royalty, as it appeared, the psychosocial influences coming from both the father side and the mother side were at odds with one another, since Elizabeth's father was relentless in teaching her to stay away from Royalty contrary to her mother's pursuits in getting her to tie the knots within Royalty. This tension became clearly visible in her refusing Prince Albert's advances to marriage in two firm occasions but finally yielding on the request at the third occasion. Her own personal predisposition to be part of social elite and the ruling class, as a hyperbolic character, must be taken to account for her final decision.

Her sense of country and duty echoed in her taking shooting lessons in preparing for resisting German attacks during WWII. The biographers further report that she was petrified by the idea of falling captive to German troops and even had her two daughters, Elizabeth II and Margaret then age 14 and 10 respectively, take shooting lessons as well. Despite the strong appeal of court life, Elizabeth nurtured no ambition of becoming queen until King George VI abdicated. It is of note that she never forgave him his abdication considering it a grave deriliction of duty to the mother country and actively worked to exile him from Britain, whereas at the outbreak of WWII she adamantly refused to leave Britain herself.

Once she became the Queen of England, albeit against her wish, she wasted no time to assume full extent of the responsibilities assigned to the Queen Consort. She played a remarkable role of support to the British people during WWII as they endured relentless and devastating German bombardments. Even when the Buckingham Palace was bombarded by the German army, she stoicly refused to live Britain when the alternative was presented to her. Unlike most other monarchs perhaps, she became commander in chief of a long list of military and paramilitary organizations. Considering her female condition, these attributions amounted to a remarkable testimony to her high combative spirits. Her stoicism was in full display when she took upon herself duties of both queen and king, upon the death of her husband.

At the same time she received a number of honorific titles during her tenure as queen in social recognition of her exemplary courage and undaunted spirits. In later years, the Queen Mother displayed unspeakable valor in the face of misfortune as the health breaks multiplied one after another and fate imposed on her the death of her daughter Margaret.

It is quite fitting to conclude that the social function represented in Royalty resulted in a perfect match with the prime qualities of the Layer-4 driven character ontologically imparted to the Queen Mother. This match made her a very suitable ruler in the spirit of Royalty at a time when the British empire had to face, on the one hand, the historical process of decolonization, with the implied social consequences, and, on the other, the formidable Nazi threat of destruction from mainland Europe.

Michael Joseph Jackson

Metamorphogenic Character

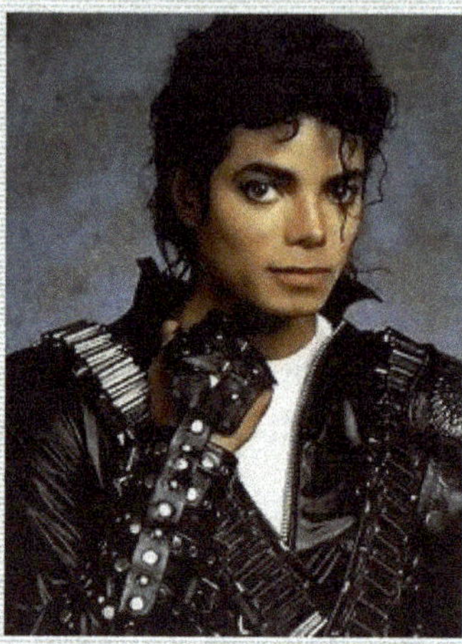

Biographyonline.net - *Michael J. Jackson (August 29, 1958 – June 25, 2009) was an American singer, dancer, entertainer, and recording artist. Michael Jackson epitomised the era of pop in the 70s, 80s and 90s, earning himself the title* the King of Pop. *He remained a global icon until his untimely death in 2009.*

Michael Jackson began his music career alongside his fellow brothers and family members in the Jackson Five. His career began in 1964, aged only 6. The group, led by Jackson's father, worked hard touring many clubs and bars performing their mix of Motown hits. They gained the attention of record labels and in 1968, signed with Motown records. It was the youngest, baby-faced Jackson, that caught the eye of reviewers. Rolling Stone magazine wrote that Michael was a ***'prodigy' with 'overwhelming musical gifts'. Michael stood out for his exceptional enthusiasm and soft, infectious musical voice.*** *The group produced four number one hit singles, including "I Want You Back", ABC and "The Lover You Save."*

Despite achieving his goal to be a music performer, Michael's childhood was far from happy. He was regularly ***beaten and threatened by his authoritarian father****. This legacy of abuse left Michael scarred throughout his adult life.*

By the late 1970s, Michael was increasingly looking to pursue a solo career. With the help of music producer, Quincy Jones, Michael produced the solo album 'Off The Wall'. The album was a great success, eventually selling over 20 million copies. The album gained much critical acclaim, and Michael secured the highest royalty rate in the music industry. (37% of album profit)

*His second solo album, Thriller, launched Michael Jackson into a position as **the most famous pop singer in the world**. With little commercial advertising and promotion, Thriller rose to number one on album sales and remained at the number one spot for a total of 37 weeks. It gained one of many Guinness World Records for Michael Jackson, attaining 110 million global sales and 29 million sales in the US. Thriller included number one hits such as Beat It, Billie Jean.*

*In March 1983, Michael Jackson performed live on Motown 25, 'Yesterday, today, forever', – a TV special. He performed **his distinctive and memorable dance move – the Moonwalk**. In the dance routine, he effortlessly moves backwards with seemingly keeping one leg perfectly straight. His performance made him a global icon of not just music, but dance. Michael Jackson **pioneered the importance of music video in promoting a pop artist**. This iconic performance has been compared to the famous Beatles' appearance on the Ed Sullivan Show in 1964. Jackson's next albums were Bad (1987) and Dangerous (1991). His final album was Invincible (2001).*

Professional Creativity

***Biography.com** - Jackson said in his memoir that he learned the [moonwalk] move from some friends, and he worked on it in the studio. Because Jackson was such a meticulous dancer — with a capacity for extreme control but also quickness — he gave the moonwalk a slick perfection.*

By doing the walk on the national television stage in 1983, Jackson was able to popularize the move in a way that groups like The Electric Booglaoos could not. As inventive and talented as dance groups at the time were, they lacked Jackson's crossover appeal to a mainstream audience.

***Jackson made the dance move a phenomenon**. - Jackson's fame cut across all demographics with the 1982 album* Thriller, *and "Billie Jean" was one of the top hits from it. In his first outing with the move, he adapted the moonwalk into his choreography at carefully selected moments within a sequence of moves: There's the moonwalk, followed by a spin and then his trademark toe-stand with its freeze-frame pose that makes the crowd go wild.*

"Michael Jackson was really good at doing the robot style and isolations. So he incorporated that into the moonwalk," said Jared Grimes, an entertainer and Broadway dancer.

Jackson made the move a national phenomenon – kids everywhere were imitating him. But the moment is a particular part of dance history because Jackson bridged the gap between West Coast street dance and the East Coast break dancers, who were part of the early days of hip-hop. The moonwalk fit perfectly into the physically demanding, almost gymnastic genre known for floor spins, fast footwork and named steps like the worm.

Even before the moonwalk, though, Jackson had changed the way that Americans interacted with dance. And the change came with the help of MTV, which launched in 1981.

Personal Life

Biographonline.net - *By the late 80s, there was an increasing number of stories speculating on Jackson's personal life, health and physical appearance. Michael Jackson underwent numerous operations of* ***plastic surgery to fix his nose and add a dimple in his chin.*** *During the 1980s,* ***his skin started to lighten****; this was due to a rare skin pigment disease, but it didn't stop a wave of speculative press stories that he was bleaching his skin colour. The press covered a range of speculative stories about Michael Jackson, including imaginary stories Michael had invented himself (such as sleeping in an oxygen tent to avoid the aging process)*

"I've been in the entertainment industry since I was six-years-old, and as Charles Dickens would say, "It's been the best of times, the worst of times." But I would not change my career... While some have made deliberate attempts to hurt me, I take it in stride because I have a loving family, a strong faith and wonderful friends and fans who have, and continue, to support me." — Michael Jackson

The press attention made Michael increasingly reclusive, spending much of his time in his 'Never Land' ranch. Speaking on the Oprah Winfrey show, Jackson addressed the issue of skin colour change:

"OK, number one. There, as I know of, there is no such thing as skin bleaching...I have a skin disorder that destroys the pigmentation of the skin, it's something that I cannot help, OK? But, when people make up stories that I don't want to be who I am, it hurts me...it's a problem for me, I can't control it."

History.com -*In the late 1980s and early 1990s, Jackson developed a reputation as an* ***eccentric recluse****. He moved to a 2,700-acre ranch called Neverland,* ***which***

***he outfitted with wild animals and a Ferris wheel.** He underwent a facelift and nose job and was rumored to have lightened his skin through chemical treatment, though he claimed his increasing pallor was due to a skin disease.*

Deep Alteration of Skin and Facial Appearance

ABC News – Why did Michael Jackson go so far to alter his appearance? *(https://abcnews.go.com/2020/MichaelJackson/story?id=7982236&page=1) - It was after the unprecedented success of 1983's "Thriller" that **Jackson's metamorphosis** became far more than an artistic statement. In the video for the mega-hit, Jackson transforms from man to werewolf to man to zombie and back to man. It was as if he was using the story to preview **the real-life drama of metamorphosis to come.***

... Lipkin said that Jackson had become addicted to plastic surgery. "Addicted, addicted to plastic surgery doesn't mean you've had 10 operations or 12," she said. "It means that no matter how much surgery you have, you're still not happy with the way you look. He kept focusing on his nose. It became, his nose became the obsession."

An obsession that led to further surgeries, leaving Jackson with barely a nose at all.

"What I think has happened recently is that something in his nose, a graft, an implant, something has now come out through the skin," Lipkin said. "And that's why he's probably got a hole in his skin. ... They're called nasal cripples. People whose nose has been done so many times that there is no nose really to breathe through. Michael Jackson has what we call an end-stage nose, a crucified nose, one that's beyond the point of no return."

...Margo Jefferson, a Pulitzer Prize-winning critic and the author of "On Michael Jackson," said, "I think he longed for some kind of peace of mind. ... He longed for what he could never possibly have back, which was some vision of a childhood. ... The little Michael Jackson, you know, who grew up struggling and suffering and ... thinking, 'I am worthless ... except when I can set this crowd going.' I think he wanted to flee that Michael Jackson completely."

It is noteworthy that Michael Jackson suffered from the vitiligo condition which causes a person to lose the skin pigment melanin. An aura of doubt always surrounded the authenticity of the condition given that Jackson seemed to pursue for himself the Caucasian canon of beauty. Note that if a person abnormally loses melanin, one avenue of treatment is to somehow seek to arrest or compensate for the loss and not necessarily accentuate the loss instead in order to acquire a white complexion. Vitiligo, for certain, gave Michael Jackson the opportunity to assert his metamorphogenic character by allowing him to transform his appearance from black to white. This urge is clearly visible in his permanent hair treatment that changed his curly hair typical of a black person, unaffected by the disease, to the straighter Caucasian type hair. While this preference in a female black artist understandably obeys mainstream cultural pressures, it was and is uncommon among male black artists who at the time wore instead puffy afro hair style. Inarguably, the tendency is to be put on account of Jackson's metamorphogenic impulses.

Love and Marital Life

Biographyonline.net. *-He married Lisa Marie Presley in 1994; it lasted two years though they remained friendly after the divorce. In 1996, he married Deborah Rowe in Sydney. Together they had two children. They divorced in 1999 and Rowe gave full custody of children to Jackson.*

Allegations of child abuse were first raised in the 1980s and re-appeared in the 1990s. This led to the trial of The People v. Jackson on 31 Jan 2005, in Sante Maria, California. After five months of high publicity, Jackson was acquitted. Though the experience left him physically weak and emotionally stressed. He departed America for the Persian Gulf Island of Bahrain.

"The minute I started breaking the all-time record in record sales—I broke Elvis's records, I broke Beatles records—the minute it became the all-time best-selling album in the history of the Guinness Book of World Records, overnight they called me a freak. They called me a homosexual. They called me a child molester. They said I bleached my skin. They made everything to turn the public against me." – Remarks at National Action Network headquarters (9 July 2002)

Towards the end of his life, he was increasingly plagued by money troubles and ill health. ***He increasingly became dependent on a variety of drugs, which was said to have contributed to his ill health and premature death****. Despite con-*

cerns over finance, he is said to have made career earnings of $500m and had assets in Sony/ATV Music Publishing catalogue worth over $300m alone.

"In a world filled with hate, we must still dare to hope. In a world filled with anger, we must still dare to comfort. In a world filled with despair, we must still dare to dream. And in a world filled with distrust, we must still dare to believe."

Charity Work of Michael Jackson

- *Michael Jackson supported many charities. This included a burns charity in Culver City, California. This followed an incident where Michael Jackson was burnt in filming a Pepsi commercial in 1984.*
- *He also supported HIV / AIDS charities at a time when it was still unfashionable.*
- *In 1984, he received an award from President Ronald Reagan for his support of charities [dedicated to helping] overcome alcohol and drug abuse.*
- *From his 1984 Victory Tour he donated all funds (around $8million to charity)*
- *In 1985, he also co-wrote the charity single "We are the World" with Lionel Richie. It sold over 30 million copies, and the proceeds were sent to the poor in the US and Africa.*
- *He continued his charity work to the end of his life supporting charity concerts such as Aid for victims of Kosovo war.*

QG Psychophysics Interpretaton

The events that unfolded throughout Michael Jackson's life very clearly profiled a phenomal metamorphogenic axis in their direction. We have opportunely highlighted the terms *metamorphosis, alteration* and others of the kind deliberately used by the biographers to qualify the temper slant behind those life events. They obviously stem from an ontological orientation of psychological character for the most part, notwithsanding the parental contribution to his particular character development.

Biographers judiciously note the negative influence of an authoritarian father in his early life and beyond who used to beat and threaten him. What is clear in Michael Jackson psychosocial development is that as a kid he had an adult life, given that at age 6 he was singing and touring with the family musical group. Arguably, he did not have the normal carefree life of a child and teenager common to most children. Likewise as an adult, Michael Jackson did not show the level of psychological maturity common to most in their adult life, displaying instead childish behavior and comradery with children whom he kept inviting to his Neverland ranch. Therefore Michael Jackson was always *other* in the two main phases of his life, true to the Layer 5 Norm of morphogenesis.

Unquestionably, life circumstances played an important role in the loss of his childhood during the developmental phase of his life. The beatings that he received from his father were also to have behavioral life-long consequences. It is clear however that a predisposed terrain is responsible for the most part for the behavior induced by those psychosocial drivers.

The castration response caused by an extremely mean and violent fatherhood relation was inarguably visible in his overly masculine vestimentation as an artist. His jackets displayed unusual rounds of ammunition, he also used to touch his groin during stage dancing, for certain a daring machist gesture by any account which apparently left most fans either indifferent or pleased by the daring. The chosen name of Neverland for his residence later on seemed to somehow echo "Disney's Wonderland"; the ferris wheel that he cared to have installed therein unequivocally speaks to this desire of still having the child's life that he was not fortunate to have. Further, "Neverland" seemed to mean the wonder land or wonder life that I "never" had as a child.

As an adult, there are other instances where Michael's behavior seemed to be reminiscent of the carelessness or immaturity typical of childhood. One such example is when he took his own child to the window of high rise and cluelessly appeared to put his life in danger. Despite the pressure borne onto him by the press at the time under the child abuse or molestation charge, it was quite difficult to make any sense of the gesture, this being the last he could possibly imagine under the circumstances.

Sexual and Marital Life

To the above psychosocial developments a form of love life typical of the metamorphogenic tempers followed suit in Michael Jackson's life, which is the trend to remain celibate or "virgin", as they are prone to refrain from the intimacy of sexual interaction. His first marriage to Lisa Marie Presley, which only lasted two years, was quite unexpected, with no known pre-couple history, and arguably seemed to have been a convenience marriage for the purpose of mending a growing negative reputation. His second marriage was not to be your typical long-nurtured relationship of intimacy either.

"Michael was still in the middle of his divorce from first wife Lisa Marie in 1996 when he befriended nurse Debbie Rowe, who worked at a dermatologist's office in Los Angeles where the singer was a frequent patient.

***Mamamia.com.au** ...It was a tumultuous time. And then, after just 19 months, Jackson's marriage to Presley crumbled. He and Rowe grew ever closer. It is unclear exactly when their friendship became more, but in her testimony at Jackson's wrongful death trial in 2013 Rowe discussed their eventual decision to have children together.*

"I was trying to help him," Rowe told the court, as reported by the Los Angeles Times. *"I said, 'What's the thing that makes you the saddest?' He said, 'I never had any children.'" She told him: "Let me have a baby with you. You can have the joy of being a parent." Rowe said that Jackson thought about her offer for a couple of weeks before agreeing.*

***While she repeatedly refused to discuss the couple's sex life**, Debbie Rowe was soon pregnant. The couple got married in November 1996, when she was six-months along. The private ceremony took place in Sydney while Jackson was on his His-tory tour.*

The least one can say, not your typical passionate love affairs.

Prodigious Artistic Vein

All critics acknowledged that Michael Jackson was a prodigious artist who innovatively blended music, dance, scenography and cinematography creating unique genres of artistic production. In that he proved to be a visionary artist with uncommon imagination and talent. It is not difficult to relate his artistic inventiveness in its very nature with the partitions germane to Layer 5 of the Foliate: Utopia, Visionary, Reformism, Chimera, Daydream, Fabulousness... The practice of his form of art saw him put tireless daily hours of composition and rehearsals into the same until he got to the point of, in his own eponymous words, “feeling the magic” out of a session, which meant reaching the pinnacle of his art. The visuals, the action and the transformational played a major part in his outwardly artistic expression as opposed to lyrism and the purely sentimental germane to artistic expression spurred by Layer 6 of the Mental Manifold. The spectacle of his finishing one of his shows in a suit that lifted him up in the air to dock into a helicopter that faded away with him in the night is unforgettable and nothing but sheer madness! He was one of these rare artists who could leave fans ravingly extatic and in awe of overwhelming outpouring of living art.

Critics unanimously acknowledge that his passage through pop culture as well as his influence on the same and the following generations of pop artists are vast, long-lasting and indelible.

Continuing Health Concerns and Problems

Michael Jackson was hard-working, extremely meticulous and disciplined in developing his artistic career. However, true to his ontological stamp, health concerns and health breaks overtook his life and career.

ABCNews - *But those close to Jackson describe a hectic lifestyle. "I think it was his lifestyle in general," said Stacy Brown, co-author of "Michael Jackson: Behind the Mask" and a family friend. "He had a lot of medical issues.* ***Most of it was brought on by himself****."*

... "When you continue to try to sustain those kind ofs standards, you can really bring unwanted stress upon yourself," McLin said. "He had been working non-stop since he was 9 years old."

But Brown described another factor that may have contributed to Jackson's failing health. "I think we will find that drugs played a major role, prescription and otherwise," Brown said. "From what I understand, there was even some heroin use. There was a lot of morphine. ***A lot of different drugs****."*

Michael Jackson concerns for issues related to his personal health, his unrelenting ingestion of drugs for one or another condition if not due to his constant modifying his body, as well as his involvement with health centers and health professionals were just overwhelming.

[Jackson collapsed in 1995 from apparent dehydration and low blood pressure]... Jackson also reportedly suffered from back pain – Jackson's health appeared to be worsening in recent years. In 2005, McLin said, Jackson was hospitalized due to "dehydration with the flu."

But Jackson's health issues that perhaps garnered the most public attention were his numerous plastic surgeries, including a widely publicized nose job... In preparation for this [last] tour, his body gave out," Brown said. "He put too much on himself, and the pressure I think took its toll. He abused himself so much for so long."

At age 50, insomnia appeared to have had the better part of him and drove him to death through abusive ingestion or inoculation of dangerous sleep-inducing opiates. *"The chief suspected cause of Jackson's death continues to be cardiac arrest."* The latter possibly caused by opiates.

Oscar Wills Wilde

Matrixial Character

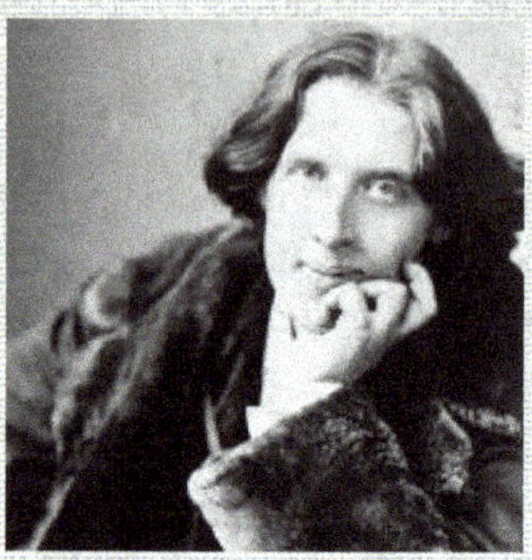

Thefamouspeople.com *– Oscar W. Wilde was a noted Irish playwright, novelist, poet and essayist, born in the middle of the 19th century into an intellectual family. While studying in Trinity, Dublin, he was influenced by the* ***aesthetic movement****, which advocated that art must be practiced only for the sake of art and soon became one of its ardent followers. Although his very first book, 'Poems' established him as an upcoming poet, he tasted real success only in the last decade of his relatively short life. But by then, despite being married with two sons, he had become entangled in a homosexual relationship and when that came into light, he was sentenced to two-year rigorous imprisonment. On coming out of prison, he went to France, where he spent the last years of his life, cut off from his family and shunned by most of his friends. By then, his books had also stopped selling and his plays were closed down. Thus he lived in poverty and ill-health till he died aged just 46.*

Childhood & Early Years

Oscar Fingal O'Flahertie Wills Wilde was born on 16 October 1854 in Dublin, Ireland. His father, Sir William Robert Wills Wilde, was a noted eye-ear surgeon. He also authored a number of books on medicine, archeology and folklore. In 1864, he was knighted for his services in the censuses of Ireland.

His mother, Jane Francesca Agnes (née Elgee) Wilde, was of Italian descent. She was a poetess, writing under the penname of 'Speranza', meaning hope. A supporter of Irish nationalist movement, many of her works were pro-Ireland and anti-British. She was also interested in Irish folktales and campaigned for women's education.

Oscar was born second of his parents' three children. His elder brother, William Charles Kingsbury Wilde, grew up to be a noted journalist and poet while his sister, Isola Francesca Emily Wilde, died of meningitis at the age of nine.

Oscar also had three half-siblings, Henry Wilson, Emily and Mary Wilde, born out of wedlock to Sir Wilde before his marriage to Jane... Up to the age of nine, Oscar Wilde was educated at home under a German governess and a French nurse. From them, he learned German and French respectively.

***Cliffnotes.com** - (https://www.cliffsnotes.com/literature/i/the-importance-of-being-earnest/oscar-wilde-biography) Wilde had two siblings: an older brother named Willie, born in 1852, and a sister, Isola, born in 1856, but who died at the age of 10. These offspring would not experience a standard, conventional childhood.*

***Poetryfoundation.org** – (https://www.poetryfoundation.org/poets/oscar-wilde) H. Montgomery Hyde reported in Oscar Wilde: A Biography, his mother was a poet and Irish revolutionary... and his father a successful eye and ear surgeon in Dublin and "author of a work which remained the standard textbook on aural surgery for many years." Though his background was literary and professional, it was anything but stable. His mother **doted on him as a child** and, according to Hyde, **"insisted on dressing him in girl's clothes."** Dr. William Wilde was a **notorious philanderer**, and, in an ironic foreshadowing of his son's famous trials, suffered public condemnation when a libel case disclosed his sexual indiscretions with a young woman named Mary Travers.*

***The famouspeople.com –** In 1864, he was enrolled at Portora Royal School, then a boarding school in Enniskillen, County Fermanagh. Here, he became especially **interested in Greek and Roman studies, receiving prizes as the best Classics student** in his last two years there.*

*Among his teachers at Trinity was John P. Mahaffy, who inspired Wilde to study Greek literature and also taught him to love "Greek things". In the year-end examination in 1872, Wilde secured **first position in Classics**.*

*Again in the year-end examination in 1873, Wilde was awarded the Foundation Scholarship. He also became a member of the University Philosophical Society, taking regular part in its proceedings. Sometime now, he was drawn towards the **theory of aestheticism** and presented a paper called 'Aesthetic Morality'.*

In 1874, he graduated from Trinity, winning the Berkeley Gold Medal, the highest medal for Greek. Thereafter, he entered Magdalen College, Oxford with a Demyship. Among his teachers here were John Ruskin and Walter Pater, who ***impressed upon him the importance of art in life****.*

Wilde was especially impressed by Pater, who advised his students "to burn always with hard, gemlike flame." He soon became famous for his role in the aesthetic movement. ***Wearing his hair long and decorating his rooms with peacock feathers, lilies, sunflowers, blue china, he openly scorned manly sports.***

This was also the time he first established himself as a poet and in 1878, won the coveted Newdigate Prize with his long poem, 'Ravenna'. In the same year, he graduated from Oxford with a double first in his B.A. of Classical Moderations and Literae Humaniores.

In London

On his graduation in 1878, Oscar Wilde returned to Dublin for a brief period. By now, his father had died virtually bankrupt. The family now sold the house and with his share of legacy Wilde moved to London, where he put up with portraitist Frank Miles, popular in London's high circle.

... Also in 1881, he secured his first job as an ***art reviewer****. However, he left it towards the end of the year, to embark on a lecture tour in the United States and Canada on the invitation of Richard D'Oyly Carte, an English talent agent and impresario.*

In the USA

Oscar Wilde reached New York City on 2 January 1882. ...During this period [one year and four months], he delivered around 140 lectures, mostly on ***aestheticism****.*

Wherever he went, he mixed with every class of people. He drank whiskey with miners in Leadville and Colorado and at the same time, visited the most fashionable salons in cities like New York, Chicago, Boston, Philadelphia, and Washington, dining with celebrities like Henry Wadsworth Longfellow and Walt Whitman.

Although the press was a little hostile to him, ***the public was intrigued by his dress code and odd character.*** *He also admired many things about America, especially its democracy and universal education. He therefore, returned to Great Britain rich, both in money matters and experience.*

Return to Great Britain

... Very soon Wilde was able to establish himself as a leading proponent of aesthetic movement and became famous for it. Apart from his literally pursuits, he began to contribute regularly as a reviewer in 'Pall Mall Gazette.'

From 1887, Wilde found employment as the editor of ***'Lady's World,' a magazine that dealt in women's fashion*** *and had lost its popularity in recent years. Soon, he was able to revive the magazine by incorporating women's viewpoints not only on art, literature and music, but also on modern life.*

In 1888, while working as editor of 'Lady's World,' Wilde published his first major work titled, 'The Happy Prince and Other Tales', a collection of children's stories. Next in 1889, he published another of his memorable works, 'The Decay of Lying'.

In July 1889, he left his job to concentrate on his literary ambition. His only novel, 'The Picture of Dorian Gray' appeared in the July 1890 edition of 'Lippincott's Monthly Magazine.'

Although the editor of the magazine had deleted roughly 500 words it was criticized by the reviewers for decadence and homosexual allusions. However, Wilde defended his work and in 1891, he had it published in book form.

Major Works

Oscar Wilde is best remembered for his last play, 'The Importance of Being Earnest', a farcical comedy in which the protagonists maintain double identities. Commended for its wits, the play has been revived many times since its premiere on 14 February 1895 at the St James's Theatre, London and thrice made into films.

Personal Life & Legacy

On 29 May 1884, Oscar Wilde married Constance Lloyd, daughter of Horace Lloyd, a wealthy Queen's Counsel. The couple had two sons, Cyril and Vyvyan.

In 1886, while Constance was pregnant with their second child, Wilde was seduced by seventeen-year-old Robert Baldwin Ross, the grandson of the Canadian reform leader Robert Baldwin. Subsequently, they developed a relationship and Ross became Wilde's first male lover.

In 1891, Wilde met Alfred Douglas, son of John Douglas, 9th Marques of Queensberry, and developed an affair with him. Unable to stop the liaison, the Marques left his calling card at Wilde's club, inscribed: "For Oscar Wilde, posing sodomite" on 18 February 1895.

Against his friends' advices, Wilde filed a suit of libel against the Marques. To protect himself, the Marques appointed detectives to find evidence about Wilde's homosexuality and planned to portray him as the older man who habitually seduced the young and innocent. Many were also coerced to give evidence against Wilde.

Imprisoned for Sodomy

As evidence against Oscar Wilde mounted, a case of sodomy and gross indecency was filed against him. The prosecution, which opened on 26 April 1895, found him guilty on 25 May 1895. He was awarded with hard labor. On the same day he was sent to Newgate Prison.

He was subsequently shifted to Pentonvile and from there to Wandsworth Prison in London. Life in the latter place was too hard for Wilde's delicate health. In early November 1895, he collapsed from hunger and illness, resulting in the rapture of his right ear drum.

On 23 November 1885, he was transferred to HM Prison Reading at the initiative of Liberal MP and reformer Richard B. Haldane and provided with reading as well as writing materials. Meanwhile his wife changed her and her sons' last name to Holland, thus dissociating themselves from Wilde's scandals.

It was here at Reading Gaol that he wrote a 50,000-word letter to Douglas. Written between January and March 1887, it was never delivered, but was partially published in 1905 as 'De Profundis' and fully published in 1962 as 'The Letters of Oscar Wilde'.

Exile & Death

Wilde was released from prison on 18 May 1887 and immediately left for France, never to return to England. Very soon, he wrote 'The Ballad of Reading Gaol', his last major work. Initially, the authorship was credited to C33, but when it became successful; his name was added to it.

Wilde lived for three more years, poor and desolate. His wife sent him three pence a week from her annual allowance. She refused to see him or allow him to see the children. Among his few friends, who remained loyal till the end, were author Reginald Turner and Robert Ross.

Sometime around 25 November 1900, Wilde developed meningitis, stemming from the ear wound he had developed in prison and died from it on 30 November 1900. Initially he was buried in the Cimetière de Bagneux outside Paris.

*Brainpickings.com – (https://www.brainpickings.org/2013/07/15/oscar-wilde-love-letters-bosie/) ... Oscar Wilde, who was imprisoned multiple times for his "crime" of homosexuality, run into bankruptcy and exile, and fell to an untimely death. But Wilde's most "sinful" quality — **his enormous capacity for passionate, profound love** — was also one of the most poetic gifts of his life.*

QG Psychophysics Interpretation

Oscar Wills Wilde was inarguably one of the greatest literary talents in the modern era. His capabilities were in display, as is oftentimes the case for remarkable figures, in his early life as a youngster. The influence of both of his parents on Oscar's upbringing and character formation is however as impacting as long-lasting.

Their decision to expose him and the other siblings to intellectuals of the time by allowing them to comingle with these figures in the literary circle that they hosted in their residence proved to have long lasting influence on the young

Oscar Wilde. Further both a French and German governesses were going to initiate him even deeper in the humanities represented in these cultures through their personal attention and spoken languages.

These factors played over the fertile ground of a native character molded by Layer 6 of the Mentation Foliate. Effectively Oscar Wilde has shown throughout his life an empathetic slant of character that made him very personable to most, despite the aristocratic standing of his family, oftentimes boasted by his mother as the biographers report, and his education mostly at the very prestigious schools in England, the many scholarships he earned and high rankings achieved. The effervescence of superiority was not part of his character and did not stick. The biographer notes that he could sit for a beer with miners in Colorado just as he could have dinner with a high class celebrity in town.

It was in the parental interaction that the psychosocial factors were going to be quite detrimental to his upbringing. His mother did dote on him as a child and, for whatever reason of her own, insisted on dressing him in girl's clothes! There is no question that an imposition of the kind was slated to influence the young boy's perception of his own gender identity and set him up for gender identity disparity. Also her constant doting on him would firmly reinforce the empathetic tendencies germane to the left-chiral partitions at Layer 6 of his Mental Body Foliate as part of an Anima Sector being already exacerbated with her imposition of feminine dressing on him. In all of that, she gave him no chance to relate to her as a boy.

Furthermore, the young Oscar must have been aware of his father's pre-marital affairs ending in 'illegitimate' children or side siblings for him. Likewise he must have been aware of his father's notoriously active philandering while married to his mother resulting in public libel. These facts could only play to settle him for greater empathetic rapprochement with his mother and greater internal emotional conflict with the father figure. Hence, a level of abatement of the Animus Sector of the Foliate in favor of the Anima Sector was for sure a contributing behavioral factor in this case.

It was thus a complex case of balance between the Anima Sector and the Animus Sector of the Foliate, which resulted in an unnatural equity balance between the two. That is why Oscar Wilde ended up finding himself with bi-sexual tendencies and behavior. He not only felt a feminine gender for himself, by reason of which he was attracted to men, but his getting married with ensuing procreation of children clearly reveals his male urges and male sexual orientation. Note well that his homesexual orientation had him in the role of a female, as clearly manifest in his vestimentation and appearance in which he displayed female fur coats, etc. In that regard, the biographer notes that the *"[American] public was intrigued by his dress code"*. His female identification and dressing choices were also hinted when he took charge of the magazine *"Lady's World", a magazine that dealt in women's fashion,* and devoted himself to its redress. More to the point, in his early adult life, he also *"openly scorned manly sports"*, per biographers' reports.

In the midst of the balance problem between the two Chiral Sectors of his Mental Foliate, mainly of psychosocial origin, it is important not to lose sight of the character or temper mark spurred by accrual of Layer 6 of his Foliate. His commitment to the arts and to culture along with his capacity for passionate love speaks to Layer 6 qualities of the Mental Foliate. As the biographer points out: *"Wilde's most "sinful" quality — **his enormous capacity for passionate, profound love** — was also one of the most poetic gifts of his life."* He was a maximum proponent of the arts and pursued the arts for their own sake. His early interests in Greek and Roman classics were a forerunner of his personal commitement to the intrinsic value of aesthetic expression per se, of which he later became a firm advocate. Useless to remind the reader that these qualities emanate from the right-chiral partitions of Layer 6 of the Mental Manifold, namely *Euphoria, Passion, Admiration* and *Sympathy*. At some point in his early adult life, he was *"wearing his hair long and decorating his rooms with peacock feathers, lilies, sunflowers, blue china..."*. A writer at Poetry Foundation finally notes:

"Wilde's love of beauty and his conception of its fleeting quality find expression in this story of a nightingale who sacrifices its life to produce the perfect rose. In the story's final satirical twist the beautiful rose is rejected because it does not match the color of a young girl's dress. In Oscar Wilde, Robert K. Miller declared that this ironic turn reveals Wilde's "ambivalence toward love" that is "related to his ambivalence about women."

Diego Armando Maradona

Paradoxical (Antagonistic) Character

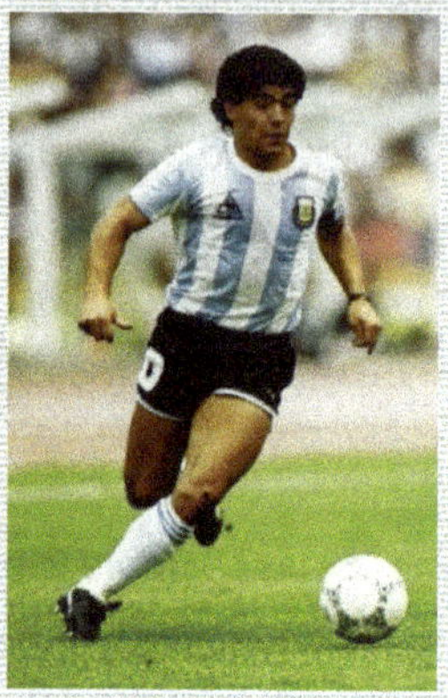

***Washington Post** – (https://www.washingtonpost.com/world/the americas/diego-maradona-death-world-reaction/2020/11/25/a1816248-2f43-11eb-bae0-50bb17126614_story.html) He was the unrepentant antihero of England's most painful soccer story, **knocking in a goal with his fist** in Argentina's 1986 victory over England in the World Cup quarterfinals.- He was the most bitter of rivals in soccer-mad Brazil, dazzling on the field and maddening off it. "Go back to the museum," he once told Pelé. - He was the outspoken supporter of the Latin American left, befriending Venezuela's socialist president Hugo Chávez and tattooing an image of Argentine-born revolutionary leader Ernesto "Che" Guevara on his left biceps and one of Fidel Castro on his left calf.*

***Biography.com** (https://www.biography.com/athlete/diego-maradona) - **Who Was Diego Maradona? -** Diego Maradona was an Argentinean soccer legend who was widely regarded as one of the best players of all time. Maradona led club teams to championships in Argentina, Italy and Spain, and famously starred for the Argentinean team that won the 1986 World Cup. However, the soccer legend's career was marred by a pair of high-profile suspensions for drug use, and he has often battled health problems in retirement.*

Early Life

Diego Armando Maradona was born on October 30, 1960, in Villa Fiorito, a province of Buenos Aires, Argentina. The fifth of eight children raised by Diego Sr. and Doña Tota, Maradona grew up in a poor but close-knit household. He received his first soccer ball as a gift at age 3 and quickly became devoted to the game. - At 10, Maradona joined Los Cebollitas, a youth team of Argentinos Juniors, one of the biggest clubs in Argentina. Showing his prodigious ability at an early age, Maradona led Los Cebollitas to an incredible 136-game unbeaten streak. He made his professional debut for the senior team shortly before his 16th birthday.

Professional Career

*A short but fearless midfielder renowned for his ability to create scoring chances for himself and others, Maradona led club teams to championships in Argentina, Italy and Spain. - The pinnacle of his career came as a member of the Argentinean national team that won the 1986 World Cup. His performance there included two memorable goals in a quarter-final victory over England. The first was scored **illegally** with his left hand, which Maradona later claimed was the work of "the hand of God" and the second required no supernatural help other than an otherworldly ability to dribble past an onslaught of defenders to find the back of the net. Altogether, Maradona played in four World Cups, and scored an impressive 34 goals in 91 international appearances for Argentina. - Despite his unquestioned brilliance on the pitch, the emotional Maradona became equally well known as a **highly controversial figure**. He became addicted to cocaine while playing in Spain in the 1980s and received a 15-month suspension after testing positive for the substance in 1991. Maradona endured another high-profile suspension three years later, this time for testing positive for ephedrine during the World Cup.*

***Wikipedia-** Maradona was notorious for his poor diet and extreme lifestyle off the pitch, including his use of **illicit drugs and alcohol abuse**, which along with personal issues, his metabolism, medication that he was prescribed, and periods of inactivity due to injuries and **suspensions**, led to his significant weight–gain and physical decline as his career progressed; his lack of discipline and difficulties in his **turbulent personal life** are thought by some in the sport to have negatively impacted his performances and longevity in the later years of his playing career...*

***Diego Maradona: Life Scandals of the Soccer Star** ... Daniel Arcucci, sports editor of La Nacion told the Associated Press, "Everything about Maradona is exaggerated — the good and the bad. As a player he was number one. He can be charming, but in his private life he broke all the rules." - During his career, he certainly found himself in trouble with the authorities often enough. - From the time he arrived in Europe to play with Barcelona, his cockiness and refusal to back down from a fight saw him clash with the club's management. - It was at this time that Diego began to take cocaine on a regular basis, although the prob-*

lem would become more apparent later. - His tenure at the club ended in disgrace after Barcelona lost the 1983-4 Copa del Rey Final. - After the full-time whistle he was the main protagonist in an all-in brawl with almost the entire Bilboa team. In footage of the incident, he can be seen launching fly kicks into numerous opposition players like a miniature martial arts expert in a 70's kung-fu movie, afro and all. - Maradona received a lengthy ban for ***his violent performance****, and decided he would rather quit Spanish football than serve out his suspension, thus facilitating his surprise move to Napoli.*

Wikipedia *- Maradona was directly involved in a violent and chaotic fight at the 1984 Copa del Rey Final at the Santiago Bernabéu stadium in Madrid against Athletic Bilbao.[40] After receiving another hard tackle by Goikoetxea, as well as being taunted with racist insults related to his father's Native American ancestry throughout the match by Bilbao fans, and being provoked by Bilbao's Miguel Sola at full time after Barcelona lost 1–0, Maradona snapped.[40] He aggressively got up, stood inches from Sola's face and the two exchanged words. This started a chain reaction of emotional reactions from both teams. Using expletives, Sola mimicked a gesture from the crowd towards Maradona by using a xenophobic term.[41]Maradona then headbuttedSola, elbowed another Bilbao player in the face and kneed another player in the head, knocking him out cold.[40] The Bilbao squad surrounded Maradona to exact some retribution, with Goikoetxea connecting with a high kick to his chest, before the rest of the Barcelona squad joined in to help Maradona. From this point, Barcelona and Bilbao players brawled on the field with Maradona in the centre of the action, kicking and punching anyone in a Bilbao shirt.[40]*

The mass brawl was played out in front of the Spanish King Juan Carlos and an audience of 100,000 fans inside the stadium, and more than half of Spain watching on television.[42] After fans began throwing solid objects on the field at the players, coaches and even photographers, sixty people were injured, with the incident effectively sealing Maradona's transfer out of the club in what was his last game in a Barcelona shirt.[41] One Barcelona executive stated, "When I saw those scenes of Maradona fighting and the chaos that followed I realized we couldn't go any further with him."[42]Maradona got into ***frequent disputes*** *with FC Barcelona executives, particularly club president Jose Luís Núñez, culminating with a demand to be transferred out of Camp Nou in 1984. During his two injury-hit seasons at Barcelona, Maradona scored 38 goals in 58 games.[43]Maradona transferred to Napoli in Italy's Serie A for another world record fee, £6.9 million ($10.48 million).*

Maradona's Drug and Legal Problems

Forbes Magazine* - Oct 18, 2013,06:02pm EDT** - *Maradona's financial problems haven't gone away either. Maradona made millions of dollars while playing around the world, including for Napoli. He amassed a tax bill in the tens of millions of dollars,* ***refusing to pay *initially because he claimed that those taxes were the team's responsibility.*

Football legend Diego Maradona has been notified by Italian tax officials that they are taking steps to freeze his assets in Italy in order to collect on his massive tax debts. Maradona, dubbed "El Pibe de Oro" *or "the Golden Boy" by his legions of fans, is said to owe nearly $53 million. The debts stem from Maradona's years playing for Napoli from 1984-91;*

The Irish Times - Tue, Jan 16, 2001, 00:00 - *In a subsequent hectic news conference Maradona explained that, as far as he was concerned, his contract with Napoli required the club to pay his income tax. - The whole business was proof of the extent to which he had been betrayed by the Napoli president (then and now) Corrado Ferlaino. - Inevitably, too, Maradona's outburst against Ferlaino ended Napoli's plans to involve him in the club's future plans. Joint president Giorgio Corbelli excluded any future deal with Maradona declaring that the ex-player's "instability" could damage the club.*

Football History (https://www.footballhistory.org/player/diego-maradona.html) *...Following the triumphant end to the World Cup, Maradona returned to club football. In his first season back, he led Napoli to a Serie A title. This was the first time that a team from the south of the country won a league title, and it happened at a time when North-South tensions were at a peak. After finishing the following two seasons as runners-up, Napoli won their second scudetto in 1990.*

Despite his success on the field, Maradona's personal life was getting worse and worse. Despite the success on the field, his personal life was getting worse and worse. In the football crazy Naples, the ball genius had become almost a semi-god but on the same time a victim for his own success with fans wanting him to as their property.

Diego started to look for refuges. He seemed to have ***vague connections with the Giuliano clan****, a powerful part of the Camorra crime syndicate and was seen* *on a party arranged by the boss Carmine Giuliano. And unbeknownst to many, he was harboring a cocaine addiction since the mid-80s. Eventually, this impeded his ability to play football, though that didn't stop him from taking Argentina to another World Cup final in 1990. West Germany was too tough of an obstacle to overcome this time. The tournament was played in Italy, Maradona's second home country at this time. When Argentina played against the home nation in Napoli, the Neapolitans were saluting their idol and many of them had a hard time to decide which team they favored.* ***Wanders-Argentina*** *- Towards the end of his time at Napoli, Maradona's performance suffered due to his drug problems, and weight gain. Eventually, in 1991, he was busted in a drug test, and received a 15-month ban, ending his days in the Italian league. - He would never return to complete his contract with Napoli, but he did continue playing, albeit with a little less magic than before.*

Rumors of close ties to the ***Neapolitan mafia****, The Camorra, followed him, and he also found time to father an illegitimate son, Diego Jr., whom he later admitted — with much insistence — to being his own. Paternity payouts and tax evasion in Italy from those days hung over him for decades after.*

Wanders-Argentina - Maradona's Life in Italy *- At the Italian club, Maradona found that though he was a god on the pitch, in real life he remained a man...*

He was still good enough to make the Argentinian team for the 1994 World Cup, despite being found guilty of firing an air rifle at journalists outside his home in the meantime. That tournament would prove to be his last at an international level, however, as he was again caught for doping, testing positive to ephedrine and promptly kicked out of the World Cup.

After scoring a superb goal in a game against Greece in the first round, he famously celebrated by running towards a TV camera screaming with elation, eyes bulging out of his head. The image has become an iconic one in Argentina, and serves as a reminder to many there about how many times Maradona, despite being the people's hero, has also frequently disappointed a great many of his fans.

Argentina failed to recover from the loss of their star, and were soon bundled out of the tournament.

Marital Problems

BBC** (https://www.bbc.com/news/world-latin-america-47500372) - **Argentina football legend Diego Maradona is to acknowledge paternity of three Cuban children, his lawyer says.

This means the 58-year-old World Cup winner, who once denied any children other than with his former wife, is now the official father of eight children. - Maradona will travel to Havana to take paternity tests and publicly recognise the children later this year, lawyer Matias Morla said. - The children, reportedly from two mothers, will be able to take his name. - Maradona spent several years in the country between 2000 and 2005 undergoing treatment for a cocaine habit. - He befriended then-President Fidel Castro during his stint in the country and got a tattoo of the leader's face on his leg.

The Star
https://www.thestar.com/sports/soccer/2013/02/27/diego_maradonas_love_life_getting_complicated.html) - BUENOS AIRES, ARGENTINA—Diego Maradona appears to have a new girlfriend. His ex-partner just gave birth to a baby he fathered. And the same ex-partner is also involved in a legal dispute with the Argentine football great's former wife. - In the last few days, local media have been awash with news and photos about a new woman in Maradona's life, who has been identified as 22-year-old Rocio Geraldine Oliva. - Maradona, 52, has declined to confirm the relationship — but he also hasn't denied it. A photo of Maradona holding a poster with the words "Rocio Te Amo" (Rocio I love you), and another photo of the two toasting each over glasses of champagne have been widely circulated in the Argentine media.

"I'm fine, relaxed and in love with Diego," Oliva said Wednesday in a television interview. "What others say means nothing to me." - Reports about the new romance surfaced two weeks ago when Maradona's long-time partner Veronica Ojeda gave birth in Buenos Aires to a baby boy who was named Diego Fernando. He has already been nicknamed "Dieguito," and Maradona — who is working in Dubai — has yet to return to Argentina to see him.

The child is the fifth known to be fathered by the former Argentine football great. He has two daughters from his marriage with Claudia Villafane — Dalma and Giannina. Maradona has two other children he has never recognized as his, although courts in paternity cases have ruled he's the father.

Ojeda seemed surprised that Maradona already had a new girlfriend — but not shocked.- "We have been separated for several months," she said. "The only thing that ties us is the baby. I want a father to be around, and therefore we have a good relationship."

Maradona's Political Views

Maradona was fascinated by Latin America's populist political leaders. One of his first tattoos, on his arm, features Che Guevara (Lynch), the Argentine revolutionary who helped to usher in the Cuban revolution. - He later added a tattoo on his shin of Fidel Castro, whom he also publicly supported. He first met Castro on a trip to Cuba in 1987. They maintained a friendship and Maradona visited in 200o to go to rehab for six months of 'detoxification' at the invitation of Castro. - He ended up living in Cuba for the better part of five years. - Maradona was also chummy with controversial Venezuelan leader, Hugo Chavez and his successor, NicolásMaduro. - He declared on the Chavez's TV program, 'Aló Venezuela,' "I hate everything that comes from the United States. I hate it with all my strength." - At the 2005 Summit of the Americas in Argentina he stood alongside Hugo Chavez to protest the presence of then U.S. President George W. Bush. - When the United States elected Barack Obama in 2012 Maradona softened his anti-American stance somewhat, but still hobnobbed with populist leaders in the Americas and even Russia's Vladamir Putin at the Kremlin.

Maradona's Rivalry with Pelé

He continued a running battle over the years with the other 'greatest player of all time,' Brazil's Pelé. - The two soccer greats trade insults regularly through the media, although the highlight (or lowlight) was probably when Pele fired a few barbs Diego's way about his low moral standards, and Maradona responded by telling Marca, "What do you want me to say? He lost his virginity to a man!" - The rivalry was put aside when Pelé appeared on Maradona's popular Argentinian TV program, La Noche de 10 (The Night of Ten, after his playing number). - The show ran for 13 episodes in television in Argentina in 2005 and scored sensational ratings. Guests included Fidel Castro, Mike Tyson and Pele. The two soccer icons were remarkably civil, even chummy, on this occasion. - The two embraced, Maradona interviewed Pelé and they kicked the ball around a bit.

Notable Language Snippets

"Go back to the museum," he once told Pelé.

"I hate everything that comes from the United States. I hate it with all my strength."

Maradona [as a coach] had overseen a typically unpredictable qualifying campaign, which saw the team suffer heavy defeats to the mighty Brazil, and the minnows, Bolivia. - Eventually in the preliminary rounds the crucial games were won, though Diego once again courted controversy by telling critical journalists that they could, "Suck it, and keep sucking it!"

Before naming his surprising final squad to take to the tournament in South Africa, Diego managed to run over a cameraman's leg in his car. Rather than stopping to apologize, he drove off shouting, "What an asshole you are! How could you put your leg under the wheel, man?"

Life after Soccer & Untimely Death

The most famous man in Argentina was never able to settle down to a quiet life of retirement since leaving football.- Drug and weight problems continued to dog him. After ballooning up to 267 pounds (121 kilograms), he underwent gastric bypass surgery in 2005. He went to drug rehab on numerous occasions, most notably in 2000 and 2004, on both occasions discovering severe damage to his heart. - Despite quitting drugs afterward, Maradona's was again admitted to hospital in 2007, after a binge of drinking, smoking cigars and eating to excessive levels he saw his body collapse once more.

Upon Maradona's death, the 80 year-old Pelé wrote on Twitter,

"I have lost a great friend and the world lost a legend. There is still much to be said, but for now, may God give strength to his family members. One day, I hope, we will play football together in heaven."

*In spite of **all his life controversy that followed him until the end,** Maradona remained immensely popular in Argentina until his death.- Argentinian psychologist and author Gustavo Bernstein wrote in his book, Maradona: Iconografia de* *la Patria (Icon of the Nation), "No one embodies our essence more. Argentina is Maradona. Maradona is Argentina."*

QG Psychophysic Interpretation

Everything about Diego Armando Maradona speaks to Antagonism, Conflicts, Disruption, Destruction and Self-Destruction, Layer 7 of his Mental Foliate, for a perfectly paradoxically-woven temper. From his choice of career, to his marital life, to his fame, to his serious health outbreaks, he was ontogenetically cut under the Paradoxical Norm which had been reinforced by important psychosocial factors.

If anyone should think that there is nothing instigative about kicking a ball into a net through one-on-one combat, metaphorically akin to a cannonball shooting round shells in a war theater, they should think twice about what the professional game of soccer is, and why its mini version in hockey turns out to be so violent. Diego Armando Maradona was so ontogenetically driven to it that he became a world sports star of the same, unquestionably one of the two universally acknowledged greatest at it.

Born in a poor slum around Buenos Aires, from a father of Amerindian descent, he was slated to bear the social fate inflicted by poverty and indigenous ethnicity in the context of a society utterly sensitive to wealth and ethnic origin, as it has always been in modern human affairs. It is by no accident that he had embraced the sporting and social cause of the city of Napoli, and felt such a deep identification with Napolitans. Says **Football History**: *"Following the triumphant end to the World Cup, Maradona returned to club football. In his first season back, he led Napoli to a Serie A title. This was the first time that a team from the south of the country won a league title, and it happened at a time when North-South tensions were at a peak. After finishing the following two seasons as runners-up, Napoli won their second scudetto in 1990."* Napolitans had him as a demigod and never withdrew their support from him till the end of his life despite the many scandals.

Maradona enjoyed world notoriety, beyond Argentina and Italy. In fame however, he was not only adored, only receiving the benefit of empathy from admirers, but hated alike, while even dividing the hearts of those who were bedazzled by his soccer talent. Unseeming personal and social behavior and a life mired in scandals with a few connections some found quite troublesome left fans all too often in reckoning.

Unconstrained, undisciplined marital and sexual life left him the fatherhood of no less than eight children from different mothers, most of whom he was conflicted about acknowledging his fathering them. For an athlete, his unending overweight problems, which degenerated into severe health conditions, were one of the greatest paradoxes of his life which fans found so difficult and painful to fathom. *"Gimnasia's first game of the season took place on Maradona's 60th birthday, October 30, 2020. - Fans were shocked when they saw Maradona come onto the field before the game. Maradona had to be helped onto the field, with two assistants on either side, aiding him to walk at a slow place. After he was presented with a cake and fireworks, he was interviewed on camera, but his voice was so weak that they had to remove his face mask so that he could be heard...*

Just a little over two weeks later, Diego Maradona had a sudden heart attack at his home in the leafy Buenos Aires suburb of Tigre. Six ambulances were rushed to the scene and healthcare workers tried diligently to resuscitate him, but it was futile."

Walter Elias Disney

Perfect Character

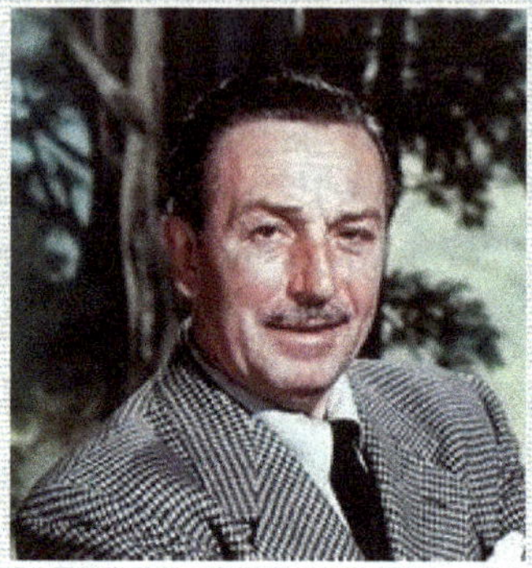

IMDb.com *- Walter E. Disney was born on December 5, 1901 in Chicago, Illinois, the son of Flora Disney (née Call) and Elias Disney, a Canadian-born farmer and businessperson. He had Irish, German, and English ancestry. Walt moved with his parents to Kansas City at age seven, where he spent the majority of his childhood. At age 16, during World War I,* ***he faked his age to join the American Red Cross****. He soon returned home, where he won a scholarship to the Kansas City Art Institute.*

Early Life and Formation

Wikipedia *- Born in Chicago in 1901, Disney developed an* ***early interest in drawing. He took art classes as a boy and got a job as a commercial illustrator at the age of 18****... The [school] schedule was exhausting, and Disney often received poor grades after falling asleep in class, but he continued his paper route for more than six years. He attended Saturday courses at the Kansas City Art Institute and also took a correspondence course in cartooning.*

IMDb *- There he met a fellow animator, Ub Iwerks. The two soon set up their own company. In the early 1920s, they made a series of animated shorts for the Newman theater chain, entitled "Newman's Laugh-O-Grams". Their company soon went bankrupt, however.*

Wikipedia *- Disneyy was a shy,* ***self-deprecating*** *and insecure man in private but adopted a warm and outgoing public persona. He had high standards and high expectations of those with whom he worked. Although there have been accusations that he was racist or anti-Semitic, they have been contradicted by many who knew him.*

***Britannica.com** - Disney's imagination and energy, **his whimsical humour, and his gift for being attuned to the vagaries of popular taste** inspired him to develop **well-loved amusements for "children of all ages" throughout the world**. Although some criticized his frequently saccharine subject matter and accused him of creating a virtual stylistic monopoly in American animation that discouraged experimentation, there is no denying his pathbreaking accomplishments. His achievement as a **creator of entertainment for an almost unlimited public** and as a highly ingenious merchandiser of his wares can rightly be compared to the most successful industrialists in history.*

Maturation of Professional Life

***IMDb** - [Ub Iwerks and Walt Disney] went to Hollywood in 1923. They started work on a new series, about a live-action little girl who journeys to a world of animated characters. Entitled the "Alice Comedies", they were distributed by M.J. Winkler (Margaret). Walt was backed up financially only by Winkler and his older brother Roy O. Disney, who remained his business partner for the rest of his life. **Hundreds of "Alice Comedies"** were produced between 1923 and 1927, before they lost popularity.*

Walt then started work on a series around a new animated character, Oswald the Lucky Rabbit. This series was successful, but in 1928, Walt discovered that M.J. Winkler and her husband, Charles Mintz, had stolen the rights to the character away from him. They had also stolen all his animators, except for Ub Iwerks. While taking the train home, Walt started doodling on a piece of paper. The result of these doodles was a mouse named Mickey. With only Walt and Ub to animate, and Walt's wife Lillian Disney (Lilly) and Roy's wife Edna Disney to ink in the animation cells, three Mickey Mouse cartoons were quickly produced. The first two didn't sell, so Walt added synchronized sound to the last one, Steamboat Willie (1928), and it was immediately picked up. With Walt as the voice of Mickey, it premiered to great success. Many more cartoons followed. Walt was now in the big time, but he didn't stop creating new ideas.

King of Simulation Entertainment

... In 1934, Walt started work on another new idea: a cartoon that ran the length of a feature film. Everyone in Hollywood was calling it "Disney's Folly", but Snow White and the Seven Dwarfs (1937) was anything but, winning critical raves, the adoration of the public, and one big and seven little special Oscars for Walt. Now

Walt listed animated features among his ever-growing list of accomplishments. While continuing to produce cartoon shorts, he also started producing more of the animated features. Pinocchio (1940), Dumbo (1941), and Bambi (1942) were all successes; not even a flop like Fantasia (1940) and a studio animators' strike in 1941 could stop Disney now.

In the mid 1940s, he began producing "packaged features", essentially a group of shorts put together to run feature length, but by 1950 he was back with animated features that stuck to one story, with ***Cinderella*** *(1950),* ***Alice in Wonderland*** *(1951), and* ***Peter Pan*** *(1953). In 1950, he also started producing live-action films, with* ***Treasure Island*** *(1950). These began taking on greater importance throughout the 50s and 60s, but Walt continued to produce animated features, including* ***Lady and the Tramp*** *(1955),* ***Sleeping Beauty*** *(1959), and* ***One Hundred and One Dalmatians*** *(1961).*

City-like Amusement Parks

In 1955 he opened a theme park in southern California: ***Disneyland****. It was a place where children and their parents could take rides, just explore, and meet the familiar animated characters, all in a clean, safe environment. It was another great success. Walt also became one of the first producers of films to venture into television, with his series The Magical World of Disney (1954) which he began in 1954 to promote his theme park. He also produced The Mickey Mouse Club (1955) and Zorro (1957). To top it all off, Walt came out with the lavish musical fantasy Mary Poppins (1964), which mixed live-action with animation. It is considered by many to be his magnum opus. Even after that,* ***Walt continued to forge onward, with plans to build a new theme park and an experimental prototype city in Florida.***

He did not live to see the culmination of those plans, however; in 1966, he developed lung cancer brought on by his lifelong chain-smoking. He died of a heart attack following cancer surgery on December 15, 1966 at age 65. But not even his death, it seemed, could stop him. Roy carried on plans to build the Florida theme park, and it premiered in 1971 under the name Walt Disney World. His company continues to flourish, still producing animated and live-action films and overseeing the still-growing empire started by one man: Walt Disney, who will never be forgotten.

QG Psychophysiscs Interpretation

Walt Disney's life course shows the analyst an undeniable stamp by the partition descriptors germane to Layer 8 of the Human Mentation Foliate. At age 16, the selflessness that he manifested in faking his age in order to enroll for World War II as an ambulance driver partakes of the inner workings of the left-chiral partitions of the Layer, in particular *humility*, *devotion* to others and the service in *subservience*. Note that he did not want or seek to join the killing part of the enterprise, however justified it could be, but strictly the life-saving part of the same.

His early educational choices before the advent of the War did show as well his personal commitment as a life mission to the business of *comedy*, *humor* and *happiness*, since he manifested henceforth keen interest in drawing and cartooning. These are pensive partition qualities pertaining to the right-chiral side of the Perfect Layer of the Foliate. It is their native overtone within the framework of his Mental Body Foliate that channeled those early life course choices.

Perhaps the secret desire of Walter Disney as an adult until the end of his life could be encapsulated in one word: *Paradise*. He relentlessy pursued fantasy, wonder and happiness as a staple to bring to others throughout all of the stages of his life. That life pursuit motorized all his enterprises and goals. It turned him into an inventor, when he modified the photographic camera for animation, when he kept inventing over decades countless number of cartoonish characters, Mickey being his most iconic one by critics, when he put his own human voice behind the cartoons. That pursuit turned him into an entrepreneur, for which he was not prepared at all, failing several of his early entrepreneurial endeavours, being abused and betrayed by other business partners. Until he realized that for the particular strain of entertainment that he wanted to bring to the world he needed to better himself at enterprising in terms of partnership and securing project financing. When he finally put himself on track to build the fantasy and wonder lands towards culminating his life realizations, he was knowledgeable enough as an entrepreneur to send staff people visit existing amusement parks around the world in order to gather the shortcomings to avoid in his projects. By the same token, it is important to realize that what Walt seeked to materialize with these themed city parks was the *ecstasy* of Paradise, for the very young, the young and the older.

Perhaps he did become the monopolist entertainer that some critics levy on his legacy. One ought to consider however the pressures from the ecosystem within which he was operating in making that judgement.

Britannica **-** *When Disneyland opened in 1955, much of Disney's disposition toward* ***nostalgic sentiment and fantasy was evident in its design and construction****. It soon became a mecca for tourists from around the world. A second Disney park, Walt Disney World, near Orlando, Florida, which was under construction at the time of his death, opened in 1971.*

Elvis Aron Presley

Asymptotic Character

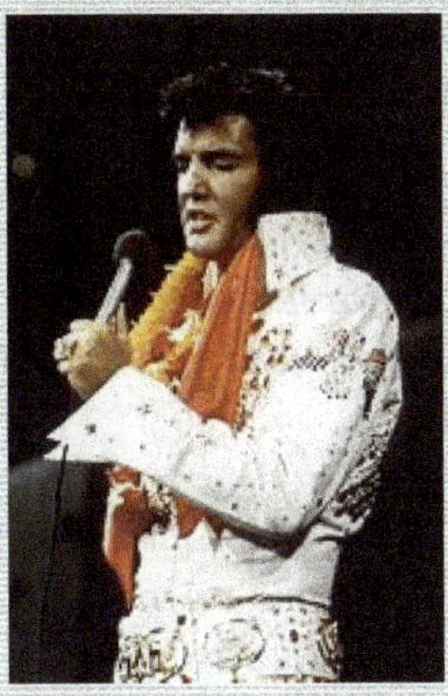

Mississipi Historical Society *- Elvis A. Presley was born in Tupelo, Mississippi, on January 8, 1935, in a two-room shotgun house in East Tupelo, then a separate municipality that some called the "roughest town in north Mississippi." Though* ***poor****, Elvis's parents, Gladys and Vernon Presley, were not unlike many others in Mississippi at that time, for the country was in the midst of the Great Depression.*

... His twin brother, Jesse Garon, did not survive, making Elvis what is called today a "twin-less twin." Elvis was cherished by his family, but psychologists say that losing a twin can deeply affect the baby's mother and the surviving twin. Elvis no doubt later yearned for a brother to help him through the rough spots of his life — of which there were many. Elvis later changed his middle name, Aaron, to Aron, to more closely ***match his twin's middle name (Garon)****. Elvis's mother — a strong and supportive presence in his life — told the young Elvis that a surviving twin gets the strength of both children, and all evidence indicates that, in this case anyway, she was right.*

The shotgun house Baby Elvis called home, the "Birthplace Home of Elvis Presley" in Tupelo, was built by his father, his uncle, and paternal grandfather... ("You can take this birthplace and put it in my living room at ***Graceland****," Elvis later said.)*

... They lost the shotgun house in 1938 when Elvis's father and two other men went to Parchman Farm—the Mississippi State Penitentiary— to serve eight months for altering a four-dollar check. Elvis and his mother moved in with relatives in Tupelo. ***His father's imprisonment was traumatic to three-and-a-half-year-old Elvis,*** *who, according to a cousin, would sit on the porch "crying his eyes out" for his daddy. Often Elvis and Gladys took the bus to Parchman on the weekends to visit him. After release from Parchman, Vernon, as a day-laborer,*

had to continue to support his mother as well as his family; as a consequence, the Presleys were to become renters, like many families, moving from one affordable space to another. ***The constant in their lives was church*** *— Vernon and Gladys had met at the Assembly of God Church and they continued to attend church there,* ***where music was becoming a big attraction to little Elvis****...*

1941: Elvis starts school

Elvis started elementary school at the East Tupelo Consolidated School on Lake Street. He was termed "sweet and average" by his teacher. His mother walked him the half mile to school each day. ***He got his first guitar lesson from Frank Smith, the new young pastor at the church they attended, and apparently Elvis took to these lessons more than he did those at school...***

Oleta Grimes, one of his teachers, was impressed by Elvis's musical talent and took him to the principal, who entered Elvis, age ten, in a radio talent contest at the Mississippi-Alabama Fair. On the appointed date, Elvis surprised his mother by going onstage and climbing up on a chair to reach the microphone to sing "Old Shep" in front of several hundred people. He won fifth prize, according to Elvis biographer Peter Guralnick. The next year, when Elvis wanted a bicycle Gladys Presley talked him into a less expensive item, a guitar for $12.95 from the Tupelo Hardware Company, not only because of its price but also because the overly protective mother feared Elvis would hurt himself on a bicycle. He began taking the guitar with him to school every day, sometimes playing a little music— ***gospel music****—for his friends.*

1948: Elvis moves to Memphis

In the fall of 1948 the Presley family was on the move again, and this time they decided to leave Tupelo and go north, to the city of Memphis, Tennessee...

Nearby were Beale Street and the Ellis Auditorium, offering national acts. The Handy Theatre was offering all the practitioners of ***"city blues"—Wynonie Harris, Bobby "Blue" Bland, and others—as well as jazz. The Blackwood Brothers, the top gospel group in America, had just moved to Memphis.***

What music was not live in Memphis was on the radio. Famed disc jockey Dewey Phillips at WHBQ was playing blues as well as rhythm and blues...

He took his guitar to school there too—when some rough kids cut the strings on it, other classmates chipped in and bought him a new set. Elvis took more guitar lessons, tagged along with his guitar teacher and played in his ban... Jerry Schilling, a friend of the teen-age Elvis, describes him as a "voracious reader," ***"very spiritual,"*** *and "a lovable rebel."*

1953: Elvis graduates high school

In April of 1953 Elvis performed as one of twenty-two acts in the Humes High "annual ***minstrel*** *show."*

... In August 1953, eighteen-year-old Elvis went down to the Memphis Recording Service on Union Avenue, home of Sun Records and run by Sam Philips, friend of disc jockey Dewey Phillips, to make a record. Like Elvis, Sam Phillips was passionate about music, especially the music ***"that white people liked but weren't sure whether they ought to or not."... Wikipedia - Phillips*** *played a major role in the development of rock and roll during the 1950s, launching the career of Presley... Phillips was the owner and operator of radio stations in Memphis; Florence, Alabama; and Lake Worth, Florida. He was also an early investor in the Holiday Inn chain of hotels and an advocate for racial equality, helping to break down racial barriers in the music industry... As a child, he picked cotton in the fields with his parents alongside* ***black laborers****. The experience of hearing black laborers singing in the fields left a big impression on the young Phillips.*

Biography.com - *... That first session didn't work out so well, but during July Elvis and guitarist Scotty Moore and bassist Bill Black—after a slow start—hit on something while they were just fooling around. It was a speeded-up version of Mississippi crooner Arthur "Big Boy" Crudup's "That's All Right," and when Phillips heard it, he interrupted them, asking "What was that?" They could not tell him exactly, so they just played it again. It was exactly the music Sam Phillips had been looking for, although he had been unable to tell them how to get there.*

Sam's brother Dewey was sold on the music too, and when he played it on his Red, Hot, and Blue *radio show at WHBQ, the listeners went wild. Dewey was kept busy on the telephone taking request after request for the song.*

When the debut single of "That's All Right" was released — with "Blue Moon of Kentucky" on the flip side — it sold like crazy, and a national phenomenon was born. Elvis was nineteen.

The group appeared for the first time on the Louisiana Hayride, *a live Saturday-night country music radio show, on October 16, 1954. The next year Elvis signed the now-famous RCA contract — for an unprecedented $40,000 — and RCA re-released the five Sun Records singles on its label.*

1956: 60 million watch Elvis on TV

... in the fall of 1956, Elvis performed twice on The Ed Sullivan Show. *The first, on September 9, 1956, drew sixty million viewers, more than eighty percent of the national TV audience.*

That year American teenagers began to buy the new portable transistor radios, a boon to spreading the new music, especially rock and roll, to young fans. When Elvis played the Mississippi-Alabama Fair in 1956, a hundred National Guardsmen were on hand to control the crowds of fans—especially the girls, who screamed out of control when Elvis sang. Scotty Moore told him why: "It was your leg, man. It was the way you were shaking your left leg." Later a reporter asked Elvis if he thought he might get rid of some of that "wiggle," and Elvis replied, "Well, sir, you take the wiggle out of it, and it's finished."

... Despite his fame — and a hot temper — his friend Schilling writes that Elvis chose "ninety percent of the time to be a nice guy."

Elvis' Love Life

Biography.com - *Elvis was stationed in West Germany during his stint in the U.S. Army. In 1959 Priscilla arrived in the country due to the Air Force transferring her father there... Elvis saw a resemblance between Priscilla and his recently deceased, and much lamented, mother, Gladys... Priscilla's age meant they couldn't go out in public, but they still saw each other often. The only thing they didn't do was fully consummate their relationship. As his time in the Army came to a close, Priscilla wanted to do so, but Elvis told her, "Someday we will, Priscilla, but not now. You're just too young."*

... In March 1960, Elvis, having finished his enlistment, left Germany. Priscilla sent letters, using pink envelopes to make them easy to locate among Elvis' fan mail... Priscilla also visited Graceland for Christmas that year. Next, Elvis asked her to finish high school in Memphis, which she was desperate to do. Her parents initially rejected the idea, but Priscilla continued to press the issue as Elvis tried to convince them that their daughter would be safely living with his father and stepmother. He also implied he wanted to marry Priscilla... Elvis valued what he saw as Priscilla's purity, so their relationship remained sexless (however, throughout his relationship with Priscilla, Elvis was with other women, ranging from girl-next-door types to Hollywood co-stars). But they were intimate in other ways... Their wedding night was the first time the couple went "all the way."

... Priscilla discovered that Elvis was reluctant to sleep with her after she'd gone through childbirth. He told her he wanted her to have time to recover, but, as Priscilla later wrote, "He had mentioned before we were married that he had never been able to make love to a woman who'd had a child." As he had before they were married, Elvis slept with other women. But Priscilla was no longer willing to simply wait for him to come home.

... Their divorce, which was finalized on October 9, 1973, was an amicable one. Priscilla would say in a 2016 interview, "I did not divorce him because I didn't love him. He was the love of my life, but I had to find out about the world."

Closerweekly.com – *Ann-Margret: "It was a very strong relationship, very intense," she wrote in her 1994 memoir* Ann-Margret: My Story. *"We both felt a current, an electricity that went straight through us... We loved our families [and] we had a strong belief in God," she once recalled to Closer.*

Connie Stevens: "Despite only dating on and off for about two years, she boldly stated Elvis was "one of the loves of my life."

Nathalie Wood: ""His mother said something like, 'Come and sit on Mama's lap,'" Lana once recalled to Closer Weekly. "They were very affectionate, and it bothered Natalie."

Linda Thompson: ".... He loved animals. He loved children. He loved people."

Ginger Alden: "He loved to play the organ [while wearing] this great jeweled robe.

QG Psychophysics Interpretation

Elvis Presley's life course was ontologically marked by the Norm of Transcentalization inherent to Layer 9 of the Mentation Foliate. We have highlighted in the above biographical reports the many elements of his life stemming from this ontology.

Transcendentalization is the experience of overcoming death. It is the end without end which we denote *Asymptotization*. At the same time it epitomizes the broadest form of space expansiveness which is infinite in scope, setting the stage for the psychological experience of both platonic interaction and spiritual manifestation.

These definitions transpire in fullness along the axis of life ontologically accorded Elvis A. Presley. His relationship with the phenomenon of death had started prenatally, having witnessed the death of his stillborn brother Garon in-utero. The biographers note that he had changed his middle name to Garon, in a clear attempt to further identify with his unborn dead brother. Note that, as Garon's twin, Elvis was ontologically both alive and dead. It was not long after birth, just age 3 ½ years, that he endured the heuristic death of his father who disappeared to state prison due to a felony. He had cried out his lungs in severance from his father for the duration. Later on the unexpected death of his mother was to further tragically deepen his personal experience with death:

"When Elvis arrived at the hospital, the AP reported he "sank to his knees beside his mother's bed and wept... "She was all we lived for," Elvis sobbed at the hospital early Thursday morning after learning of his mother's death... The AP reported that Elvis Presley was "near hysteria" at his mother's funeral services yesterday. Elvis, 23, and his father, Vernon, 48, "wept throughout the service" at National Funeral Home in Memphis."

Elvis also had an overwhelming experience with maternity within the context of transcendentalization. We already mentioned the eventful life in utero with a twin brother who was to become stillborn later. The latter resulted in a strong bond between his mother and him due to the lost consanguine life in twin brother Garon. The biographers expressly note her words of consolation and support to him for the circumstance. It was also in her company that the infant Elvis used to visit his incarcerated father. This shared ontological and psychosocial development overall thus turned mother Gladys into overprotectiveness for Elvis, on one hand, and, on the other, brought Elvis to the level of a spiritual experience with mother Gladys, beyond the Oedipus complex situation. Absent this understanding, the analyst will remain unable to decipher the peculiarities of his marital, courtship and sexual life. To put it in one word, the ontological and psychosocial experience with his mother had predisposed him to a Marian experience with every woman. Hence his reluctance to engage in sexual penetration of his beaus and refusal of sexual interaction altogether should the woman become pregnant or give birth to a child, as it occurred with his one-time wife Priscilla. For the same likely reasons he happened to name his ranch **Grace**land, as much as he had turned teenager fiancée Priscilla, by probable own election, to the **Immaculate Conception** High School when she joined him in Memphis and needed to finalize her high school education.

The Layer-9 trend to transcendent spirituality was profound in Elvis Presley and as a mold shaped the entirety of his rock and roll music. Gospel chants and the blues took him for certain to rock and roll, and at the same time it is the transcendent strain of his character that made this strain of music highly attractive to him. His extremely expressive body activity on the stage and in particular the incessant leg wiggling during his stage performances must reminisce of the transport common in religious trance. With good reason he reportedly said "if you take the wiggle out of it, it's finished." Elvis also played on stage, as part of his charm, this goodhearted *cluelessness* and mimics of self-detachment that were then quite unusual in a performer.

It may well be that Elvis could never overcome the untimely death of his dear mother (age 46), his "best girl" as he called her, and sought in a myriad of other women the deep human connection with spiritual overtone that he had maintained with her throughout their common lives. This unsolvable likely delivered him to the potent opiate drugs that tragically took his life at the equally early age of 42. Nevertheless, the King of Rock and Roll rocked and solaced America and the World at a historical moment of geopolitical turmoil, deep material deprivation and moral distress in the modern era.

Leonardo Da Vinci

Hyper-Egocentric Character

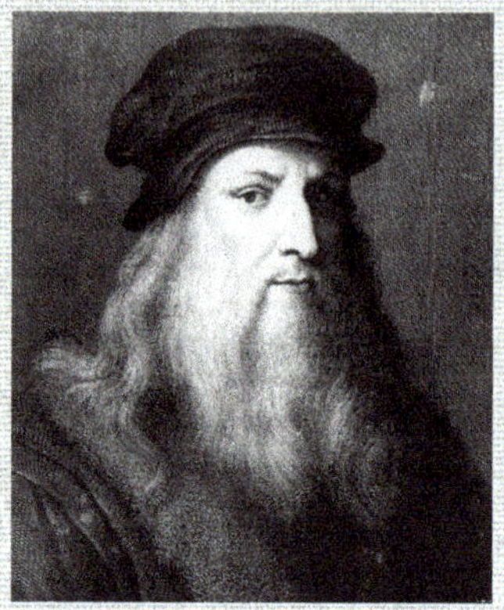

Celebrities-galore.com *- Da Vinci was born in a farmhouse outside the village of Anchiano in Tuscany, Italy (about 18 miles west of Florence) on April 15, 1452.*

Born out of wedlock to respected Florentine notary Ser Piero and a young peasant woman named Caterina, da Vinci was raised by his father and his stepmother.

At the age of five, he moved to his father's estate in nearby Vinci (the town from which his surname derives), where he lived with his uncle and grandparents... ***[Notablebiographies.com]*** *when he was fifteen, his father apprenticed him to Andrea Del Verrocchio (1435–1488), the leading artist of Florence and the early Renaissance. Verrocchio, a sculptor, painter, and goldsmith, was a remarkable craftsman. He had great concern for the quality of execution in expressing the vitality of the human figure. These elements were important in the formation of Leonardo's artistic style. It should be noted that much in* ***Leonardo's approach to art originated from using tradition****, rather than rebelling against it...* ***[Biography.com]*** *According to Lives of the Most Excellent Painters, Sculptors and Architects, written around 1550 by artist Giorgio Vasari, del Verrocchio was so humbled by the superior talent of his pupil that he never picked up a paintbrush again. (Most scholars, however, dismiss Vasari's account as apocryphal.)... At the age of 20, da Vinci qualified for membership* ***as a master artist*** *in Florence's Guild of Saint Luke and established his own workshop. However, he continued to collaborate with del Verrocchio for an additional five years.*

... In 1478, after leaving Del Verrocchio's studio, Da Vinci received his first independent commission for an altarpiece to reside in a chapel inside Florence's Palazzo Vecchio.

Three years later the Augustinian monks of Florence's San Donato a Scopeto tasked him to paint "Adoration of the Magi." ***The young artist, however, would leave the city and abandon both commissions without ever completing them.***

Maturation of Professional Life

[Celebrities-galore.com] *[Da Vinci became] a polymath, painter, sculptor, architect, musician, mathematician, engineer, inventor, anatomist, geologist, cartographer, botanist, and writer, who is considered to be one of the greatest painters of all time...* ***Leonardo da Vinci is practical, down to earth with strong ideas about right and wrong.*** *He is orderly, organized, systematic and controlled, and once committed - he employs decisive and methodical steps to problems solving, without giving up easily... Leonardo seeks to* ***establish a solid foundation,*** *and would rather use hard work and long hours...*

Although da Vinci is known for his artistic abilities, fewer than two dozen paintings attributed to him exist. One reason is that his interests were so varied that he wasn't a prolific painter. Da Vinci's most famous works include the "Vitruvian Man," "The Last Supper" and the "Mona Lisa."... Based on accounts from an early biographer, however, the "Mona Lisa" is a picture of Lisa Del Giocondo, the wife of a wealthy Florentine silk merchant. The painting's original Italian name — "La Gioconda" — supports the theory, but it's far from certain. Some art historians believe the merchant commissioned the portrait to celebrate the pending birth of the couple's next child, which means the subject could have been pregnant at the time of the painting.

If the Giocondo family did indeed commission the painting, they never received it. For da Vinci, the "Mona Lisa" ***was forever a work in progress****, as it was his attempt at perfection, and he* ***never parted with the painting****.*

... ***He abandoned the "Battle of Anghiari" project*** *after two years when the mural began to deteriorate before he had a chance to finish it.*

... In 1482, Florentine ruler Lorenzo de' Medici commissioned da Vinci to create a silver lyre and bring it as a peace gesture to Ludovico Sforza. After doing so, ***da Vinci lobbied Ludovico for a job*** *and sent the future Duke of Milan a letter that barely mentioned his considerable talents as an artist and* ***instead touted his more marketable skills as a military engineer.***

Using his inventive mind, da Vinci sketched war machines such as a war chariot with scythe blades mounted on the sides, an armored tank propelled by two men cranking a shaft and even an enormous crossbow that required a small army of men to operate.

The letter worked, and Ludovico brought da Vinci to Milan for a tenure that would last 17 years. During his time in Milan, da Vinci was commissioned to work on numerous artistic projects as well, including "The Last Supper."

... Ludovico Sforza also tasked da Vinci with sculpting a 16-foot-tall bronze equestrian statue of his father and founder of the family dynasty, Francesco Sforza. Da Vinci sculpted a life-size clay model of the statue, but the project was put on hold when war with France required bronze to be used for casting cannons, not sculptures. After French forces overran Milan in 1499 — and shot the clay model to pieces — ***da Vinci fled the city along with the duke and the Sforza family.***

Ironically, Gian Giacomo Trivulzio, who led the French forces that conquered Ludovico in 1499, followed in his foe's footsteps and commissioned da Vinci to sculpt a grand equestrian statue, *one that could be mounted on his tomb. After years of work and numerous sketches by da Vinci, Trivulzio decided to scale back the size of the statue,* ***which was ultimately never finished.***

... ***Da Vinci returned to Milan in 1506 to work for the very French rulers who had overtaken the city seven years earlier and forced him to flee.***

... In 1502 and 1503, da Vinci also briefly worked in Florence as a military engineer for Cesare Borgia, the ***illegitimate son of Pope Alexander VI*** *and commander of the papal army. He traveled outside of Florence to survey military construction projects and sketch city plans and topographical maps.*

He designed plans, possibly with noted diplomat ***Niccolò Machiavelli,*** *to divert the Arno River away from rival Pisa in order to deny its wartime enemy access to the sea. [Note that Machiavelli] wrote* The Prince, *a handbook for politicians on the use of ruthless, self-serving cunning, inspiring the term "Machiavellian" and establishing Machiavelli as the "father of modern political theory"...* ***he earned a reputation for deviousness,*** *enjoying shocking his associates by appearing more shameless than he truly was."*

... Amid political strife and the temporary expulsion of the French from Milan, da Vinci left the city and moved to Rome in 1513 along with Salai, Melzi and two studio assistants. Giuliano de' Medici, brother of newly installed Pope Leo X and son of his former patron, gave da Vinci a monthly stipend along with a suite of rooms at his residence inside the Vatican.

... Along with Melzi, da Vinci departed for France, never to return. He lived in the Chateau de Cloux (now Clos Luce) near the king's summer palace along the Loire River in Amboise. As in Rome, da Vinci did little painting during his time in France. One of his last commissioned works was a mechanical lion that could walk and open its chest to reveal a bouquet of lilies.

Sexual Life

[Da Vinci] was repulsed by female sexuality. Historian Elizabeth Abbott in a lecture she delivered at Carleton University in Ottawa quotes [Da Vinci]: 'the sexual act of coitus and the body parts employed for it are so repulsive, that were it not for the beauty of the faces and the adornment of the actors and the pent-up impulse, nature would lose the human species.' She points to a sketch da Vinci drafted of heterosexual intercourse as a prime example of his revulsion... "The woman is only represented by her cavities — there is no face, or head, or torso," Abbott observed in conversation with IDEAS host, Nahlah Ayed..." He referred to [sexual intercourse] as repellent... Meanwhile, he drew countless beautiful sketches of the phallus and anus... "His sort of male sexuality was understood and accepted," said Abbott. "He preferred the company of and the beauty of men... ***Indeed, homosexuality was such a fact of artistic life in Renaissance Florence that the word "florenzer" became German slang for "gay." ...*** *But what was despised [in Renaissance Italy] was sodomy. Why? It was probably because it was considered by the Church to be unnatural. Sex was supposed to be for procreation only."*

In 1476, Leonardo da Vinci was arrested by the Office of the Night under the accusation of sodomy. The Office of the Night was the moral policing unit in Florence. While eventually acquitted, the experience was so humiliating for him that Abbott argues da Vinci vowed himself to live a life of celibacy.

... Da Vinci died of a probable stroke on May 2, 1519, at the age of 67. He continued work on his scientific studies until his death; ...For centuries after his death, thousands of pages from his private journals with notes, drawings, observations and scientific theories have surfaced and provided a fuller measure of the true "Renaissance man."

QG Psychophysics Interpretation

Per the above biographical notes, sheer force, overpower, overwhelming, self-serving superego are the key words to circumscribe Leonardo Da Vinci's life course, in accordance with the Hyper-Egocentric stamp of his character. He also displayed a notable mercenary spirit resulting from his focus on self-service and personal satisfaction. To the latter there is likely a strong contributing factor from the psychosocial dimension of his early childhood.

Effectively, being born out of wedlock from a peasant mother from whom he was apparently completely severed through the course of his upbringing robbed him the chance to learn empathy with the world and others from a nurturing mother. One must expect impact in one way or another on psychological formation by a situation where he was born and to be treated as a "nobody" in an aristocratic society, totally severed from interaction with his biological mother due to social class segregation. We do not know enough of his relationship with his stepmother to assess the same either as a possible positive compensating factor or an even more negative contribution in that sense. Nevertheless at age 5 he was already shipped to the grandparents' home to live with them and an uncle. His little sympathy for women and women's body probably had much to do with this squint and uneasy, if any, maternal nurture. Effectively to see ugliness in a woman's vagina as he did is to forget at the first place that all human lives come to be through that anatomical formation. It is our opinion that it is a non sequitur to value life and not value the vagina.

Likewise the presence, exemplification and guidance from a close father were almost never there for Leonardo. Instead the only exemplification was that of a trespassing or social norm violation, of which he was rather painfully the product. The realization that his life must have been an element of embarrassment to his father must have never left him.

Furthermore, resolute departure from the constraints of the medieval era dominated by an abusive Catholic Church constituted to a large extent the atmosphere which drove the Renaissance period and contributed for sure in Leonardo's defying and dismissing the moral virtues predicated by the Church. The very popes of the time could present to the world illegitimate children of their own!

It is thus fair assessment that the psychosocial elements absorbed by Leonardo Da Vinci in his developmental years fluidly played into his self-serving superego predisposition as a Hyper-Egocentric character. Note that he could not be judged for an amoral character however, since he understood the value in higher qualities despite his inability to fully live by them. Attributed to him is the following quote which gives a glimpse in his way of thinking: *"I love those who can smile in trouble, who can gather strength from distress, and grow brave by reflection. 'Tis the business of little minds to shrink, but they whose heart is firm, and whose conscience approves their conduct, will pursue their principles unto death."* His understanding that conscience is the ultimate arbiter of morality is an important insight. However the quote reveals at the same time his commitment to strength, absolute resolve and overpower.

Leonardo Da Vinci was determined to make something big and compelling out of himself at all costs. As the biographer notes, he did not rebel against tradition but rather anchored his creativity on traditions and institutions to affirm his personal worth and make himself best possible living. Note that many of his commissioned works were left unfinished. Most importantly, he mustered the strength and persistence to become the most polyfaceted professional of the Renaissance period, which earned him the title "the Renaissance man". As noted by the biographer, he became polymath, painter, sculptor, architect, musician, mathematician, engineer, inventor, anatomist, geologist, cartographer, botanist, and writer, and the greatest painter of all time. By all accounts an impressive set of skills, which he equally and willfully put at the service of the virtuous and the non virtuous as well as those at both sides of a conflict.

Mona Lisa was a painting he worked on and never departed throughout his professional life, albeit a commissioned workpiece. It is perhaps the most famous world painting and which so much has been written about. It may well be that the notoriously cryptic smile on Mona Lisa's face has only been telling the world the underpinnings of Da Vinci's spirit in the terms herein exposed. Who knows?

Rosa Louise Parks

Hyper-Hyperbolic Character

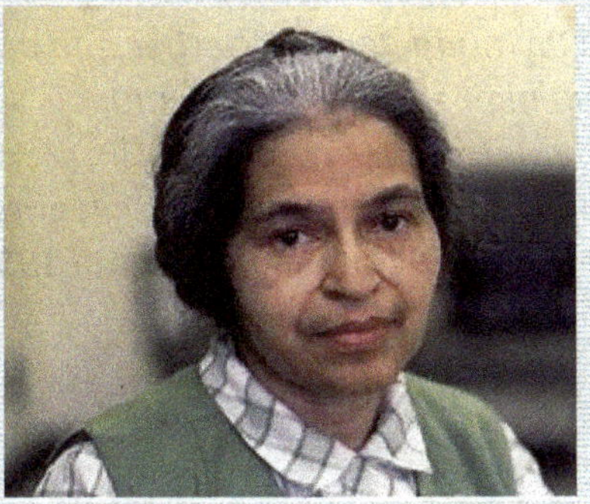

Biography.com *- Parks was born Rosa Louise McCauley on February 4, 1913, in Tuskegee, Alabama. Her parents, James and Leona McCauley, separated when Parks was two. Parks' mother moved the family to Pine Level, Alabama, to live with her parents, Rose and Sylvester Edwards. Both of Parks' grandparents were formerly enslaved people and strong advocates for racial equality; the family lived on the Edwards' farm, where Parks would spend her youth.*

Parks' childhood brought her early experiences with racial discrimination and activism for racial equality. In one experience, ***Parks' grandfather stood in front of their house with a shotgun while Ku Klux Klan members marched down the street.***

Education

Throughout Parks' education, she attended segregated schools. Taught to read by her mother at a young age, Parks attended a segregated, one-room school in Pine Level, Alabama, that often lacked adequate school supplies such as desks. ***African American students were forced to walk to the first through sixth-grade schoolhouse****, while the city of Pine Level provided bus transportation as well as a new school building for white students.*

Beginning at age 11, Parks attended the city's Industrial School for Girls in Montgomery. In 1929, while in the 11th grade and attending a laboratory school for secondary education led by the Alabama State Teachers College for Negroes, ***Parks left school to attend to both her sick grandmother and mother back in Pine Level****.*

Parks didn't return to her studies. Instead, she got a job at a shirt factory in Montgomery. After marrying in 1932, she earned her high school degree in 1933 with her husband's support.

Marriage

In 1932, at age 19, Parks met and married Raymond Parks, a barber and an active member of the NAACP. After graduating high school with Raymond's support, Parks became actively involved in civil rights issues by joining the Montgomery chapter of the NAACP in 1943, serving as the chapter's youth leader as well as secretary to NAACP President E.D. Nixon — a post she held until 1957. The couple never had children.

Activism

History.com - Parks was not the first African American woman to be arrested for refusing to yield her seat on a Montgomery bus.
Nine months before Parks was jailed, 15-year-old Claudette Colvin was the first Montgomery bus passenger to be arrested for refusing to give up her seat for a white passenger. (Parks was involved in raising defense funds for Colvin.) Three other African American women—Aurelia Browder, Mary Louise Smith and Susie McDonald—also ran afoul of the bus segregation law prior to Parks. The four were plaintiffs in the Browder v. Gayle case that resulted in the Supreme Court ruling bus segregation unconstitutional.

Parks was a civil rights activist before her arrest.
Parks was a long-time member of the Montgomery chapter of the National Association for the Advancement of Colored People (NAACP), which she joined in 1943. At the time of her arrest, she was a secretary of the local NAACP chapter, and the previous summer she had attended a workshop for social and economic justice at Tennessee's Highlander Folk School. Her political activism continued through the boycott and the rest of her life.

Her act of civil disobedience was not pre-meditated.
Although Parks knew that the NAACP was looking for a lead plaintiff in a case to test the constitutionality of the Jim Crow law, she did not set out to be arrested on bus 2857. Parks wrote in her autobiography that she was so preoccupied that day that she failed to notice that Blake was driving the bus. "If I had been paying attention," she wrote, "I wouldn't even have gotten on that bus."

Parks did not refuse to leave her seat because her feet were tired.
In her autobiography, Parks debunked the myth that she refused to vacate her seat because she was tired after a long day at work. "I was not tired physically," she wrote, "or no more tired than I usually was at the end of a working day. I was not old, although some people have an image of me as being old then. I was forty-two. ***No, the only tired I was, was tired of giving in."***

Biography.com - *The police arrested Parks at the scene and charged her with violation of Chapter 6, Section 11, of the Montgomery City Code. She was taken to police headquarters, where, later that night, she was released on bail.*

Due to the size and scope of, and loyalty to, boycott participation, the effort continued for several months. The city of Montgomery had become a victorious eyesore, with dozens of public buses sitting idle, ultimately severely crippling finances for its transit company. With the boycott's progress, however, came strong resistance.

... Decades would pass before Parks' role in the boycott made her a respected figure across the country; between the bus boycott and widespread recognition for her work, Parks' life encompassed both difficulties and triumphs.

Parks and her husband lost their jobs after the boycott

Soon after the Montgomery bus boycott began, Parks lost her job as a tailor's assistant at the Montgomery Fair department store. Her husband Raymond also had to leave his job as a barber at ***Maxwell Air Force Base*** *because he'd been ordered not to discuss his wife.*

Yet the boycott's conclusion didn't make it easy for either of them to get back to earning a living — Parks was too identified with the protest for her or her husband to land another regular job in Alabama.

Parks had been a dedicated volunteer for the Montgomery Improvement Association (MIA), a local group that had helped coordinate the boycott, but the organization didn't hire her, nor did any other civil rights group. Despite contributions such as traveling to give talks about the boycott to raise funds for the MIA and the NAACP, ***male leadership did not identify with Parks' needs.***

There was also jealousy among locals over the amount of attention Parks had received. In the end, she decided her only choice was to leave Alabama with her husband and mother.

Her family moved to Detroit, hoping to find work

In 1957, Parks and her family went to Detroit, where her brother and cousin lived. Unfortunately, finding work there still wasn't easy, either. Parks soon headed to Virginia to take a job as a hostess at the Hampton Institute's Holly Tree Inn. But when promised accommodation for her mother and Raymond never came through, Parks returned to Detroit at the end of the 1958 fall semester.

Back in Detroit, Raymond had to go through required training before he could become a barber and Parks could only find piecework sewing jobs. ***Then she had an operation for an ulcer (a condition that had developed under the stress of the bus boycott), and needed to have a throat tumor removed.***

Medical costs and the difficulties of working while ill pushed Parks and her family to the edge. In July 1960, Jet *magazine described her as a "tattered rag of her former self — penniless, debt-ridden, ailing with stomach ulcers, and a throat tumor, compressed into two rooms with her husband and mother."*

Parks worked closely with Martin Luther King Jr. and Malcolm X

Having worked with Martin Luther King Jr. on the bus boycott, Parks truly admired the civil rights leader. At the Southern Christian Leadership Conference's annual convention in 1962, she saw a man attack King — and experienced how King made sure the attacker faced no retaliation afterward. Following his assassination in 1968, she traveled to Memphis to support a sanitation workers' march that King had been involved in before proceeding to King's funeral.

Yet Parks also found much to appreciate in Malcolm X's leadership. Her beliefs more closely aligned with Malcolm's, and differed from King's, on the limits of non-violence.

In a 1967 interview, Parks stated, "If we can protect ourselves against violence it's not actually violence on our part. That's just self-protection, trying to keep from being victimized with violence."

She eventually got a job as an assistant to Congressman John Conyers

After moving to Detroit and despite her hardships, Parks remained committed to helping her community. She joined neighborhood groups that focused on everything from schools to voter registration.

In 1964 she volunteered for John Conyers' congressional campaign. The candidate appreciated her support and credited her with getting King Jr. to come to Detroit and provide an endorsement. After Conyers won the election, he hired Parks as a receptionist and assistant for his Detroit office. She started in 1965 and remained until her retirement in 1988.

The job was a boon for Parks' financial situation, as it offered a pension and health insurance. ***And Parks excelled at work that ranged from aiding homeless constituents to joining Conyers in protesting a General Motors decision to close local plants.*** *Plus her past wasn't forgotten; Conyers once remarked, "Rosa Parks was so famous that people would come by my office to meet her, not me."*

Years after the boycott, Parks was still a target

Unfortunately, Parks was not always universally admired. For many white people who wanted to maintain the racist status quo, she'd been a hated figure since the Montgomery bus boycott. During that action, they'd made menacing calls and sent death threats. ***The attacks had been so venomous that Parks' husband Raymond suffered a nervous breakdown.***

Though the boycott had ended in 1956, hateful missives continued to be sent to Parks into the 1970s. She was accused of being traitor and of harboring Communist sympathies. (Racists often felt African Americans were not capable of organizing on their own and had to be getting outside help.)

Even working for Conyers, she remained a target; rotten watermelons and hate mail arrived for her at his office when she started there. ***Yet, as always, such cruel attacks didn't keep Parks from doing her job.***

Autobiography and Memoir

In 1992, Parks published Rosa Parks: My Story, *an autobiography recounting her life in the segregated South. In 1995, she published* Quiet Strength, *which includes her memoirs and focuses on the role that religious faith played throughout her life.*

Accomplishments and Awards

Parks received many accolades during her lifetime, including the Spingarn Medal, the NAACP's highest award, and the prestigious Martin Luther King Jr. Award.

On September 15, 1996, President Bill Clinton awarded Parks the Presidential Medal of Freedom, the highest honor given by the United States' executive branch. The following year, she was awarded the Congressional Gold Medal, the highest award given by the U.S. legislative branch.

TIME *magazine named Parks on its 1999 list of "The 20 Most Influential People of the 20th Century."*

... Also in February 2013, President Barack Obama unveiled a statue designed by Robert Firmin and sculpted by Eugene Daub honoring Parks in the nation's Capitol building. He remembered Parks, according to The New York Times, *by saying "In a single moment, with the simplest of gestures, she helped change America and change the world. . . . And today, she takes her rightful place among those who shaped this nation's course."*

QG Psychophysics Interpretation

Consistent with a character rooted on the Hyper Quadratic Operator, Rosa Park's life has unquestionably been one of very tall stoicism and heroism in the unrelenting pursuit of implanting the social norm of racial equality in the USA. Having witnessed how her grandfather used to adopt a strong stance against Alabama's Klu Klux Klan and with great grandfathers that were slaves, she was already firmly driven psychosocially to the life of prominent civil right and social activism that she was predisposed for by her character type. It further appears that with a grandfather like hers, the complete absence of her father through the course of her life did not lessen the paternal drive to develop personal instigative abilities throughout her upbringing. In addition, the very active presence of both a mother and grandmother in her life certainly accorded her a strong precapacity for empathy.

These conditions seemingly contributed to a level of equilibrium in her political activism whereby we see her espousing to a certain extent Malcolm X's views of opposing violence with violence, but engaging instead in the practices of passive resistance advocated and executed by Martin L. King.

The following chronicle drawn from the excerpts aims at highlighting those acts and events impulsed by hyperactive right-chiral pensive qualities in Layer 4 of Rosa's Mental Body as well as the deep shame fomented in her by racial segregation. Perhaps these unexpressed feelings of shame partly informed her decision to remain childless. Yet late in her life, as childless as she was, she expressed that *"Racism is still with us. But it is up to us to prepare our children for what they have to meet, and, hopefully, we shall overcome."* Also note that before that day when she decided to refuse giving up her seat, she had given in in previous accasions time and time again and must not have felt good about herself for doing so to say the least.

"Parks' grandfather stood in front of their house with a shotgun while Ku Klux Klan members marched down the street.

Parks' mother moved the family to Pine Level, Alabama, to live with her parents, Rose and Sylvester Edwards. *Her parents, James and Leona McCauley, separated when Parks was two.*

African American students were forced to walk to the first through sixth-grade schoolhouse, while the city of Pine Level provided bus transportation as well as a new school building for white students.

Parks [courageously] left school to attend to both her sick grandmother and mother back in Pine Level.

After marrying in 1932, she earned her high school degree in 1933 with her husband's support.

Parks was a civil rights activist before her arrest. Parks was a long-time member of the Montgomery chapter of the National Association for the Advancement of

Colored People (NAACP), which she joined in 1943. At the time of her arrest, she was a secretary of the local NAACP chapter, and the previous summer she had attended a workshop for social and economic justice at Tennessee's Highlander Folk School. Her political activism continued through the boycott and the rest of her life.

[About the contravening slender that wanted Parks to just have been tired when she refused to give in to the bus driver, she writes:] *"I was forty-two. No, the only tired I was, was tired of giving in."*

Yet the boycott's conclusion didn't make it easy for either of them to get back to earning a living — Parks was too identified with the protest for her or her husband to land another regular job in Alabama.

... [civil right] male leadership did not identify with Parks' needs.

In the end, she decided her only choice was to leave Alabama with her husband and mother.

In 1957, Parks and her family went to Detroit,... ***Then she had an operation for an ulcer (a condition that had developed under the stress of the bus boycott), and needed to have a throat tumor removed.*** *In July 1960,...* Jet *magazine described her as a "tattered rag of her former self — penniless, debt-ridden, ailing with stomach ulcers, and a throat tumor, compressed into two rooms with her husband and mother."*

Parks also found much to appreciate in Malcolm X's leadership. Her beliefs more closely aligned with Malcolm's, and differed from King's, on the limits of nonviolence.

After Conyers won the election, he hired Parks as a receptionist and assistant for his Detroit office.

And Parks excelled at work that ranged from aiding homeless constituents to joining Conyers in protesting a General Motors decision to close local plants.

Years after the boycott, Parks was still a target. *The attacks had been so venomous that Parks' husband Raymond suffered a nervous breakdown.*

Though the boycott had ended in 1956, hateful missives continued to be sent to Parks into the 1970s. She was accused of being traitor and of harboring Communist sympathies. (Racists often felt African Americans were not capable of organizing on their own and had to be getting outside help.)

Even working for Conyers, she remained a target; rotten watermelons and hate mail arrived for her at his office when she started there. ***Yet, as always, such cruel attacks didn't keep Parks from doing her job."***

" Parks received many accolades during her lifetime, including the Spingarn Medal, the NAACP's highest award, and the prestigious Martin Luther King Jr. Award. On September 15, 1996, President Bill Clinton awarded Parks the Presidential Medal of Freedom, the highest honor given by the United States' executive branch. The following year, she was awarded the Congressional Gold Medal, the highest award given by the U.S. legislative branch. TIME *magazine named Parks on its 1999 list of "The 20 Most Influential People of the 20th Century." ... Also in February 2013, President Barack Obama unveiled a statue designed by Robert Firmin and sculpted by Eugene Daub honoring Parks in the nation's Capitol building. He remembered Parks, according to* The New York Times, *by saying "In a single moment, with the simplest of gestures, she helped change America and change the world."*

Elizabeth Taylor

Hyper-Asymptotic Character

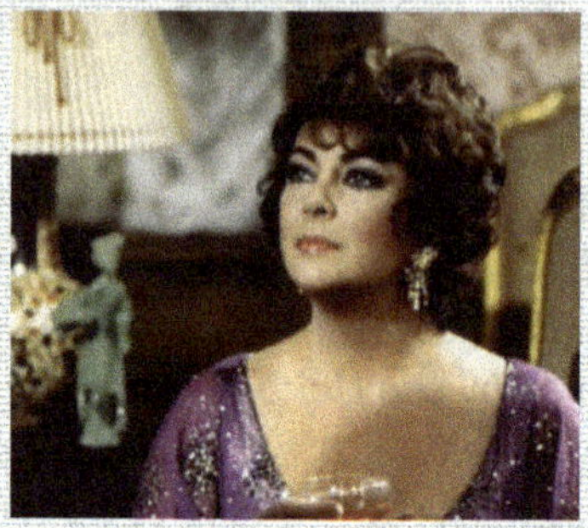

The Guardian *- Elizabeth Taylor evokes more images than the number of husbands she had. She was the breathtakingly beautiful child who ... seemed to slip into adulthood unscarred by her precocious professional success; the sultry dramatic actress; the compulsive bride, who went through husbands like fashion trends; the scarlet woman who broke up America's sweethearts, Eddie Fisher and Debbie Reynolds; the female half of what can very legitimately be described as the greatest love affair of the 20th century; the most beautiful woman in the world; front-page stalwart of the National Enquirer; star of some of the best movies of her era; star of some of the worst celebrity perfume adverts; the gay rights campaigner; the defender of Michael Jackson...*

Even towards the end of her life, Taylor, despite near incapacitation, still not only understood the increasingly ridiculous celebrity world, but proved that – to paraphrase a quote from her most photographed role – age could not wither her. She was one of the most mature users of Twitter and her Twitter feed was so Tayloresque as to be nigh-on parodic, mixing passionate defences of Jackson with shout-outs to reality TV android Kim Kardashian and the occasional – and necessary – denials that she had re-re-re-re-re-re-re-re-remarried ("Jason is my dearest friend!" she tweeted last year, at the age of 78, with an understandable giggle).

...“My troubles all started because I have a woman's body and a child's emotions,” she also said, according to ABC News

Biography.com.- *Throughout her life, Taylor wed seven men in eight marriages (she married Richard Burton twice), but by the time she died on March 23, 2011, she hadn’t been married since 1996, almost 15 years. Here’s a complete list of Taylor’s husbands:*

Taylor met Conrad "Nicky" Hilton, the son of hotelier Conrad Hilton (and future great-uncle of Paris Hilton), in October 1949 at Mocambo nightclub in Los Angeles — and they were wed on May 6, 1950, at Beverly Hills' Church of the Good Shepherd with 600 guests in attendance and an additional 3,000 fans outside. She wore a $3,500 gown at the ceremony, which MGM paid for since her film Father of the Bride was coming out. Even though Taylor was only 18 at the time of her first marriage, it wasn't her first engagement. She had been previously engaged to football player Glenn Davis and billionaire Bill Pawley.

Michael Wilding *(Married February 1952 to January 1957)*

Barely a year after her divorce from Hilton, Taylor wed British actor Michael Wilding who was 20 years her senior and also on marriage number two. During their five years together, Taylor gave birth to two sons, Michael Jr. and Christopher. Christopher told Hollywood Reporter that growing up, he and his brother could play with Taylor's Golden Globes, but not her Oscars. Eventually, as Taylor's career skyrocketed, the couple's relationship soured.

Mike Todd *(Married February 1957 to March 1958)*

By the time Taylor married entertainment producer Mike Todd ... a month after her divorce from Wilding, she was pregnant with their child, Liza. Todd was known to shower the young star with gifts, like the time he set up an entire display of Van Cleef & Arpels jewelry in their yard or the time he had a meal flown in from Paris. Tragically Todd was killed in a plane crash in 1958 — Taylor was supposed to travel with him, but had opted out since she had a cold. "I was the happiest with Mike Todd," Taylor said during her later years.

Eddie Fisher *(Married May 1959 to March 1964)*

Devastated by the tragedy of Todd's death, Taylor turned one of their closest couple friends, Debbie Reynolds *and her husband* Eddie Fisher, *one of the 1950s most popular singers. (Fisher had been a best man at Taylor and Todd's wedding.) But soon Taylor and Fisher started an affair and Fisher left Reynolds. "I divorced Debbie and married Elizabeth the day I finished my run at the Tropicana, " Fisher said,* according to **Vogue**. *"It was a typical two-rabbi Jewish ceremony. As usual, Elizabeth was late for her own wedding... We were married under the chuppah, a canopy, and as is traditional, at the end of the ceremony, I stomped on a wine glass." Taylor had said, "Our honeymoon will last 40 years,"* **according to ABC News**. *Five years later, they divorced.*

Richard Burton *(Married March 1964 to June 1974 and October 1975 to August 1976)*

Taylor was still married to Fisher when she reconnected with Burton on the **Cleopatra** *set in 1962 (they had met at a party a decade before that). "When I saw him on the set of* **Cleopatra**, *I fell in love and I have loved him ever since, practically my whole adult life," she wrote in* People. *Their romance was so passionate, it often* ignited into fights. *Ironically, after starring together in a 1973 TV movie* Divorce His, Divorce Hers, *they actually divorced a year later. But by October 1975, they remarried — though it didn't even last a whole year. "Even when we could no longer live together, we continued to love each other," she continued in 1988. "To this day, my feelings for him are so strong I cannot speak about him without being overcome with emotion."*

John Warner *(Married December 1976 to November 1982)*

After her double marriage to Burton, Taylor turned to politics — for love, that is. She wed former U.S. Secretary of the Navy John Warner, who later became a five-term U.S. Senator for Virginia. The two met at a Washington, D.C., dinner for Queen Elizabeth II, at which Warner was asked to escort Taylor. Even though he's a Republican and she was a Democrat, they connected, especially over their shared love of horses. "I found her very interesting, fascinating. She is a great conversationalist, and she is just a lot of fun," he told **People**. *They remained friendly until her 2011 death.*

Larry Fortensky *(Married October 1991 to October 1996)*

Taylor's final marriage was to a construction worker who she met during her time in rehab at the Betty Ford Clinic in 1988. "Elizabeth was in there for pills, I was in there for beer," he told **People**. *"I knew who she was, of course, but I can't tell you that I remember watching any of her films. She was funny and sweet, and the more I got to know her, the sweeter she became...we had an instant physical attraction." They wed at Michael Jackson's Neverland Ranch and while they had playful moments together, ultimately the spotlight was too much. "Those cameras everywhere... Elizabeth was used to it. I never got used to it," he said. "I have wonderful memories of my time with Elizabeth, and I will treasure her memory forever... I love her. I always will. And I know she loved me too." They also kept in touch for the remainder of her life.*

Those born in the 40s will probably remember her as the wife of Richard Burton and the actor who radiated sex without ever being as coarsely upfront with her assets as, say, Monroe or Jane Russell. Those born in the 70s will have the slightly less erotic image of Taylor as the wife of the unforgettably named Larry Fortensky, sporting makeup, jewellery and hair that makes Russell Brand today look a bit low-key. Yet she was equally famous to those born in either decade, and this is not just because of her ever fluid image but her fearlessness at breaking social mores.

Her close friendships with gay actors – most notably Rock Hudson and Montgomery Clift – showed her to be more open-minded than most in an age when homosexuality was career-threatening. Taylor did more than pretty much anyone in her era by helping to remove the stigma of both homosexuality and, tragically, Aids by her loyalty to Hudson when he was dying from the disease.

Just as scandalous in its way was Taylor's relationship with Burton. Both were married when they met and neither made any attempt to hide not just their love for one another but their lust. Now divorce is as common among actors as undeserved Oscars but Taylor and Burton still look red-blooded next to today's anaemic Hello! wedding spreads. The publication last year of Furious Love: Elizabeth Taylor, Richard Burton and the Marriage of the Century, by Sam Kashner and Nancy Schoenberger, truly puts to shame today's pretenders, not least with its inclusion of Burton's love letters to Taylor. But there was one letter even Taylor, the consummate celebrity, couldn't share with the public: the last one Burton wrote to her just before his death in 1984, saying he wanted to come home, and Taylor was home. That letter remained where it has ever since she received it: in her dressing table drawer, next to her bed.

Carrie Fisher compares her mother, Debbie Reynolds, and her father, Eddie Fisher, to Brad Pitt and Jennifer Aniston, with Taylor – who made Fisher her husband number four – playing the Angelina Jolie role. It is a smart riff, neatly evoking the media hysteria that accompanied Fisher and Taylor's affair while he was still with Reynolds and the ensuing marriage (and, inevitably, divorce – there was no way little Fisher could ever compete with the mountain of machismo that was Richard Burton).

...Taylor had the life, the looks, the movies, the smarts and the talent, and she ... looked as if she not only enjoyed the occasional plate of pasta but my God, to watch her eat it would have been an experience in itself. As they say in Hollywood, it's the films that got small.

QG Psychophysic Interpretation

The center axis of observable behavior in Elizabeth Taylor's life had been the exaggerated, the big and bigger than life, the incommensurate, in one word, the asymptotic! The great constant of her life had been love-match, or sexuality. Her sexual life, however, had been overtaken by the central trend in her character, the incommensurate. Her spectacular beauty easily seduces many men, and of note is the fact that her sexuality did not take the likes of behavior identifiable with the Matrixial character, that is to say, love-passion with its share of deep wrenching commotion leading to despair, grief and profound turmoil when the losses and sentimental aggravations occur.

Instead, she seduces her match and engages with him in legal matrimony for the exercise of her female attributes and faculties, in sexual enjoyment and much desired maternity. She wrote of herself in young age:

"As I learned how to perfect my screen image, I determined to find an area where I could comfortably move into independent adulthood. I soon realized the only way I could escape was through marriage." She also wrote:

"I am sorry I did not fully understand the reasons driving me into early matrimony. At the time, I just knew I ached to become a real woman, a wife."

After a few years of marriage, she will shut down the matrimony while keeping a quasi loving relationship with her ex husbands **in the distance,** or platonically, if you will. She never referred with animosity to any of them. She said of Todd that he was her best love. She even provided financial assistance to ex husband Larry Fortensky at his several requests. She confessed her unending love for Richard Burton, whom she married twice, and who may have been her only true love, by her own admission.

Her extrapolating overture and overboard sensitiveness are not only expressed in seducing her match, but in further driving him to idolizing her. Often, she and her husband of the moment take hospitality in not only one luxurious hotel suite but include the entire floor above and below as well for the duration of their stay! All of which goes in hand with the incommensurate of her character as well.

Enemy of the petty, she remained in defiant defense of her friend Michael Jackson who the media and the entertainment establishment took, in the view of many, to ridicule and vilify for many years. She even celebrated one of her marriages in his ranch. She also remained in open support of her homosexual friends, Rock Hudson and Montgomery Clift, affected by AIDS, at the time at the risk of harming her own celebrity status. She further instituted a foundation to provide assistance to those affected by the disease. Arguably, it is also in defense of what she saw as the pettiness and narrow scope of social customs that she made no secret of her involvement with married men she fell in love with until a divorce freed them up for her. In the process, she gained for herself the attention and idolatry of an entire planet!

Finally, the lack of practical sense is incontrovertibly clear in the fact of eight consecutive marriages, remarriage with the same person, an early marriage with a man 20 years older and an endless list of romances. To many her love life qualified as dysfunctional. If one can never judge the profound ontological meaning in every life as predetermined by character, however dysfunctional they may appear, one can at least see where common sense is strikingly missing.

Chapter 4

A UNIQUE DISEASE MODEL FOR ALL MENTAL DISORDERS

The broadest categorization of mental pathologies in psychology was until recently the duplet consisting in *neurosis* and *psychosis*, which has been submitted to reconsideration in the last decade. Notwithstanding their pinpointing to a class-level classification, these terms do not currently convey consensually stringent definitions in psychology and psychiatry. In building a disease model toward unraveling the etiologies of the entire spectrum of Mental Disorders of psychological origin for better diagnosis, it is important to address and rigorize their definitions from a theoretical viewpoint. The etiologies of most mental diseases are knowingly not at all understood in allopathic psychiatry, as gathered in the glossary of clinical mental disorders exposed in the next Chapter per current research literature and common clinical practice in the field. While analytic psychology apportions answers to how mental disease occurs, predominantly from unconscious drives and inner conflicts, the deeper understanding of why unconscious transactions occur generically the way they do, which spells out authentic clues to adequate etiological interpretations, is not at all understood. In this chapter, we present the psychophysics etiological foundations of the entire spectrum of known Mental Disorders, to be followed by a compendium view of each of these Disorders in the next Chapter. This effort aims at providing the psychotherapist with an insightful comprehension of the etiological mechanisms underlying every clinical mental disorder for best practice. In this cast of our study, we stay clear of neurologic presentations and elaborations, given our antimonist position that it is only possible to intelligibly and parsimoniously elicit observable expression of the central nervous system on the psychological plane through complete segregation of neurologic functions from the functional Architecture of Mentation in its fullness.

4.1 Curing Imprecise Definitions of Neurosis

The use of the term *neurosis* (originally *psychoneurosis*) in psychological literature is frankly quite disparate in alloted semantics. Many psychotherapists utilize the term to describe a spectrum of mental illnesses outside of psychotic disorders. It was originally coined in the 18th century to label a range of psychological disorders that could not be attributed to a physical cause. Modern psychologists and psychiatrists today have come to utilize the term neurosis to qualify anxious symptoms and behaviors. Pioneering psychoanalysts Sigmund Freud and Carl G. Jung inarguably made a completely different use of the term when they applied it to the description of mentation processes themselves.

Therefore no unique definition of the term neurosis exists. Accordingly, the official science deprecated the term neurosis for etiological reports in 1980, setting a diagnosis of *Depression* or *Anxiety* Disorder for what mental disease was previously understood to be a neurosis. Until then, psychotherapists had arrived at the minimal consensus that a neurosis was a diagnosable psychological Disorder which degrades quality of life *without disrupting the individual's perception of reality*. Albeit fallen in disuse, many psychotherapists further acknowledge the importance of the concept in understanding modern therapies applied to psychological disorders.

We are going to further analyze the concept in what appeared to have garnered consensual acknowledgment. It is important to highlight at the outset that neurosis or psychoneurosis is a not an individual disease descriptor but a class descriptor of diseases. The commonality in that class of mental diseases had been explored over the centuries, per recount below.

1. First to have coined the term in 1769, Dr. William Kullen, from Scotland, claimed the meaning of term to be*"disorders of sense and motion caused by a general affection of the nervous system."* Dr. Kullen included in his definition epilepsy and coma disorders.

2. According to the German-British psychologist Hans Jürgen Eysenck (1916-1997), *neurosis is defined by emotional instability.*
3. For the founder of Psychoanalysis, neurologist Sigmund Freud (1856-1939), neurosis is a *coping strategy in response to repressed emotions* from unpleasant past experience that may or may not have been altogether contained within the unconscious.
4. The Swiss psychiatrist Carl Gustav Jung (1875-1961) who founded analytic psychology from Freudian advances believed that a neurosis was *a clash of conscious and unconscious events* in the mind.
5. More recently, neurosis has come to refer to *the group of mental disorders that do not interfere with rational thought or the individual's ability to function*, even though they may cause distress.

In highlight in these definitions are: ability to still function properly in **conscious** daily living despite the morbid symptoms, clash between **conscious awareness/rationale** and unconscious drives, a conscious **coping strategy** to respond to repressed emotions, an emotional instability experienced during **conscious** daily living. All of which is in accord with the squint consensus reached about a definition of neurosis as a diagnosable psychological Disorder which degrades quality of life *without disrupting the individual's perception of reality.*

In seeking a fitting umbrella for this characterization within our psychophysics framework, it is important to recall what we have outlined in our mathematical-physics definition of the Conscious v. the Unconscious in Chapter 1: "*Viewed from the covariant vantage between the two orthogonal variables... it is because our conscious thoughts feature dominance of volition over presentation/motivation that they acquire the constricted quality that characterizes them. They are sober and constrained thoughts, so to speak,* ***with a realistic quality to them... The conscious language only bears one dimension in that every term means one thing****, synonyms and homonyms being a few exceptions to the rule.*"

It is equally important to recall in this context our definition of Self-Awareness:

Self-Awareness is the invariant discrete bundle of Sense of Self and adjoint Self-Effector which remains preserved under emotional alterations, exercise of rea-

son and purposeful activity as well as across changing developmental stages during the lifecycle. It is expressed both during the mental states of arousal and during the phases of nocturnal sleep eliciting dreaming activity.

In further pursuing our mathematical-physics rendition of mental phenomena for utmost objectivity and accuracy, we define neurosis on the basis of geometric symmetry in the following manner:

Definition 1a: *A neurosis is the paroxysmal transformation in the intensity level of the pensive partitions of one Layer of the Mental Foliate, whether partial, half chiral or total, while the conscious Sense of Self and adjoint Self-Effector remain invariant or unaltered.*

Definition 2a: *A neurosis may also be a paroxysmal transformation in the density level of the hypocursor as a monolith while remaining invariantly captive within the boundaries of the conscious cognos.*

As a reminder, the *hypocursor* is a designation for the mentation cursor as it sojourns within the boundaries of the Conscious cognos (Layer 1 through Layer 3).

The above definitions, notably Definition 1a, gather what has been consensually known to neuroses as previously indicated, while providing an objective measurable basis for this class of mental impairment. We have shown the preliminary basis for that measure in Chapter 3 in the characterization of a metric for Layer intensity paroxysm. We will soon show the specifics of its application to neurosis and psychosis. Further advantage of this approach is to provision the etiological primitives that consistently define a coherent taxonomy of mental diseases and to elucidate the nature and reason of their particular semiology and nosology. Accordingly, we are departing from the categorizations of mood disorder and personality disorder, which our psychophysics mental Foliate does not quite support in the way they are generally presented.

4.1.1 Taxonomic Impropriety of the Mood Label for Disorders

Psychologically, a mood is an affective state of mind created by inner feelings accompanied with facial and physiognomic expressions or attitudes respectively. At the forefront of the construct of mood is emotion with which it is interchangeable to some extent. Except for the mentation partitions of Layer 3 in the Foliate map, most of the other partitions in the map, if not all, show a certain connotation attributable to mood, some in greater measure than others. For instance, it is difficult to deny moody fit or attitude altogether to a stingy person bent on cupidity most of the time or an envious individual prone to begrudge others' possessions at the slightest chance. Even in the Layer 3 partition of Aberration, in the case of a person prone to aberrant personal opinions, one may discern a certain emotional moody fit in discourse expressing those viewpoints. Inasmuch as mood is associated with emotions, it becomes a property assimilable to the *t*-axis of the QG coordinate system and as such attributable to all the mentation partitions of the Foliate. Therefore on the basis of the normalization inherent to the Foliate map, we do not find systematic support for the taxonomic use of the construct of mood in mental disorders in the rather unspecific and imprecise manner in which it is generally presented. We will later show how to usefully redimension this notion within the QG psychophysics context.

4.1.2 Impropriety of the Personality Disorder Category

Likewise we find improper the notion of personality disorders. Personality is defined in psychiatry to be *"the way of thinking, feeling and behaving that makes a person* ***different from other people****. A personality disorder is a way of thinking, feeling and behaving that deviates from the expectations of the culture, causes distress or problems functioning, and lasts over time."* Because it is at times so difficult to determine the boundaries between illness and normality, some disorders appearing to be an exaggeration of normal and socio-dependent behavior, it is quite understandable for official mental science to attempt to establish a continuum between behavior or personality typified to be normal, on one hand, and morbidity on the other hand. By the same token, establishing the objective basis for defining human personalities will not be exempt of subjectivity if estranged from pure mathematical characterization as a strict warrant of rigor. Furthermore, it may not be quite realistic and proper to establish a standard of *"difference from other people"* when seeking to establish types that are expected to taxonomically gather all possible groups in a population distribution.

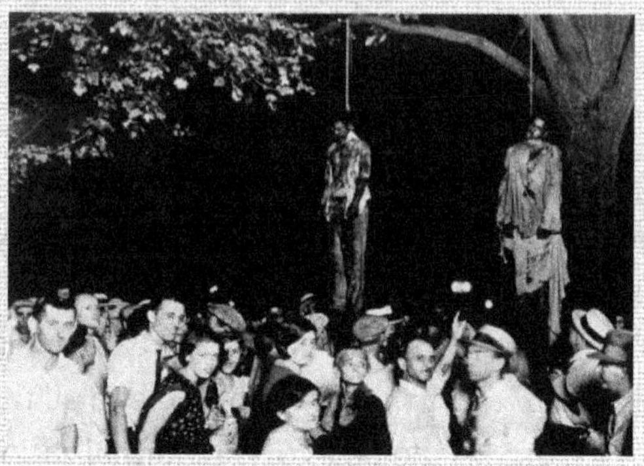

What's more, sociocultural references to define normality or the acceptable is outright improper, albeit understandable in the lack of better insight, because collective abnormality did play an integral part in mankind's history and cannot therefore be disregarded. Examples of this collective folly are centuries of dehumanization of African blacks through bondage, genocidal antisemite Nazism or the past Austral apartheid regime. The standard of psychological normality must not be dependent on sociocultural convenience or codes but mandatorily based on detached mathematical descriptors or mathematical-physics formalism, if it is to be as objective a measure as might be. Suffice it to remember that medicine would not accept a standard of cultural norms to qualify and diagnose serious physiological conditions, i.e. cancer or diabetes, no more than human mentation abnormalities should be, at best effort, coded in reference to social norms.

4.2 Curing Imprecise Definitions of Psychosis

In official psychological and psychiatric science, a clear and rigorous definition of psychosis has not been reached to date. Hence a differential diagnosis method is still at the tentative phase as acknowledged by the APA (American Psychiatric Association) in an open petition to clinicians and researchers to apportion continuous clinical data to that aim (Fig. 4.1):

" The APA is offering a number of "emerging measures" for further research and clinical evaluation. These patient assessment measures were developed to be administered at the initial patient interview and to monitor treatment progress. They should be used in research and evaluation as potentially useful tools to enhance clinical decision-making and not as the sole basis for making a clinical di-

agnosis. Instructions, scoring information, and interpretation guidelines are provided; further background information can be found in DSM-5. The APA requests that clinicians and researchers provide further data on the instruments' usefulness in characterizing patient status and improving patient care at http://www.dsm5.org/Pages/Feedback-Form.aspx."

The diseases of mania and depression, whether individually considered or in their joint syndromal manifestation, represent two more important markers for the diagnosis of psychosis. This proposition imputes that any one of these two disorders, including the bipolar expression, is to be considered an expression of psychosis. Avolition elicited in the absence or marked diminution of emotional expression is also proposed as a symptom of psychosis. It is important to realize that what the proposition infers is that if mania, depression or manic depression (bipolar disorder) is a diagnosis, then the condition is to be qualified a psychotic one. So the other proposed symptoms ought to be interpreted as well, should they present with a moderate or severe level. In other words, the proposition seems to essentially pose that psychosis is a pathological class, not an individual disease per se, and to which certain mental disorders may belong. We are further driven to this conclusion when we consider that most practicing clinicians consider schizophrenia i.e. to be a psychosis. By the same token, we must recognize that if psychosis is a pathological class, then it cannot be an individual disease at the same time, as it appears, lest a serious taxonomic and etiological interpretation problem arises.

One other important proposed marker for psychosis is the level of severity of psychomotor manifestion. In other words, when there is clear involuntary motion, we are not strictly dealing with the conscious but largely the unconscious. Although tics are involuntary motion that may be present in neuroses, there is the recognition that such severe involuntary motion as hand wriggling or catatonia must be symptomatic of deeper unconscious impairments. To this nosological count of the involuntary component, we must join the addition of avolition in the diagnostic proposition. The proposition recognizes that the lack of emotional expression, a void in facial expressivity, lack of personalized gestures and most importantly absence of self-initiated behavior are characteristic of avolition and count toward a psychosis diagnosis.

Clinician-Rated Dimensions of Psychosis Symptom Severity

Name:______________________ Age:______ Sex: [ ] Male [ ] Female Date:______________

Instructions: Based on all the information you have on the individual and using your clinical judgment, please rate (with checkmark) the presence and severity of the following symptoms as experienced by the individual in the past seven (7) days.

Domain	0	1	2	3	4	Score
I. Hallucinations	❑ Not present	❑ Equivocal (severity or duration not sufficient to be considered psychosis)	❑ Present, but mild (little pressure to act upon voices, not very bothered by voices)	❑ Present and moderate (some pressure to respond to voices, or is somewhat bothered by voices)	❑ Present and severe (severe pressure to respond to voices, or is very bothered by voices)	
II. Delusions	❑ Not present	❑ Equivocal (severity or duration not sufficient to be considered psychosis)	❑ Present, but mild (little pressure to act upon delusional beliefs, not very bothered by beliefs)	❑ Present and moderate (some pressure to act upon beliefs, or is somewhat bothered by beliefs)	❑ Present and severe (severe pressure to act upon beliefs, or is very bothered by beliefs)	
III. Disorganized speech	❑ Not present	❑ Equivocal (severity or duration not sufficient to be considered disorganization)	❑ Present, but mild (some difficulty following speech)	❑ Present and moderate (speech often difficult to follow)	❑ Present and severe (speech almost impossible to follow)	
IV. Abnormal psychomotor behavior	❑ Not present	❑ Equivocal (severity or duration not sufficient to be considered abnormal psychomotor behavior)	❑ Present, but mild (occasional abnormal or bizarre motor behavior or catatonia)	❑ Present and moderate (frequent abnormal or bizarre motor behavior or catatonia)	❑ Present and severe (abnormal or bizarre motor behavior or catatonia almost constant)	
V. Negative symptoms (restricted emotional expression or avolition)	❑ Not present	❑ Equivocal decrease in facial expressivity, prosody, gestures, or self-initiated behavior	❑ Present, but mild decrease in facial expressivity, prosody, gestures, or self-initiated behavior	❑ Present and moderate decrease in facial expressivity, prosody, gestures, or self-initiated behavior	❑ Present and severe decrease in facial expressivity, prosody, gestures, or self-initiated behavior	
VI. Impaired cognition	❑ Not present	❑ Equivocal (cognitive function not clearly outside the range expected for age or SES; i.e., within 0.5 SD of mean)	❑ Present, but mild (some reduction in cognitive function; below expected for age and SES, 0.5–1 SD from mean)	❑ Present and moderate (clear reduction in cognitive function; below expected for age and SES, 1–2 SD from mean)	❑ Present and severe (severe reduction in cognitive function; below expected for age and SES, > 2 SD from mean)	
VII. Depression	❑ Not present	❑ Equivocal (occasionally feels sad, down, depressed, or hopeless; concerned about having failed someone or at something but not preoccupied)	❑ Present, but mild (frequent periods of feeling very sad, down, moderately depressed, or hopeless; concerned about having failed someone or at something, with some preoccupation)	❑ Present and moderate (frequent periods of deep depression or hopelessness; preoccupation with guilt, having done wrong)	❑ Present and severe (deeply depressed or hopeless daily; delusional guilt or unreasonable self-reproach grossly out of proportion to circumstances)	
VIII. Mania	❑ Not present	❑ Equivocal (occasional elevated, expansive, or irritable mood or some restlessness)	❑ Present, but mild (frequent periods of somewhat elevated, expansive, or irritable mood or restlessness)	❑ Present and moderate (frequent periods of extensively elevated, expansive, or irritable mood or restlessness)	❑ Present and severe (daily and extensively elevated, expansive, or irritable mood or restlessness)	

Note. SD = standard deviation; SES = socioeconomic status.

Copyright © 2013 American Psychiatric Association. All Rights Reserved.
This material can be reproduced without permission by researchers and by clinicians for use with their patients.

Fig. 4.1 A tentative classificatory proposal by the American Psychiatric Association toward diagnosis of psychotic dysfunction severity

The diagnosis of severity of **Cognitive impairment** begs some discussion from our psychophysics viewpoint. Cognition is generally understood to be *the mental action or process of acquiring knowledge as well as comprehending through thought, experience and the senses, all with the support of memory*. All in all, teleology stands for a quite fitting generic philosophical construct to sum up content of cognition.

Cognitive impairment is spelled out as trouble learning new things, concentrating, remembering or making practical decisions affecting one's standing in every day life. Cognitive impairment is acknowledged to be manifest in:

- Mental Confusion
- Poor motor coordination
- Identity confusion
- Tenuous or deficient judgment
- Loss of short-term or long-term memory

In cognitive science and psychology, cognition is generally understood to be an attribution of the Conscious. It is openly at play in the process of learning where the faculty of reasoning plays a key role. However, as much as teleology is integral to cognition, it is not possible to advocate its absence in several high profile mental disorders such as Mania, Bipolar Disorder in the manic phase, Schizophrenia, etc. It is well known that there exists a high level of insightfulness in Mania and Bipolar Disorder to the point that they can inspire masterpieces in artistic expression, including literary intellectual authoring. Schizophrenia may inspire some of the most heightened painting expressions verging on symbolism. Patients with Mania or in the manic phase of Bipolar Disorder may be able to exercise acute judgement allowing them to keenly pick personality defects of their relatives or peers on which they can return very abusive and disparaging language. A differential diagnosis in this case becomes problematic because the inclusion of those diseases for the qualification of psychosis becomes mutually exclusive with Cognitive Impairment.

4.3 Redimensioning the Notion of Delusion

1.- A delusion is a disorder whereby a person has an *unshakable belief in something untrue,* according to some common dictionaries fed by literature from the science. Another Dictionary definition of ***delusion***: *"an idiosyncratic belief or impression that is firmly maintained despite being contradicted by what is generally accepted as reality or rational argument, typically a symptom of mental disorder."*

A delusion may more precisely be defined as a form of distorted mental representation whereby elements of reality take a factitious overtone in conforming opinion or a consciously held belief by an individual. In this form of representation the mind has partially departed reality, in that it dresses reality in a partially different way than commonly assumed. It is still however making contact with reality, in past or present. In the Conscious Cognos, the Human Mind constantly makes discrete anticipating projections. Nonetheless, the Conscious Cognos is endowed with the faculty to distinguish or discriminate between perceived and memorized elements of reality and unreal self-projections. All 3 layers of the Conscious Mind are infused with this capacity. From the intense motivation to *possess* (Layer 1) elements of reality to the intense motivation to *capture* or *inquest* (Layer 2) elements of reality to the intense motivation to *associate* (Layer 3) elements of reality, the Conscious Cognos imprints this reality-oriented vector to the Hypocursor and so informs its ingrained Self-Awareness and Self-Identity.

When somebody who appears to be otherwise quite normal firmly believes that reality around himself/herself is fake or does not exist, or that his brain cells are fake along with all the other cells and atoms and electrons that make up his body, the subject's mind is certainly edging the state of delusion. To believe that reality around oneself is fake or false, one must already acknowledge the perception of that reality. Hence what the mind does in this case is to simply deny that reality, having lost the imperative of sound criteria to assess the same.

Furthermore, should we acknowledge the basis of collective recognition invoked in the definition, because **everybody else** believes that the person's body and being and habitat **are real and exist**, despite the person's wish, that individual's thought comes to fully meet the criteria of the definition for being delusional. So it is because the basis of external reality would be given in common collective acknowledgment of the same. In this case, even other non human forms of the living agree on the nature of discrete perceptions of the natural world: gazelles and deers run away when tigers and other predators are running after them to have a meal as we humans may equally witness! They don't seem to think that the predators are innocuous imagined ghosts. Although different forms of the living may physically perceive one 3D reality, whether object or event, in different ways, they generally agree in cognition and behavior that the elements of that reality are not observer-dependent but observer-independent.

Should an adult individual feel an intense or compulsive love for animals or so much wants to protect them that he is willing to trespass into a zoo tiger den to be with the dangerous animal, that individual is most probably delusional. This news story may exemplify better:

Man Who Jumped into Bronx Zoo Tiger Den Gets Year in Mental Health Facility[12]

NEW YORK DAILY NEWS | Oct 15, 2013 at 3:21 PM

The man who wanted to become "one with the tiger" will become a one-year patient in a mental health facility.

David Villalobos, who survived a September 2012 leap into the Bronx Zoo's tiger den, pleaded guilty Tuesday to trespassing in the strange case, the Bronx district attorney said.

Under a plea bargain deal, Villalobos must complete a one-year stay in a mental health facility as part of his conditional discharge.

Villalobos, 26, managed to pet the 400-pound beast before the tiger mauled the former real estate agent.

---

[12] *https://www.nydailynews.com/new-york/bronx/man-jumped-bronx-zoo-tiger-den-year-mental-health-facility-article-1.1486473*

The defendant, who jumped from a passing monorail and scaled a fence to reach the pit, suffered a broken right shoulder, right ankle, rib and pelvis along with a punctured lung.

Villalobos was critically injured by 11-year-old Bachuta, a male Amur tiger, before zoo workers used fire extinguishers to drive the big cat away.

The state of delusion may rather be labeled an extreme form of neurosis, since conscious awareness is not lost in this form of impairment, for one. From the QG psychophysics viewpoint, the cursor in that state (hypocursor) still sweeps the 3 layers of the Foliate which delimit Consciousness or the Conscious Cognos. We can see in the example related in the above news chronicle that the elements of reality are fully acknowledged by the individual. It is the form of belief they nurture in the individual's conscious cognos, a subjective creation, that are *unrealistic or untrue to nature*. It is still possible to employ reason to temporarily dissuade someone from delusional thoughts or behavior, albeit obviously not to cure the impairment. We are thus on firm grounds to conclude that delusions are rather neurotic in nature, in accord with our definitions for neurosis. Therefore, we would discard delusion for inclusion in the set of criteria for psychosis as proposed.

4.4 Redimensioning the Notion of Hallucination

Hallucination is an experience involving the apparent perception of something that is not present or real. For instance, to keep a conversation with somebody that is not there, by reason of a projection of one's mind that puts the unreal person in the physical reality around, is to be hallucinating.

"When hallucinating, the patient hears a third party talk about him, hears a voice telling him i.e. that death is imminent, or that he is about to be put on death row. He "sees" the guillotine. He may even see the ghost of the dead recriminating his infamous conduct."

In hallucination, the mind perceives during the state of wake an unphysical reality with the likes of what is customarily physical or observable, and appears to create its own phenoma in a physically inexistent world. It is not possible at all to reason a hallucinating person.

Should a subject believe that he or she is the head of state of his/her country or has the grand power of resuscitating the dead, these forms of impaired thoughts outgrow the criteria for delusion because the object of the thought or the phenoma taken for granted is not factually part of reality. The mind, in those cases, has already completely stepped outside of reality and created its own or its own illusory world. These forms of thoughts are one step beyond delusion and outright qualify as hallucinations.

The state of hallucination must definitely be labeled an expression of psychosis, since conscious Awareness is completely lost in this form of impairment and gives way to unconscious Awareness. From the QG psychophysics viewpoint, the cursor in that state (hypercursor) is limited to sweep the 5 layers of the Foliate that delimit the Unconscious or the Unconscious Cognos.

Hence the following psychophysics definitions for psychosis:

Definition 1b: *A psychosis is the highest paroxysmal transformation in the intensity level of the pensive partitions of one Layer of the Mental Foliate, partial, half chiral or total, while the unconscious Sense of Self and adjoint Self-Effector remain invariant or unaltered.*

Definition 2b: *A psychosis may also be the highest paroxysmal transformation in the reciprocal density level of the hypercursor as a monolith while remaining invariantly captive within the boundaries of the Unconscious cognos.*

As a reminder, the *hypercursor* is our designation for the mentation cursor as it sojourns within the boundaries of the Unconscious cognos (Layer 5 through Layer 9).

4.5 Neurosis v. Psychosis

Our approach etiologically elucidates at a stroke the important fact that there is no difference in the nature of symptoms between these two classes of Dysfunction but essentially a difference in intensity of the symptoms. Research had long corroborated this commonality in the phenomal nature of associated symptoms. Ian Kelleher and Mary Cannon write in 2014[13]:

"The breakdown of traditional divisions between psychosis and neurosis has been on the horizon for some time. Claridge, for example, in 1972, argued that psychotic symptoms, rather than being qualitatively distinct from neurotic symptoms, represented extremes of cognitive and personality characteristics. There is now much evidence that psychotic symptoms are a common feature of neurotic disorders, and recent population research has demonstrated substantial covariation of mood and psychotic symptoms. Indeed, in 2 independent community studies, we recently found that a large majority of young people who reported psychotic symptoms had at least 1 nonpsychotic Axis-1 psychiatric disorder, demonstrating that where psychotic symptoms occur, they do so more commonly in the context of neurosis than of psychosis proper. In fact, psychotic symptoms were shown to be strong markers of risk for multimorbid neurotic disorders, with their prevalence increasing in a dose-response manner with the number of Axis-1 disorders. Psychosis, then, rather than being distinct from neurosis, can, in fact, reflect important features of, and inform about, neurotic psychopathology."

We have reached this redress by redimensioning key nosological elements of mental illness, in particular those proposed for rating psychosis symptom severity. The layered architecture along with normalized partition distribution inherent to the Mentation Foliate of our psychophysics model is key to this redress. It naturally provides two group cover classes, as known in mathematical Representation Theory, to fittingly absorb psychosis and neurosis, through QG typological categorization. Therefore every mental disease instigated by activity of a mentation Layer will have two forms of expression, either a neurotic one or a psychotic one. Other dimensions of classification with correlated pathologies are forthrightly predicted by the model, which we will address shortly. This categorization is an important dent in taking down the undesirably high multimorbidity rate in the current classification of mental pathologies.

---

[13] *Schizophrenia Bulletin*, Volume 40, Issue 2, March 2014, Pages 266–268, https://doi.org/10.1093/schbul/sbt230

A direct consequence of our model is that while all disorders based on Layer 5 through Layer 9 may present both forms of impairments (psychosis or neurosis), those based on Layer 1 through Layer 3 can only possibly present the neurotic form of impairment. So it is because it is not possible to lose contact with reality while the Conscious Cognos is in action, even more so when its activity is accrued. Due to the primacy of volition over representation/motivation, which percolates into the partitions making up the three sets of pensive Layers of this mentation province, the Conscious Cognos holds an almost unbreakable bond with reality. For the same reason, the projections realized by this Cognos, in order to develop the moment-to-moment activity undertaken by the individual, are of short spread. In effect, we must anticipatively project in our minds in a representational form what we want to do in order to successively undertake the activities of the day. For the most part, the elements of these micro projections are direct duplicates of elements of the natural world, before we imprint volitional dynamics to them. Further, there is a very short span or lag between these tight reality-driven projections and their execution by the Conscious Self-Effector.

If the impairment progresses to the scenario predicted in *Definition 1a*, insomnia will ensue as the Hypocursor will be unable to transition into the Unconscious Cognos by transforming into a Hypercursor. The association between many neuroses and their corresponding psychoses are well known in the field for many disorders, albeit officially unsettled thus far, akin to the association between characterological types and neuroses. For instance, Cyclothymia is well acknowledged to be the neurotic version of the psychosis of Bipolar Disorder. Paranoia i.e. had long been recognized as a *"deformation of character"* (Pierre Daco, 1960). The *schizoid character* knowingly predisposes to schizophrenia (Pierre Daco, 1960). It is clear that the axis that profiles a neurosis with its correlating psychosis equally traverses a particular defined character or temperament within our framework. As previously mentioned, we contemplate three accrual levels for each of the 9 axial Layers of the Foliate. We show in Fig. 4.6 how the association between neuroses and psychoses are construed based on etiology governed by Layers of the Mentation Foliate.

We will now attempt to resolve the very controversial subject of Pathological Lying in clinical mental science, the status of which as a psychosis or a neurosis has parked unending thorny debates. Likewise, we will subsequently address the discordant note that Mental Confusion, which is currently classified as a psychosis, seems to strike in our etiological framework.

4.6 Accrual Metric for Psychological Disorders

In Chapter 3, we have posited for the foundation of psychological character a natural level of predominance of one mental Layer over all others in terms of the intensity of its root partitions along with its superimposed representations and processes. Every human psyche experiences a predominance of **one** or another mental normal with respect to all others. Whenever the natural predominance of the one mental normal forming psychological character becomes disproportionate, mental dysfunction ensues. At the end, a dysfunctional mind is thus exactly like a normal or healthy mind insofar as the organization of structural components of the Mental Body. Hence the following principles:

Definition 1c: *The dynamics associated with one and only one mental normal account for the condition of an abnormal mind affected by a neurosis or a psychosis. Never two or more.*

Definition 2c: *The predominance associated with abnormality is always a sum up to that of the Layer responsible for the individual's psychological character to produce an absolute Level 4 or Level 5 paroxysm.*

Definition 3c: *An absolute Level 4 paroxysm defines a neurosis while an absolute Level 5 paroxysm defines a psychosis.*

According to the metric defined in Chapter 3 for Layer paroxysms, we obtain the equations below defining accrual levels for neurosis. We must remember that layer accruals at the level of psychological character or temperament were already asymmetric due to asymmetric gender characterization at the chiral sides of the normal Layer. I_{2L} is the intensity on the left-chiral side for Character setting and I_{2R} or the intensity on the right-chiral side for Character setting. We thus obtain the following set of equations for neurosis:

For Females: $I_{3L} = I_{2L} + \Delta_{A2} = 7+3=10$ and $I_{3R} = I_{2R} + I_0 = 5+1=6$ *(2)* ,
where I_{3L} is be the intensity level for neurosis oncome for left chirality, I_{3R} for right chirality and Δ_{A2} the set increment of 3 for all accruals.

For Males: $I_{3L} = I_{2L} + I_0 = 5+1=6$ and $I_{3R} = I_{2R} + \Delta_{A2} = 7+3=10$ *(3)* ,
where I_{3L} is the intensity level for neurosis oncome for left chirality and I_{3R} for right chirality.

Likewise in psychosis:

For Females: $I_{4L} = I_{3L} + \Delta_{A2} = 10+3=13$ and $I_{4R} = I_{3R} + I_0 = 6+1=7$ *(2)* ,
where I_{3L} is be the intensity level for neurosis oncome for left chirality, I_{3R} for right chirality and Δ_{A2} the set increment of 3 for all accruals.

For Males: $I_{4L} = I_{3L} + I_0 = 6+1=7$ and $I_{4R} = I_{3R} + \Delta_{A2} = 10+3=13$ *(3)*,
where I_{4L} is the intensity level for psychosis oncome for left chirality and I_{4R} for right chirality.

ACCRUAL LEVEL	FOLIATE ELEMENT	PENSIVE CONDITION	INTENSITY EMULATION
Ground Level 0	*Foliate's Left Chiral Sector or Foliate's Right-Chiral Sector*	*ASEXUALITY*	
Ground Level 1	*Foliate's Left Chiral Sector or Foliate's Right-Chiral Sector*	*GENDER IDENTITY*	
Paroxysm Level 1	*Any of the 9 Primitive Layers*	*CHARACTER DETERMINATION*	
Paroxysm Level 2	*Any of the 9 Primitive Layers*	*NEUROTIC DISORDER*	
Paroxysm Level 3	*Any of the 9 Primitive Layers*	*PSYCHOTIC DISORDER*	

Table 4.1 Hierarchy of the Mental Foliate's accretion with 5 absolute levels.
The **Intensity Emulation** column attempts to emulate the pulsive intensity of implicated flows in terms of incandescence of a light bulb.

It is important to stress, as stated in the definitions, that the syndromal expression of a disorder may be limited to any one of the chiral sides of a Layer, either for the entire duration of a disease or in a prodromal progress of the same. It may even be limited to just a few partitions of the Layer, albeit infrequently so.

4.7 Resolving the Identity Problem of Lie Representations

The question of the definition of Lying, most commonly conceived to be insistent Lying as inferred in the nomer of Pathological Lying, has been a long-time unsolved problem in mental science. Ill understood and poorly researched, with no psychological test to diagnose it, Pathological Lying has been forever at the fringes of clinical psychological and psychiatric practice. For most practitioners, it has inarguably become more of a mental disorder than mere behavioral excess. What the general public understands to be lying is well captured in the common dictionary definitions of the term: *"an untrue statement with intent to deceive."* In clinic, however, the behavior far outgrows the confines of deceipt, since there is an observable omnipresent component of compulsion or irresistibility to the symptom and in many cases absence of observable intent of self-benefit or even a psychological motive. Pathological Liars even lie to purposely incriminate or otherwise cause damage to themselves. Therefore, to establish Aristotelian logic as the standard to comprehend the pensive nature of Lying, a long adopted stance among analysts, is deemed to be an inadequate and misplaced assessment criterion, since logic does not seem to be a part of it at all.

From the vantage of our psychophysics Foliate, the question before us is simple: what is the Cognos that produces the mental state or process of Lying? Is it the Conscious Cognos or the Unconscious Cognos? Our answer is unequivocal: assuredly the Unconscious Cognos. The principles of Logic are not a part of it at all, since Logic is entirely a construction of the Trinary Mentation Layer (Layer 3) emanating from the QG Association norm. The very first characteristic of a lie is its departure from reality. It is a fabrication or a factitious mental act. We can therefore see it in the predominance of representational potentiality and motivational latency over the volitive directive, which characterizes the Unconscious Cognos, all taken over the coordinate system over which the Mentation Foliate develops. In that very particular condition, a lie is exactly equivalent to a delusion or a hallucination.

One way to represent the mentation quality resulting from the *m-t* plane incarnating representational and motivational latencies is to think of it in terms of the psychological notion of *suggestibility*. It is important to grapple this QG *Quintessential* quality of suggestibility because it is intimately associated with the notion of *belief*. Due to the preeminence of the fact of representation in the Unconscious Cognos, the Mind makes no distinction between fact or artifact and passively accepts or certifies the intelligence or payload incrusted in the representation that it either receives or projects itself. That is how *belief* arises from the *suggestible* Unconscious Cognos. By the same token, it is very much this quintessential quality of the Unconscious Cognos that makes both hypnosis and autohypnosis possible. So therefore it is not so much that a Hypnotist is imposing commands to a subjugated mind as it is that he/she uses a modus operandi that exploits the suggestible quality of the Unconscious Cognos, both to fray a direct access path to it and to interact with it. Both the representations that make it into the Unconscious Cognos and those that it projects for itself are altogether taken by that Cognos at their very face value. The Unconscious Cognos does not reason them but automatically admits them with no aposteriori instance of validity assessment, again because of the supremacy of representation/motivation over volition.

We find all these significant elements in the behavior of insistent, impulsive or compulsive lying. When a person incurs an occasional lie in the act of daily living in order to procure a self-benefit of any class, the act most commonly originates from the Unconscious Cognos, imposing the factitious representation in the lie to the Conscious Cognos, through an orthoflow. The latter will at the end deliberate or make a decision about proceeding with it or not. So it is even though most people, including analysts thus far, may believe that the act has been fomented by logical decision of the Conscious Cognos. Aside from deliberation, all the Conscious Cognos does is to acknowledge the representation and, most importantly, impose the implicit principles of reality check in order to maintain the lucidity that the representation in the lie is fictional or factitious.

The next level up in this hierarchy is when the impulses are frequent enough to impose these factitious representations to the Conscious Cognos time and time again in the daily course of living and drives the subject to form serial chains of lies. This corresponds to a Foliate with a Layer 7 with the paroxysmal level that determines Character (Paradoxical Character). One of the most glaring examples of this particular case is given in what the culture has come to term *bigo-*

try[14]. Bigots, in their interactions with peers and the rest of society, typically denature reality and choose to believe – and attempt to lead others to positively believe – in what they originally well knew to be patently untrue. However, you will be hard pressed to determine the line between factitious belief in those concepts and genuine belief in the same in the bigot mind. Because of the paroxysmal level of these factitious projections coming in from the Unconscious Cognos, the lying mind has lost the Conscious discriminating capacity for reality check vis-à-vis these impulses and becomes simply unable to disbelieve its own fabrications. It is fair to say that the more recidivist liars repeat their factitious statements to themselves, to peers and the rest of society, the more they are indeed engaging themselves in autohypnosis or autosuggestion of these bigot claims or beliefs.

The next level up of paroxysm delivers the Pathological Liar with a well-known nosology in clinical milieu. They are not only repetitive in the act of lying but completely unable to control their behavior, which gives their factitious fabrications the true tone of delusions. They incur in false accusations of others with no tangible benefits for themselves, they even purposelessly self-incriminate themselves. Despite the clearly negative consequences to the habitual liar's reputation and livelihood, of which the liar is well aware, the lies will not stop and outright qualify as compulsive and uncontrollable. The crimes associated with the behavior of Pathological Lying include in order of significance plagiarism, forgery, swindling and outright theft. A few pathological liars manage to be successful professionals without any public record of crime. To that extent, those are no different than other neurotic subjects, who appear to be quite normal in behavior by socially managing the external expression of their morbidity.

Some analysts have mistakenly argued that *"the blurring of fact and fiction that occurs in Pathological Lying is not the same as the absolute conviction that occurs in persons with delusions."* They have failed to understand the important

---

[14] A common Dictionary definition of bigotry: *"Obstinate or unreasonable attachment to a belief, opinion, or faction; in particular, prejudice against a person or people on the basis of their membership of a particular group," i.e. ethnicity.* Such beliefs are unreasonable because they do not correspond to reality, often applying a blanket damning characterization to an entire group without any exception.

fact that the lie is in itself a fiction, that by going around telling it the individual reveals that he/she is upholding it as his/her truth, that he/she will go the extra lengths of making significant changes to their lives, i.e. moving town, in order to uphold these lies as their truths to society, that he/she may construct an entire string of confabulations to uphold these lies altogether as truth. Finally, these subjects are notably under an eponymous *"irresistible impulse"* to produce all these lies. For all intent and purposes, the pathological liar is living in his/her own world of lies and confabulations. That, in some cases, he/she may concede to his/her factiousness when heavily pressed to acknowledge the same really makes no difference, because there is no longer any basis to ascertain that the individual is sincere and truly able to discern between what is real and what is confabulated, especially in view of the fact that he/she has been autosuggesting himself/herself that the fables are true.

Furthermore, one ought to remain cognizant that the norm in operation here is Paradox. In other words, the habitual liar is caught in a world of *paradoxical delusions* that has him/her play a game of falsity vs. truth, whereby what is true is morbidly viewed and sensed as false and what is false morbidly taken and offered for truth. The analyst must keep in mind that all lies play out on a duplet tenet, which is a representation of fact or reality on one hand and, on the other, an antithetic factitious projection to the fact. Morbidity as a paradoxical delusion starts when the Mind bijectively interchanges the attributes of the two tenets and makes the factual representation something of a fiction and the factitious projection (aka the lie) something asserted to be real. As this inversion becomes stronger and stronger, the subject soon lands into the psychosis world. Some analysts have controversially seen in the behavior of the pathological liar a *"wish psychosis"*. To the extent that the evoked bijective inversion is fully realized in the Mind, that label is well justified. Many minds in Nazi Germany, such as philosopher Martin Heidegger, exemplified this form of psychosis in our view.

The nihilist philosopher infamously wrote: *"Truth cannot be out there—cannot exist independently of the human mind—because sentences cannot so exist, or be out there. The world is out there, but descriptions of the world are not.* ***Only descriptions of the world can be true or false.****"*

In parsing the piece, for M. Heidegger, the entire natural world out there has no essential truth to it, it is false. It is indeed a specious argument to be looking for truth out there and conclude that there is no truth out there, because it is obvious that truth is a human concept borne out of the human mind. What is out there as the natural world – objects and events – exists in and of itself, independent of human beings' assessment or rendition known as truth or fiction. This form of reasoning constitutes a specious or fallacious argument proper to nihilists as their first step towards negation of reality. Further, what is true for M. Heidegger is only the human spoken word, which he understands to not be out there. So what does not materially exist is true, and what materially exists is unimportant, a negligible quantity at very least and false at most. Michael Wheeler, a historian of this day, explains some aspects of Heidegger's writings as follows *(Stanford University's Plato Encyclopedia)*:

"...In words that we have just met, it is language and not biology that, for Heidegger, constitutes the house of Being. So the German Volk *are a linguistic-historical, rather than a biological, phenomenon, ...* **Heidegger suggests that while Africans (along with plants and animals) have no history** (in a technical sense understood in terms of heritage), the event of an airplane carrying Hitler to Mussolini is genuinely part of history (see Polt 1999, 155)."

So therefore, for the philosopher, the biological manifestation of Man is a physical reality that is unimportant and does not partake of Heidegger's *"House of Being"*. What is important is the ethereous existence of language or simply *words* as he put it, which of course are not out there to be grabbed. And so he found that at the end the German people is no more than a linguistic-historical category! Be that nonetheless as it may, he did not find that Africans were speaking creatures akin to the German people... because unlike the German people, they are for him equivalent to plants and animals and cannot manifest history!

What he believed of the essence of the German people, he reportedly expressed in an address to German university students: *"Not theorems and ideas be the rules of your being. The Fiihrer himself and alone is the present and future German reality and its law. Learn ever deeper to know that from now on each and every thing demands decisions, and every action, responsibility. Heil Hitler!"*

Did he not place the House of Being in the empire of words (as vehicles of ideas) for theorems and ideas all of a sudden not be the rules of the students' beings anymore? And you further have to wonder if the Fiihrer was the only human who could speak or utter words in Germany, because he alone made up Germany!

These rambles of course, and despite Heidegger's surprisingly widespread contemporary influence in the West as a philosopher, have no more value than the drivels coming out of a mind that has sunk in deep drunkenness and with which they are totally interchangeable. What in the world is this *"House of Being"* metaphor, if it is only a metaphor? Paradoxes abound in his clearly nihilist and bigot thinking. It is no wonder that he died demented, in psychosis, that is (aka madness in vernacular language)? Many philosophical minds of the kind which inhabited the province of these paradoxical incoherences, otherwise known as negation of reality in many regards, i.e. Soren Kierkegaard and Friedrich Niestche, had equally experienced a prodromal evolution to psychosis.

Perhaps, one of the best ways to represent this pathological state is to picture a deeply inebriated person that hypothetically has not succumbed to psychomotor unbalance. He would be as such engaging in one of the most prominent intrapsychic symptoms of alcohol intoxication: disjoint language. Very characteristically, drunkenness severely impacts the ability to put fluent language out there but very peculiarly disparate *words*: the two or three words that the drunken individual is able to put together at a time are markedly slurred, frequently fumbled, and almost always incoherent, although their attitude is antagonistically argumentative leaning to defiance and violence.

Verbal and physical aggression towards others, very particularly loved ones, while hallucinating (seeing or hearing things that are unreal or projected – or unable to see physical reality for what it is) are well known manifestations of the state of deep inebriation. When it comes to M. Heidegger, everyone knows of the level of violence and madness there was behind the infamous *"Heil Hitler"* salute to which he was not at all estranged with a mind that saw Hitler to be materially all of Germany. It is anybody's guess what kind of refined form of extermination he may have mentalized for those Africans who in his book were patently not human beings and only had an existence comparable to plants and animals unlike the Aryan people!

Finally, when one makes an entire intellectual career on these confabulations and disjunctions, pathological lying probably finds itself at its best "house".

4.8 Factitious Disorder as a Variant of Pathological Lying

Factitious Disorder is a serious mental disorder in which someone blatantly attempts to deceive others by feigning sickness or by purposely getting sick or even with the aid of self-injury. The morbid behavior of falsely presenting others, such as children, as being ill, injured or impaired, equally qualifies as Factitious Disorder. Even caregivers are not immune from this disease. In making up symptoms, the person may tamper with medical tests to convince others that treatment, such as high-risk surgery, is needed to treat them.

Sufferers of Factitious Disorder go to great lengths to hide their deception. Therefore, it may be difficult to peers, family members or caregivers to assess whether or not the syndrome these subjects experience qualify as morbidity from a serious mental health disorder. The affected insistently continue with their deception, even without receiving any visible benefit or reward or when faced with objective evidence that counters their claims.

It is important to point out that even though sufferers are fully cognizant they are themselves causing their symptoms or illnesses, they may not understand the reasons for their behavior or identify the behavior as a morbid problem. We see here again the inner workings of the suggestible mind discussed in Pathological Lying. When it comes to the variant of presenting others as being ill or somehow impaired, we face the bigot behavior that characterizes as well Pathological Lying. The affected by this variant present another person as sick, injured or having problems functioning, and claims urgency of medical attention. Usually this type of sufferer is knowingly a parent with the express intent of harming a child. It is clear that this form of abuse can put a child in serious danger of injury or unnecessary medical care.

The extent to which Factitious Disorder symptoms may go in the attempt to deceive others can become quite alarming in their seriousness. These symptoms may involve:

- Using fake names to seek treatment from many different doctors or hospitals.
- Making up health histories, and presenting loved ones, health care professionals or support groups with a false medical history, such as claiming to have had cancer or AIDS. Or they may have falsified medical records to indicate a particular illness.
- Outright faking or exaggerating symptoms, such as stomach pain, seizures or passing out.
- Causing self-harm to become sick, i.e. by injecting themselves with bacteria, milk, gasoline or feces. They may injure, cut or burn themselves. They may take medications, such as blood thinners or drugs for diabetes, in order to mimic diseases. They may also interfere with wound healing as they intently reopen or infect cuts.
- Skewing results by tampering with medical instruments, such as heating up thermometers, contaminating their urine samples with blood or other substances in order to falsify lab tests.

Let's conclude by pointing out that the inner workings of the mentation partitions at Layer 7 of the Foliate are undoubtedly fueling this type of morbidity.

4.9 The Confusion about Mental Confusion

The impairment of Mental Confusion in clinical mental science is defined to be a sudden change in mental status in which a person becomes unable to think with his/her usual clarity and instead thinks in a dissociative manner. The condition exhibits a significant loss of ability to associate and coordinate, leading to a foggy mental fit of disorientation incapable to tell time and dates, identify and recognize locations and even relatives, friends and acquaintances. In that state of mind, the individual tends to mumble for speech or say things that are disconnected, generally qualified to be nonsensical.

It is a regrettable error in clinical psychopathology that other symptoms have been lumped with the above, by virtue of the fact that they appear to be the same mental condition from a cognitive standpoint. Said symptoms follow:

- Loss of conscious awareness
- Perception of things that are not real
- Getting upset or worked up for no apparent reason
- Exhibiting delirium tremens

It is clear that these symptoms are tightly related to alcohol intoxication. Further, avoiding at all cost ingestion of alcohol is an express clinical prophylactic recommendation against these symptoms. One may then justifiably infer that these inebriation symptoms constitute the basis in official science for considering alcohol intoxication a common cause of Sudden Confusion (aka Mental Confusion). From an ultrastructural analytic standpoint, however, one can see an irreducible distinction between the two symptom sets, in that the first is based on cognitive intellection impairment and the second on paradoxical cognition as visualized in our psychophysics approach.

Furthermore, it is mainly on account of the second symptom set that Mental Confusion is generally considered to be a psychosis. Should that set be discounted from the nosology of Mental Confusion as we effectively do, the disorder loses at a stroke the psychotic character usually associated with it. From our perspective, the most legitimate set of symptoms of Mental Confusion relates it to the cluster of disorders fomented by Layer 3 of the Mentation Foliate. Heuristically, Mental Confusion is best understood cognitively as Down Syndrome without the genetic, physiological and anatomic caveats associated with it. The newer nomenclature captures this cognitive impairment under the label Mental Retardation or Intellectual Disability.

It would seem that at the summit of hypointellection, formerly denoted *stuporous confusion* in psychology, the state of the mind becomes similar to or interchangeable with the psychosis of delirium. In fact, the mental partition of *Aberration* pertaining to Layer 3 of the Foliate perfectly accounts for this fit of the mind as it reaches a paroxysmal level in its expression. The pensive partition of *Aberration* at ground level already stands for an extreme deficit in synthetic or logical thinking. The accrual in the set of partitions pertaining to the Left-Chiral side of Layer 3 *(Aberration, Idiocy, Disorientation and Doubt)* gives a full and accurate account of the pensive primitives that develop the nosology consisting of the 1st symptom set reported for the disorder as its legitimate basis. In this context, Mental Confusion becomes one more disorder within the cluster of Intellection Disorders, next to Mental Retardation or Intellectual Disability. There is not a loss of contact with reality per se therein, but an extreme deficit in associating synthetically the elements of reality as well as self within reality, the latter otherwise known as personal coordination. Consequently, Mental Confusion is neither a psychosis, nor a loss of consciousness, but only a neurosis. Most clinicians would not acknowledge that Down Syndrome in its strict psychological aspects is a psychosis, therefore no more so Mental Confusion.

4.10 Dysfunctional Language in Mental Confusion

Two newly identified forms of disorder, namely Communication Disorder and Language Disorder, may help reinforce the intellection perspective that we uphold in regards to Mental Confusion.

4.10.1 Language Disorder

Language Disorder is a communication disorder whereby the affected person has persistent difficulties in learning and using various forms of language (i.e., spoken, written, sign language). Individuals with *Language Disorder* show language abilities significantly below expectation for their age. This impairment limits their ability to communicate or effectively participate in many a social, academic, or professional endeavor.

Children with Language Disorder are typically delayed in learning or speaking their first words and phrases. Whenever they speak, their sentences are shorter and less complex than expected for their age. Individuals with Language Disorder typically incur grammatical errors, exhibit limited vocabulary, and may notably have trouble finding the right word at times. They are generally unable to provide proper information about key events they witnessed or experienced or tell a story coherently.

It is reportedly common for deficits in intellectual comprehension to be underestimated, because people with *Language Disorder* may be good at finding strategies to cope with their language deficits, such as using context to infer meaning. However hypointellection in terms of a deficit in mental associativity is clearly at the basis of this dysfunction. The Left-Chiral partitions of Layer 3, which are responsible for Mental Confusion, are responsible alike for the associative drawbacks causing Language Disorder.

4.10.2 Social Communication Disorder

Social Communication Disorder is mainly characterized by difficulties in understanding and using language for social purposes (for example, having conversations and telling stories). Children with Social Communication Disorder may experience difficulties with:

- Understanding and applying the many different "rules" circumscribing the varied social situations they are confronted with (talking in a classroom is different than talking on a playground, i.e.).
- Interpreting and using non verbal communication, (eye contact, gestures, and facial expressions).
- Infering things that are implicitly understood but not directly stated, i.e. humor, metaphors, and words with more than one meaning.

These artifacts all imply relational mentation abilities which are eclipsed when the disorder has set in, and involve prevalent exercise of the Left-Chiral partition set at Mentation Layer 3.

In Language Disorder and Social Communication Disorder, note well that these subjects' minds are not completely bereft of higher intellection, which is the province of the Right-Chiral set of mentation partitions at Layer 3. Effectively, they are able to consciously adopt strategies to cope with their disease, particularly in Language Disorder. The patient with Language Disorder is lucid enough to consciously self-censor himself or herself in producing speech: when the subject feels emotionally safe, i.e. while at home, he or she will freely speak, but not at school where peer pressure or learning pressure under instructors creates enough tension to contribute to an intentional muting of all communication.

From its condition of foremost vehicle of communication, Language is Quanto-Geometrically typed as an interrelational artifact obeying the Association Norm regimenting Layer 3 of the Mentation Foliate. Its direct connection and involvement with the mental fits of that Layer come to no surprise.

4.11 Subjacent States of Agitation and Depression in All Mental Disorders

Data accumulated over more than half a century seems to suggest that Agitation and Depression are two generalized components of all mental disorders. However, the effort to find their appropriate dimension in the current official disease model has left many dissatisfied because it has no more than worsened the multimorbidity problem. It is Ian Kelleher and Mary Cannon who wrote:

"The strong interrelationships emerging between psychosis, neurosis, and mood instability, together with the ebb and flow of diagnoses over time, force us to question established ideas about traditional divisions and distinctions right across the psychiatric diagnostic spectrum."

Identification of the super classes in psychiatric and psychological etiology has long remained an unsolved problem which hampers the effectiveness of psychotherapies in very significant ways. We have shown above the foundational basis for the broad classes of neurosis and psychosis. Psychiatrists Xiaohua LIU and Kaida JIANG tangentially and indirectly raise the same question of appropriate classes for Depression and Agitation which seem to hold multiform expression as an undesirable wide variety of mental disorders.

They write for the Shanghai Archives of Psychiatry in relation to Depression:

"Depressive disorder has been variously sub-typed in a wide variety of ways depending on its clinical features and presumed etiology: endogenous or reactive depression, organic or psychogenic depression, retarded or agitated depression, anxious depression, depression with psychotic symptoms, mixed depression, atypical depression, and so forth...

... the bewildering array of proposed diagnostic subtypes – which seem to change at least once a decade – confounds the diagnostic process. In most cas-

es, clinical psychiatrists diagnose the subtype of depression as part of a comprehensive evaluation of a depressed patient and are expected to use information about the presumed subtype to decide on the treatment plan that is most likely to effectively treat the symptoms and relieve patient distress. But which of the proposed classifications of subtypes are most clinically useful?"

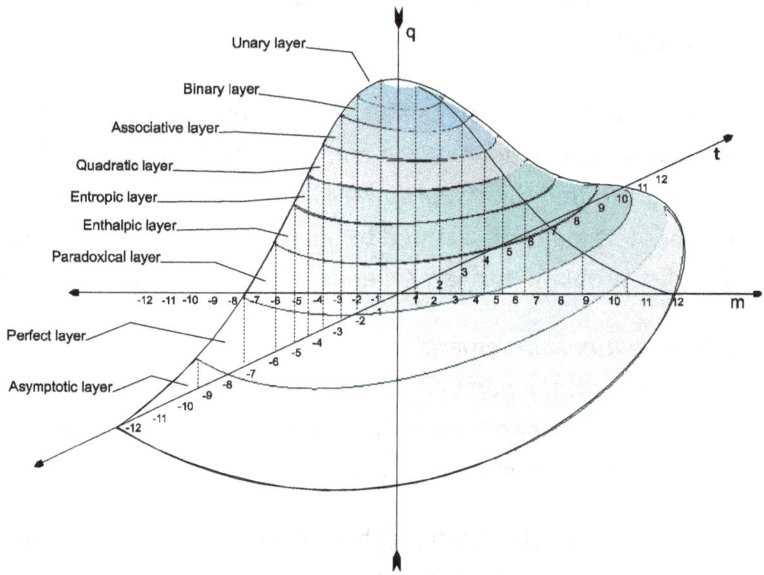

***A.**- The Quanto-Geometric 3D Manifold with equated binary distribution along the t-axis and across the m-axis*

PASSIVE LATENCY - ANIMA					ACTIVE LATENCY - ANIMUS			
-4	-3	-2	-1		1	2	3	4
Dramatism	Pessismism	Negativity	Disapproval	Hybrid	Assent	Optimism	Assurance	Excitement
Timidity	Introversion	Solitude	Indifference	↑ ↓	Conservatives:	Possessiveness	Competitivenes	Cupidity
Inquisitiveness	Curiosity	Superficiality (In	Credulity	↑ ↓	Sincerity	Mirroring	Duplicity	Authoritarianism
Aberration	Idiocy	Disorientation	Doubt (Perple:	↑ ↓	Discernment	Perspicacity	Clairvoyance	Lucidity
Remorse	Guilt	Shame	Regretfulness	↑ ↓	Presumption	Audacity	Stoicism	Heroism
Delirium	Hallucination	Fabulousness	Daydream	↑ ↓	Chimera	Reformism	Visionary	Utopia
Despair	Sadness (Disapp	Sorrow	Pity	↑ ↓	Sympathy	Admiration	Euphoria	Passion
Terror	Fear (Anguish)	Angst	Anxiety	↑ ↓	Resentment	Repugnance	Wickedness	Fury
Subservience	Devotion	Humility	Laziness	↑ ↓	Equity	Hope	Happiness	Ecstasy
Inanity	Cluelessness	Austerity	Patience	↑ ↓	Temperance	Endurance	Tenacity	Resilience
PARALYSIS					PURPOSEFULNESS			

***B.**- QG qualities and sub-qualities infused in the Binary Group division of the Mental Manifold as shown in A*

Fig. 4.2 Tabular Map of the Binary grouping of the Mentation Manifold

Because of the very serious impact of the derived comorbidity problem on diagnostics and choice of applicable treatments, this classificatory and etiological deficiency has created a state of generalized dissatisfaction if not staunch critical reactions among practitioners.

We are next going to show that, in the QG Mental Foliate, a fitting dimension exists for Depression and Agitation that is consistent with all the other characterizations from the model directly applicable to psychopathology. A preeminent feature of the QG Mental Foliate is the *m-axis* inherent to the coordinate system that grandfathers the ontological qualities distilled in the variables of the Function, and on which the graph develops. We have asserted that the positive *m-axis* stands for intent or intentionality inherent to Motivation, whereas the quality of passiveness or paralysis maps to the negative side of the Motivational *m-axis*.

PASSIVE LATENCY					ACTIVE LATENCY			
-4	-3	-2	-1		1	2	3	4
Dramatism	**Pessimism**	**Negativity**	**Disapproval**		**Assent**	**Assurance**	**Optimism**	**Excitement**
Timidity	Introversion	Solitude	Indifference	↑ ↓	Conservativenes	Possessiveness	Competitivenes	Cupidity
Inquisitiveness	Curiosity	Superficiality (In	Credulity	↑ ↓	Sincerity	Mirroring	Duplicity	Authoritarianism
Aberration	Idiocy	Disorientation	Doubt (Perple	↑ ↓	Discernment	Perspicacity	Clairvoyance	Lucidity
Remorse	Guilt	Shame	Regretfulness	↑ ↓	Presumption	Audacity	Stoicism	Heroism
Delirium	Hallucination	Fabulousness	Daydream	↑ ↓	Chimera	Reformism	Visionary	Utopia
Despair	Sadness (Disapp	Sorrow	Pity	↑ ↓	Sympathy	Admiration	Euphoria	Passion
Terror	Fear (Anguish)	Angst	Anxiety	↑ ↓	Resentment	Repugnance	Wickedness	Fury
Subservience	Devotion	Humility	Laziness	↑ ↓	Equity	Hope	Happiness	Ecstasy
Inanity	Cluelessness	Austerity	Patience	↑ ↓	Temperance	Endurance	Tenacity	Resilience
PARALYSIS					**PURPOSEFULNESS**			

Fig. 4.3 Conflation in the Mental Manifold between 1) Passive Latency and Paralysis and 2) Active Latency and Purposefulness

This metric is capital in understanding the phenomena of Depression and Agitation as they translate those high-level primitives to the psychological or mentation plane (Fig. 4.3). The quality of paralysis or passive latency is quite ostensible in the entire set of root mentation partitions pertaining to the left side of the distribution, i.e. terror, despair, inanity, aberration, etc. The quality of purposefulness or active latency is for itself quite ostensible in the entire set of root mentation partitions pertaining to the right side of the distribution, i.e. fury, tenacity, heroism, cupidity, passion, etc. These two antisymmetric qualities each exist at one or the other chiral side of the Distribution in every partition composing a wing.

It is critical to identify those two potentialities, namely paralysis and purposefulness, to be the qualities responsible for the notorious states of Depression and Agitation respectfully. It is thus predictable that they will become transparent and functionally effective to every chiral segment of a Mentation Layer throughout the entire Foliate. Since those two qualities subtend each one of the two chiral sets of a Layer, they thus become quite ostensible symptomatically when pathological accrual occurs in the referred Layer. One can accordingly see the cross dimensional layout of Depression as a paralysis constraint and Agitation as an intentionality pressure in all psychopathologies involving Layer intensity accrual, and as an underlying condition.

More granular analysis of the states of Agitation and Depression in disorders should give us a number of different gradations that map to the threads of the QG distribution per the nomenclature at the top of each of the 8 threads. For Depressions, these threads or longitudes are:

1. Dramatism **[-4]**
2. Pessimism **[-3]**
3. Negativity **[-2]**
4. Disapprobation **[-1]**

Whereas for Agitation, these threads or longitudes are:

1. Assent **[1]**
2. Assurance **[2]**
3. Optimism **[3]**
4. Excitement **[4]**

Unfortunately, despite all the field reports and research in psychology and psychiatry, science of the mental has not garnered sufficient comprehensive data about Depression and Agitation as they symptomatically appear across the spectrum of mental disorders to carry out analysis at that granular level. It is possible though to draw some distinction in intensity of these states between one disorder and another in the same group. A qualitative distinction between the same is nonetheless not possible in the current categorization of the referred impairments, let alone one that straightforwardly rises to the level of azimuthal symmetry inherent to the QG Mental Foliate model, as inherited from the physical theoretical primitives. Be that as it may, we will nevertheless later attempt to map those categories as best appropriate. Following is an exhaustive list of officially categorized Depressive disorders:

- Major Depression
- Minor Depression (Dysthymia)
- Bipolar Disorder
- Melancholic Depression
- Catatonic Depression
- Seasonal Affective Disorder
- Psychotic Depression
- Recurrent Depression
- Recurrent Brief Depressive Disorder
- 'Situational' Depression
- Atypical Depression
- Peripartum (Postpartum) Depression
- Premenstrual Dysphoric Disorder
- Depression associated with Dementia (Alzheimer's)
- Depression associated with Schizophrenia
- Depression with ADHD
- Depression with Obsessive Compulsive Disorder
- Depression with Anxiety Disorder

It is interesting that such cases as Asthenia or Burnout Syndrome, which are legitimate disorders fueled by excessive psychogenic exhaust, are not officially categorized as members of the extensive family. Associate Professor of Psychiatry Masaru Mimura (Showa Univ., School of Medicine, Dept of Psychiatry – Japan) writes:

"A recent review of patients with depression indicated that some type of personality disorder was present in 20–50% of inpatients and 50–85% of outpatients with depression. Among these patients, relatively frequent types of personality disorders were borderline (10–30%), histrionic (2–20%), anti-social (0–10%), and obsessional (0–20%), showing a great deal of diversity. Although the comorbidity of depression and personality disorder is of clinical importance, it is not an un-

complicated problem. It needs to be borne in mind that the prognosis and treatment policy will vary according to the type of comorbid personality disorder."

The picture that emerges from this state of affairs is that depression may clinically accompany a very high percentage of mental disorders, independently of their nature, consistent with our theoretical vision that it must ultrastructurally subtend a large array of mental disorders.

4.12 Bijective Causation between Mental Disorders and Depression-Agitation

One the most interesting features of mental disorders of all nature is their covariant relationship with Depression, deficiently captured in the science under the nomer of comorbidity, to mean an individual psychopathology involving multiple typified impairments or dysfunctions. It is also noteworthy that Depression may not just coexist with these otherwise qualified disorders, as it may alternatively precurse them as much as they may be forerunners to Depression. The above cited author further writes:

"A second issue is the temporal relationship between depression and other comorbid mental disorders. There are three ways of considering the order of onset:

1) When depression precedes the other disorder, depression may serve as a causative factor for the subsequent disorder;

2) when the other disorder precedes depression, that disorder may serve as a causative factor for depression; and

3) when depression and the other disorder occur simultaneously, the symptoms of these two diseases may be considered attributable to a different cause(s).

In general, in patients with co-morbid depression, the other mental disorder often precedes the initial episode of depression (secondary depression), and this is particularly so when the patient is male."

We must add to this account the fact that such external factors as psychotropic agents may accidentally revert the primary disease, i.e. Bipolar Disorder, to Depression–Agitation, whenever these pharmacological agents are not prescribed or administered with sufficient parcimony. Masaru Nimura writes:

"The response of mixed depression to antidepressants could be a useful tool for studying the anxiety versus the bipolar nature of its "hypomanic" symptoms, as a bipolar nature would be supported by a worsening of these symptoms by antidepressants. There are few specific studies on this topic. In a combined bipolar I disorder and bipolar II disorder sample, mixed depression treated by antidepressants was more likely to switch than nonmixed depression. In major depressive disorder, low-dose fluoxetine improved mild irritability and psychomotor agitation, but imipramine led to many discontinuations due to central nervous system (CNS) side effects. The impact of antidepressants on mixed depression may thus be related to different biochemical effects, increasing norepinephrine apparently being more likely to worsen mixed depression. However, in major depressive disorder, high-dose fluoxetine was also found to induce psychomotor agitation (in 40% of cases)."

The author acknowledges that hypomanic symptoms configure a form of depression that pertains to Bipolar Disorder as a disease in its own right. She also acknowledges the existence of other depressive symptoms (anxiety) pertaining differentially to Mixed Depression when she writes: *"The response of mixed depression to antidepressants could be a useful tool for studying the* ***anxiety versus the bipolar nature*** *of its "hypomanic" symptoms, as a bipolar nature would be supported by a worsening of these symptoms by antidepressants."* Very explicitly, the author acknowledges that antidepressants may paradoxically worsen the depressive hypomanic phases of bipolar disorder but not the depressive symptoms of Mixed Depression. Other studies bring up even more evidence of the switching from one depression type to the other under the influence of antidepressants:

"We considered 12 studies of patients initially thought to have unipolar MDD who required a new diagnosis of bipolar disorder, usually with verification by occurrence of spontaneous mania or hypomania. Such diagnostic changes occurred in 3.3% within 5.4 years, or 5.6 times less than the rate of mood switching

with antidepressants. If the relatively low rates of new bipolar diagnoses are not due to under-reporting, ***their marked difference from rates of antidepressant-associated mood switching leaves open the possibility that direct pharmacological, mood-elevating actions of antidepressants may be involved in mood switching, in addition to hypothesized "uncovering" or perhaps even "causing" of bipolar disorder.*** *Of particular concern is that these ambiguous possibilities leave specifically uncertain the potential value of long-term treatment with antimanic or putative mood-stabilizing agents." … "Cumulative risk of mood switching increased up to 24 months of antidepressant treatment."* [15]

In a study published in 2018, Gioia Baggiani, Luca Ambrosiani, et al show the influence of some psychotropic drugs in reverting one conjugate state of a disease to the other such as in Bipolar Disorder when used in mono-drug therapies, which has become certified in mainstream psychiatry as they write after Bauer and Gitlin:

"…the second-generation antipsychotics now dominate the pharmacotherapy of acute mania. This reflects both their clear efficacy as shown in studies and meta-analysis, their ease of administration, relatively more benign side effect profiles (certainly compared to first-generation antipsychotics), and their rapidity of response compared to lithium.

However, the ideal mood stabilizer has to be effective against both mania and depression, without any risk of increasing the incidence of opposite episodes. Unfortunately, ***some antipsychotics can increase the risk of depression*** *and antidepressants can trigger mania if used as monotherapy. This problem is sometimes overlooked in the context of acute episodes, because the aim may be the short-term response."*

Before we address the counterpart of generalized Depression, Agitation, that is, a few remarks about diagnosis based on gender definition are in order. The discussion about Agitation follows thereafter.

---

[15] **"Switching" of Mood From Depression to Mania With Antidepressants,** Gioia Baggiani,1 Luca Ambrosiani,1 Pierfranco Trincas,2 Caterina Burrai,3 and Alberto Bocchetta1,* https://www.psychiatrictimes.com/view/switching-mood-depression-mania-antidepressants

4.13 Differential Syndrome Diagnosis of Depression Based on Gender Definition

It is predictable from our psychophysics Foliate model that women will generally present with a higher tendency for Depression than men do owing to the natural prevalence of the left-chiral pensive partitions of the entire Foliate in women, in accordance with the metric that we have established to elicit gender and abnormality definitions. Effectively, Psychiatrist Masaru Nimura writes:

"Almost twice as many women as men have major or clinical depression; hormonal changes during puberty, menstruation, pregnancy, miscarriage, and menopause, may increase the risk."

It is easy to understand that proneness of behavior based on the inner tendency seminally inherent to the left-chiral partitions of the entire mentation spectrum strongly predisposes women to the emotional depletion or, in fact, paralysis characteristic of Depression. As to the second part of the statement, we must remember that in general a "pathological risk factor" only infers an observation concerning noticed correlation between a condition of whatever nature and a specific pathology, but has not the value of an identified direct causal relation. Therefore the cited endocrine factors should not be taken as etiological causes of gender distribution of the disease but circumstantial factors that may accompany the onset of Depression in women. We will later see that gender prevalence, in fact, plays out in the distribution of many a mental pathology other than Depression. The ultimate cause is nothing else than the modality in which gender prevalence is ontologically realized as profiled in and measured by our metric framework.

4.14 Agitation as a Morbid Symptom

Agitation, in which we include impulsiveness and tremors, is a derivate of the active-motivational primitive that animates the right-chiral Sector of the Mentation Foliate as postulated. These conditions are found in many mental disorders, notably:

- Mood disorders
- Burnout
- ADHD
- Autism
- Alcohol intoxication and withdrawal
- Grief Reaction
- Work and School-related Stress Disorders
- Peer pressure morbidity

Agitation is quite notable as a psychomotor impairment in one Disorder generally considered organic for the most part: the disorder of *Parkinson's Disease*. It is of great import to highlight the psychomotor manifestations in Parkinson's Disease whose organic causes have yet to been found, towards redimensioning its etiological roots. The following generic symptoms and risk factors are known for the disease, noting that they are different in amount in every specific case:

1. *Symptoms often begin on* ***one side of the body*** *and usually remain worse on that particular side, even after they begin to affect both sides.*
2. ***Men*** *are much more likely to develop Parkinson's disease than women are.*
3. *Patients experience characteristic* ***tremors****. A tremor, or shaking, usually begins in a limb, quite often the patient's hand or fingers. The patient may rub his/her thumb and forefinger back and forth, in what is known as a* ***pill-rolling tremor****. Hand may tremble while at rest.*
4. *Affected patients may experience cognitive problems (dementia) and thinking difficulties. These usually occur in the later stages of Parkinson's disease. (Such cognitive problems are staunchly intractable to known medications).*
5. *Obsessive-Compulsive behavior is very common among patients affected with Parkinson's Disease.*
6. *Affected patients experience depression and anxiety at a very high rate*[16]*, sometimes in the very early stages of the disease.*

---

[16] Nicoletti, A., Luca, A., Raciti, L., Contrafatto, D., Bruno, E., et al. (2013). Obsessive compulsive personality disorder and Parkinson's disease. *PLoS ONE* 8(1): e54822. doi:10.1371/journal.pone.0054822

7. *Cognitive impairment in **Parkinson's** disease (50% of cases) is said to be characterized by predominant executive function deficits, attention difficulties, visuospatial dysfunction, slowed thinking, difficulties in word-finding, in resolving situations that implicate making choices, and in learning and remembering information.*
8. *Slowed movement (bradykinesia). Over time, Parkinson's disease may slow limb motion, making simple tasks difficult and time-consuming. Steps may become shorter when walking. Affected individual may drag his feet when walking. Just getting out of a chair may become quite difficult.*
9. *Muscle rigidity may occur in any part of the body. The stiff muscles can be painful and limit the range of motion, becoming mainly responsible for:*
    - *Impaired posture and balance. Patient's posture may become stooped, or else he exhibits balance problems.*
    - *Loss of automatic movements. Decreased ability to perform unconscious movements, including blinking, smiling or swinging the arms when walking.*
    - *Speech changes showing soft or quick enunciation or slur. The patient may show hesitation before talking and a monotone accent devoid of the usual inflections.*
10. *Acting out nightly dreams in relatively frequent nightmares.*

The above symptom set is clear evidence that there is a strong component of mental dysfunction in Parkinson's Disease, which makes the disease both of a psychomotor and psychogenic nature. That assessment holds despite the fact that cognitive impairment may be mild in some cases, in the sense that it may not affect the performing of tasks of a normal life. At this effect, we must remember, however, that many neuroses do not visibly disrupt normal living either.

It is worth highlighting the compulsive-obsessive form of the psychogenic impairment in the disease, which is no less than a translation of the Agitation or Impulsiveness factor inherent to the pensive forms of the right-chiral Sector of the Mental Foliate. Further, in the words of Parkinson's specialists, the disease affects what they have termed "predominant executive functions", which is a nomer for motivational mentation. However, the termed "deficit" in those functions constitutes a misperception of what is really occurring in the manifestion of those functions. When the patient is ostensibly unable to talk, it may be instead an instance of a compulsive concurrence of ideas hampering the choice of proper words. Therefore, locution compulsion may well be what composes the common cognitive impairment of word finding in the disease. Note accordingly that these patients are knowingly dysfunctional in most circumstances of life that require choices. The motivational level may run so high that the body is unable to remain below the threshold of limb activity during the state of sleep, causing physical enactment of dreams.

In addition to these features, there is intense and prolonged unilaterality or asymmetry in the brain, or in fact the central nervous system, in terms of one predominant chiral side of the body manifesting the impairments. On the mental plane, this indirectly corresponds to one Sector of the Mental Manifold being at the front wheel. This condition is further strongly supported, on the basis of our psychophysics framework, by the fact that the statistics give males a much greater proneness to this Disorder than females, evidencing accrued hyperactivity of the Animus Sector of the Foliate, already naturally in accretion in the male Foliate. The monist perspective which dominates psychiatric medicine and medical science in general leads researchers to enlist a suite of physiological factors in the etiological hypotheses for the Disease, such as possible drop in the level of the neurotransmitter dopamine, credited to regulate movement as well as cognition, memory, learning, attention, and sleep. Researchers believe that changes in levels of acetylcholine and norepinephrine could be linked to memory and executive function loss in Parkinson's disease. Nevertheless, it is acknowledged that the cognitive changes possibly associated with dopamine decline, the most probable contributing factor among the suspected neurotransmitters, are typically mild and limited. The direct physiological cause of Parkinson's disease is therefore unknown, even though the biochemical agents developed for its therapy may be more or less effective in palliating some of its known symptoms. Our etiological exegesis bears on the following:

1. Overaccretion of the Right-chiral pensive Sector of the entire Mental Foliate, beyond character determination accrual.
2. Complete swings or binary flips of the hyperactive state from one chiral Sector of the Foliate to the other.
3. Conversion from the psychogenic elements of the various dysfunctions of the Mental Body (or Foliate) in the Disorder to motor elements in the biological body, setting a psychosomatic nature to the Disorder.

Proposition 2 accounts for the entire set of depletion symptoms in the disease, both psychological such as Depression, and biological such as the slowness in motion, muscle stiffness and inability to deploy fully developed movements. Of course, the characteristic limb tremors represent the conversion of the compulsive/impulsive drives in motivational mentation as a primitive. So therefore, the two major Sectors of the Foliate are permuting in hyperintensity in the prodromal evolution of the Disease, while projecting onto the biological counterparts.

Noting that dopamine, acetylcoline, and epinephrine are, along with GABA and serotonin, the molecules par excellence that mediate implementation of motion by the nervous system, it is a remarkable fact that they only have mild and limited effects in the expression of a disease where motion is so significantly impaired in one way or another. The major feedback chains underlying permanent activity of the hormonal system, which includes noradrenergic neurons themselves, have not been found implicated in this Disorder either. These two facts alone strongly advocate for the psychosomatic nature of the disease.

Finally, it is worth noting that the state of Depression which we studied earlier as a component or underlying condition in many mental Disorders was duly rooted on the Left-chiral set of partitions pertaining to the Layer responsible for the Disorder. In Parkinson's Disease, Depression is instead rooted on the entire Left-chiral Sector of the individual's mentation Foliate. It is always accompanied with feelings of anxiety, fear and loss of motivation. Consistent with our psychophysics attribution, the following conditions are also part of Parkinson's Disease, their ultimate cause being otherwise unknown in allopathic medicine:

1. Fatigue - Many people with Parkinson's disease lose energy and experience fatigue, especially later in the day.
2. Pain - Some people with Parkinson's disease experience pain, either in specific areas of their bodies or throughout their bodies. Unmotivated anxiety and fear are also part of this symptomatic frameset.
3. Sexual dysfunction - Some people with Parkinson's disease duly notice a decrease in libido or sexual performance.

Etiologically, the 1st is a Layer 8 contribution to the disease in the Left-chiral partition group, the 2nd a Layer 7 contribution to the disease equally in the Left-chiral partition group, and the 3rd is caused by an accrual flip of an entire Sector of the Foliate which will naturally and intrinsically hamper or disrupt sexual expression, both in orientation and libido, in addition to performance, as we shortly discuss.

4.15 True Nature and Root Causes of Paraphilic Disorders

Whilst many sexuality-related disorders have been incontroversially classified in mental science thus far with clear consensual diagnostic elements, the particular group dubbed Paraphilias has posed enormous classificatory and diagnosis problems that have divided the community. Paraphilic disorders were formerly denoted sexual perversion or deviant behavior. At which point does an unusual or culturally uncommon sexual behavior become an outright paraphilic disorder is the question at the nexus of the controversy. There are even advocates in the social corpus for a total ban on all qualified sexual disorders, which allopathic medicine of the day is not about to submit to. In the West, homosexuality and lesbianism have recently been declassified as sexual mental disorders under social pressure reflecting in permissive political legislation. There is no doubt that latest advances in medical science about the knowledge in the chromosomic basis and endocrine regime that sustains human sexuation at the biological level have firmly contributed to the deflation of the emotional charge surrounding male and female homosexual behavior in Western Culture. Our ambition in this presentation is to plant a stake that flags the same markers in mental science in order for psychotherapy to present judicious and rational choices to individuals in distress about their sexual behavior in general, both for better living in self-satisfaction and for cure. We have discussed in Chapter 2 one of the most important among these markers, which is the dissection of the Mental Manifold in two lateral antisymmetric mentation regimes which primarily define human sexuation at the mental level. Each of the two regimes features a specific pensive accrual level with respect to the antisymmetric par, which determines binary gender differentiation.

As a principle:

> *Firstly, all human sexuality disorders arise at first order from a gender identity and expression crisis portended by one or the other chiral regime of the entire Mental Manifold (Anima or Animus Sector).*
>
> *Secondarily, the Layer that naturally accrues for the determination of character in the Foliate contributes to higher morbid paroxysm with the chiral set of partitions that are also part of the lateral sub-spectrum defining the individual's gender (Anima or Animus Sector).*

Therefore, setting aside the gender identity dysfunctions that we have discussed in Chapter 2, in virtually every sexual disorder, two pathological components feeding into one another ought to be contemplated: one is the sexuation regime and the other is a specific mentation Layer in over accrual. In the very particular case of paraphilias, Layer 7 is to be identified with the morbid paroxysm. Below a short hierarchical list of sexual mental disorders:

Sexual Disorders

- Female Orgasmic Disorder (Frigidity)
- Erectile Disorder
- Ejaculation Disorder (Delayed and Premature)
- Male Hypoactive Sexual Desire Disorder
- Female Sexual Interest Arousal Disorder

Paraphilias

- Sexual Masochism
- Sexual Sadism
- Exhibitionism

- Transvestism
- Voyeurism
- Frotteurism
- Fetichism
- Pedophilia

In Pedophilia i.e., the individual registered a sexual identity/expression crisis during an early phase of development as a child. Translate that the sexuation subspectrum registered a morbid accrual level, never to be resolved. Many studies with samples as large as about 1000 individuals have interestingly correlated Pedophilia with handedness, specifically non-right-handedness (which equates left-handedness plus ambidextrous). Results of a handful of such studies[17] *"showed that the relations between pedophilia and lower IQ, lesser education, and **increased rates of non-right-handedness** were the same in homogeneous groups referred by lawyers or parole and probation officers as they were in a heterogeneous group referred by a miscellany of other sources."*

Other more conclusive findings are reported in detail by the study cited below.

"A sample of 404 adult men underwent assessment[18] following illegal or clinically significant sexual behaviors or interests. Patients' assessments included: administration of a modified version of the Edinburgh Handedness Inventory; recording of patients' phallometric (penile) responses to erotic stimuli depicting adults, pubescent children, and prepubescent children of both sexes; and a tabulation of the numbers of patients' victims, ages 0–11, 12–14, 15–16, and 17 and older, of both sexes. In Study 1, patients' right-handedness scores correlated negatively with their phallometric responses to stimuli depicting prepubescent children and positively with stimuli depicting adults, replicating the pattern described in a previous report (Cantor et al., 2004). Unlike the previous study, however, patients' handedness scores did not significantly correlate with their numbers of prepubescent victims. To explore this discrepancy, Study 2 combined the patients from this replication sample with those in the previously reported sample, categorizing them by the sex and age group of greatest erotic interest to

---

[17] Intelligence, Memory and Handedness in Pedophilia, APA Pscyharticles, American Psychological Association, https://doi.org/10.1037/0894-4105.18.1.3

[18] Handedness in Pedophilia and Hebephilia, Springer, 2005, James M Cantor et al.

them. ***The odds of non-right-handedness in men offending predominantly against prepubescent children were approximately two-fold higher than that in men offending predominantly against adults and three-fold higher after eliminating those men with intrafamilial (i.e., incest) offenses.*** *Handedness differences between men erotically interested in males versus females were not statistically significant.* ***These results indicate that the rates of non-right-handedness in pedophilia are much larger than previously suggested*** *and are comparable to the rates observed in pervasive developmental disorders, such as autism, suggesting a neurological component to the development of pedophilia and hebephilia."*

Psychoanalytic orthodoxy will note that the (male) pedophile's heightened sexual arousal and attraction to prepubescent children are related to unresolved oedipal issues which cause inability to relate to adult females. Etiological exegesis in this analytic stream also expressly notes the presence of emotional congruence between a pedophile and young children in terms of low self-esteem and tendency to submissiveness in interpersonal relations. It is interesting to note that this interpretation, which mainly derives from the role played by psychosocial development in psychoanalysis, is incidentally a characterization of the Anima sector of the Mentation Foliate. As such, it rejoins the "asymmetric" or chiral tendency of "non-right handedness" that clinical research has uncovered in the male expression of the Disorder.

Further, and very importantly, depression is almost always part of the symptom set of pedophilia. By adding depression to low self-esteem, to tendency to submissiveness, to non-right-handedness, to inability to sexually relate to females in many cases, one can see the sketch of definite exacerbated imprint of an entire side of the Mental Foliate which is here no other than the Anima sector. The culprit for the disorder is most likely a disparity between the gender of the Mental Body and gender of the biological body as discussed in Chapter 2. This hypothesis is further strongly supported by the existence of a pedophilic variant, so-called unofficially *virtuous pedophilia*, or *pedophilia Obsessive Compulsive Disorder*, in which the patient is alarmed or distressed by the very fact of experiencing sexual attraction to children, has no intention of acting upon such urges and genuinely manifests greastest aversion to the possibility of harming them. The patient in this case almost considers himself a victim of his own estranged feelings. Compare with the sentiment of a transvestite who mentally feels and experiences the intellection of his gender as genuinely female and is so driven to the alarming and distressing feeling that he is trapped in a male body. We must also remember that, similar to *virtuous pedophiles*, a category of transvestites do not experience any urge at all to make good sexually on their self-acknowledged gender, being content to only represent it in their vestimenta and personal physiognomic presentation. We are therefore most likely facing here only two different responses to the same root cause, a disparity between biological gender and mentation Foliate gender. The differential is likely due, in one part, to psychosocial development factors, and, for the other part, possibly to the gradient of exacerbation of the Anima sector in each case as well.

It is important to highlight that, in the case of female pedophilia, the exegesis effort calls for an outright overaccrual of the left-chiral side of the Foliate from the accrual level already present in the female Foliate for gender determination, in lieu of a gender disparity between Mental Foliate and biological body, to be the culprit in the disorder. In any case, this exegetical effort gives the analyst a glimpse of the panoply of cohesive and valid interpretations brought about in this framework to support an insightful analysis of these particularly intricate dysfunctions, a vast subject that we cannot address here in totality. It may well be that more targeted studies, now unfortunately unavailable, are required to conduct the analysis to even greater depth, granularity, and thoroughness. Nevertheless, a squint extension to these views is offered in the specific presentation of Pedophilia Disorder in Chapter 4.

4.16 Authentic Dimensional Nature of Obsessive-Compulsive Disorders

In the introduction to their 2020 study of Obsessive-Compulsive Disorder (OCD) Dan J. Stein, Daniel L. C. Costa, et al write[19]:

"Obsessive–compulsive disorder (OCD) is a highly prevalent and chronic condition that is associated with substantial global disability. OCD is the key example

---

[19] Obsessive-Compulsive Disorder, Nat Rev Dis Primers. ; 5(1): 52. doi:10.1038/s41572-019-0102-3, July 2020

of the 'obsessive–compulsive and related disorders', a group of conditions which are now classified together in the Diagnostic and Statistical Manual of Mental Disorders, Fifth Edition, and the International Classification of Diseases, 11th Revision, and which are often underdiagnosed and undertreated... Although OCD is a relatively homogenous disorder with similar symptom dimensions globally, individualized assessment of symptoms, the degree of insight, and the extent of comorbidity is needed."

Let us observe at the outset that if *"Obsessive-Compulsive and Related Disorders"* is a pathology class label, the question of why it should not have a higher hierarchical generic denomination is well granted. If that higher hierarchical denomination cannot be found from derivation from a primitive or first principle, one ought to conclude that the notion under the label is probably theoretically flawed, taxonomically deficient and therefore formally unacceptable, at the very least deemed subject to revision.

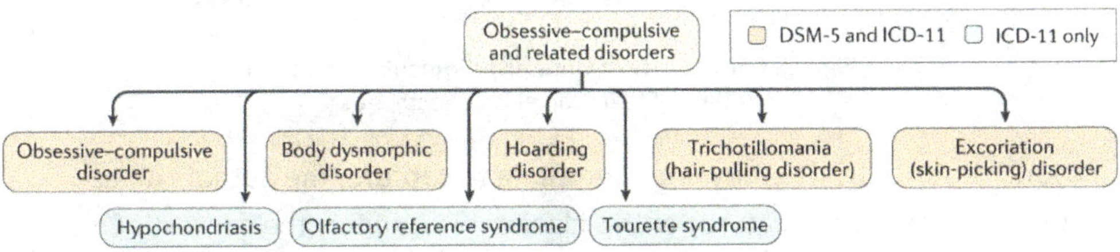

Fig. 4.4 Obsessive-Compulsive disorder tree by Dan J. Stein, Daniel L. C. Costa, et al

Analytic scrutiny will undoubtedly find the Disorders grouped together in this class quite arbitrary from a fundamental mentation viewpoint. Illustration in Fig. 4.4 shows the restricted group of (8) Disorders arranged under this class. Depending on one's definition of obsession and compulsion, these features may be found in virtually all mental disorders. One ought to wonder why the very impairments of *Suicidal Obsession* or *Approval Compulsion* are not direct members of this class or why *Bulimia Nervosa*, featuring patients who are obsessed with activity of their digestive system, is not a prime member either, and so on and so forth.

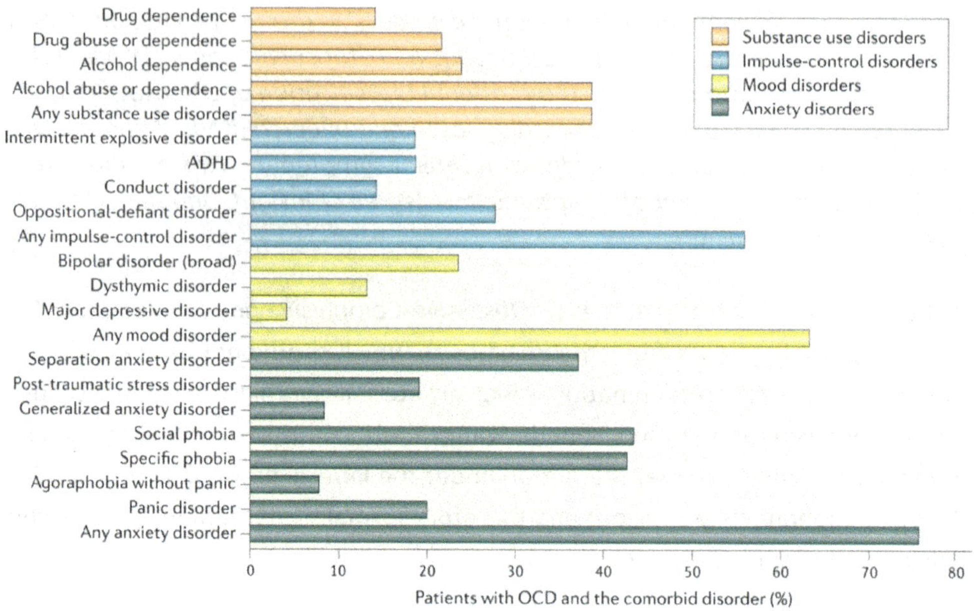

Fig. 4.5 Comorbidity in Obsessive-Compulsive disorder
by Dan J. Stein, Daniel L. C. Costa, et al

Beyond the specificities they are attempting to capture, the authors do acknowledge the global features of this class of disorders in the context of mental pathology in general. Of Obsessive Compulsive Disorder in particular they write:

"Common sets of obsessions and compulsions in patients with OCD include concerns about contamination together with washing or cleaning, concerns about harm to self or others together with checking, intrusive aggressive or sexual thoughts together with mental rituals, and concerns about symmetry together with ordering or counting. Failing to discard items is characteristic of hoarding disorder, but hoarding to prevent harm, for example, can also be seen in OCD. These symptom dimensions have been observed around the world, indicating that in some ways OCD is a seemingly homogenous disorder. Nevertheless, OCD can present with a range of less common symptoms, including scrupulosity, obsessional jealousy and musical obsessions. Avoidance is another key feature of OCD; individuals might curtail a range of activities to avoid obsessions being triggered."

As a side remark, the confusion of OCD, presumably one disorder of its own, and the class itself is quite notable in this proposition. A clearer picture of the globality of the syndrome is offered by the authors under the comorbidity view of the same (Fig. 4.5):

"OCD is characterized by substantial comorbidity. In the NCS-R, 90% of respondents with lifetime OCD (based on DSM-IV diagnostic criteria) met the diagnostic criteria for another lifetime disorder in DSM-IV; of these disorders, the most common were anxiety disorders, mood disorders, impulse-control disorders and substance use disorders. Tic disorders and other OCRDs also commonly co-occur with OCD. In 79.2% of cases, OCD began after the comorbid anxiety disorders, whereas OCD was about equally likely to begin before or after a mood disorder, and began after comorbid impulse-control and substance use disorders in 92.8% and 58.9% of cases, respectively. In addition, some evidence suggests increased comorbidity of general medical disorders in individuals with OCD."

We make it our challenge in this treatise to debunk and substantially discharge the notion of comorbidity in psychiatry. At this effect, it is interesting and paramount to stress here the parallel between the duplet Depression-Agitation, previously discussed, and the duplet Obsession-Compulsion. The passive inevitability trend animating Obsession and the active impulsive trend animating Compulsion are beyond argument. On that account Obsession tightly relates to Depression in terms of passive mentation that presents itself to the conscious mind as a non called for representation and Compulsion relates to Agitation as active motivational intentionality. Just as we have shown that the duplet Depression-Agitation is subjacent to every mental disorder, so is the duplet Obsession-Compulsion on account of both the Anima and the Animus Sectors of the Foliate. These two well formally defined Sectors of our psychophysics Manifold model of the Mental Body represent the primal classes that the proposed taxonomy has not ascertained. Consequently, there is no reason at all why the entire list of known psychogenic mental disorders should not be reported in the illustration in Fig. 4.5.

Perhaps the only judicious dimension of this class, we find from our psychophysics perspective, is the stereotypical aspect of behavior in a limited number of syndromes. This dimension is represented in the tic syndromes, which are incidentally instantiated by Layer 7 of the Mental Foliate. Consequently Layer 7 would stand for the corresponding class, which makes tics the manifestation of what the duplet Depression-Agitation becomes at Layer 7 of the Mental Foliate.

Trichlotillomania and Excoriation are two such tic syndromes. It is our assessment that tic mannerisms in themselves represent a low-level transversal subclass but not a vertical class in the Disorder hierarchy.

4.17 Redimensioning the Notion of Mood in Analytic Psychology

Let's start with the following Dictionary definition of the notion of Mood (same across the board):

"In psychology, a mood is an affective state. In contrast to emotions or feelings, moods are less specific, less intense and less likely to be provoked or instantiated by a particular stimulus or event. Moods are typically described as having either a positive or negative valence." - Wikipedia

In this attempt to frame the notion, we recognize:

- Typification of an affective state
- Claim of unspecificity in its very affective quality and causes
- Lesser affective intensity
- Endowed with an algebraic positive or negative descriptor

Perhaps, from our viewpoint, the most important descriptor here is that which assigns an algebraic sign to the notion in terms of an either positive or negative emotional state. To that categorization, we would next add the sense of gradation marked in lesser or greater intensity of feelings. Therefore, this characterization is for the most part directly translatable to the azimuthal symmetry feature of our model as discussed in Chapter 1. At the same time, in doing so we are curing the vagueness generally associated with the notion.

The notion of emotion and feeling in all cultures do not present qualifiable gradation in nature but in intensity. Although these categories are known, they are not generally attributed in their entirety to the notion of emotion. Because our mathematical-physics framework dictates these variables, we are going to posit their existence according to the specifications of the model and qualify them accordingly.

We are going to assign the longitudes or threads of the Foliate to the mood notion, resulting in the existence of 8 forms of mood or mood states, namely 4 positive ones and 4 negative ones in algebraic terms. There is further a differential quality to each of these mood states that is easily observable. One can easily understand that they are equally antisymmetric to one another as dictated by the model, in accordance with the azimuthal symmetry category.

Therefore, we have:

Disapprobation	**[-1]**	◄=►	**[1]**	Assent
Negativity	**[-2]**	◄=►	**[2]**	Assurance
Pessimism	**[-3]**	◄=►	**[3]**	Optimism
Dramatism	**[-4]**	◄=►	**[4]**	Excitement

In short, the Disapprobation mood is arguably that which is typically displayed by what we call a moody person, to describe the fact that he/she lives in chronic *displeasure*. It runs opposite to the smiley mood of someone who is mostly *acquiescent*.

The negativity mood is the one displayed by someone who reacts with a constant *"no"* to everything with or without any justification, whereas the Assurance mood is one that shows *confidence* as a matter of course.

The pessimism mood is one that we generally see in a person that is in the constant expectation of the *worse* to happen, whilst the optimism mood is in display when somebody is in a *cheering* attitude.

The Dramatism mood is that one which we probably qualify with the word *distress* to describe the attitude of making a drama about everything. It runs in opposition to the mood of *excitement* which qualifies the feeling of "being excited" about something with or without justification.

Fig. 4.6 All-Encompassing Foliate Model

	PASSIVE LATENCY - ANIMA					ACTIVE LATENCY - ANIMUS						
	-4	-3	-2	-1		1	2	3	4			
	Dramatism	Pessimism	Negativity	Disapproval	Hybrid	Assent	Assurance	Optimism	Excitement	QG CHARACTER	PSYCHA. PERSONALITY	MORBIDITY TYPE
1	Timidity	Introversion	Solitude	Indifference	← →	Conservativenes	Possessiveness	Competitivenes	Cupidity	EGOCENTRIC	*Janet's Jealous self*	*Only neuroses (No known form of psychoses)*
2	Inquisitiveness	Curiosity	Superficiality (In	Credulity	← →	Sincerity	Mirroring	Duplicity	Authoritarianism	REALISTIC		
3	Aberration	Idiocy	Disorientation	Doubt (Perple	← →	Discernment	Perspicacity	Clairvoyance	Lucidity	INTELLECTUAL	*Adler's inferiority complex*	
4	Remorse	Guilt	Shame	Regretfulness	← →	Presumption	Audacity	Stoicism	Heroism	HYPERBOLIC	*Super-Ego*	*Neuro-psychoses*
5	Delirium	Dystopia	Fabulousness	Daydream	← →	Chimera	Reformism	Visionary	Utopia	UTOPIAN	*Shadow - Alter Ego*	*Neuroses and Psychoses*
6	Despair	Sadness (Disapp	Sorrow	Pity	← →	Sympathy	Admiration	Euphoria	Passion	MATRIXIAL	*Id*	
7	Terror	Fear (Anguish)	Angst	Anxiety	← →	Resentment	Repugnance	Wickedness	Fury	PARADOXICAL	*Personal Unconscious*	
8	Subservience	Devotion	Humility	Laziness	← →	Equity	Hope	Happiness	Ecstasy	PERFECT	*General Unconscious*	
9	Inanity	Cluelessness	Austerity	Patience	← →	Temperance	Endurance	Resilience	Tenacity	ASYMPTOTIC	*Collective/Archetypical Unc*	

4.18 Connecting Pathological Analytic Psychology with QG Psychophysics Etiology

There are a number of pensive mechanisms traditionally identified in Analytic Psychology as *defense mechanisms,* whose function is to bring appeasement to a subject as a result of anxieties, feelings of angst and dissatisfaction of personal desires. In general, the science of Psychoanalysis has ascribed these mental patterns to the instance of the Unconscious Mind designated the *Personal Unconscious*. QG psychophysics framework largely supports this view and establishes the following principle or generalization:

All psychological pathological mechanisms are essentially rooted in the mentation root sublayer and informed by the superimposed representations. Dynamically, these mechanisms develop through normal transflows, and seek to achieve or restore equilibration in the Mental Foliate whenever it undergoes a local geometric deformation as a result of life events internally experienced in the representational sublayer at an extremum level.

One may liken this facsimile with a balloon bearing a spotty bump. The inflated bloat is a result of an increase in representational process intensity and/or density of the subtending root partitions. Pensive mechanisms are how partitions on a normal relate to one another, notably through azimuthal symmetry (anti-symmetry) inherent to the trigonometric chirality of the distribution and the invariant dictate of equilibration. Any form of representation or set thereof in a partition that would tend to create a symmetric imbalance due to its accrued intensity will end up causing a reaction by the antisymmetric partition on the Layer to counter-balance the abnormality. Paroxysmal representations of anxious-paradoxical nature in the negative quarter, for instance, may trigger a denial response emerging from the antisymmetric Repugnance partition of the Layer.

At the same time, it is also important to understand that the pensive mechanism seminally represents the expression of an intelligence informed by the inherent Norm of the Layer and its partitioned components (Fig. 4.6). There is a true persona associated with each mental normal in the sense that each has its own form of reaction and projection, within the global operational pattern of the Mind. Human personality types exist and become visible in a human sociocultural context because of this innate mentation Layer intelligence. We have seen in Chapter 3 how this disposition comes to materialize characterologically in the temper defining a human psychological type; in other words, how each temper type takes its roots in a specific mental normal.

Each Mental Norm thus represents a way to think or a pensive modality that is further reflected in all the partitions making up that normal altogether. As an example, all the partitions in the paradoxical Layer represent a visualization of negation, opposition or annihilation either in the form of instigation (positive quarter) or in the form of victimization (negative quarter).

The above is what undergirds the Analytic Psychology demarcation of inner selves, which in the Freudian Model are represented by the Id, the Ego and the Super Ego. As a reminder, in Freudian theory the Id is given to be the primitive and instinctual part of the mind which contains sexual and aggressive drives as well as hidden memories, the Super Ego stands for moral conscience, and the Ego is the realistic (conscious) part that mediates between the desires of the Id and the Super Ego. There is also the Alter-self or the Shadow, which is given as another form of the Ego in a sort of personality split. We present in Fig. 4.6 the correspondence between the inner selves as viewed by the many different psychological schools and Layers of our psychophysics Mentation Foliate.

What emerges from this correspondence is that each major thinker has indeed captured and interpreted an important part of the human psyche in its configuration and operation. Where they missed the mark is in the persistent attempt to explain the fullness of human behavior from that singular set of personality expression and faculties. They had also failed to uncover the correct spectrum of personality types, along with the relationship between those types and the singular selves or personas promoted by their individual vision of the human psyche.

1.- Janet's Psychology

Pierre M. F. Janet had a sense of the importance of the Egocentric pole of the psyche and built a psychology of jealousy as the core promoter of human behavior. His visualization maps to a highlight of the Egocentric or Monolithic mentation Layer of our psychophysics framework.

2.- Behaviorism

The behaviorists, led by Pavlov and later John B. Watson in the same vein, have priviledged the stimulus-response feature in all of psychic activity. They ascertained that human mental activity is primarily based on reflexive reactions in response to object or event perception. A dog will start to salivate at the **view** of even that customary feeding recipient (with no actual food within) or even the person who usually brings the recipient with food (while still omitting to bring it over). They generalized all human mental activity to be based on such perceptually driven reflexes or stimuli. Their view maps to the Binary or Ambivalent mentation Layer which prominently hinges on the perception of Reality.

3.- Adler's Individual Psychology

Alfred Adler promoted an individual psychology in which inferiority complex, superiority complex and style of life played a major role. He influentially coined the very term *inferiority complex* which remained an important concept in psychology. His visualization put the highlight on the Intellection Layer of our Mental Foliate, Layer 3, that is, which becomes an irrefutable attribution when the partitions of that Layer are individually considered.

The above three attributions inarguably incarnate the Ego evoked in Freudian psychoanalysis in the embodiment of the conscious self with the mission of harnessing reality.

4.- Roger's Self Theory

It is fitting to include in this rubrique of the conscious self the interesting Carl Roger's Self Theory. This theory centers around the concept of the phenomenal self, in other words the image of oneself that each individual uniquely perceives through the senses. The phenomenal self relates to our ontological Sense of Self-Awareness, which is an objective entity in that it cannot falter in any mental Foliate and stands as an invariant. Roger's phenomenal self is a dependency of the conscious Self-Awareness, could not exist without it and represents a variable through the course of life. To the limit, one may consider it to be part of the variance or transformation inherent to the Symmetry that profiles Self-Awareness, per our original definition. Effectively, the phenomenal self does not necessarily represent the real self, as posited by Carl Rogers: many people who are very successful professionally and highly respected in their circles still consider themselves abject failures, although, we argue, they still conserve their sense of Self-identity. Therefore, Roger's phenomenal self justifiably maps in part to the Hypocursor of the mentation Foliate.

5.- Social Learning Theorists

Other psychoanalysts who objected to Freud's so-called pansexualism and sought elsewhere than the personal unconscious the profound motives of human behavior include those who give prime relevance to social factors in human behavior. In that vision, society with its practices and norms heavily conditions individual behavior. Social learning theorists have expressly put considerable emphasis on rewards and punishments. One might argue that it is necessarily through internalization of social principles that the sense of reward and punishment cognitively arises in the mental. In reward and punishment transpires the manicheic duplet of good and bad, hero or villain, etc. typical of the typological Norm animating the Quadratic Mental Layer.

One can also easily see that this attribution matches the Freudian Super Ego entity as well.

6.- Jung's Creative Shadow Entity

We have already mentioned in this study several important aspects of Jungian psychology. One entity brought about by that view of the Mental is what has been designated the *Shadow*, a sort of *alter-self* that every individual bears at the unconscious level. Carolyn Kaufman had this to say about the Jungian Shadow entity *"...in spite of its function as a reservoir for human darkness—or perhaps because of this—the shadow is the seat of creativity;" so that for some, it may be that "the dark side of his being, his sinister shadow...represents the true spirit of life as against the arid scholar."* [20] For Jungian psychoanalysts, the process of accepting one's Shadow and integrating it to one's personality despite its *alter* character is a capital step toward reaching mental harmony in psychotherapy.

From our psychophysics vantage, the Jungian Shadow entity is in fact nothing but the Metamorphogenic persona construct in the QG Mentation distribution, in view of the freedom and creativity traits that Jungians ascribe to it – a complete match with the pensive partitions that the Metamorphogenic Layer consists of.

7.- Freud's Id Construct

In the Freudian Id construct, we recognize that we have in fact two different Foliate layers: the Matrixial Layer and the Paradoxical Layer. The Libidinal aspect of the construct is an outright match to the Matrixial Layer, while the Aggressive Drive aspect included in the notion is a direct match to the Paradoxical Layer.

While there has historically been a number of objections to Freud's attempt to make libido the single central motive of all human normal and morbid behavior, it is universally acknowledged that libido represents an important factor in the

---

[20] Kaufman, Carolyn. "**Three-Dimensional Villains: Finding Your Character's Shadow**" *Archetype Writing: The Writer's Guide to Psychology.*

expression of human behavior in general, both normal and pathological. In other words, libido is universally acknowledged to be a functional instance of Mind. The Matrixial Layer in our psychophysics model provides that standing in its most adequate and equanimous dimension. That said, we must not forget the cross-match cross-spectrum dimension of love on the basis of the binary distribution of the Foliate, on which we profusely elaborated in previous Chapters.

As to the Aggressive Drive, visible in vital survival instincts, it is incontrovertibly located in the province of the Paradoxical Layer. Most of the mechanisms put forth in Freudian psychoanalysis to explain the dynamics of the psyche pertain to the activity of that Layer. We provide further down a broad interpretation of said mechanisms.

8.- Reconciling Freudian Id and Jungian Personal Unconscious within the Layered Foliate

It is important to relate the Freudian Id entity to the Jungian Personal Unconscious in this review. The **Freudian Id** is a part of the Unconscious and represents the impulsive aspect of the psyche which responds directly and immediately to basic urges, needs, and desires, including libidinal urges. It is not conceived to be affected by or concerned with logic and external reality of the natural world. In analytic psychology, the **Personal Unconscious** stands for Carl G. **Jung**'s designation for the Freudian **Unconscious**, as contrasted with the **Jungian** concept of the **Collective Unconscious**. In the mapping represented in Fig. 4.6, we have ascribed the Id to Matrixial Layer with the clear understanding that this match only concerns the Libidinal aspect of the Id. Part of Jung's Personal Unconscious is also a match to the Matrixial Layer inasmuch as it acknowledges sexual urges. To the other inflexible urges and needs contemplated in both visions, we reserve the Paradoxical Layer.

It is clear that a correct and systematic demarcation between unconscious desires, urges, needs and instincts has not been properly realized in both the Freudian and the Jungian visions. This lack of a stringent systematization in these unconscious elements is for certain responsible for the dissatisfaction among following psychoanalysts, leading them to promote other visions of psychological transactions. Nevertheless, we provide below following this review an extensive analysis of the particular mechanisms associated with the two aforementioned Freudian and Jungian entities, of broad traditional acceptation in psychology to date, and as viewed under our psychophysics critical vantage.

9.- Horney and Fromm's Connectedness Instance

Psychologists Karen Horney and Erich Fromm also count amongst the many psychoanalytic revisionists in psychology and proposed a different theory of fundamental human motives in which they enlisted:

- Relatedness
- Transcendence
- Rootedness
- Identity
- Frame of Orientation

In the first three elements one can see the connectedness element which is another nomer for Collectiveness. Fromm advocates for a society *"in which man relates to man lovingly, in which he is rooted in bonds of brotherliness and solidarity... which gives him the possibility of transcending nature by creating rather than by destroying, in which everyone gains a sense of self by experiencing himself as the subject of his powers rather than by conformity."* Fromm argues that individual mental sickness is borne out of modern society, which runs opposite to these prescriptions and so provides the first causal factor of individual frustrations leading to abnormality. It is not difficult to see in this depiction the image of Jung's Collective Unconscious, which all map to the Perfect Layer of our Mentation Foliate.

4.19 Psychic Equilibration through Layer Transflows

From the QG analytic perspective, when it comes specifically to defense mechanisms, we posit that these are strictly developed by the Paradoxical Normal Layer, well in accordance with the combative or conflictive character evoked in the term *defense* originally chosen to designate them. Below is a list of such processes. No other layer is involved in the formation of these so-called defense mechanisms.

Repression, for certain one of the most impacting and most extensively studied among these mechanisms, is a form of containment taking place within the Paradoxical mental normal as a blockage within intralayer activity between the layer's inner partitions. Very importantly, it is not to be considered, as customarily postulated in Psychoanalytic Theory, a multilayer phenomenon involving an upper layer squashing back down a pensive orthoflow as it surges from the depth of the Unconscious. Instead, it is strictly a phenomenon obeying the Paradoxical Norm of the layer in the portrayal of opposition or conflict between the representations of two or more partitions therein. In that condition, it is an ondulatory flow with longitudinal back and forth travel akin to the eternal sinusoid model.

Denial is an equilibration reaction that is equally typical of the Paradoxical Persona per its very Norm. It is not a rational, consciously reasoned determination as perceived by the conscious self. It originates from the Paradoxical Persona, in reaction to angst imbuing an internalized life situation. As a pensive flow it circulates through the Paradoxical layer in the form of a partition-to-partition transflow. Denial occurs in very disturbing life situations, whereby the Paradoxical Persona simply resorts to denial of reality in the refusal to believe that those situations have effectively occurred in order to abate the ensuing anguish.

Rationalization, Intellectualization, Projections, Identification and so-called Reactive Formations are all reverse or antithetic reactions used by the Paradoxical persona to deal with frustrations or dissatisfied representational motives imbued in its partitions. A brief analytic presentation of each follows.

In ***rationalization***, the frustration of having been refused a work-related position for instance emerges as the false satisfaction that it was a bad position anyway and that the actor illusively saved himself/herself another frustrating situation. The antagonistic character between the motive and the failure to realize it constitutes what mediates the nature of the pretense called upon to dissolve the pain or frustration experienced by the subject. The term rationalization elected to designate this pensive pattern is probably ill-chosen in that it fails to properly characterize the true motive at work in the mechanism.

In *intellectualization*, the subject displays a want that he yearned for and at the same time an undesirable about the same motive that he did not wish: he/she declares having not really wanted what he/she was actively seeking to obtain, after having been refused the object of his/her motives. The conflicting character of the pensive pattern is very clearly portrayed here as well and might benefit from a more appropriate designation than intellectualization.

In ***projections***, the subject foists off or projects onto others the negative qualifications that he/she judged for himself/herself as a result of anxiety imbuing the desires or motives fostered at the level of his/her Paradoxical mental normal. To talk about the libertinage of the young generation or mankind's blanket dishonesty may be a concealment of one's own sexual desires causing anxiety and frustrations or one's own treacheries respectively. The motives of these pensive patterns are germane to the Paradoxical layer and the fact that they emerge through *antithetic* orthoflows is just another artifact of the Paradoxical Norm.

In ***identification***, the subject assumes or robs the identity of a superior who is responsible for his frustrations and anxieties, in an attempt to tamper the same through usufruct of the role of instigator. The subject imitates his superior's attitudes or mannerisms and repeats his word phrasings. The identification in this case may report to any figure of superior qualities or groups with higher abilities in the instigative usufruct attempt. It is important to understand this mechanism not just as an identification but as a forceful or audacious grab of someone's identity for the motive of self-appeasement.

In ***reaction formation,*** the Paradoxical Persona attempts to resolve the hostility that he feels vis-à-vis the world around by showing a hypertrophied sense of cordiality that overtakes the subject's overall behavior in life. It is in fact a form of dupery to be understood as an attempt by the Paradoxical Persona to make believe that he/she is amenable to everything and everyone when in fact he/she caters feelings of hostility towards them. He/she props open the door to everyone, endlessly saying "Yes, sir – Yes, Madam", holding a big smile, being agreeable like no one else and profusely apologetic for the slightest mistake.

These mechanisms are the ones at work in the development of many a dysfunction. They ought to be primarily understood as the workings of the Paradoxical

Persona according to its very Quanto-Geometric Norm of Paradox. It is certain that not all forms of abnormality are germane to the Paradoxical mental normal. Because the science of Analytic Psychology has not hitherto ascertained keen insight into the specific granular elements of the Architecture of mind, it has sought in these specific mechanisms the cause of the vast majority of mental dysfunctions. That may well be the reason why we see psychoanalysis overanalyze in many instances of mental disorder, as noted in Chapter 2. Such is, in particular, the case of what had been known in European psychology in the francophone vein as In-Depth Analytic Psychology *(La Psychologie des Profondeurs).*

4.20 Psychic Equilibration through Antisymmetric Flips

We lay down below a few examples of flips resulting from paroxysmal life situations that overexcite partitions at one or the other chiral side of the antisymmetric *normals* (or Layers). The reaction occurs as an equilibration mechanism seeking to maintain the natural par symmetry (or azimuthal symmetry) dictated by the trigonometric geometry of the normal Layers composing the Mental Foliate. In conventional Analytic Psychology, this mechanism has been dubbed *compensation mechanism*. Although it is understood to be a form of defense mechanism, we declassify it as a compensation mechanism and instead recognize its belonging to a mentation class rather, given the origin of its etiological dynamics. It is thus the parity (+, -) of the distribution of partitions on a mentation Layer that instantiates the compensation swings. Obviously, the subject experiences in conscious awareness these compensation drives, not knowing their origin and the reason for their particular nature.

PASSIVE-LATENCY PAROXYSMS

1. If you physically look very different from your peers causing an expression of shyness and you are being bullied, you may extemporaneously flip to staunch aggressiveness as a restoration reaction.

2. If you feel abused by others unduly putting their nose in your personal business (as in subreptitiously inquiring and gossiping about things happening in your personal life), you may flip to the extremum of bossing

people about how to do everything in their lives.

3. If you are always confused and in doubt about yourself, your capacities and your work (inferiority complex), you may come to flip to the compulsion of appearing to know everything, to be overly sure of yourself and always perfect in your conduct and occupations.

4. If you are feeling disloyal or remorseful of your acts or feelings with respect to social norms, you might flip to heroic attitudes of a champion of good manner and enforcer of social norms, as well as stringently self-imposed discipline or stoicism.

5. If you feel that your body or the world is in shambles and constant disorder, you may flip to the advocacy of radical changes even where they are not at all needed, i.e. in devotional venues and their practices.

6. If you feel unattractive and unable to generate attraction, you may flip to the compulsion of showing passion left and right, i.e. excessive dating, etc.

7. If you are feeling angst due to a conflict that is either constant or insolvable in your life, you may flip to actively inflict punishment through offensive and wicked behavior all around you.

8. If you are suffering from mistreatment as if reduced to subservience, you might flip to complete reliance on Providence or false joy/exaltation as provided by the habit of narcotics ingestion.

9. If you feel that life has driven you into incomprehensible situations dramatically forcing you to helplessness and austerity, you might react by compulsively switching to a display of the greatest endurance and resilience going forward in your life.

ACTIVE-LATENCY PAROXYSMS

1. If you are a cupid that is given to accumulate material possessions, you may suddenly one day become worried about losing it all or feeling quite insecure about your ability to keep all your possessions.

2. If you have been embarrassed or disparaged by people you feel were foolish, superficial or inconsiderate, you may one day turn to stingy comedy or satire in order to embarrass foolishness or heedlessness, wherever they may be coming from.

3. If you like displaying cleverness by being a perfectionist in your main occupation, you may become overly worried or obsessed about displaying sloppy work that paints you as an idiot in your mind.

4. If you are an extremely generous a person that displays "grandeur d'âme" as a matter of course, you may become suddenly convinced of being persecuted for your deeds and personal grandeur.

5. If you keep dreaming about or in constant visualization of a utopian better world, you may suddenly start unduly believing the present world is nothing but dystopia everywhere.

6. When you are profoundly in love and intensely live your passion over time, you may become wary about what is next to happen to put you in despair about this deep and intense sentiment.

7. If you are a wicked person who always seeks to harm other people, you may suddenly wake up with the angst of being destroyed or harmed yourself, or with the conviction that others are actively seeking to harm you.

8. If you are a champion of hope, good luck and belief in Providence, you may suddenly flip to the belief that the devil is everywhere to put you in

misery and defeat, in making you lose favor with Providence.

9. If life puts you time and time again to the test of endurance and you strive to overcome obstacles by being resilient, you may suddenly become a champion of procrastination and defer almost everything, or else you may suddenly find yourself in the utter withdrawal of inanition.

We will later see that these sorts of flips occur in virtually every mental disorder involving both chiral sides of a mentation Layer and have been denoted mood swings in the current disease nomenclature. The current official disease model has not recognized the universality of the flip mechanism in mental disorders, limiting it to the so-called mood disorders. This misunderstanding is clearly reflected in the label of bipolar disorder expressly and specifically given to the disorder of Manic Depression, thereby putting in evidence ignorance of the nature and origin of bipolar swings per se in mental dysfunctions.

4.21 Delinquent Conduct vis-à-vis Psychopathology

Delinquency is understood to be unlawful conduct by any individual within any social class in a political democracy, but not a psychiatric mentation disorder per se. It is a tricky subject in that oftentimes the ones who propose and directly or indirectly impose defining criteria for particular delinquent or unlawful conducts are the first to breach them. For instance, in the 2008 worldwide depression, the credit rating companies, as self-appointed raters of goodwill and responsible behavior, and which are admittedly the first to stick the epithet of "delinquent" to the citizenry, were found to have committed egregious unethical acts in the conduct of business in connivance with banking executives. Certainly, in that arena, one of the most difficult concepts to grapple with is the omnipresence of evil in all of human culture and history. The overwhelming manifestation of evil permeates the entire set of human institutions, from Health to Church to Legislature. It is even difficult to estimate at which point in the history of mankind evil has culminated its predatory manifestations. Indeed, from incarceration of little children forced to remain in cages with their wastes in recent times, to human beings chained in their nakedness at the bottom of transatlantic slave trade boats in past times, to priests of all time defiling women and children or advocating genocide, to care givers knowingly and self-servingly prescribing lethal agents, the problem of evil is ageless and omnipresent among Men. It might be the biggest problem faced by Men in the course of our evolution, much beyond ignorance.

Evil manifests in many different forms, and there are many words for evil: hatred, crime, genocide, bigotry, homicide, lie, fear, arson, suicide, slander, death, Devil, etc. Dr.Gerald L. Kovacich, Dr. Andy Jones, wrote in 2006 in a forensic analysis piece[21]:

"Crime has never been the sole possession of any one race, religion, society, community, or nation, and a pervert has always been a pervert, seeking sexual gratification by illegal means and in illegal ways."

Perhaps the most important way to understand and grapple with evil is not through the opposition stance of rejecting it outright through moral, philosophical or legislative prescriptions or decrees. It is paramount to comprehend and come to terms with the fact that evil is a Norm. It is one among the nine foundational Norms framed in the crucible that molds the expression of physical reality. It is a peculiar norm that does not respect or harmonize with the other Norms of the primitive canon and as such qualifies as the antinorm Norm. We have termed it in this treatise[22] the Paradoxical Norm or the Norm of Destruction, incarnated in Layer 7 of the Mentation Foliate.

In that sense, the evil of Death is not the opposite of life, as we commonly have it. Death is a constant part of life. It is not the end of life and it is not outside of life. In fact, in our human bodies, there is knowingly an entire system of orchestration of Death, both at the cellular level and the functional physiological level that is an integral part of homeostasis. Further, such structures as the human skeleton, hair and nails long outlive clinical death of the human body. The norm that perpetrates evil is thus an integral part of the functional framework of the living. In culture and institutional health care, we have proved not at all intent in keeping with this clarity in our world vision.

---

21 High-Technology Crime Investigator's Handbook (Second Edition), *2006*

22 The same lexicon is used for this Norm throughout QGT.

The first victory of evil over Man is to have succeeded in making us believe in our cogitations that the above is untrue, that all of that which is outside of evil is either unimportant, untrue or unreal, and that because evil is everywhere Absolute Bounty does not and cannot exist. Evil makes us believe in the dystopia of a world forever mired in inescapable evil. However, the Norm of Evil is only part of the primitive canonical stack, has its place and only place within the stack, and as such it is functionally subject to the entire protocol represented in and by the canonical novena stack. Evil is irrevocably subject to Bounty (the entire stack and its protocol) and at the service of Bounty. And that is why, despite evil, Absolute Bounty does exist.

To at once oppose evil is to play its game and ineluctably fall at its feet, whether it is the one inside or the one we might see outside. It is strictly by following the Hierarchy of Norms, or the foundational primitive Norms, that one can successfully interact with evil. And it is only by following the higher Norms to the Norm of Evil that one can successfully control and eventually defeat evil at will. Therefore, only the Perfection Norm and the Transcendental Norm, both situated higher up in the canonical primitive stack over the Paradoxical Norm, bear the inner faculties for controlling and defeating evil. The first is the Golden Rule:

> ***Do not do onto others what you would not like them to do onto you. Only treat others as you would treat yourself.***

This cardinal principle is about the state of Bounty and individual freedom. It proposes that one cannot define the Good or what is good from self. No one can define how to be a good human being in and of oneself. You can only define Good or Bounty in relation to others. What is good for you is only what will be good for others as well. What is not virtuously good for you is not good for others either. Hence the State of Goodness or Bounty is a collective ontological state that transcends the self. It is far and away from an Abstraction, it instead dictates collective experience at the same time that it arises from collective experience. Further, it is Totalitarian. The Golden Rule definition emanates from the Perfection Norm at Layer 8 of the QG Normal Primitive Stack, which embodies a higher form of degree of freedom, translatable in a *degree of freedom from self*, or universal connectedness.

One of the most genuine expressions of this form of degree of freedom from self is observable in the human axis of self-detachment that goes from laughter to orgasm to extasis. Consequently, in the quest to overcome evil whose common agency is fear, should one oppose laughter to fear, whether internal or externally borne out by a threat, the fear is duly neutralized and eventually overcome. Fearlessness is a due attribute of Perfection.

The second cardinal principle to control and overcome evil is the ***principle of No Reaction or Inanition*** (or Yield), an emanation of the higher Transcendental Layer of the QG Primitive Stack, Layer 9, that is. In religious canon, it is given as the Sabbath. Some inspired political leaders in recent history have found a partial translation of this cardinal principle in the political creed of Non Violence, which had nevertheless scored two enormous political successes in world history vis-à-vis colonialism (1930) and apartheid (1990).

What is important to recognize is that it is only by exercising means and faculties emanating from the two Higher Norms of Perfection and Trancendentalization that evil can be controlled and vainquished when necessary. Useless to say that institutional legislation outside of the framework of these two Norms in the societal context is not going to dent human evil. The human institution of Justice has been putting behind bars through *law enforcement* the evil in identified social delinquents, who permeate all layers of society indistinctly, throughout the entire course of human history. Perhaps psychiatric science may contribute to bring this pursuit at the level of the individual citizen's psyche, which is where the awareness and comprehension of this affair must be experienced in order for the evolution of mankind to enter the phase of assertively controlling and dominating Evil.

Although the problem of evil verges into psychopathology, very particularly with the Disorders rooted on Layer 7 of the human Mentation Foliate, which propend outright criminal behavior in many cases as we shall see, it is more likely that contribution of Psychatric science to the resolution of this enormous human problem will come from a humanistric approach via the knowledge of Mind and its framework of operation in normalcy. It is so much more so when it comes to young Minds in development as regards to the important societal issue of *Juvenile Delinquency*.

4.22 Underpinnings of Sleep Disorders

Attempts to explain the sleep paradigm in human culture date back at least four millennia, precisely to the Egyptians who, by all accounts, count among the first known dream psychoanalysts.

4.22.1 Brief History of the Study of Sleep

Effectively, the Egyptians' belief system was pre-Jungian in the practice of visualizing the workings of an alter-self in the interpretation of nightly dreams as well as the use of universal symbols in their interpretation. They further seemed to have achieved an understanding of the metaphysics of nocturnal dreams since they pursued a form of clairvoyance by which prophecies were often sought from nightly dreams they considered premonitory. Given the fantastic material achievements that we witness today from the ancient Kemetic civilization through continued archeological findings, these visualizations shall not be altogether disregarded by today's science of the mental, and psychophysics itself must take notice.

The Greeks followed in suit with Democritus who laid out the first formal theory of precognition of dreams. There was no doubt that his approach to dreams was laid on a physical basis towards elucidating the possible metaphysical embodied in nightly dreams. Around Century IV BC, Alcmaeon described sleep as a state of unconsciousness, while Aristotle upheld the contrasting view of suspension of consciousness. Aristotle noticed that sleeping happens with closed eyes, and thus assumed it consists of an absence of overall sensorial perception. Obviously, he erroneously did not consider the sensorial thresholds beyond which sleep could be interrupted, which might indicate concurrent perception does influence sleep content to some extent. Nevertheless, Aristotle was the first to emphasize the role played by closed eyes during the sleep state, intuitively inferring the REM form of sleep. The Romans took the understanding of sleep to a new dimension insofar as the arrangement of sleeping spaces, environment conditioning as well as sleep-related behaviors. In the meantime, for the next two millenia, mankind kept sleeping, quite literally and figuratively.

The Renaissance period saw the emergence of one of the best diagnosticians of sleep disorders before the modern era, in the figure of a literary genius by no other name than William Shakespeare. As Yury Furman, MD, put it in an article about Shakespeare and sleep disorders[23]:

"...Shakespeare also recognized the psychological problems often underlying recurrent nightmares and other disorders such as sleepwalking and sleeptalking..."

Shakespeare, admittedly, heeded and vividly described several other major sleep disorders that he intently observed, among them sleep apnea and insomnia.

Beginning with the Enlightenment period that followed, there has been no shortage of sleep disorder depiction in the psychological and neurological literature in development. Let's opportunely evoke the famous fairy tale "The Sleeping Beauty" based upon the Little Briar-Rose (by The Grimm Brothers, 1812), originally La Belle au Bois Dormant by Charles Perrault (1697), in which the fairy's curse spell upon the princess condemns her to sleep for one hundred years, only to be eventually awaken by a prince who shall kiss her for such. This story recognizes the important fact that perception of the environment during sleep does continue on and inform sleep content, notwithstanding the perception thresholds that will cause arousal when crossed. The sleeping princess will perceive the rocking lip touches from the prince which will ultimately cause her to awake.

4.22.2 Biological Factors Influencing the State of Sleep

It has become well known that indigestible food that turns up the digestive system will induce nightmarish dreams, as much as noise and smells perceived by a sleeping brain will transpire in ongoing dreams within the symbolic representations of their imageries. By the same token, very strong smells such as the smell of the chemical agent chloroform and other hypnoids may quite swiftly induce seizure or sleep. There is no doubt that perception has a direct and complex connection with sleep, no less than the hormonal system does. The sedative or sleep-inducing power of French kisses has been linked by recent research to oxytocin. Philematology or the science of kissing has demonstrated that a kiss can increase the level of oxytocin in circulation. In several research studies at

---

[23] October 1997 issue of Neurology - *Shakespeare and Sleep disorders,* https://doi.org/10.1212/WNL.49.4.1171

Rudgers University (New Jersey, 2009) and Lafayette College (Pennsylvania, 2009), blood and saliva tests showed that men in the kissing group of the study had a burst of oxytocin, while cortisol levels, the stress hormone, registered a decline in both men and women. Whether those findings give credit to the old time fairy tale in which the prince's kisses end up awakening the long sleeping princess remains an interesting question[24].

During the 19th and 20th centuries, progress in neuroanatomy has paved the way for better understanding of the biological underpinnings of the sleep function. From hypothalamus activity to the thalamus recently spotted to be a control center for the sleep-wake cycle or circadian rhythm, we have come one step closer to the unraveling of this rather mysterious function of life. The pineal gland has proven to play an irrevocable role in sleep pattern control. Melatonin, a pineal hormone, synthesized from tryptophan and serotonin via acetylation and methylation reactions respectively, is known to have a pivotal role in the establishment of the circadian rhythm. The pituitary gland complements this production during the sleep state by releasing the growth hormone, which assists the body in the vital functions of repair and developmental growth. Aforementioned oxytocin, so-called "love" hormone, is mainly produced in the hypothalamus, where it is released into the blood stream via the pituitary gland, and other parts of the brain and spinal cord, where it binds to oxytocin receptors in order to act as a sleep promoter, and influence behavior in general. A 2003 study by Ellison states that *"this link [with sleep inducement] makes sense because oxytocin counters the effects of cortisol, which is known as the stress hormone."*

4.22.3 Characterizing and Monitoring Sleep via EEG

The invention of the electroencephalogram (EEG) in the early 1900's allowed for recording of electrical brain activity and proper identification of wave patterns in various normal sleep phases and sleep disorders alike. Following the revolutionary development of EEG recording, Eugene Aserinsky took the study of the sleep function one step further with the discovery of REM (Rapid Eye Movement) Sleep. REM sleep is characterized by lack of response of the body volun-

---

[24] http://www.popten.net/2009/02/a-kiss-is-a-mechanism-for-mate-assessment/

tary muscles with persistent dreaming, except of course for the ocular muscles, whereas the Non-REM sleep implements the opposite. In other words, when the closed eyes move (REM), the body is stagnant; when the closed eyes are stagnant (Non-REM), the body moves. Note that dreamers usually enter REM sleep about 90 minutes after falling asleep. It lasts for about 10 minutes. As the state of sleep proceeds, each REM period becomes longer than the previous, finally lasting up to about an hour.

Important though all these developments might be in the knowledge of how the sleep function is exercised, it is fair enough of an assessment to strictly constrain them to the arena of physiological conditioning and monitoring of sleep. Quite in opposition to the monist perspective, physiological expression of sleep is not to be conflated with the immanent psychogenic nature of the state of sleep. The functional neural perspective says little about the configuration of the psyche during sleep and the dynamics of one of the two most critical aspects of sleep, which is the dream dimension of the same. As the founder of modern time psychoanalysis in its structured form, Sigmund Freud tapped into the vast universe of dreams, and took to insightfully unveil the unseen: profound libidinal and aggressive thoughts as it were in course throughout nocturnal dreams, which decisively underpin human behavior ultimately. He recognized early on the importance of this extraordinary content of sleep and declared *"dreams [to be] the royal road to the Unconscious."* If the overdrive of the digestive system may provoke nightmarish dreams, it does not dictate the specifics of the content of those dreams in the framework of mentation activity and history as much as symbolic representational code proper to the Unconscious alter selves or personae. No more than oxytocin is going to tell who one loves.

From a mentation vantage, sleep is a tête-à-tête with dreams. As though this type of exercise was still needed after Freud and Jung , Michael Schredl explains how the wake-like issues are reflected in dreams, in support to the link between awake thoughts and dreams[25].

---

[25] Dreams in patients with sleep disorders, *DOI:* 10.1016/j.smrv.2008.06.002

"...Overall, the findings support the arousal-retrieval model of dream recall but also clearly indicate that other factors like cognitive impairment or micro-arousal might affect the dreaming process. The content analytic findings support the continuity hypothesis of dreaming which states that waking-life issues are reflected in dreams. The number of studies in this field is still very small, however, and further research is needed to confirm and expand the reviewed findings."

4.22.4 Lucid Dreams

Most interesting is the exotic breed of dream denoted *lucid dream*, first experienced and described by Tibetan Buddhists in the form of Sushupti yoga, in which the monk can be fast asleep and awake for a few seconds without being able to identify the self with the body. It is paramount to underscore that patients who experience lucid dreaming and self-induced hypnotic states are well able to describe their experiences in minute detail. Lucid dreaming is a state whereby the dreamer remains aware of his/her own non real dreaming activity while being asleep. During a lucid dream, the dreamer may or may not gain relative control over the represented dream characters, narrative, and environment. He/she is aware that the scrolling events through the mind are not matter-of-factly happening, nonetheless the dream will feel very vivid and real to the lucid dreamer. There are also instances of paroxysm in nightly dreams where one expresses to oneself that *"this is only a dream, this is not happening"* in order to do away with the emotional stress one is circumstantially undergoing in the act of dreaming. It is more likely that these instances of dreaming activity qualify as lucid dreams as well because of the meta-consciousness experienced in those cases, the awareness of self-awareness, that is. Effectively, lucid dreaming belongs to an even higher dimensional metric of Mentation than common dreams. It equates looking at oneself in a front mirror from another smaller mirror placed at head rear. In this case, you would see an embedding succession of images of self in the front mirror, each being comparable to a different physical metric dimension. Comparatively, in a lucid dream one of these self-images, the second one in line, acquires a certain level of independence.

Researchers believe that frequent lucid dreaming is rare, with only 23 percent of people experiencing lucid dreams at least once a month and about 55 percent experiencing one or more lucid dreams in their lifetime. Like most dreams, lucid dreaming usually happens during REM sleep.

4.22.5 QG Psychophysics Etiology of Sleep and Sleep Disorders

Our psychophysics Theory for sleep disorders poses the principle that they all primarily originate in accrual dynamics proper to the Mentation Cursor, as a reflection of triplet QG Quintessence in the very Mentation dimensional metric. There is for sure an influence of the cosmic alternation resulting from Sun-Earth gravitational interaction on biological sleep processes in the living. At the biological level this influence is majorly mediated by the pituitary gland which regulates the circadian rhythm. The circadian rhythm is also jointly influenced by the variations in the metabolic/energy level of the body. We hypothesize the existence of a corresponding vector at the Mentation metric level acting in a parallel fashion to tailor the dynamics of the Mental Cursor.

The concepts of awareness and Mental Cursor as preliminarily discussed in Chapter 1 are paramount to the exegesis of Sleep disorders. What we have stipulated for all disorders other than sleep-related is threefold:

- If the patient is aware of his symptoms and acknowledges their abnormality, then Awareness is Conscious, for a Neurotic type of Disorder.
- If the patient is unaware of his symptoms, then Awareness is Unconscious, for a Psychotic type of Disorder.
- If the patient is vaguely aware of the abnormality of his symptoms, then Awareness is Semiconscious, for a quasi Neurotic or quasi Psychotic type of Disorder.

We have further ruled that whenever the Cursor is located or sojourning in the Conscious Cognos (Layers 1, 2, 3), the Mental is in the Awake state, and we then designate the Cursor a Hypocursor. Whenever the Cursor is located or sojourns in the Unconscious Cognos (Layers 5, 6, 7, 8 and 9), the Mental is in the Sleep state, and we then designate the Cursor a Hypercursor. Whenever the Cursor is located on or spanning Layer 4, the Mental is in a Semiconscious or Semiunconscious state and we then designate the Cursor a Quadratic Cursor or Quadracursor.

When it comes to sleep-related disorders, it is principally the quality and specific dynamics of the Mental Cursor as incarnation of Awareness or Self-Awareness that characterize the Disorder. Akin to the instances of accrual for the pensive partitions of a Layer in producing neuroses and psychoses, there are also states of accrual for the Cursor. Unlike Layer accrual however, we have restrictively set only 1 level of accrual for the Mentation Cursor.

When the Hypercursor is accrued, we thus have a morbid state of Sleep. When the Hypocursor is accrued, we have insomnia (morbid state of wake). When the Quadracursor is accrued, then we have a disturbed, sleep-like state of wake. As a reminder, the Cursor sweeps over the Layers from one partition to the next with no admissible interstitial positioning between partitions, and superimposes the partition it is resting on. It may be physically considered a Manifold inside a Manifold (the discrete partitions). Its accretion is responsible for both the abnormal forms of sleep and the paranormal ones (including hypnosis).

To be clear, when people experience difficulty to sleep, it is an abnormal situation whereby they remain stagnantly conscious all the while. It is a condition that may arise from accrual of any one of the 3 Layers making up Consciousness. The Hypocursor is then so to speak bombarded by the pulses coming from these partitions, so gaining "inertia" that prevents it from drifting away across Layer 4 into the larger region of the Unconscious. Alternatively, the Hypocursor may simply become accrued on its own and accuse the same dysfunctional dynamics causing the morbidity of insomnia.

The problems with the Hypercursor when in accretion tend to be instead persistent (or chronic) state of sleep or morbid somnolence. The accretion in the Hypercursor keeps it in sojourn within the Unconscious Cognos (Layer 5 through 9), causing the persistent morbid somnolence issues. Just as the Hypocursor, accretion in the Hypercursor may either result from over accretion in the dynamics of a particular Layer of the Unconscious Cognos (Layer 5, 6, 7, 8 or 9), or from autogenic dysfunction, both of which will hold the Cursor captive or stagnant within the Unconscious realm.

The Quadracursor may experience the exact same types of problems from Layer dynamics accretion or autogenic paroxysm, the concerned Layer here being Layer 4.

An important pathological state of the Mentation Cursor in any of its three modes is a fixed or akinetic condition by which it remains stagnant by over accretion on a *single* partition within the captive Layer, unable to drift away or doing so in very slow motion. This level of over accretion of the Cursor must be understood in terms of an extremely high extremum in intensity.

At the end, QG psychophysics Theory proves both Alcmaeon and Aristotle right as it pertains to Sleep and Sleep disorders, which are disorders of Consciousness, Semiconsciousness, and Unconsciousness (i.e., Insomnia, Sleep-wake disorders, Hypersomnia, and so-called Parasomnias).

4.23 Parasomnias and the REM and NREM Taxons

"Parasomnia" is a term invented to regroup the variety of unusual behaviors people experience in relation to sleep or somnolence, in particular prior to falling asleep, during sleep, or during the arousal period from sleep back to wakefulness. The considerable variation in symptom characteristics, dysfunctional severity, and dysfunction frequency covered by the term makes it taxonomically and psychotherapeutically unhelpful and inauspicious alike.

The taxonomy that has been put under the term parasomnia distinguishes three symptomatic groups for diagnosis: NREM-related, REM-related, and "other." The created taxons are therefore defective in that they do not ascertain a valid criterion for cross-class differentiation. Effectively, "other" is as vague and eclectic a nomer as anyone may wish and there are important sleep traits that are common to both NREM and REM sleep as we shall shtortly see.

This picture is further complicated by a view among some researchers that beyond psychopathology the phenomena covered by parasomnias are transition states undergirded by the brain in the process of awakening or falling asleep, as well as transition states between rapid eye movement (REM) and non rapid eye movement (NREM) sleep cycles. They seem to remove the focus for the parasommnia qualifier from the very state of sleep itself.

REM sleep first occurs about 90 minutes after falling asleep, as previously mentioned. If most of our dreaming imageries occur during REM sleep, a portion of them does occur during Non-REM sleep. Therefore dreams are not an exclusive property of REM sleep. The more important question is why certain dreams seem to echo a prime visual experience and others do not. Further, the question of why the visual cortex would feel compelled to ignite a vivid visual experience on its own that seems completely purposeless, and even at counter purpose with the recovery and atonic experience of sleep as an objective, is another important interrogation.

What's more, as rapid eye movement sleep occurs after the first four NREM stages of the night sleep, following this first complete sleep cycle, NREM and REM stages will repeat in a cyclical fashion every 90 minutes or so for the rest of the night virtually as a program. The person's eyes will move rapidly or jitter underneath the eyelids during REM sleep while the body experiences faster breathing and the heart rate and blood pressure increase. The characteristic trait of REM sleep is not just the constant eye jitter under the lids but a diurnal-like physiological posture as described, which seems comparable to some extent with the alert posture that is the province of the Conscious Cognos. We must remember that we do not go to sleep to be active but to be as passive as possible in the hopes of recovery from fatigue and functional rebalance. In this context, the cycling of NREM sleep appears to be a recovery response to the REM sleep phases as well, not just to the physiological expense of diurnal activity.

Furthermore, an important functional consideration is that deep sleep in which the body is extantly inactive and has been shown to help strengthen the immune system does not occur during the REM phase. Most neuroscientists agree that while stages 1 to 4 and REM sleep are all important, deep sleep is the most essential of all for feeling rested and staying healthy. The estimate is that average healthy adult gets about 1 to 2 hours of deep sleep per 8-hour period of night sleep. Therefore why is REM sleep necessary? We assert that the full elucidation of the REM-NREM sleep constraint and their alternation in a virtual program constitute a promise to a fundamental insight in deeper human ontology. Why do blind-born people who have never "seen" a single thing or object of any sort have the exact same visual experience in REM dreams as sighted people do? Brain imaging monitoring shows the exact same neural circuit activity in both cases. A question for the monists to keep busy figuring.

It remains that refurbishing the parasomnia notion is slated to bring more clarity to our vision of sleep-related dysfunctions. The "unusual" character that the notion is based on covers too many of an eclectic string of facts, especially when scrutinized from our perspective, for the notion to be of any defining usefulness. We are going to segregate, or break into different groups wherever applicable, the many syndromes that are generally gathered under this nomer, consistent with our definitions for the distinct principled categories inherent to the Mental Foliate visualization. An etiologic exegesis for more successful diagnosis and towards better cure will naturally emerge from this taxonomic redress. We propose the following taxons for the sleep disorders that have been identified with a more or less REM relationship:

Turbulent Sleep Disorders

- Aggressive REM Sleep Disorder (REM Sleep Behavior Disorder)
- Nightmare Disorder (Dream Anxiety Disorder) – (REM)
- Sleep-Related Bruxism (REM)
- Night Terrors (NREM)
- Sleep-Eating Disorder (Comorbid to Binge Eating Disorder) (NREM)
- Exploding Head Syndrome
- Sleep-Related Enuresis (NREM)

Sexomanic Sleep Disorder (NREM)

Confusional Arousal (NREM)

Sleepwalking (NREM)

We take the step to coin the new disorder label *Turbulent Sleep Disorder* only because our psychophysics framework does showcase an opportune key to meaningfully cluster all the related variants under this label taxonomically. Certainly, it does no good to multiply classificatory variants without being able to recognize common denominators which could be meaningful from a treatment standpoint. In the Sleep disorder section of the next Chapter, we will discuss in detail the etiologies that make this taxonomic adjustment convenient, as we expose a more detailed analysis and a systematic approach to each specific disorder. Following is a brief description of the involved syndromes.

REM Sleep Behavior Disorder (RSBD) is characterized by odd vocalizations or movements during REM sleep, aggressiveness manifest in violence against a bed partner (fist hits or strangulation), often as a reaction to a dream. It is usually attributed to dysfunction in the muscles responsible for skeletal muscle atonia in the extremely relaxed state concurrent to the REM stage.

Nightmare Disorder is characterized by vivid dreams defined by threats to survival or security generally resulting in fatigue, distress, reduced cognition. Nightmare disorder frequently accompanies Post Traumatic Stress Disorder (PTSD). Motor activity is often limited during nightmare episodes. In children, it is to be associated with severe psychosocial stressors.

Night Terror (or Sleep Terror) essentially differs from Nightmare Disorder in that it is a NREM sleep disorder. Those dreamers often scream in their sleep. Most are unresponsive to outside stimuli and keep no memory of the source or origin of their terror upon waking. Most night terror episodes reportedly last between 30 seconds and 3 minutes.

In **Sleep-Eating Disorder**, the dreamer moves away from the bed, still in the unconscious state, and serves himself or herself food and starts eating. It is a disorder that is co-morbid to Binge Eating Disorder and other related Disorders.

Sleep-Related Bruxism is an abonormal condition in which the dreamer takes to grind or clench his or her teeth causing a characteristic audible noise perceivable by others.

Sleep-Related Enuresis is your familiar nightly bed wetting disorder, which may be a sign of significant psychosocial stressors.

Sexomanic Sleep Disorder, colloquially known as "sexsomnia," is characterized by unusual sexual behaviors during sleep, such as aggressive masturbation, initiation of sexual intercourse with a partner, and utterance of sexual noises.

Confusional arousals: The sleeper exhibits mental confusion or confused behavior in bed. The affected display very little autonomic arousal in the form of mydriasis (dilated pupils), tachycardia (accelerated heartbeat), tachypnea (accelerated breathing), or perspiration. Confusional arousals are also known as Elpenor syndrome.

Sleepwalking or Somnambulism occurs when people get out of bed while still asleep and exhibit limited awareness or responsiveness to their surroundings. They may further engage in other complex or involved activities such as sorting clothes, street wandering, etc. Sleepwalking may become dangerous to safety and cause injuries should the individual lose balance or collide with other objects.

It is important to remain clear that there is more to sleep than REM or NREM distinction, as important as the REM phase of sleep might be. Beyond the REM/NREM characterization, the above recount already gives us a glimpse at the subjacent typological phenoma that permeate the expression of these disorders. These psychophysics typological undercurrents will become very clear when we next put these disorders under the QG etiological magnifier at end of the next Chapter. By and large, it cannot be overstated that sleep disorders are first and foremost a dysfunction of the Mentation Cursor in nature, very particularly in its Hypercursor and Quadracursor modes. Should the term Parasomnia remain in use, the mentioned representation is the only meaningful attribution it may be accorded.

4.24 Comorbidity with Sleep-Related Disorders

A final word on Sleep-Related Disorders in comorbidity with other mental Disorders is very much granted. Sleep-related dysfunctions perhaps represent the most legitimate dimension of comorbidity in psychiatry. They are knowingly present in a vast array of Disorders.

The main reason for this form of multimorbidity is the fact that over accrual of pensive partitions in a Foliate's normal Layer tends to be covariant with Cursor over accrual as the normal Layer tide may entrain and constrain the Cursor's sojourn. Even though we have not formally established a metric for Cursor accrual, it clearly follows from the implications and consequences of our psychophysics framework that the cursor as a spotlight monolith is subject to at least three discrete gradients of intensity variation: one ground-level gradient which defines the state of normality for all three modes of the cursor, one overaccrual gradient which determines the three Hyper Character types and one other higher gradient which majorly determines the impairments in Sleep Disorder. Other gradients of the Mentation cursor do exist which apply to artificial or provoked (paranormal) forms of sleep; we will not however engage this ultrastructural level of analysis in this Treatise.

It is finally well worth reiterating that over-excitation of the Mentation Cursor must be understood to be the very prime factor responsible for sleep disorders. This makes for a seminal duplet factor contributing to sleep disorder syndromes: an over tidal normal Layer joined to an over tidal Mentation Cursor as the major. At the end, the imperious behavior that transpires through the directive of the tidal Cursor is nothing else than the particular phenomenology spurred by the causal pensive partitions inherent to the Layer in question as an extrapolation of sorts.

4.25 Conclusion

What we have accomplished in this Chapter is to redimension the mental disease model by showing the objective etiological foundations of mental pathology. One must recognize that to avoid setting a clear disease model in psychopathology by desisting to characterize behavior as pathology is already a judgemental subjective attitude, no matter the motivating good intentions of avoiding stigma. We have shown that the primitives and fundamental Norms to undergird such an undertaking do exist. That is what our psychophysics model profusely confers to the enterprise by putting the entire science of psychology and psychiatric psychotherapy within the strictness of the same physical framework utilized to address physical law in the natural world or the study of matter. Thus, our Psychophysics approach has ably shed light on this taxonomy through emphasizing a Theoretical perspective based on innovative Quanto-Geometric constructs cast as a special application to Psychiatry and Psychology. The formulation encompassed background of Quanto-Geometric Theory with bridging to both Clinical Psychological Problems (CPP) and current psychiatric diagnosis. Cognition, behaviors, emotions and morbidity were all viewed from a novel QG perspective emphasizing pathological categories deriving from the QG model's physical categories, and encompassing the entire universe of mental pathologies and their mechanisms.

We have catered to the principle that one only mental Layer of the Foliate is responsible for the nosology and etiology of a particular disorder. To further generalize, the distinction between one mental disorder and another is essentially based on the set of partitions that is accrued in the disease, either cross spectrum (entire chiral side of the Foliate distribution), specific subset within one particular Layer of the spectrum, levels of accrual in pensive flow and partition density according to a clearly defined metric, or affectation of the mental cursor dynamics. For sleep related disorders, it is the dynamics of the Mentation Cursor that are principally at stake.

We have also redimensioned within this context the traditional psychoanalytic mechanisms such as projections, drives, compensation, etc, in terms of dynamics innate to the Foliate and par symmetry categories inherent to the Foliate.

This psychophysics functional anatomy of the Mental allows us to cure at a stroke the dreadful and so much decried problem of multimorbidity which has long mired psychotherapy and hampered its effectiveness alike. In the next Chapter, we are going to show at large the many benefits of this approach by undertaking detailed etiological analysis of the entire universe of known mental disorders, the vast majority of which has remained completely unknown in allopathic medicine to this day.

Chapter 5

DIAGNOSIS AND ETIOLOGY OF EVERY PSYCHOGENIC MENTAL DISORDER

We present in the following an exhaustive and detailed study of virtually every registered psychiatric disorder which we have found to have an intrinsic psychogenic origin. We have purposely excluded neurologic diseases which would need to be preferentially addressed in the context of an analysis of the functional anatomy of the central nervous system in particular. In the previous Chapter we have proposed a unique disease model for all mental disorders. Our goal in the current one is to engage a thorough description of each mental disorder by framing them in a canvas format based on the formulated QG Psychophysics-driven template of the Mental. A peremptory emphasis has been placed on the etiology of mental disorders, the vast majority of which are admittedly without a known cause at all in Allotropic Medicine. The descriptive canvasses each showcase a palette of sections, namely: (1) a defining introduction, (2) a symptom block, (3) a variant block, and other blocks displaying (4) usual language clinically witnessed, (5) noticeable behavioral flips or swings, (6) derived disabilities in family and social settings, (7) the mentation layer-partitions responsible for the disorder, (8) characterological filiation of the disorder, (9) relevant epidemiologic statistics, (10) an insights block of analytic tenure, and lastly (11) a pathological affiliate extension gathering other disorder(s) belonging to the same dysfunctional taxon as the main.

We have especially engineered this canvas presentation in order to finally cure the single most important and debilitating deficiency in psychiatric medicine, which is the complete ignorance of the root causes of the vast majority of psychological mental disorders. This eminent criterion has guided the choice of blocks and their arrangements in the presentation, determined as we are to provide clear and extensive diagnostic exegesis to mental pathology at the most fundamental level. The *INSIGHTS* block further exposes the basis which grounds expression of the disorder within our QG psychophysics framework and explains the theoretical primitives that appropriately frames the same, in complete accordance with the observed clinical nosology.

5.1 Introduction and Identity Block

In this block we present and discuss the common DSM label and identity of the disorder. It is understandable that the innovative psychophysics perspective that we bring to the table will not always concord with the traditional taxonomic perspective held in the science for many disorders.

One main challenge has been to develop an unbiased approach to reconcile the nomenclature and taxonomy differences in the various fields of Psychology, Psychiatry, and Psychophysics. Given the broad application of the Mental Foliate as formulated, these correlations started to come together in a very elaborate process. Currently, however, there is no express correlation between the DSM-5 disorder classes, and the QG filiation and Manifold partitions sustaining the reported disorders.

Be all that as it may, we have intently refrained from presenting new disorder labels or modifying existing ones in order to avoid logistical disruptions in clinical practice from the diagnosis standpoint. Only a few exceptions we have made where the diagnostic exegesis demanded a slight remassage or re-composition of an existing disorder label for the name to be meaningful and concordant with the etiology.

An overwhelming amount of clinical psychological patients do not admittedly receive a clear and appropriate diagnosis because the predefined criteria and categories in Psychiatry and Psychology cannot thoroughly accommodate the nosologic spectrum of their specific impairments. The clinician shall keep that important fact in mind when evaluating the taxonomic changes that we have introduced, consequential with the newly uncovered etiologic dictates. We are certain that our approach will remedy this serious caveat, as soon as the phenotypic nature of the problematic symptoms is fully weighed, elucidated and judiciously dimensioned within the canvas formulation.

5.2 Symptoms Block

This block showcases a dual winglet designed to extol at once the *PASSIVE-RESPONSIVE* symptom subset and the *ACTIVE-REACTIVE* symptom subset proper to a disorder, consistent with the binary Gaussian distribution inherent to the Mentation Foliate model. This formulation directly supports and paves the way to the psychophysics exegesis of the disorder delivered in full in the *INSIGHTS* block. Quite frequently, one can foresee from the narrative size in the two nosology winglets which side of the Foliate, if any, is going to be prevalent in the expression of the disease.

5.3 Variants Block

This block gathers the other known disorders associated with the main label whereby there is only a slight or horizontal distinction in the expression of the disease, i.e. *Delayed Sleep-Wake Phase Disorder* and *Advanced Sleep-Wake Phase Disorder* in the Sleep-Wake Disorder class.

5.4 The Language Block

We have made every attempt to present therein as much as possible the actual clinical language that practitioners witness from the mentally impaired in clinical interviews or what others report to have typically or eponymously heard from them.

Beyond the obvious semiologic interest, there exists a correlation between linguistic structures and mental agency, which we profusely elicit in the last Chapter of this Treatise as we discuss psychometric methods for mental disorder diagnosis.

5.5 Behavioral Flips Block

This important block highlights the behavioral flips or swings observed in a very large number of mental pathologies. Except in very few cases, such as Bipolar Disorder, where mood swings are frequently noted, the clinical or research literature does not usually call out these swings which exist in virtually every mental disorder involving the participation of a full mentation Layer, if one takes the time to look for them. To extol those flips or swings brings vigorous support to the foundations of our psychophysics theory as well as a solid contribution to better understanding and diagnosing of mental pathology.

5.6 Derived Disabilities Block

We report here the consequential disabilities experienced by the impairment sufferer in settings that official science denotes “important areas of functioning”, i.e. family setting, work settings and other broader social settings. The effects of these disabilities usually become opportune when it comes to impairment treatments.

5.7 QG Layer-Partitions Block

This block underscores the Layer, Partitions, Foliate Sector and/or Mental Cursor Mode that are responsible for the disorder. When we represent in grey tone individual partitions or a Left-Chiral or Right-Chiral subset of partitions, it means a prevalence of the other Chiral set of partitions in causing the dysfunction. The represented palette of partitions is an exact match to the phenomenological report in the nosology block. Per the Mental Manifold model, the elements at the Left-Chiral side have been labeled with a negative number due to their majorly passive quality, whereas the elements at the Right-Chiral side have been labeled with a positive number. Included is the numeric identifier of the relevant Layer as well. As a reminder, this number is not an ordinal number, nor does it have an arithmentic value, despite the fact that the numeric presentation mimics an algebraic-like format. The referred number indicates instead a normal QG type and has the value of an operator.

5.8 Characterological Filiation Block

This block aims at eliciting the fluid relationship between character (or personality) and dysfunction, a fact well-known in psychology and psychiatry specifically in relation to the so-called Personality Disorders in DSM. In the disease model we have generalized this relationship to all mental pathologies and echo this link here at every step in an attempt to stamp its etiologic importance within the clinical cadre.

The next Chapter will unveil a few psychometric tests destined to extol character type in both normal and mentally impaired individuals affected with neurosis.

5.9 Statistics Block

We make every attempt to represent the most reliable statistical figures from authoritative institutions. We must keep in mind however that there are no broad consensual or official statistical figures in psychiatry despite a periodic international effort to classify mental disorders. The statistical figures are especially important in that in many instances they support and validate the exegetic propositions emerging from the psychophysics pathological model.

5.10 Insights Block

This block delivers the bulk of our diagnostic exegesis for every disorder. While we understand that psychoanalysis or analytic psychology in general endeavours to investigate the underlying motivations and drives spurring every mental disorder, it is also clear that the structural roots of mental illness in relation to an architechure and dynamic model of the Mind have not been rigorized to any psychophysics extent that we know. It is that dissatisfaction which has led to the falling out with psychoanalysis in official psychiatry, which the DSM-III definitively cemented. At the same time, psychiatric medicine has been notably unable to identify to any extent at all the neural structures or circuits that could have been responsible for the dysfunctions in mental pathology of pure psychological nature, leaving them bereft of any etiology whatsoever, except for the vague invocation of genetic factors in some cases.

Note that we have made use of several analytic psychology entities such as projections and conversions which have received a perfect legitimation by and seating within our psychophysics approach. We have also shown how mood swings and other transactions generally understood to be compensation mechanisms have been systematized within our framework as behavioral flips generalized to all mental disorders.

5.11 Pathological Affiliates Block

This block shows the vertical affiliation that relates mental disorders to one another, as opposed to the horizontal connection shown in the Variants category. It displays the many entities pertaining to a class along with the main Label, whereas the entities in the Variants section constitute a subclass. Expect all Pathological Affiliate entities in a class to share the same Mentation Layer, whether the full spectrum of partition on sthe Layer or simply a Chiral subset thereof.

5.12 Indexes

The compendium of Disorders is flanked by two glossaries for the reader's convenience, one at the front end and the other at the back end. The head glossary, which precedes the compendium, is arranged by alphabetical order of the diagnoses in order to help easily further locate them individually within the compendium. The second glossary which follows the Disorder compendium is arranged by QG Layer to facilitate prospection of a Disorder by Layer class. It is the closest hierarchy yet to a QG Taxonomy of mental disorders.

The following keys are displayed in the glossaries for each disorder: *DSM Label, Alternative Labels, Filiation, In-Foliate Locus, QG-Layer, QG Partition, Allotropic cause, QG Psychophysics Etiology, ICD-10-CM code,* and *Page number*. Their meaning is self-evident. What we designate Filiation is a taxon characterizing the identity of the disorder, which is directly placed subsequent to the Layer level. The first-level entity in that class is denoted "Principal" to mean a first-order entity (Fig. 5.1). Thus, under one Layer denomination there will be many "Principals". Subsequent to the "Principal" species, there will be "Variants" of the Principal. The third tier of the Taxonomy is the "Pathological Affiliates" level.

Pathological affiliate disorders usually present a lesser amount of features than the Principal. In some limited cases the Affiliate may show a more direct relationship with a Variant than the Principal. It is important to realize that, notwithstanding a few adjustments in disorder Labels and nosologic reports that we have undertaken, this taxonomic hierarchy is established upon the existing nomenclature and nosologic characterization thus far instituted in psychiatry, in estrangement with the fundamental etiologic roots of mental disorders. We have already explained the practical reasons for electing to peg to this compliance.

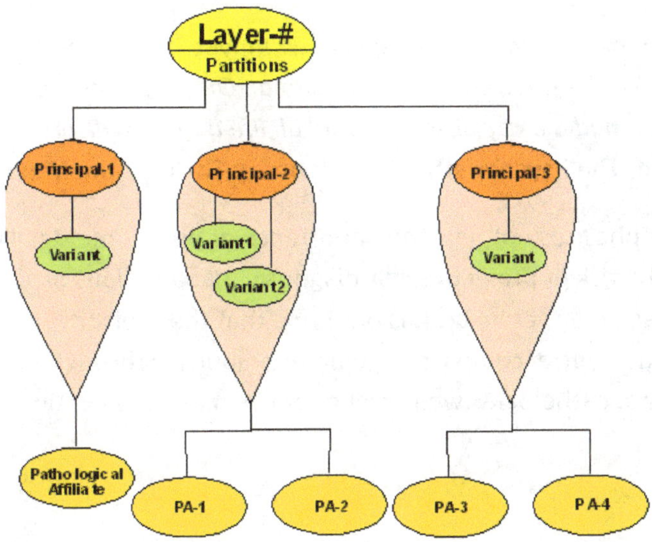

Fig. 5.1 Taxonomic structure of QG psychopathology

Consequently, no one should expect this hierarchy to be perfect, despite the high level of discipline it establishes within the existing classification. The most genuine and systematic Taxonomy deriving from the QG Psychophysics framework would demand stringent and extensive adjustments to the existing classificatory identity labels, a large number of which derive from classes and groups frequently incongruent and loose, along with corresponding nosologic adjustments in the clinical report spectra. Such a Hierarchy would strictly cater to Layers, Partitions, antisymmetric longitudes, Foliate Sectors as well as Cursor Modes driving the dynamics of mental disorders. A taxonomic redress this kind would amount to nothing less than a profound revolution in the pathological nomenclature and taxonomic structures. Despite the appeal of such drastic changes for the benefit of accuracy, we believe that gradual modifications to the current Hierarchy may be better indicated from the practical clinical standpoint.

Lastly, in addition to the glossaries, we offer a ***Commented Bibliography*** at the end of this Chapter, a convenience to directly bring to the clinician the original sources we have consulted in order to support some of the unusual facts or unconventional propositions brought about by this study.

"I was much crazier than I had imagined. Or maybe it was a bad idea to read DSM-IV when you're not a trained professional. Or maybe the American Psychiatric Association had a crazy desire to label all life a mental disorder."
— Jon Ronson, The Psychopath Test: A Journey Through the Madness Industry

The above emphasizes not only the importance of proper mental illness diagnosis, but also the risk of projective self-diagnosis that a zealous professionally-driven approach may yet incur. It is our hope that the tools that follow provide clinicians a true neutral compass to guide their journey through the very bushy forest of mental pathologies while being totally immersed within.

Analytic Compendium of Psychogenic Mental Disorders

Glossary of Disorders

-A-

Abulia
Alternative Labels: None
Filiation: PA to Burnout
In-Foliate Locus: Left+Right
Foliate Layer: **[1]**
Partitions: 1 [(-4, -3, -2, -1) (+1, +2, +3, +4)]
Allotropic Cause: Unknown
Psychophysics Etiology: Complete
IC-10-CM: R68.89
Page No: 360

Acrophobia
Alternative Labels: Fear of Heights
Filiation: Variant of Phobia
In-Foliate Locus: Left-Chiral
Foliate Layer: **[7]**
Partitions: 7 [(-4, -3, -2, -2) (+1, +2, +3, +4)]
Allotropic Cause: Unknown
Psychophysics Etiology: Complete
IC-10-CM: F40.241
Page No: 436

Acute Stress Reaction
Alternative Labels: Stress
Filiation: Variant of PTSD
In-Foliate Locus: Left-Chiral
Foliate Layer: **[7]**
Partitions: 7 [(-4, -3, -2, -1) (+1, +2, +3, +4)]
Allotropic Cause: Unknown
Psychophysics Etiology: Complete
IC-10-CM: F43.0
Page No: 556

Adjustment Disorder
Alternative Labels: None
Filiation: PA to Bipolar Disorder
In-Foliate Locus: Left+Right
Foliate Layer: **[6]**
Partitions: 6 [(-4, -3, -2, -1) (+1, +2, +3, +4)]
Allotropic Cause: Unknown
Psychophysics Etiology: Complete
IC-10-CM: F43.23
Page No: 366

Agitation Disorder
Alternative Labels: None
Filiation: Principal
In-Foliate Locus: Left+Right
Foliate Layer:
Partitions: [Right-Chiral Sector] of Foliate
Allotropic Cause: Unknown
Psychophysics Etiology: Complete
IC-10-CM: R45.1
Page No: 269

Agoraphobia
Alternative Labels: Fear of Open Spaces
Filiation: Variant of Phobia
In-Foliate Locus: Left-Chiral
Foliate Layer: **[7]**
Partitions: 7 [(-4, -3, -2, -2) (+1, +2, +3, +4)]
Allotropic Cause: Unknown
Psychophysics Etiology: Complete
IC-10-CM: F40.01
Page No: 436

Agressiveness
Alternative Labels: Intermittent Explosive Disorder
Filiation: Principal
In-Foliate Locus: Left+Right
Foliate Layer: **[1]**
Partitions: 1 [(-4, -3, -2, -1) (+1, +2, +3, +4)]
Allotropic Cause: Unknown
Psychophysics Etiology: Complete
IC-10-CM: R45.6
Page No: 378

Alzheimer's Disease
Alternative Labels: Dementia
Filiation: Principal
In-Foliate Locus: Left+Right
Foliate Layer: **[9]**
Partitions: 9 [(-4, -3, -2, -1) (+1, +2, +3, +4)]
Allotropic Cause: Trauma, Vascular
Psychophysics Etiology: Partial
IC-10-CM: G30.9
Page No: 526

Animal Phobia
Alternative Labels: None
Filiation: Variant of Phobia
In-Foliate Locus: Left-Chiral
Foliate Layer: **[7]**
Partitions: 7 [(-4, -3, -2, -2) (+1, +2, +3, +4)]
Allotropic Cause: Unknown
Psychophysics Etiology: Complete
IC-10-CM: F40.218
Page No: 435

Anorexia Nervosa
Alternative Labels: BAN syndrome
Filiation: Variant of BAN
In-Foliate Locus: Left+Right
Foliate Layer: **[7]**
Partitions: 7 [(-4, -3, -2, -1) (+1, +2, +3, +4)]
Allotropic Cause: Unknown
Psychophysics Etiology: Complete
IC-10-CM: F50.0
Page No: 568

Anxiety Syndrome
Alternative Labels: None
Filiation: PA to PTSD
In-Foliate Locus: Left-Chiral
Foliate Layer: **[7]**
Partitions: 7 [(-4, -3, -2, -1) (+1, +2, +3, +4)]
Allotropic Cause: Unknown, Biological
Psychophysics Etiology: Complete
IC-10-CM: F41.9
Page No: 559

Approval Compulsion
Alternative Labels: None
Filiation: Principal
In-Foliate Locus: Left+Right
Foliate Layer: **[3]**
Partitions: 3 [(-4, -3, -2, -1) (+1, +2, +3, +4)]
Allotropic Cause: Unknown
Psychophysics Etiology: Complete
IC-10-CM: F42
Page No: 406

Asthenia
Alternative Labels: Neurasthenia
Filiation: Variant of Burnout Syndrome
In-Foliate Locus: Left-Chiral
Foliate Layer: **[8]**
1[(-4, -3, -2, -1), (+1, +2, +3, + 4)]
Allotropic Cause: Unknown
Psychophysics Etiology: Complete
IC-10-CM: F48.8
Page No: 358

Attention Deficit/Hyperactivity Disorder
Alternative Labels: None
Filiation: Principal
In-Foliate Locus: Left (Inattentive)
Right (Hyperactive)
R+L (Combined type)
Foliate Layer: **[2]**
Partitions: Combined type 2 [(-4, -3, -2, -1) (+1, +2, +3, +4)]
Allotropic Cause: Biological, Substance use in pregnancy, Neurologic
Psychophysics Etiology: Complete
IC-10-CM: F90.0
Page No: 351

Authoritarianism
Alternative Labels: None
Filiation: Principal
In-Foliate Locus: Right-Chiral Layer 1
Foliate Layer: **[2]**
Hyper-Quantum Operator
Allotropic Cause: Unknown
Psychophysics Etiology: Complete
IC-10-CM: N/A
Page No: 541

Autism
Alternative Labels: None
Filiation: PA to Schizophrenia
In-Foliate Locus: Left+Right
Foliate Layer: **[8]**
Partitions: 8 [(-4, -3, -2, -1) (+1, +2, +3, +4)]
Allotropic Cause: , Genetic
Psychophysics Etiology: Complete
IC-10-CM: F84.0
Page No: 446

Autogynephilia
Alternative Labels: Eonism, Automonosexuality
Filiation: Variant of Transvestic Disorder
In-Foliate Locus: Left+Right
Foliate Layer: **[7}**

Partitions: 7 [(-4, -3, -2, -1) (+1, +2, +3, +4)]
Allotropic Cause: Unknown
Psychophysics Etiology: Complete
IC-10-CM: F65.1
Page No: 463

Avoidant Personality Disorder
Alternative Labels: None
Filiation: PA to Social Anxiety Disorder
In-Foliate Locus: Left-Chiral
Foliate Layer: **[1]**
Partitions: 1 [(-4, -3, -2, -1) (+1, +2, +3, +4)]
Allotropic Cause: Unknown
Psychophysics Etiology: Complete
IC-10-CM: F60.6
Page No: 378

Avoidant/Restrictive Food Intake Disorder
Alternative Labels: None
Filiation: Variant of Bulimia – Anorexia Nervosa
In-Foliate Locus: Left Chiral
Foliate Layer: **[7]**
Partitions: 7 [(-4, -3, -2, -1)]
Allotropic Cause: Not well known
Psychophysics Etiology: Complete
IC-10-CM: F50.82
Page No: 573

-B-

Binge Eating Disorder
Alternative Labels: Clastomania
Filiation: Variant of Bulimia -Anorexia Nervosa
In-Foliate Locus: Right-Chiral only
Foliate Layer: **[7]**
Partitions: 7 [(+1, +2, +3, +4)]
Allotropic Cause: Unknown
Psychophysics Etiology: Complete
IC-10-CM: None
Page No: 569

Bipolar Disorder
Alternative Labels: Manic Depression
Filiation: Principal
In-Foliate Locus: Left+Right or either Right or Left-Chiral only
Foliate Layer: **[6]**
Partitions: 6 [(-4, -3, -2, -1) (+1, +2, +3, +4)]
Allotropic Cause: Unknown, Biological
Psychophysics Etiology: Complete
IC-10-CM: F31
Page No: 366

Blood-Injection-Injury Phobia
Alternative Labels: Hemophobia
Filiation: Variant of Phobia
In-Foliate Locus: Left-Chiral
Foliate Layer: **[7]**
Partitions: 7 [(-4, -3, -2, -2) (+1, +2, +3, +4)]
Allotropic Cause: Unknown
Psychophysics Etiology: Complete
IC-10-CM: F40.23
Page No: 436

Body Dysmorphic Disorder
Alternative Labels: Dismorphophobia
Filiation: Principal
In-Foliate Locus: Left+Right
Foliate Layer: **[6]**
Partitions: 6 [(-4, -3, -2, -1) (+1, +2, +3, +4)]
Allotropic Cause: Unknown
Psychophysics Etiology: Complete
IC-10-CM: F45.22
Page No: 535

Body Integrity Identity disorder
Alternative Labels: Apotemnophilia
Filiation: Principal
In-Foliate Locus: Left+Right
Foliate Layer: **[7]**
Partitions: 7 [(-4, -3, -2, -1) (+1, +2, +3, +4)]
Allotropic Cause: Unknown
Psychophysics Etiology: Partial
N/A
Page No: 375

Borderline Personality Disorder
Alternative Labels: None
Filiation: PA to Bipolar
In-Foliate Locus: Left+Right
Foliate Layer: **[6]**
Partitions: 6 [(-4, -3, -2, -1) (+1, +2, +3, +4)]
Allotropic Cause: Unknown
Psychophysics Etiology: Complete
IC-10-CM: F60.3

Page No: 366

Bulimia-Anorexia Nervosa (BAN)
Alternative Labels: BAN Syndrome
Filiation: Principal
In-Foliate Locus: Left+Right
Foliate Layer: **[7]**
Partitions: 7 [(-4, -3, -2, -1) (+1, +2, +3, +4)]
Allotropic Cause: Unknown
Psychophysics Etiology: Complete
IC-10-CM: F50.2
Page No: 568

Bulimia
Alternative Labels: BAN syndrome
Filiation: Variant of BAN
In-Foliate Locus: Left+Right
Foliate Layer: **[7]**
Partitions: 7 [(-4, -3, -2, -1) (+1, +2, +3, +4)]
Allotropic Cause: Unknown
Psychophysics Etiology: Complete
IC-10-CM: F50.2
Page No: 568

Burnout syndrome
Alternative Labels: Asthenia, Neurasthenia
Filiation: Principal
In-Foliate Locus: Left+Right
Foliate Layer: **[1]**
Partitions: 1 [(-4, -3, -2, -1) (+1, +2, +3, +4)]
Allotropic Cause: Unknown
Psychophysics Etiology: Complete
IC-10-CM: Z73.0
Page No: 357

Cataplexy
Alternative Labels: None
Symptom of Narcolepsy Type 1
Hypercursor over accrued
Foliate Layer: **[9]**
Layer 9 Overaccrued
Allotropic Cause: Unknown
Psychophysics Etiology: Complete
IC-10-CM: F47.411 - F20.2
Page No: 601

Catatonia
Alternative Labels: None
Filiation: Principal
In-Foliate Locus: Left+Right
Foliate Layer: **[6]**
Partitions: 6 [(-4, -3, -2, -1) (+1, +2, +3, +4)]
Allotropic Cause: Unknown
Psychophysics Etiology: Complete
IC-10-CM: F06.1
Page No: 611

-C-

Chronic/Persistent Vertigo
Alternative Labels: Dizziness
Filiation: PA to Burnout
In-Foliate Locus: Left-Chiral
Foliate Layer: **[1]**
Partitions: 1 [(-4, -3, -2, -1) (+1, +2, +3, +4)]
Allotropic Cause: Little known, Biological
Psychophysics Etiology: Incomplete
R42.0
Page No: 359

Claustrophobia
Alternative Labels: Fear of closed spaces
Filiation: Variant of Phobia
In-Foliate Locus: Left-Chiral
Foliate Layer: **[7]**
Partitions: 7 [(-4, -3, -2, -2) (+1, +2, +3, +4)]
Allotropic Cause: Unknown
Psychophysics Etiology: Complete
IC-10-CM: F40.240
Page No: 436

Compulsive Gambling Disorder
Alternative Labels: None
Filiation: Principal
In-Foliate Locus: Left+Right
Foliate Layer: **[5]**
Partitions: 5 [(-4, -3, -2, -1) (+1, +2, +3, +4)]
Allotropic Cause: Unknown
Psychophysics Etiology: Complete
IC-10-CM: F63.0
Page No: 432

Conduct Disorder
Alternative Labels: None
Filiation: Principal
In-Foliate Locus: Right-Chiral Only
Foliate Layer: **[7]**

Partitions: 7 [(+1, +2, +3, +4)]
Allotropic Cause: Unknown
Psychophysics Etiology: Complete
IC-10-CM: F91.9
Page No: 565

Copromania
Alternative Labels: None
Filiation: PA to Schizophrenia
In-Foliate Locus: Left+Right
Foliate Layer: **[7]**
Partitions: 7 [(-4, -3, -2, -1) (+1, +2, +3, +4)]
Allotropic Cause: Unknown
Psychophysics Etiology: Complete
IC-10-CM: N/A
Page No: 632

Cotard's syndrome
Alternative Labels: Delire des Negations
Filiation: Principal
In-Foliate Locus: Left+Right
Foliate Layer: **[7]**
Partitions: 7 [(-4, -3, -2, -1) (+1, +2, +3, +4)]
Allotropic Cause: Unknown
Psychophysics Etiology: Complete
IC-10-CM: F22.0
Page No: 397

Couvade Syndrome
Alternative Labels: None
Filiation: PA to Pseudocyesis
In-Foliate Locus: Left+Right
Foliate Layer: **[5]**
Partitions: 7 [(+1, +2, +3, +4)]
Allotropic Cause: Unknown
Psychophysics Etiology: Complete
IC-10-CM: F44.89
Page No: 498

Cyclothymia
Alternative Labels: None
Filiation: PA to Bipolar Disorder
In-Foliate Locus: Left+Right
Foliate Layer: **[6]**
Partitions: 6 [(-4, -3, -2, -1) (+1, +2, +3, +4)]
Allotropic Cause: Unknown
Psychophysics Etiology: Complete
IC-10-CM: F34.0
Page No: 366

Delayed Ejaculation Disorder
Alternative Labels: Male Orgasmic Disorder
Filiation: PA to Erectile Disorder
In-Foliate Locus: Left-Chiral Side
Foliate Layer: **[7]**
Partitions: 7 [(-4, -3, -2, -1) (+1, +2, +3, +4)]
Allotropic Cause: Unknown
Psychophysics Etiology: Complete
IC-10-CM: N53.11
Page No: 484

-D-

Dependant Personality Disorder
Alternative Labels: None
Filiation: Principal
In-Foliate Locus: Left+Right
Foliate Layer: **[6]**
Partitions: 6 [(-4, -3, -2, -1) (+1, +2, +3, +4)]
Allotropic Cause: Unknown
Psychophysics Etiology: Complete
IC-10-CM: F60.7
Page No: 538

Depersonalization Disorder
Alternative Labels: None
Filiation: PA to Cotard
In-Foliate Locus: Left+Right
Foliate Layer: **[7]**
Partitions: 7 [(-4, -3, -2, -1) (+1, +2, +3, +4)]
Allotropic Cause: Unknown
Psychophysics Etiology: Complete
IC-10-CM: F48.1
Page No: 397

Depressive Disorders
Alternative Labels: Depression
Filiation: class Disorder
In-Foliate Locus: Left-Chiral Only
Foliate Layer: **[6]**
Partitions: 6 [(-4, -3, -2, -1)]
Allotropic Cause: Unknown, Biological
Psychophysics Etiology: Complete
IC-10-CM: F33.0
Page No: 269

Derealization Disorder
Alternative Labels: None

Filiation: PA to Cotard
In-Foliate Locus: Left+Right
Foliate Layer: **[7]**
Partitions: 7 [(-4, -3, -2, -1) (+1, +2, +3, +4)]
Allotropic Cause: Unknown
Psychophysics Etiology: Complete
IC-10-CM: F48.1
Page No: 397

Dermatillomania
Alternative Labels: Excoriation
Skin picking
Filiation: Principal
In-Foliate Locus: Right-Chiral
Foliate Layer: **[7]**
Partitions: 7 [(-4, -3, -2, -1) (+1, +2, +3, +4)]
Allotropic Cause: Unknown
Psychophysics Etiology: Complete
IC-10-CM: F42.4
Page No: 579

Developmental Coordination Disorder
Alternative Labels: None
Filiation: Principal
In-Foliate Locus: Left+Right
Partitions: 3 [(-4, -3, -2, -1)]
Allotropic Cause: Unknown
Psychophysics Etiology: Complete
IC-10-CM: F82
Page No: 585

Disinhibited Social Engagement Disorder
Alternative Labels: None
Filiation: Principal
In-Foliate Locus: Right-Chiral
Foliate Layer: **[6]**
Partitions: 6 [(-4, -3, -2, -1) (+1, +2, +3, +4)]
Allotropic Cause: Unknown
Psychophysics Etiology: Complete
IC-10-CM: F94.1
Page No: 546

Dissociative Amnesia
Alternative Labels: None
Filiation: PA to Split PD
In-Foliate Locus: Left+Right
Foliate Layer: **[5]**
Partitions: 5 [(-4, -3, -2, -1) (+1, +2, +3, +4)
Allotropic Cause: Little known, Biological, Trauma
Psychophysics Etiology: Complete
IC-10-CM: F44.0
Page No: 430

Dysruptive Mood Dysregulation Disorder
Alternative Labels: None
Filiation: PA to Bipolar
In-Foliate Locus: Left+Right
Foliate Layer: **[6]**
Partitions: 6 [(-4, -3, -2, -1) (+1, +2, +3, +4)]
Allotropic Cause: Unknown
Psychophysics Etiology: Complete
IC-10-CM: F34.81
Page No: 561

Dysthymia
Alternative Labels: None
Filiation: Principal
In-Foliate Locus: Left-Chiral sector of Foliate
Allotropic Cause: Unknown, Biological, Trauma
Psychophysics Etiology: Complete
IC-10-CM: F34.1
Page No: 372

-E-

Enuresis
Alternative Labels: Bedwetting
Filiation: Variant of Turbulent Sleep Disorder
In-Foliate Locus: Left+Right
Foliate Layer: **[7]**
Partitions: 7 [(-4, -3, -2, -1) (+1, +2, +3, +4)]
Allotropic Cause: Unknown, Biological
Psychophysics Etiology:
Page No: 628

Epilepsy
Alternative Labels: Seizures
Filiation: Principal
In-Foliate Locus: Left+Right
Foliate Layer: **[9]**
Partitions: 9 [(-4, -3, -2, -1) (+1, +2, +3, +4)]

Allotropic Cause: Unknown, Biological, Trauma
Psychophysics Etiology: Complete
Page No: 515

Erectile Disorder
Alternative Labels: Impotence
Filiation: Principal
In-Foliate Locus: Left-Chiral Side
Foliate Layer: **[7]**
Partitions: 7 **[**(-4, -3, -2, -1) (+1, +2, +3, +4)**]**
Allotropic Cause: Unknown
Psychophysics Etiology: Complete
IC-10-CM: N52.9
Page No: 480

Exhibitionistic Disorder
Alternative Labels: None
Filiation: Principal
In-Foliate Locus: Left-Chiral Only
Foliate Layer: **[7]**
Partitions: 7 **[**(+1, +2, +3, +4)**]**
Allotropic Cause: Unknown
Psychophysics Etiology: Complete
IC-10-CM: F65.2
Page No: 450

-F-

Factitious Disorder
Alternative Labels: None
Filiation: PA to BIDD
In-Foliate Locus: Left+right
Foliate Layer: **[7]**
Partitions: 7 **[**(-4, -3, -2, -1) (+1, +2, +3, +4)**]**
Allotropic Cause: Unknown
Psychophysics Etiology: Complete
IC-10-CM: F68.10
Page No: 264

Female Orgasmic Disorder
Alternative Labels: Frigidity
Filiation: PA to Female Sexual Interest-Arousal Disorder
In-Foliate Locus: Left-Chiral Side
Foliate Layer: **[7]**
Partitions: 7 **[**(-4, -3, -2, -1) (+1, +2, +3, +4)**]**
Allotropic Cause: Unknown
Psychophysics Etiology: Complete
IC-10-CM: F52.31
Page No: 478

Female Sexual Interest-Arousal Disorder
Alternative Labels: Frigidity
Filiation: Principal
In-Foliate Locus: Left-Chiral Side
Foliate Layer: **[7]**
Partitions: 7 **[**(-4, -3, -2, -1) (+1, +2, +3, +4)**]**
Allotropic Cause: Unknown
Psychophysics Etiology: Complete
IC-10-CM: F52.22
Page No: 474

Fetishism
Alternative Labels: none
Filiation: Principal
In-Foliate Locus: Left-Chiral
Foliate Layer: **[2]**
Partitions: 2 **[**(-4, -3, -2, -1) (+1, +2, +3, +4)**]**
Allotropic Cause: Unknown
Psychophysics Etiology: Complete
IC-10-CM: F65.0
Page No: 392

Frotteuristic Disorder
Alternative Labels: None
Filiation: PA to Exhibitionistic Disorder
In-Foliate Locus: Left-Chiral Only
Foliate Layer: **[7]**
Partitions: 7 **[**(+1, +2, +3, +4)**]**
Allotropic Cause: Unknown
Psychophysics Etiology: Complete
IC-10-CM: F65.81
Page No: 453

-G-

Gender Identity Disorder
Alternative Labels: Gender Dysphoria
Filiation: Principal
Either Left or Right Chiral
Foliate Layer: **[X]**
Entire L-Chiral or R-Chiral side of the foliate
Allotropic Cause: Unknown
Psychophysics Etiology: Complete
IC-10-CM: F64.9

Page No: 459

Generalized Anxiety
Alternative Labels: None
Filiation: PA to Separation Anxiety
In-Foliate Locus: Left+Right
Foliate Layer: **[7]**
Partitions: 7 [(-4, -3, -2, -1) (+1, +2, +3, +4)]
Allotropic Cause: Unknown, Biological
Psychophysics Etiology: Complete
IC-10-CM: F41.10
Page No: 438

Grief reaction
Alternative Labels: Sadness
Filiation: Principal
In-Foliate Locus: Left-Chiral Only
Foliate Layer: **[6]**
Partitions: 6 [(-4, -3, -2, -1)]
Allotropic Cause: Unknown
Psychophysics Etiology: Complete
IC-10-CM: F43
Page No: 425

Guilt syndrome
Alternative Labels: None
Filiation: Principal
In-Foliate Locus: Left+Right
Foliate Layer: **[4]**
Partitions: 4 [(-4, -3, -2, -1) (+1, +2, +3, +4)]
Allotropic Cause: Unknown
Psychophysics Etiology: Complete
IC-10-CM: N/A
Page No: 422

-H-

Histrionic Personality Disorder
Alternative Labels: None
Filiation: Principal
In-Foliate Locus: [Right Chiral Sector] of Foliate
Foliate Layer: [6]
Partitions: 6 [(+1, +2, +3, +4)]
Allotropic Cause: Unknown
Psychophysics Etiology: Complete
IC-10-CM: F60.4
Page No: 499

Hoarding
Alternative Labels: None
Filiation: Principal
In-Foliate Locus: Left+Right
Foliate Layer: **[1]**
Partitions: 1 [(-4, -3, -2, -1) (+1, +2, +3, +4)]
Allotropic Cause: Unknown
Psychophysics Etiology: Complete
IC-10-CM: F42.3
Page No: 466

Homosexuality/Lesbianism (when causing distress)
Alternative Labels: None
Filiation: Principal
In-Foliate Locus: Left+Right
Foliate Layer: **[7]**
Partitions: 7 [(-4, -3, -2, -1) (+1, +2, +3, +4)]
Allotropic Cause: Unknown, Genetical
Psychophysics Etiology: Complete
IC-10-CM: N/A
Page No: 282

Hypersomnia
Alternative Labels: Hypersomnolence
Filiation: Principal
Hypercursor over accrued
Foliate Layer: **[9]**
9 Overaccrued
Allotropic Cause: Unknown, Biological
Psychophysics Etiology: Complete
IC-10-CM: G47.10
Page No: 596

Hypochondria
Alternative Labels: Illness Anxiety Disorder
Filiation: Principal
In-Foliate Locus: Left+Right
Foliate Layer: **[5]**
Partitions: 5 [(-4, -3, -2, -1) (+1, +2, +3, +4)]
Allotropic Cause: Unknown
Psychophysics Etiology: Complete
IC-10-CM: F45.21
Page No: 442

Hypomania
Alternative Labels: Mania

Filiation: PA to Bipolar
In-Foliate Locus: Right-Chiral
Foliate Layer: **[6]**
Partitions: 6 [(-4, -3, -2, -1) (+1, +2, +3, +4)]
Allotropic Cause: Unknown, Biological
Psychophysics Etiology: Complete
IC-10-CM: F31.0
Page No: 366

Hysteria
Alternative Labels: Conversion Disorder
Filiation: Principal
In-Foliate Locus: Left+Right
Foliate Layer: **[5]**
Partitions: 5 [(-4, -3, -2, -1) (+1, +2, +3, +4)]
Allotropic Cause: Unknown
Psychophysics Etiology: Complete
IC-10-CM: F44.4
Page No: 354

-I-

Impostor Syndrome
Alternative Labels: Fraud syndrome, Neurosis of Failure
Filiation: Principal
In-Foliate Locus: Left+Right
Foliate Layer: **[3]**
Partitions: 3 [(-4, -3, -2, -1) (+1, +2, +3, +4)]
Allotropic Cause: Unknown
Psychophysics Etiology: Complete
IC-10-CM: N/A
Page No: 363

Infantile Neglect Disorder
Alternative Labels: None
Filiation: Principal
In-Foliate Locus: Right-Chiral
Foliate Layer: **[6]**
Partitions: 6 [(-4, -3, -2, -1) (+1, +2, +3, +4)]
Allotropic Cause: Unknown
Psychophysics Etiology: Complete
IC-10-CM: T74.02
Page No: 547

Inferiority Complex
Alternative Labels: None
Filiation: Principal
In-Foliate Locus: Left+Right
Foliate Layer: **[3]**
Partitions: 3 [(-4, -3, -2,-1) (+1, +2, +3, +4)]
Allotropic Cause: Unknown
Psychophysics Etiology: Complete
IC-10-CM: N/A
Page No: 412

Insomnia
Alternative Labels: None
Filiation: Principal
Hypocursor over accrued
Foliate Layer: **[1,2,3]**
Layers 1,2,3 Overaccrued
Allotropic Cause: Unknown, Biological
Psychophysics Etiology: Complete
IC-10-CM: G47.00
Page No: 592

Insufficient Sleep Syndrome
Alternative Labels: Sleep deprivation
Filiation: PA to Insomnia
Hypocursor over accrued
Foliate Layer: **[1, 2, 3]**
Layers 1, 2, 3 Overaccrued
Allotropic Cause: Unknown, Biological
Psychophysics Etiology: Complete
IC-10-CM: F51.12
Page No: 594

Intellectual Disability
Alternative Labels: Mental Retardation
Filiation: PA to Inferiority Complex
In-Foliate Locus: Left+Right
Foliate Layer: **[3]**
Partitions: 3 [(-4, -3, -2, -1) (+1, +2, +3, +4)]
Allotropic Cause: Unknown
Psychophysics Etiology:
F70-F79
Page No: 414

Intermittent Explosive Disorder
Alternative Labels: None
Filiation: Principal
In-Foliate Locus: Left+Right
Foliate Layer: **[7]**
Partitions: 7 [(-4, -3, -2, -1)(+1, +2, +3, +4)]
Allotropic Cause: Unknown
Psychophysics Etiology: Complete

IC-10-CM: F63.81
Page No: 382

-J-

Juvenile Delinquency
Alternative Labels: None
Filiation: Principal
In-Foliate Locus: Right-Chiral Only
Foliate Layer: **[7]**
Partitions: 7 [(+1, +2, +3, +4)]
Allotropic Cause: Unknown, Biological
Psychophysics Etiology: Complete
IC-10-CM: Z72.810
Page No: 565

-K-

Kleine-Levin Syndrome
Alternative Labels: Sleeping beauty syndrome
Filiation: PA to Hypersomnia
Hypercursor over accrued
Foliate Layer: **[9]**
9 Overaccrued
Allotropic Cause
Psychophysics Etiology: Complete
IC-10-CM: G47.13
Page No: 598

Kleptomania
Alternative Labels: Pathological stealing
Filiation: Principal
In-Foliate Locus: Left-Chiral Only
Foliate Layer: **[7]**
Partitions: 7 [(-4, -3, -2, -1)]
Allotropic Cause: Unknown
Uncontrollable impulse
Psychophysics Etiology: Complete
IC-10-CM: F63.2
Page No: 389

-L-

Language Disorder
Alternative Labels: None
Filiation: PA to Social Anxiety disorder
In-Foliate Locus: Left-Chiral
Foliate Layer: **[6]**
Partitions: 1 [(-4, -3, -2, -1) (+1, +2, +3, +4)]
Allotropic Cause: Unknown
Psychophysics Etiology: Complete
IC-10-CM: F80
Page No: 267

Logorrhea
Alternative Labels: Excessive Talking
Filiation: various
In-Foliate Locus: Left+Right
Foliate Layer: **[3] mainly – [6] or [9] secondarily**
Partitions: X [(-4, -3, -2, -1) (+1, +2, +3, +4)]
Allotropic Cause: Unknown, Biological
Psychophysics Etiology: Complete
IC-10-CM: R47.89
Page No: 631

-M-

Male Hypoactive Sexual Desire Disorder
Alternative Labels: None
Filiation: PA to Erectile Disorder
In-Foliate Locus: Left-Chiral Side
Foliate Layer: **[7]**
Partitions: 7 [(-4, -3, -2, -1) (+1, +2, +3, +4)]
Allotropic Cause: Unknown
Psychophysics Etiology: Complete
IC-10-CM: F52.0
Page No: 483

Malignant Catatonia
Alternative Labels: None
Filiation: Variant of Catatonia
In-Foliate Locus: Left+Right
Foliate Layer: **[6]**
Partitions: 6 [(-4, -3, -2, -1) (+1, +2, +3, +4)]
Allotropic Cause: Unknown
Psychophysics Etiology:
F06.1
Page No: 611

Melancholy
Alternative Labels: None
Filiation: PA to Bipolar Disorder

In-Foliate Locus: Left+Right
Foliate Layer: **[6]**
Partitions: 6 [(-4, -3, -2, -1) (+1, +2, +3, +4)]
Allotropic Cause: Unknown
Psychophysics Etiology: Complete
IC-10-CM: F32.9
Page No: 366

Mental Confusion
Alternative Labels: Delirium
Filiation: Principal
In-Foliate Locus: Left+Right
Foliate Layer: **[3]**
Partitions: 3 [(-4, -3, -2, -1) (+1, +2, +3, +4)]
Allotropic Cause: Little known, Biological, Neurological
Psychophysics Etiology:
R41.0
Page No: 265

Mythomania
Alternative Labels: Pseudologia Fantastica
Filiation: Principal
In-Foliate Locus: Left+Right
Foliate Layer: **[4]**
Partitions: 4 [(-4, -3, -2, -1) (+1, +2, +3, +4)]
Allotropic Cause: Unknown, low self-esteem
Psychophysics Etiology: Complete
IC-10-CM: N/ or F69
Page No: 385

-N-

Narcissistic Personality Disorder
Alternative Labels: None
Filiation: Principal
In-Foliate Locus: Right-Chiral Only
Foliate Layer: **[1]**
Partitions: 1 [(+1, +2, +3, +4)]
Allotropic Cause: Unknown
Psychophysics Etiology: Complete
IC-10-CM: F60.81
Page No: 502

Narcolepsy Type 1 and 2
Alternative Labels: None
Filiation: PA to Hypersomnia
Hypercursor over accrued
Foliate Layer: **[9]**
9 Overaccrued
Allotropic Cause: Unknown, Biological
Psychophysics Etiology: Complete
IC-10-CM: G47.419
Page No: 601

Narcomania
Alternative Labels: Drug addiction
Filiation: PA to Bipolar
In-Foliate Locus: Left+Right
Foliate Layer: **[7]**
Partitions: 7 [(-4, -3, -2, -1) (+1, +2, +3, +4)]
Allotropic Cause: Unknown, Biological
Psychophysics Etiology: Complete
IC-10-CM: F19.10
Page No: 457

Natural Environment Phobia
Alternative Labels: None
Filiation: Variant of Phobia
In-Foliate Locus: Left-Chiral
Foliate Layer: **[7]**
Partitions: 7 [(-4, -3, -2, -2) (+1, +2, +3, +4)]
Allotropic Cause: Unknown
Psychophysics Etiology: Complete
IC-10-CM: F40.228
Page No: 435

Neglect Syndrome
Alternative Labels: Hemispatial Neglect, Unilateral Neglect, Hemi-inattention, Hemineglect
Filiation: Principal
In-Foliate Locus: Left+Right
Foliate Layer: **[7]**
Partitions: 7 [(-4, -3, -2, -1) (+1, +2, +3, +4)]
Allotropic Cause: Neurological
Psychophysics Etiology: Complete
R41.4
Page No: 409

Nightmare Disorder
Alternative Labels: Dream Anxiety Disorder
Filiation: Variant of Turbulent Sleep Disorder
Hypercursor over accrued
Foliate Layer: **[7]**
Partitions: 7 [(-4, -3, -2, -1) (+1, +2, +3, +4)]
Allotropic Cause: Unknown

Psychophysics Etiology: Complete
IC-10-CM: F51.5
Page No: 628

Non-Rapid Eye Movement Sleep Arousal Disorder
Alternative Labels: None
Filiation: Variant of Turbulent Sleep Disord-er
Hypercursor over accrued
Foliate Layer: **[7]**
Partitions: 7 [(-4, -3, -2, -1) (+1, +2, +3, +4)]
Allotropic Cause: Unknown
Psychophysics Etiology: Complete
IC-10-CM: G47.5
Page No: 627

Nymphomania
Alternative Labels: Don Juanism, Satyriasis, Erotomania, Hypersexuality
Filiation: Principal
In-Foliate Locus: Left-Chiral in Women and female-oriented Homosexual Men
In-Foliate Locus: Right-Chiral in Men and male-oriented Lesbian
Foliate Layer: **[7]**
Partitions: 7 [(-4, -3, -2, -1) **or** (+1, +2, +3, +4)]
Allotropic Cause: Unknown
Psychophysics Etiology: Complete
IC-10-CM: F52.8
Page No: 487

-O-

Obsessive Disorders
Alternative Labels: Depression-Agitation Disorders
Filiation: class Disorder
In-Foliate Locus: Left-Chiral Sector
Foliate Layer: [Any one Layer in accretion]
Partitions: [(-4, -3, -2, -1)] or [(+1, +2, +3, +4)]
Allotropic Cause: Unknown
Psychophysics Etiology: Complete
IC-10-CM: F42
Page No: 286

Obsessive-Compulsive Personality Disorder
Alternative Labels: None
Filiation: PA to Dependent PD
In-Foliate Locus: Left+Right
Foliate Layer: **[6]**
Partitions: 6 [(-4, -3, -2, -1) (+1, +2, +3, +4)]
Allotropic Cause: Unknown
Psychophysics Etiology: Complete
IC-10-CM: F60.5
Page No: 286

Oppositional Defiant Disorder
Alternative Labels: None
Filiation: Principal
In-Foliate Locus: Right-Chiral
Foliate Layer: **[7]**
Partitions: 7 [(-4, -3, -2, -1) (+1, +2, +3, +4)]
Allotropic Cause: Unknown
Psychophysics Etiology: Complete
IC-10-CM: F91.3
Page No: 555

-P-

Panic Disorder
Alternative Labels: None
Filiation: PA to PTSD
In-Foliate Locus: Left-Chiral
Foliate Layer: **[7]**
Partitions: 7 [(-4, -3, -2, -1) (+1, +2, +3, +4)]
Allotropic Cause: Unknown, Biological
Psychophysics Etiology: Complete
IC-10-CM: F40.10
Page No: 559

Paranoia
Alternative Labels: Megalomania
Filiation: Principal
In-Foliate Locus: Left+Right
Foliate Layer: **[4]**
Partitions: 4 [(-4, -3, -2, -1) (+1, +2, +3, +4)]
Allotropic Cause: Unknown, Neurological, Biological
Psychophysics Etiology: Complete
IC-10-CM: F23
F60
Page No: 439

Paranoid Personality Disorder
Alternative Labels: None
Filiation: PA to Paranoia
In-Foliate Locus: Left+Right
Foliate Layer: **[4]**
Partitions: 4 [(-4, -3, -2, -1) (+1, +2, +3, +4)]
Allotropic Cause: Unknown
Psychophysics Etiology: Complete
IC-10-CM: F60.0
Page No: 439

Parasomnia
Alternative Labels: none
Filiation: Class taxon
In-Foliate Locus: Left+Right
Foliate Layer: All
Partitions: All on Layer
Mental Cursor overaccrued
Allotropic Cause: Unknown, Biological
Psychophysics Etiology: Complete
IC-10-CM: F47.50
Page No: 315

Passion Blues
Alternative Labels: Prolonged Grief
Filiation: PA to Grief
In-Foliate Locus: Left-Chiral Only
Foliate Layer: **[6]**
Partitions: 6 [(-4, -3, -2, -1)]
Allotropic Cause: Unknown
Psychophysics Etiology: Complete
IC-10-CM: F43.0
Page No: 426

Pedophilic Disorder
Alternative Labels: None
Filiation: Principal
In-Foliate Locus: Left-Chiral Sector of Foliate
Foliate Layer: **[7]**
Partitions: 7[(-4, -3, -2, -1) (+1, +2, +3, +4)]
Allotropic Cause: Unknown
Psychophysics Etiology: Complete
IC-10-CM: F65.4
Page No: 470

Perfectionism
Alternative Labels: None
Filiation: Principal
In-Foliate Locus: Left+Right
Foliate Layer: **[3]**
Partitions: 3 [(-4, -3, -2, -1) (+1, +2, +3, +4)]
Allotropic Cause: Unknown
Psychophysics Etiology: Complete
IC-10-CM: R46.89
Page No: 400

Periodic Limb Movement Disorder
Alternative Labels: None
Filiation: PA to RLS
In-Foliate Locus: Left-Chiral, Quadracursor
Foliate Layer: **[4]**
Partitions: 4 [(-4, -3, -2, -1) (+1, +2, +3, +4)]
Allotropic Cause: Unknown, Biological
Psychophysics Etiology: Complete
IC-10-CM: G47.61
Page No: 605

Peripartum Dysphoria
Alternative Labels: None
Filiation: PA to Bipolar
In-Foliate Locus: Left+Right
Foliate Layer: **[6]**
Partitions: 6 [(-4, -3, -2, -1) (+1, +2, +3, +4)]
Allotropic Cause: Pregnancy
Psychophysics Etiology: Complete
IC-10-CM: F53.0
Page No: 371

Phobia
Alternative Labels: None
Filiation: Principal
In-Foliate Locus: Left-Chiral
Foliate Layer: **[7]**
Partitions: 7 [(-4, -3, -2, -2) (+1, +2, +3, +4)]
Allotropic Cause: Unknown
Psychophysics Etiology: Complete
IC-10-CM: F40.00
Page No: 435

Post Traumatic Stress Disorder
Alternative Labels: None
Filiation: Principal
In-Foliate Locus: Left-Chiral
Foliate Layer: **[7]**
Partitions: 7 [(-4, -3, -2, -1) (+1, +2, +3, +4)]
Allotropic Cause: Unknown
Psychophysics Etiology: Complete
IC-10-CM: F43.10

Page No: 555

Postpartum Dysphoria
Alternative Labels: None
Filiation: PA to Bipolar
In-Foliate Locus: Left+Right or either Right or Left-Chiral only
Foliate Layer: **[6]**
Partitions: 6 [(-4, -3, -2, -1) (+1, +2, +3, +4)]
Allotropic Cause: Hormonal
Psychophysics Etiology: Complete
IC-10-CM: F53.0
Page No: 371

Postpartum Psychosis
Alternative Labels: None
Filiation: PA to Bipolar
In-Foliate Locus: Left+Right or either Right or Left-Chiral only
Foliate Layer: **[6]**
Partitions: 6 [(-4, -3, -2, -1) (+1, +2, +3, +4)]
Allotropic Cause: Hormonal
Psychophysics Etiology: Complete
IC-10-CM: F53.1
Page No: 371

Premature Ejaculation
Alternative Labels: None
Filiation: PA to Erectile Disorder
In-Foliate Locus: Left-Chiral Side
Foliate Layer: **[7]**
Partitions: 7 [(-4, -3, -2, -1) (+1, +2, +3, +4)]
Allotropic Cause: Unknown
Psychophysics Etiology: Complete
IC-10-CM: F52.4
Page No: 484

Premenstrual Dysphoria
Alternative Labels: PMS, PMDD
Filiation: PA to Bipolar Disorder
In-Foliate Locus: Left+Right
Foliate Layer: **[6]**
Partitions: 6 [(-4, -3, -2, -1) (+1, +2, +3, +4)]
Allotropic Cause: Hormonal
Psychophysics Etiology: Complete
IC-10-CM: F32.81
Page No: 370

Pseudocyesis
Alternative Labels: False Pregnancy, Phantom Pregnancy
Filiation: Principal
In-Foliate Locus: Left+Right
Foliate Layer: **[5]**
Partitions: 5 [(-4, -3, -2, -1) (+1, +2, +3, +4)]
Allotropic Cause: Unknown
Psychophysics Etiology: Complete
IC-10-CM: F45.8
Page No: 496

Psychogenic Stuttering
Alternative Labels: Stammering
Filiation: Principal
In-Foliate Locus: Left+Right
Foliate Layer: **[6]**
Partitions: 6 [(-4, -3, -2, -1) (+1, +2, +3, +4)]
Allotropic Cause: Not well known, Neurological in Neurogenic form
Psychophysics Etiology: Complete
IC-10-CM: F80.81
Page No: 403

Purging
Alternative Labels: None
Filiation: Variant of Bulimia/Anorexia
In-Foliate Locus: Left+Right
Foliate Layer: **[7]**
Partitions: 7 [(-4, -3, -2, -1) (+1, +2, +3, +4)]
Allotropic Cause: Unknown
Psychophysics Etiology: Complete
IC-10-CM: F50
Page No: 568

Pyromania
Alternative Labels: Fire setting
Filiation: PA to Antisocial Personality Disorder
In-Foliate Locus: Right-Chiral Only
Foliate Layer: **[7]**
Partitions: 7 [(+1, +2, +3, +4)]
Allotropic Cause: Unknown
Psychophysics Etiology: Complete
IC-10-CM: F63.1
Page No: 514

-R-

Rapid Eye Movement Sleep Behavior Disorder
Alternative Labels: None
Filiation: Principal
Hypercursor over accrued
Foliate Layer: All
Partitions: All on Layer
Allotropic Cause: Unknown
Psychophysics Etiology: Complete
IC-10-CM: G47.52
Page No: 315

Reactive Attachment Disorder
Alternative Labels: None
Filiation: Principal
In-Foliate Locus: Left-Right
Foliate Layer: **[6]**
Partitions: 6 [(-4, -3, -2, -1) (+1, +2, +3, +4)]
Allotropic Cause: Unknown
Psychophysics Etiology: Complete
IC-10-CM: F94.1
Page No: 551

Restless Legs Syndrome
Alternative Labels: None
Filiation: Principal
In-Foliate Locus: Left-Chiral
Quadracursor
Foliate Layer: **[4]**
Partitions: 4 [(-4, -3, -2, -1) (+1, +2, +3, +4)]
Allotropic Cause: Unknown, Biological
Psychophysics Etiology: Complete
IC-10-CM: G25.81
Page No: 602

Rumination Disorder
Alternative Labels: None
Filiation: PA to Bulimia
In-Foliate Locus: Left+Right
Foliate Layer: **[7]**
Partitions: 7 [(-4, -3, -2, -1) (+1, +2, +3, +4)]
Allotropic Cause: Unknown, Biological
Psychophysics Etiology: Complete
IC-10-CM: F98.21
Page No: 573

-S-

Sadistic (Antisocial) Personality Disorder
Alternative Labels: Psychopathy, Sociopathy
Filiation: Principal
In-Foliate Locus: Right-Chiral Only
Foliate Layer: **[7]**
Partitions: 7 [(+1, +2, +3, +4)]
Allotropic Cause: Unknown
Psychophysics Etiology: Complete
IC-10-CM: F60.2
Page No: 506

Schizoid Personality Disorder
Alternative Labels: None
Filiation: PA to Social Anxiety Disorder
In-Foliate Locus: Left-Chiral
Foliate Layer: **[8]**
Partitions: 8 [(-4, -3, -2, -1) (+1, +2, +3, +4)]
Allotropic Cause: Unknown
Psychophysics Etiology: Complete
IC-10-CM: F60.1
Page No: 448

Schizophrenia
Alternative Labels: Dementia precox
Filiation: Principal
In-Foliate Locus: Left+Right
Foliate Layer: **[8]**
Partitions: 8 [(-4, -3, -2, -1) (+1, +2, +3, +4)]
Allotropic Cause: , Trauma, Genetic
Psychophysics Etiology: Complete
IC-10-CM: F20.9
Page No: 445

Schizotypal Personality Disorder
Alternative Labels: None
Filiation: PA to Schizophrenia
In-Foliate Locus: Left+Right
Foliate Layer: **[8]**
Partitions: 8 [(-4, -3, -2, -1) (+1, +2, +3, +4)]
Allotropic Cause: Unknown
Psychophysics Etiology: Complete
IC-10-CM: F21
Page No: 448

Seasonal Dysphoria
Alternative Labels: Winter blues

Filiation: PA to Bipolar
In-Foliate Locus: Left+Right
Foliate Layer: **[6]**
Partitions: 6 [(-4, -3, -2, -1) (+1, +2, +3, +4)]
Allotropic Cause: Unknown
Psychophysics Etiology: Complete
IC-10-CM: F39
Page No: 366

Selective Mutism

Alternative Labels: None
Filiation: PA to Social Anxiety Disorder
In-Foliate Locus: Left-Chiral
Foliate Layer: **[1]**
Partitions: 1 [(-4, -3, -2, -1) (+1, +2, +3, +4)]
Allotropic Cause: Unknown
Psychophysics Etiology: Complete
IC-10-CM: F94.0
Page No: 380

Separation Anxiety

Alternative Labels: None
Filiation: Principal
In-Foliate Locus: Left-Chiral
Foliate Layer: **[6]**
Partitions: 6 [(-4, -3, -2, -1) (+1, +2, +3, +4)]
Allotropic Cause: Unknown
Psychophysics Etiology: Complete
IC-10-CM: F93.0
Page No:

Sexual Masochistic Disorder

Alternative Labels: Masochism
Filiation: Principal
In-Foliate Locus: Left-Chiral Only
Foliate Layer: **[7]**
Partitions: 7 [(-4, -3, -2, -1)
Allotropic Cause: Unknown
Psychophysics Etiology: Complete
IC-10-CM: F65.51
Page No: 490

Sexual Sadism Disorder

Alternative Labels: Sexual Sadism
Filiation: Principal
In-Foliate Locus: Right-Chiral
Foliate Layer: **[7]**
Partitions: 7 [(-4, -3, -2, -1) (+1, +2, +3, +4)]
Allotropic Cause: Unknown
Psychophysics Etiology: Complete
IC-10-CM: F65.52
Page No: 455

Shift Work Type Sleep Disorder

Alternative Labels: None
Filiation: Variant of Sleep-wake disorders
In-Foliate Locus: Left+Right
Foliate Layer: **[4]**
Partitions: 4 [(-4, -3, -2, -1) (+1, +2, +3, +4)]
Allotropic Cause: Unknown
Psychophysics Etiology: Complete
IC-10-CM: G47.26
Page No: 619

Sleep Paralysis Disorder

Alternative Labels: None
Filiation: PA to Sleep-Wake Disorders
In-Foliate Locus: Left+Right
Foliate Layer: **[4]**
Partitions: 4 [(-4, -3, -2, -1) (+1, +2, +3, +4)]
Allotropic Cause: Unknown
Psychophysics Etiology: Complete
IC-10-CM: G47.53
Page No: 623

Sleep-Wake Disorders

Alternative Labels: None
Filiation: Principal
In-Foliate Locus: Left+Right
Foliate Layer: **[4]**
Partitions: 4 [(-4, -3, -2, -1) (+1, +2, +3, +4)]
Allotropic Cause: Unknown, Biological
Psychophysics Etiology: Complete
IC-10-CM: G47.20
Page No: 619

Sleepwalking

Alternative Labels: Somnambulism
Filiation: Principal
In-Foliate Locus: Left+Right
Hypercursor overaccrued
Foliate Layer: **[5]**
Partitions: 5 [(-4, -3, -2, -1) (+1, +2, +3, +4)]
Allotropic Cause: Unknown
Psychophysics Etiology: Complete
IC-10-CM: F51.3
Page No: 608

Social Anxiety Disorder
Alternative Labels: Timidity, Social phobia
Filiation: Principal
In-Foliate Locus: Left-Chiral
Foliate Layer: [1]
Partitions: 1 [(-4, -3, -2, -1) (+1, +2, +3, +4)]
Allotropic Cause: Unknown
Psychophysics Etiology: Complete
IC-10-CM: F40.10
Page No: 378

Social Communication Disorder
Alternative Labels: None
Filiation: PA to Schizophrenia
In-Foliate Locus: Left-Chiral
Foliate Layer: [3]
Partitions: 3 [(-4, -3, -2, -1) (+1, +2, +3, +4)]
Allotropic Cause: Unknown
Psychophysics Etiology: Complete
IC-10-CM: F80.82
Page No: 268

Somatic Symptom Disorder
Alternative Labels: None
Filiation: PA to Hysteria
In-Foliate Locus: Left+Right
Foliate Layer: [5]
Partitions: 5 [(-4, -3, -2, -1) (+1, +2, +3, +4)]
Allotropic Cause: Unknown
Psychophysics Etiology: Complete
IC-10-CM: F45.9
Page No: 356

Specific Learning Disorder
Alternative Labels: None
Filiation: Principal
In-Foliate Locus: Left+Right
Foliate Layer: [3]
Partitions: 3 [(-4, -3, -2, -1) (+1, +2, +3, +4)]
Allotropic Cause: Unknown, Biological
Psychophysics Etiology: Complete
IC-10-CM: F81.0
Page No: 418

Specific Phobia
Alternative Labels: None
Filiation: Sub-class Phobia Variants
In-Foliate Locus: Left-Chiral
Foliate Layer: [7]
Partitions: 7 [(-4, -3, -2, -2) (+1, +2, +3, +4)]
Allotropic Cause: Unknown
Psychophysics Etiology: Complete
IC-10-CM: F40.2
Page No: 435

Split Personality Disorder
Alternative Labels: Dissociative Identity Disorder, Multiple PD
Filiation: Principal
In-Foliate Locus: Left+Right
Foliate Layer: [5]
Partitions: 5 [(-4, -3, -2, -1) (+1, +2, +3, +4)]
Allotropic Cause: Not well known, Trauma and Abuse
Psychophysics Etiology: Complete
IC-10-CM: F44.81
Page No: 428

Stereotypic Movement Disorder
Alternative Labels: None
Filiation: PA to Trichotilomania-Dermatilomania
In-Foliate Locus: Right-Chiral
Foliate Layer: [7]
Partitions: 7 [(-4, -3, -2, -1) (+1, +2, +3, +4)]
Allotropic Cause: Unknown
Psychophysics Etiology: Complete
IC-10-CM: F98.4
Page No: 583

Stupor
Alternative Labels: None
Filiation: Variant of Catatonia
In-Foliate Locus: Left+Right
Foliate Layer: [6]
Partitions: 6 [(-4, -3, -2, -1) (+1, +2, +3, +4)]
Allotropic Cause:
Psychophysics Etiology: Complete
IC-10-CM: R40.1
Page No: 611

Suicidal Obsession
Alternative Labels: None
Filiation: Principal
In-Foliate Locus: Left-Chiral
Foliate Layer: [7]
Partitions: 7 [(-4,- 3, -2, -1) (+1, +2, +3, +4)]
Allotropic Cause: Unknown

Psychophysics Etiology: Complete
IC-10-CM: F42.0
Page No: 531

-T-

Tics Disorders
Alternative Labels: None
Filiation: PA to Obsessive-Convulsive Disorder
In-Foliate Locus: Left+Right
Foliate Layer: **[7]**
Partitions: 7 [(-4, -3, -2, -1)(+1, +2, +3, +4)]
Allotropic Cause: Unknown
Psychophysics Etiology: Complete
IC-10-CM: F95.9
Page No: 289

Transvestic Disorder
Alternative Labels: None
Filiation: Principal
In-Foliate Locus: Left+Right
Foliate Layer: **[7]**
Partitions: 7 [(-4, -3, -2, -1) (+1, +2, +3, +4)]
Allotropic Cause: Unknown
Psychophysics Etiology: Complete
IC-10-CM: F65.1
Page No: 462

Transvestic Fetishism
Alternative Labels: None
Filiation: PA to Transvestic Disorder
In-Foliate Locus: Left+Right
Foliate Layer: **[7]**
Partitions: 7 [(-4, -3, -2, -1) (+1, +2, +3, +4)]
Allotropic Cause: Unknown
Psychophysics Etiology: Complete
IC-10-CM: F65.1
Page No: 395

Trichotillomania-Dermatillomania
Alternative Labels: None
Filiation: Principal
In-Foliate Locus: Left+Right
Foliate Layer: **[7]**
Partitions: 7 [(-4, -3, -2, -1) (+1, +2, +3, +4)]
Allotropic Cause: Unknown
Psychophysics Etiology: Complete
IC-10-CM: --
Page No: 575

Trichotillomania
Alternative Labels: Hair-Pulling
Filiation: Principal
In-Foliate Locus: Left-Chiral
Foliate Layer: **[7]**
Partitions: 7 [(-4, -3, -2, -1) (+1, +2, +3, +4)]
Allotropic Cause: Unknown
Psychophysics Etiology: Complete
IC-10-CM: F63.3
Page No: 575

-V-

Voyeuristic Disorder
Alternative Labels: None
Filiation: Principal
In-Foliate Locus: Left-Chiral Sector overaccrued
Foliate Layer: **[2] or [7] optionally**
Partitions: 2 or 7 [(-4, -3, -2, -1) (+1, +2, +3, +4)]
Allotropic Cause: Unknown
Psychophysics Etiology: Complete
IC-10-CM: F65.3
Page No: 493

Attention Deficit/Hyperactivity Disorder (ADHD)

ADHD is a mental dysfunction whereby the ability to exercise attention span in a controlled manner is quite severely impaired. The perception and capture of the objects of Reality peremptorily impose on the subject's mind, causing incontrollable hyperactivity in pursuit of ever more perceptions in a ubiquitous Reality.

PASSIVE –RESPONSIVE SYMPTOMS

Attention span tends to spread inhomogenously causing random disparate perceptions. Easily distracted, i.e. looking at window or glance at a clock when being addressed. Frequently forgets daily tasks. Prone to lose belongings due to inattention during their manipulation.

ACTIVE-REACTIVE SYMPTOMS

Hyperactive, always on the go. Children are constantly running or climbing. Adults stand up when they should be seated, always moving feet and hands. All seem literally powered by an internal engine and experience internal restlessness that feels painful. Many also exhibit twitches.

KNOWN VARIANTS

Inattentive Type, Hyperactive Type and Combined Inattentive-Hyperactive Type.

LANGUAGE

Extremely talkative. Finish people's sentences. Can't wait to speak and too frequently talk over people in conversations. Generally loud and disruptive.

BEHAVIORAL FLIPS

Known Mood swings in the Combined Type.

DERIVED DISABILITIES

Tend to take forever to complete assignments of any kind. School performance tends to be alarmingly poor. Inability to follow step-by-step instructions at workplace. Resist, postpone or procrastinate obligatory tasks requiring sustained attention and continued mental engagement.

AWARENESS

Conscious self-awareness: only neurotic form of the dysfunction known.

CHARACTEROLOGICAL FILIATION

Reality-Driven Type

QG LAYER-PARTITIONS

Inattentive Type: **2[-4, -3, -2, -1]**

Hyperactive Type: **2[+1, +2, + 3,+ 4]**

Combined Type: **2[(-4, -3, -2, -1), (+1, +2, + 3, + 4)]**

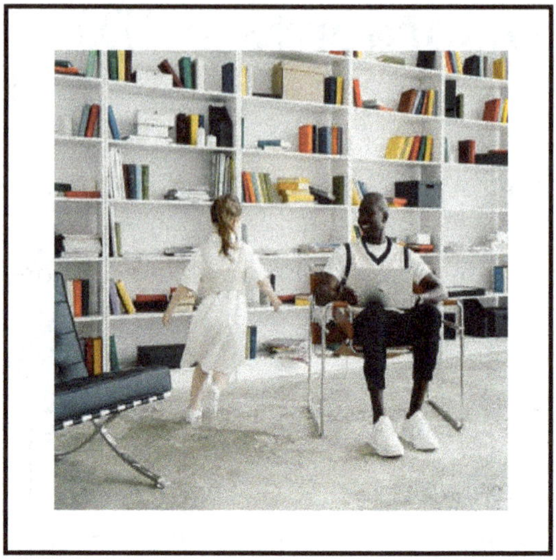

STATISTICS

8.4% of children – 2.5% of adults

INSIGHTS

The Quanto-Geometric Binary Norm that informs normal layer **2** is key to an understanding of the reason for the symptoms in ADHD. What the ADHD mind is doing is constantly *pairing* with *Reality* or the objects thereof in a binary fashion through the act of perception whose modus operandi is *imaging*. The subject does not lose attention; it is a misconception to interpret the ADHD or ADD state of mind as a deficit of attention. What there is in ADHD is a disparate spread of attention or attention focused elsewhere than the desired or due spot for the required duration. That is clearly visible when the subject's attention is captured by something else as he/she looks through the window or stares at a clock while he/she is being addressed. Because the objects of reality are so many, on the active-latent mode the subject's attention is motivationally pursuing their perception one after another, and so he/she ends up exhibiting hyperactivity.

Note that 20% of children with ADHD exhibit twitching, which can be confused with autism symptomatology, for the claim of co-morbidity. Twitching is a direct production of the *Mirroring* mind fit, which makes the subject repeat cadence sounds, or reproduce with persistent eye blinking something he/she might have perceived that is construable as such.

Lastly, the mood swings that are part of the nosology of ADHD, which put the subject on a flip between inattention and hyperactivity, are well described by the antisymmetric feature inherent to the Quanto-Geometric normal layer characterization.

Hysteria

The term *Hysteria*, synonymous with *Hypochondriasis*, had been deprecated since 1980 in favor of three different denominations covering different aspects of this condition: *Conversion Disorder, Illness Anxiety Disorder* and *Factitious Disorder*. The typical symptoms formerly attributed to Hysteria are now mostly classified under Conversion Disorder, which is alternatively designated Somatoform Disorder or Histrionic Personality Disorder. Effectively, the theatrical or drama-playing aspect of this condition in general is a prominent trait that accompanies the apparent physiological disorders these patients claim to suffer from. *Hysteria* is etymologically rooted in the Greek word for *uterus (hustera)*, chosen by virtue of the observed prevalence of this condition in women ever since old age.

PASSIVE –RESPONSIVE SYMPTOMS

Consecutively, violent migraines, vomiting, limb paralyses, extreme sensory symptoms such as partial or complete loss of skin sensation, blindness, deafness, aphonia, diplopia, and globus (sensation of a lump in the throat), or an epileptic-like seizure of pure psychogenic nature. The somatic symptoms always represent bodily sensations without an underlying recognizable medical basis.

ACTIVE-REACTIVE SYMPTOMS

Crises of commotion, tremor or dystonia, convulsions, spasms and contractures, gait abnormalities. Bizarre skin eruptions (stigmata). Also, feigning of symptoms in Factitious Disorder. Some would atrociously mutilate or burn themselves without experiencing any sensation of pain. Disproportionate levels of concern, in fact motivation, for organic dysfunctions. Sexual forwardness.

KNOWN VARIANTS

Illness Anxiety Disorder, Conversion Disorder, Factitious Disorder.

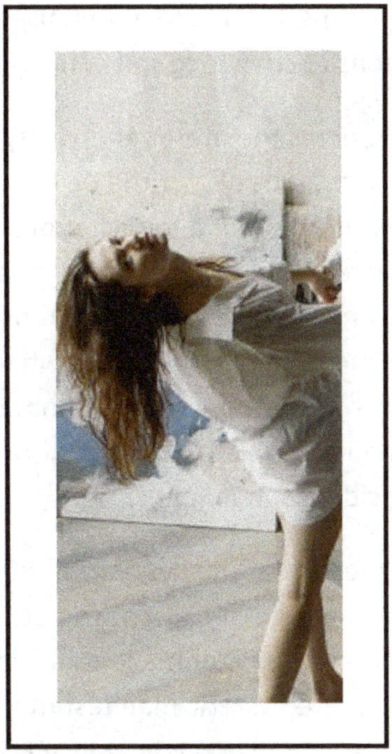

LANGUAGE

Dysarthria (slurred slow speech), abundant flow of words, laments sometimes in yelling, sexual profanities, hollers, insults and curses.

BEHAVIORAL FLIPS

Torrents of tears and laughter. Vociferating laments and insults in a row.

DERIVED DISABILITIES

Insomnia. Focused attention on bodily symptoms leads to incessant bodily checkups, maladive excess seeking of medical help and laboratory testing.

AWARENESS

Conscious (Neurotic Disorder) – With hallucinations, psychotic. In noted variants, Awareness is Conscious (Neurotic Disorders).

CHARACTEROLOGICAL FILIATION

Metamorphogenic Personality

QG LAYER-PARTITIONS

5[(-4, -3, -2, -1) (+1, +2 ,+3 ,+4)]

STATISTICS

5-7% prevalence in the general population, with much higher incidence in females.

INSIGHTS

The Quanto-Geometric Norm of Disorder or Metamorphosis, together with the partitions making up normal Mental Layer **5** of the Mentation Foliate which it informs, are uniquely responsible for the string of blustering alterations storming the Hysteric patient's mind. Further, the Entropic Mental layer materializes these dysfunctional alterations through the *endocrine system* which it totally governs. Unable to materially transform the material world, it reports these visions of change to self soma or the somatic universe of self.

Whereas the uterus knowingly represents an *endocrine organ* whose secretions are responsible for the development of pregnancy and preparation of the *mammary gland* for lactation, evidence now exists that the nonpregnant uterus secretes a hormone that regulates *pituitary function*. The secreted protein entering the bloodstream is transported to the pituitary gland, brain-based master gland of the human body, where it *constantly* acts as an inhibitor of prolactin secretion. There lies the momentous reason, hitherto misjudged perhaps by medical science, why this disorder affects women in a disproportionately higher incidence than men.

Where does the hysteric brain's power to materialize deafness, blindness and the barrage of phsychosomatic alterations come from? The simple answer: the metamorphogenic agent of change embodied in the endocrine system in total. Why are hysteric manifestations so strikingly similar to hypnosis, as noted in all time cognitive science since Freud? Because they are motorized by the same Mentation Layer **5** in the unconscious Foliate, first layer of Mind which awareness migrates to when we transition into sleep, whether natural or artificial.

PATHOLOGICAL AFFILIATES

Somatic Symptom Disorder

Somatic Symptom Disorder is characterized by an extreme disparaging focus on physical symptoms — such as pain or fatigue. In most cases, these symptoms do not have a diagnosable underlying medical condition. The preoccupation is overblown and morbid, causing frenzy for medical care, while significantly affecting the sufferer's day-to-day living. Constant worry about potential illness and incessantly checking the body for abnormalities make up a significant part of these patients' daily distressful living.

Burnout Syndrome

Burnout Syndrome is a state of generalized mental and nervous exhaustion as a result of prolonged duress imposed on mentalization functions in terms of quasi uninterrupted work of intellectual nature and lack of repose and sleep. The state of fatigue is deep and abnormal in that the organism is unable to recover or renew its levels of energy due to nervous and possibly muscular intoxication and the breakdown of the very physiological mechanisms of recuperation. In particular, nerve cells within the peripheral and central nervous system become unable to store energy and eliminate built up toxicity accumulated during their activity.

PASSIVE –RESPONSIVE SYMPTOMS

Sensation of overwhelming fatigue. Hypersensitivity in the senses of touch and contact at hands and feet. Sensations of excruciating pain upon minimal contact. Dizziness that may progress into vertigo. Drop or limited scope of attention. Headaches and sensations of heaviness and roughness in the forehead. Pain at back of the neck. Remain in state of generalized loss of interest, indifference and oftentimes bedridden. Loss of appetite and possible weight loss. Pain and sensation of looseness in limb joints.

ACTIVE-REACTIVE SYMPTOMS

Sluggishness, undecisiveness, visible incapacity to act. Loss of concentration ability, dispersion of willpower. Tremor from fatigue and otherwise normal activity becomes agitation and overdrive. Severe drop in the psychological tension and impression that thoughts are slowing down.

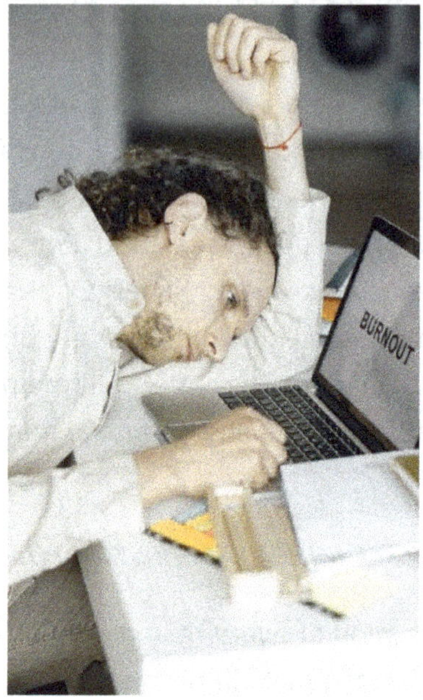

KNOWN VARIANTS

Asthenia, Psychasthenia, Neurasthenia – *not to be confused with Stuporous or Catatonic Depression.*

LANGUAGE

May experience difficulty to comprehend spoken and written language or to express oneself. Tend to withdraw from speaking.

BEHAVIORAL FLIPS

Known swings between state of relaxation (fatigue) and agitation. Psychogenic tremor occurring from the state of rest.

DERIVED DISABILITIES

Marked loss of mnemonic capacity. Maladive fear of losing one's mind to derangement. Unmotivated melancholy. Depressed libido. Suffer from light and short sleep periods to severe insomnia.

AWARENESS

Conscious (Neurotic Disorder)

CHARACTEROLOGICAL FILIATION

Unary

QG LAYER-PARTITIONS

1[(-4, -3, -2, -1), (+1, +2, +3, + 4)]

STATISTICS

Accounts for 60% of work absenteeism.

INSIGHTS

Under the Unary Norm, the passive-responsive partitions of Normal Layer **1**, namely *Timidity, Indifference, Solitude and Introversion*, which fuel an important aspect of this Disorder, inoculate in the dysfunctional behavior a marked consciousness of Self tilted toward self-devaluation. Accordingly, self-esteem is down, the individual thinks that he or she is of no good to anyone, and good for nothing. The feeling of oneself being a failure, particularly rooted in the partition of *Timidity* with accrual (self-reservation and self-devaluation), comes back unrelentingly, making him or her think that he/she does not deserve his/her family life, that the attention and love that others manifest toward him/her is unjustified. The individual retrieves in deep *Solitude* and nurtures sentiments of uselessness and even abandonment by loved ones. He almost does not address anyone, as if having nothing to say that might interest them.

Frequently, the drop in psychological tension and mentalization functions, emanating in fact from a profound state of *Indifference,* is so severe that it overtakes the body and shows an individual with a completely rendered humanity, with head either lying on the desk and dropped arms hanging in the air, or head held in the hands in a show of unmitigated wash of energy and negativity.

PATHOLOGICAL AFFILIATES

Chronic Persistent Vertigo (Dizziness)

Chronic Persistent Vertigo is equivalent to *Dizziness* and stands for a condition manifested by repetitive spells of positional dizziness. There exist four different facets of this condition: vertigo, disequilibrium, pre-syncope, and lightheadedness. In the type of persistent postural-perceptual dizziness or disequilibrium, it can be triggered by standing, walking, looking at traffic or even sitting in a busy restaurant. One form or another of these symptoms, if not the full set, is almost always a nosologic component of *Burnout Syndrome*.

PASSIVE - RESPONSIVE SYMPTOMS

Lightheadedness (feeling of disconnectedness from the environment) or fainting, wooziness or heavy-headedness, nausea, tinnitus or ringing in the ear. A certain sense of floating. May be accompanied by headaches, blacking out (losing sense of conscious awareness).

ACTIVE - REACTIVE SYMPTOMS

A false sense of motion or spinning (vertigo). Disequilibrium (feeling unsteady) and tendency to stumble. These balance problems are frequently accompanied with vomiting and at times nystagmus (uncontrollable eye movements).

QG LAYER-PARTITIONS

1[(-4, -3, -2, -1), (+1, +2, +3, + 4)**]**

INSIGHTS

We consider Vertigo a Pathological Affiliate to Burnout Syndrome. The Ego standing is deeply affected in Vertigo as the sensation of lightheadedness becomes more severe and possibly culminates in loss of conscious awareness. There is also a tilt of the weight of experienced symptoms to the *PASSIVE-RESPONSIVE* side of the Layer's pensive palette.

Abulia

Abulia is a motivational deficiency whereby the the affected subject finds it difficult to exercise willpower in order to undertake normal daily activities. It is characterized by an apparent decrease in thought content or pensive representations, spontaneous initiatives of active conduct and even communication, as well as a profound disinterest in elements of daily living. It may be either mild or severe.

PASSIVE - RESPONSIVE SYMPTOMS

Persistent passivity, reduced interest in usual pastimes, reduced emotional responsiveness and spontaneity. Delayed response time to questions and circumstances requiring a response. Marked disinterest in things that are happening around. Lack of personal emotional preferences about things of life, other people, and avoidance of others. Emotional remoteness. Extreme quietness and muteness. Chewing food for long period of time without swallowing them.

ACTIVE - REACTIVE SYMPTOMS

Difficulty in initiating and sustaining purposeful movements or actions, such as completing projects or important tasks. Inability to exercise willpower and withdrawal from events and activities. Indecisiveness displayed in difficulties in making decisions or plans. Lack of spontaneous movement, reduced spontaneous speech, reduced social interactions. Very disminished interpersonal communication.

QG LAYER-PARTITIONS

1[(-4, -3, -2, -1), (+1, +2, +3, + 4)**]**

INSIGHTS

We consider Abulia a Pathological Affiliate to *Burnout Syndrome* due to the important commonality in their nosologic elements, in particular as relates to the depletion or exhaustion of the Ego's positive faculties and abilities. There is also a narrow similarity with the symptoms that appear in *Chronic Persistent Vertigo.* These symptoms, dominated by exhaust and depletion of energy and what we normally call willpower, are instigated by left-chiral partitions of Layer **1**, *Timidity, Indifference, Solitude and Introversion,* that is. We have to remember that it requires a lot of Ego or Egocentrism to be *indifferent*, or to be a *loner* or *introverted.* In fact what appears to be a depletion in energy and willpower by the Ego as pertains to the right-chiral pensive side of motivation (+ side of *m*-axis) is to be forthrightly judged as an accrual in the left-chiral pensive side of motivation (- side of *m*-axis). The binary division of symptoms as represented in the Symptom block clearly bears out this characterization in that most of the reported *ACTIVE-REACTIVE* symptoms are formulated as lacks, which tilts the scales to the *PASSIVE-REACTIVE* side.

Note that, in this family of disorders, there is no configurational impairment of the psyche whereby the willpower axis (*t*-axis) would be impaired or compromised, as the common language lexicon might suggest. In the behavior showcased in exhaust, lack of energy and willpower, the individual will remain in deep personal withdrawal, in solitude and staunchly introverted (little communication). And that says it all.

Furthermore, it is worth noting that official science rightfully cautions not to confuse abulia with depression. It is admitted that while they share some common features, abulia and depression are two different disorders. People living with abulia typically do not exhibit such signs as sadness or suicidal thoughts that may be found in some forms of depression. Instead, they only exhibit a lack of concern about the world around them while remaining centered on self.

Impostor Syndrome

People with *Impostor Syndrome* or *Fraud Syndrome* struggle to accept that their performance and success in their varied undertakings are a result of true achieved expertise and competence. While they are intelligent enough to achieve a broad personal culture or a high level of professional qualification as well as objective successes, they are invaded by sentiments of incompetence, inferiority, and self-minimization. These feelings make them putatively unworthy of appreciation and any merit in their own eyes, driving them to believe they only live to be exposed as a "fraud" or impostor.

PASSIVE –RESPONSIVE BEHAVIOR

Fear of failure, low self-esteem. Dubious of own competency and skills. Because success entails questioning their own merits, they also live in the fear of success. Always in doubt about authenticity of their good results, which they tend to attribute to serendipity. Self-sabotaging is common as an idiotic behavioral expression geared at justifying their own perceived worthlessness.

ACTIVE-REACTIVE BEHAVIOR

In order to prove their worth, tend to work much harder and longer or overwork due to the persistent feeling of not having truly earned their title (despite numerous degrees and achievements). Hyper organized and overdriven: overboard on tasks, goal setting and multitasking. Overly sensitive to racial discrimination and negative stereotypes.

KNOWN VARIANTS

Inferiority complex – *Perfectionism* are disorders of the same class *(see Commented Bibliography)* - Neurosis of Failure

LANGUAGE

"What gives me right to be here?... My success must be due to my self-torture."

BEHAVIORAL FLIPS

Termed flips between intense feelings of low self-esteem and broad intellectual engagements resulting in over-achievements.

DERIVED DISABILITIES

Depression and anxiety commonly ensue due to effects of being hyper organized, overdriven, constant morbid doubts about self capacities and achievements, as well as fear of being unmasked.

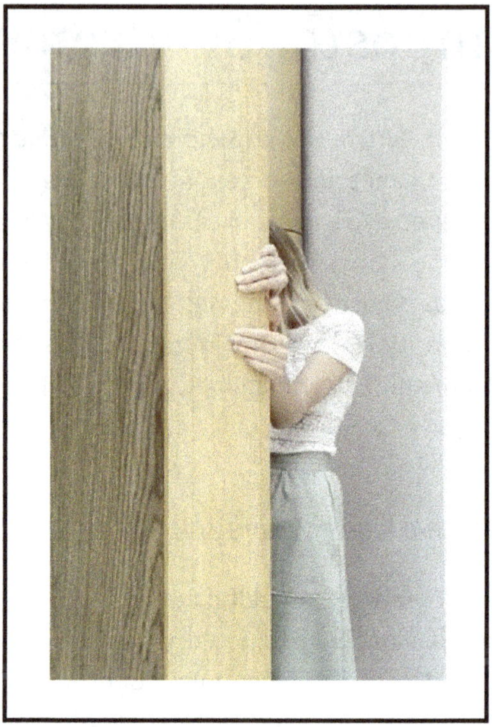

AWARENESS

Fully conscious and aware of symptoms – No known psychotic form.

CHARACTEROLOGICAL FILIATION

Trinary

QG LAYER-PARTITIONS

3 [(-4,-3,-2,-1) (1, 2, 3, 4)] - Neurosis of failure: **3 [(-4,-3,-2,-1)]**

STATISTICS

Prevalence varies between 9-8.2% of the population.

INSIGHTS

Currently, *Impostor Syndrome* is not an officially recognized psychiatric disorder: neither featured in the *DSM-5* nor listed as a diagnosis in the *International Classification of Diseases (ICD10).* However, it is profusely present in the rest of the literature, so reflecting a real or persistent psychological dysfunction among the population globe wide.

These feelings of low self-esteem exist among men and women across a range of age groups from adolescents to late-stage professionals, within many professional settings, and among multiple ethnic and racial groups. We find complete support for this syndrome as a type of mental dysfunction in the QG framework, a reason of import for its explicit inclusion in our classification. Impostor syndrome is often reported to be comorbid with burnout among various employee populations including clinicians. This comorbidity must be understood, however, as a product of external impositions non-organically related to the essential ontogenic stream or type of the illness itself.

Bipolar Disorder

Bipolar Disorder is very common mental illness affecting both men and women, in which the patient experiences periods of high mood excitement, high level of excitability, unmotivated euphoria, upbeat and high energy, and frequently exhibiting short temper and misbehaving. At other times, the mood is completely down, subsumed in feelings of distress, lack of energy and desire, loss of tite, withdrawing from activities and friends. In the period of high excitement or mania, the mood may tone down to become hypomania.

PASSIVE –RESPONSIVE SYMPTOMS

Depressed mood, feelings of sadness, emptiness and hopelessness. Tearful and prone to suicidal thoughts in the form of planning or outright attempts of suicide. Unreasonable negative prospects for the future. Hyperreligiosity on the themes of pain and sacrifice, implorations. Lack of interest in activities once enjoyable. Chanting of sad themes and extreme sensitivity to melancholic music. Poor appetite and weight loss.

ACTIVE-REACTIVE SYMPTOMS

Euphoric and highly upbeat. Undertaking endless simultaneous tasks without completing them. Elicit passionate urges possibly leading to promiscuity. Prone to seduction through attractiveness and over-adorning their environment. Unusual talkativeness with praises for known figures in pop culture and history. Racing thoughts and poor judgement in decision making. High irritability, intractability and restlessness. Obsession with order, lush and light.

KNOWN VARIANTS

Bipolar Disorder I, Bipolar Disorder II, Bipolar NOS Disorder per DSM-5, Cyclothymia. Hypomania, Borderline Personality Disorder. Seasonal Dysphoria, Melancholy (Melancholic Depression). Long-Term Adjustment Disorder.

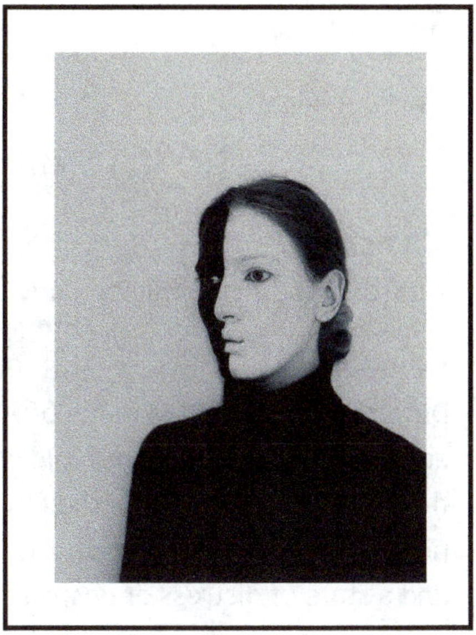

LANGUAGE

Clang associations, i.e.*"the train brain tainted me",* are common. Use of words with rhyme or pun. Neologisms are common, so is echolalia (repeating one's words). Speech is disorganized by jumping from one topic to another, and by using word salad (words hard to understand). The speech is pressured and loud.

BEHAVIORAL FLIPS

May experience major depressive episodes *before* and *after* the manic episode. In addition, bipolar symptoms may swing in their polar expression with seasons of year.

DERIVED DISABILITIES

Trouble sleeping and not feeling tired after sleep loss. Severe insomnia in the form of complete or significant lack of sleep over prolonged period of time (manic phase), or excessive amount of sleep (depressive). Substance abuse, alcoholic addiction.

AWARENESS

Unconscious in hallucinatory Bipolar Disorder (hearing voices, talking to self, etc.), which is psychotic in nature. Unconscious as well when self-denial of illness and/or refusal of medication are present. Otherwise awareness is conscious and disorder qualifies as neurosis and quasi equivalent to Cyclothymia.

CHARACTEROLOGICAL FILIATION

Matrixial

QG LAYER-PARTITIONS

6[(-4, -3, -2, -1), (+1, +2, +3, +4)]

6[(-4, -3, -2, -1)]

6[(+1, +2, +3, +4)]

6[(-4, -3, -2, -1), (+1, +2, +3, +4)**]**

6[(-4, -3, -2, -1), **(+1, +2, +3, +4)]**

STATISTICS

2.8% of US adults (5 million individuals) are affected.

INSIGHTS

Despite the alternative name of Manic Depression, in fact its originally designated label, it is important to avoid confounding the low phase of this illness with the class of depression marked by authentic fatigue and exhaustion as experienced i.e. in Burnout Syndrome. In the low down mood of the dysfunction, we find a state of distress or despair which if long sustained may lead the patient to suicide. It is because of the element of despair or distress in the soul, so to speak, in the low-down mood that suicidal thoughts ensue, which seldom if ever occur in the feelings of exhaust and overwhelming fatigue that accompany the class of disorders pertaining to Asthenia.

It is important to understand the "mood" element in this disorder as a tonal feeling associated with the heart or expressions of heart, otherwise considered sentimental fits amply evoked and celebrated in all-time lyric literature. It is for this very reason that some of the greatest world writers, intellectuals and artists, were knowingly affected by Bipolar Disorder. The illness in fact heightens the expression of sentimental fits, well expressed in the suite of partitions pertaining to Layer **6** of the Mental Foliate with Passion at the top of the suite.

It is worth scrutinizing further the Bipolar NOS (Not Otherwise Specified) category mentioned as the 3rd variant in the Disorder. Albeit a contentious category, Bipolar NOS is otherwise commonly regarded as a precursor to either Bipolar I or Bipolar II Disorder. It applies in the following situations:

1. The subject meets the criteria for Bipolar Disorder I or II, but there is a concern that the symptoms may be caused by recreational drugs, alcohol or a neurological disorder, instead of being of psychological origin.

2. The patient has experienced both hypomania and depression, but the episodes are too short to qualify as a cyclothymic disorder. Hypomania is a qualified mild level of manic behavior (elation that does not reach euphoria).
3. The subject has experienced alternating manic or depressive symptoms, but the episodes are too short to meet the criteria for Bipolar I or Bipolar II.
4. The subject may have had multiple episodes of hypomania but no depressive episode.
5. The patient has had a manic or mixed episode after having been previously diagnosed with either schizophrenia or a psychotic episode.

It is likely that in case 5, there is instead a Depressive Disorder involving the entire Anima sector of the Foliate, per our etiological analysis of mixed Depression dysfunction.

In case 2, the differentiation with Cyclothymia is indeed inconsequential, because the duration of the swings is of no particular significance from root etiology perspective. It is the pensive strength of the symptoms that is of paramount import. So it is in our judgment because no neurochemical agent has yet been developed with granular effectiveness arising from an understanding of the intimate neurochemistry that is implicated in the psychotherapy of this case or in general. Therefore, from our pensive root etiological perspective, and intensity gradient metric, Cyclothymia qualifies as the neurotic level of full spectrum Bipolar as a psychotic syndrome. In that context, Hypomania ought to be viewed as equivalent to the manic phase of Cyclothymia, the neurotic version of full spectrum Bipolar Disorder.

In case 3, if the differential criteria is based on the frequency of mood swings as to whether they occur within days or weeks or months, the difference is etiologically meaningless from the point of view of the nature and root cause of the disease. We have to remember that, unbeknownst to mental science of this day, swings occur in the vast majority of mental disorders. We have sought to make this feature crystal clear in this treatise. Furthermore, in the case of this particular disease there are environmental factors, specifically of astronomic nature as reflected in the seasonal variations of the year, that impact the cyclicity and prodromal course of the dysfunction. Therefore, to be fundamental, diagnostic rules must go beyond these factors.

Our psychophysics framework offers a better umbrella for an insightful comprehension of the many different nosologies of Bipolar Disorder, including those complex instances of the disease where, within the bipolar alternation, there seems to be a prevalence of depression over mania, or a prevalence of mania over depression. The last two palettes of root partitions depicted under the *QG LAYER/PARTITIONS* key perfectly model this situation.

Case 4 is another one of these peculiar facets of the disease which we may readily elucidate by invoking accretion strictly in the activity of the right-chiral set of partitions in the implicated Layer **6** of the Foliate. The etiology of this case is depicted in the 3rd palette of partitions listed under the *QG LAYER / PARTITIONS* block. We have highlighted under that block the distinct sets of individual pensive roots responsible for the different variations of the disease.

PATHOLOGICAL AFFILIATES

Premenstrual Dysphoria

Premenstrual Dysphoria takes the form of either *Premenstrual Syndrome (PMS)* or *Premenstrual Dysphoric Disorder (PMDD)* depending on the number of symptoms present, per official DSM-5 psychiatry. At least five of the symptoms mentioned below during the week preceding the onset of menses are nominally required for the disorder to qualify as PMDD. Same holds for the one-week period starting from end of the menses. PMS is usually characterized by a lesser amount of symptoms. Again, these differential diagnostic criteria based on an arbitrary number of symptoms, albeit innocuous in this case, are not fundamental.

PASSIVE –RESPONSIVE SYMPTOMS	***ACTIVE-REACTIVE SYMPTOMS***
Mood lability, dysphoria, sadness, sensitivity to rejection, hopelessness, feeling anxious or edgy. Decreased interest in usual activities. Bloating sensation, weight gain, breast tenderness. Insomnia or Hypersomnia.	Irritability or anger. Appetite change or cravings for specific foods. Decreased concentration.

INSIGHTS

One may notice the similarity in the nature of the above symptom set with a subset of those manifest in Bipolar Disorder in general, which jusfifies our taxonomic affiliation of this Disorder with the latter. Heightened appetite and cravings must be linked to the elation in the partitions of *Euphoria* and *Passion*. Irritability, akin to Bipolar Disorder, appears secondarily if the euphoric attitude is somehow countered by a peer or close one in the least amount.

Finally, in concluding this section it is worth noting that in the francophone culture Bipolar Disorder is instead labeled *"Manie Dépressive"*, a nomer that specifically spells and joins Mania (Excitement) to Depression. This alternative nomer very explicitly and faithfully renders the mentation characteristics of the disease, at the same time that it helps straightforwardly capture the reasons for the affiliation of certain other diseases to the mentation roots of this Disorder. Such is the case for: *Peripartum Dysphoria, Postpartum Dysphoria* and *Postpartum Psychosis – Maternity Blues.*

Dysthymia

Dysthymia is also called *Persistent Depressive Disorder* and represents a chronic long-term form of depression whereby the patient loses interest in normal daily activities, and remains imbued in feelings of hopelessness, low self-esteem and an intimate sense of personal inadequacy. The person finds it hard to be upbeat even on happy occasions in social or personal circumstances. These feelings last for years and will significantly interfere with personal relationships, school and work. To others the affected individual displays a gloomy temper that is just capable of having fun and much given to constant complaining.

PASSIVE –RESPONSIVE SYMPTOMS

Loss of interest in daily activities. Sadness, emptiness or feeling down. Hopelessness. Tiredness and lack of energy. Low self-esteem, self-criticism or feeling incapable. Feelings of guilt and worries over the past. Sleep problems.

ACTIVE-REACTIVE SYMPTOMS

Difficulty concentrating and trouble making decisions. Irritability or excessive anger. Decreased activity and productive effectiveness. Avoidance of social activities. Poor appetite or overeating.

KNOWN VARIANTS

Belongs to the family of Mixed or Major Depression.

LANGUAGE

Languagecan be hesitant, less colorful, and depicts inner state of sadness. Overall, it may have a depressive prosody.

BEHAVIORAL FLIPS

Tendency to overdo things in a bid to compensate for the maladive discomfort of paralysis and deep sadness. Attempting at times to flip to enthusiasm by using inappropriate humor.

DERIVED DISABILITIES
Lack of productivity at work.

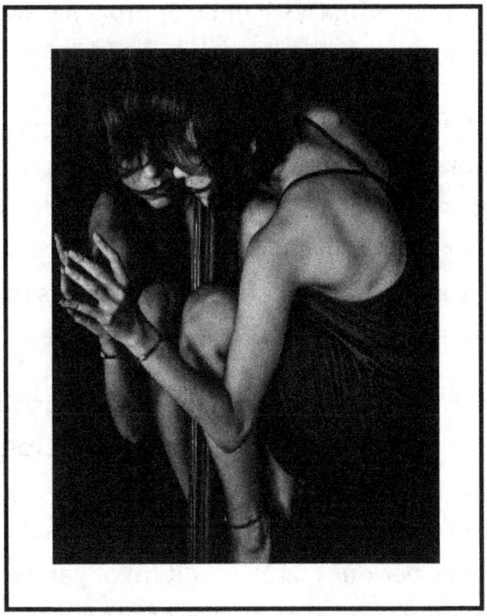

AWARENESS
Conscious (Neurotic Disorder)

CHARACTEROLOGICAL FILIATION
None

QG LAYER-PARTITIONS
[Left-Chiral Sector] of Foliate

STATISTICS
Women are up to **3 times** more likely to develop Dysthymia than men. At any point in time, 3% of the population remain affected by Dysthymia, while over the course of a lifetime, up to 6% of the general population may become sufferers.

INSIGHTS
Judging by the nosologic elements of Dysthymia, there is a tight association between Major or Mixed Depression and Persistent Depressive Disorder which appears to be a minor of the former. More than one left-chiral palette of partitions appears to show in the Disorder. The Indifference of Layer 1, feelings of guilt of Layer 4, worries over the past typical of nostalgic sorrow or despair of Layer 6 as much as the constant gloomy mood, low self-esteem and feelings of personal incapacity proper to disorientation and doubt of Layer 3, are all indication of an accrued Left-Chiral Sector of the Foliate. The elements of lack appearing in the *ACTIVE-REACTIVE* block of symptoms, such as avoidance of social activities, must be attributed to lexicon that in fact reflects a rather passive attitude in miss or withdrawal, not a forthright projective incline. Further, as with Major Depression, traumatic events such as the loss of a loved one, financial problems or a circumstantial high level of stress are known triggers to *Persistent Depressive Disorder* in some people. It is also known that among those positively

diagnosed with Dysthymia, approximately 10% will go on to develop Major Depression.

Therefore the relationship between the two Disorders in terms of a major and a minor of Depression is clear and supported by the *normals* or *normalization* of their symptom sets. This relationship does not dwell in the order of neurosis versus psychosis however, because in each of the two disorders both of the Conscious and the Unconscious Cognos (pertaining to the Left-Chiral Sector) are implicated.

Despite and against the common notion that a "personality disorder" may spur Dysthymia, we have noted no characterological affiliation for this Disorder, because there is essentially no single Layer prevalence in the expression of the dysfunction. The filiation would have to be instead associated with gender prevalence per our Chiral definition of gender, which characterizes prevalence of the entire Left-Chiral Sector of the Foliate to spur or create female sexuation. And effectively we have to predictably observe the glaring statistical fact that **3 times** more women than men are found with this Disorder, according to official statistics!

This outcome speaks to the accuracy of our psychophysics etiological framework.

Body Integrity Identity Disorder

Body Integrity Identity Disorder (BIID or Apotemnophilia) is a rare, infrequently studied and highly secretive condition in which there is an intense desire to amputate a major limb or to become paralyzed, i.e. through the severing of the spinal cord. Subjects suffering from BIID usually experience symptomatic onsets of the illness in early childhood. A related condition designated Somatoparaphrenia shares a subset of the symptoms presenting in Apotemnophilia which emerge mainly after occurrence of right-hemisphere brain damage. Somatoparaphrenia is most often characterized by a delusion of disownership of left-sided body parts and is often brought about by extensive right-sided lesions of the brain. Therefore while Apotemnophilia is of psychological/psychiatric nature, Somatoparaphrenia is of strictly neurologic nature.

PASSIVE –RESPONSIVE SYMPTOMS

Peculiar masochistic desire to be paralyzed. Simulating paralysis through factitious use of paraplegic devices such as wheelchairs. Unjustified belief that the patient's body limbs do not belong to self. Intense distress. Fascination for perception or company of disabled people or people with amputed limbs. Impressions of asymmetry or monolaterality of the body (i.e. sensation of left leg being too long, or one leg is not theirs).

ACTIVE-REACTIVE SYMPTOMS

Peculiar sadistic desire of limb amputation, most commonly one leg or one arm and more infrequently both. Peculiar desire to have the limb preferentially amputated at a very particular level. Experience deep sadistic satisfaction to have their limbs effectively amputated, even if the amputations causes impairment in ambulation. Sadism arises from the fact that patients do not acknowledge self-ownership of the limb that amputation is desired for. It is stranger to them.

KNOWN VARIANTS

Somatoparaphrenia is a neuropsychological variant. BIID is tightly related to Cotard's Syndrome.

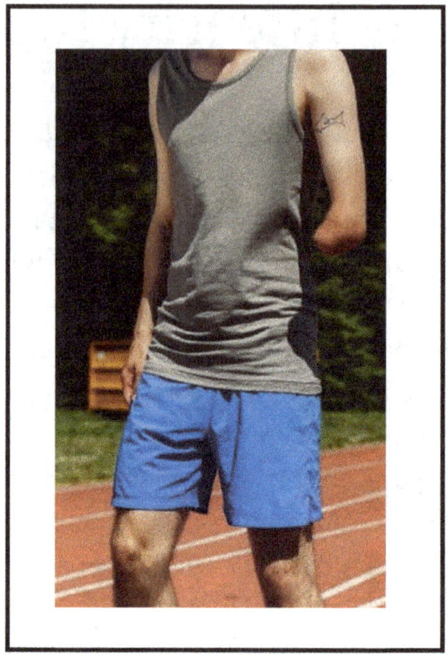

LANGUAGE

"I have this limb that should not be."
"...would feel complete with leg amputation!" Lamenting is common.

BEHAVIORAL FLIPS

Peculiar desire of limb amputation characteristic of Apotemnophilia can flip to give way to the other no less peculiar desire to be paralyzed or pretension to be so by factitiously using a paraplegic device (Bruno RL, 1997).

DERIVED DISABILITIES

BIID is associated with disruption in social, family life, and work. Post amputation, the patient may require a prosthetic leg to improve ambulation.

AWARENESS

Conscious (Neurotic Disorder).

CHARACTEROLOGICAL FILIATION

Paradoxical

QG LAYER-PARTITIONS

7[(-4, -3, -2, -1), (+1, +2, +3, +4)]

STATISTICS

Higher incidence in men, very rare condition or unreported due to secrecy.

INSIGHTS

The partitions represented in Layer **7** of the Mental Foliate in our analysis are clearly responsible for producing the etiology of this illness, since they clearly reflect the weight ofmasochistic-sadistic desires for amputation and paraplegy. A growing number of studies tend to show that the morbid desire to become paraplegic is an important aspect of the nosologic panorama of this illness. For instance, there are reports that patients with paraplegy-oriented morbidity do not experience amputation urges. However, this fact has not been sufficiently understood thus far to prompt the creation of another classificatory variant from the nosology of this illness as would be required.

Once the nosology is understood in terms of expression of two different modes of behavior (passive-responsive and active-reactive) one is on better footing to understand gender distribution of the illness that effectively puts it more on the side of men. Clearly the desire for amputation is an expression of castration (here a sadistic urge), which requires the mental body to be sensitive to mono-laterality and its identification with the virile member. A single limb is definitely an asymmetry that is similar to the virile member as an asymmetric organ of the body. Patients' bizarre fixation with the length of limb to be left by the amputation is reminiscent of male sensitivity to the length of the growing penis during development. The illness is accordingly prevalent in the male same-sex orientated population. The debate on the role of sexual components in apotemnophilia/BIID is an open one, and remains more theoretical than experimental.

Social Anxiety Disorder

As a psychiatric illness, *Social Anxiety Disorder*, formerly known as *Timidity*, made a second debut in 1980 as Social Phobia. The understanding of the disorder was later redefined and took on the current designation of Social Anxiety Disorder. It is associated with apprehension, lack of self-confidence, and awkwardness when a person is in proximity to or approached by other individuals, especially in new situations with unfamiliar people. Social Anxiety Disorder is usually associated with low birth weight.

PASSIVE –RESPONSIVE SYMPTOMS

Feeling very self-conscious in front of other people, feeling embarrassed or awkward. Physically withdraws in shyness and systematically staying away from places where other people have convened. Feeling *"their mind going blank"*. Show more reserve and caution than a situation demands, with fear of being scrutinized. Frequently ruminating failures of conduct. Lack of forthrightness may manifest as love shyness toward potential partners.

ACTIVE-REACTIVE SYMPTOMS

Show rigid body posture, stiff walk and make little eye contact. Experience rapid heart rate during episodes and butterflies in stomach. Frequent bursty reactions. During episodes, experience cold sweats and even trembling and blushing (if white complexion). Slow to develop interpersonal relationships, in particular of sexual nature. At times disinhibited behavior can manifest, such as risk taking and bullying aggresivessness.

KNOWN VARIANTS

Erethism (Mercury poisoning) manifesting as shyness, embarrassment, timidity and self-consciousness, as well as lack of self-confidence and social phobia. Avoidant Personality Disorder. Compensatory Aggressiveness.

LANGUAGE

Anxious prosody, hesitant enunciation. Vehement language in the Aggressive mode: *"I was a hell of a shy person. One day I reacted and became heavy-handed for good as I should have always been."*

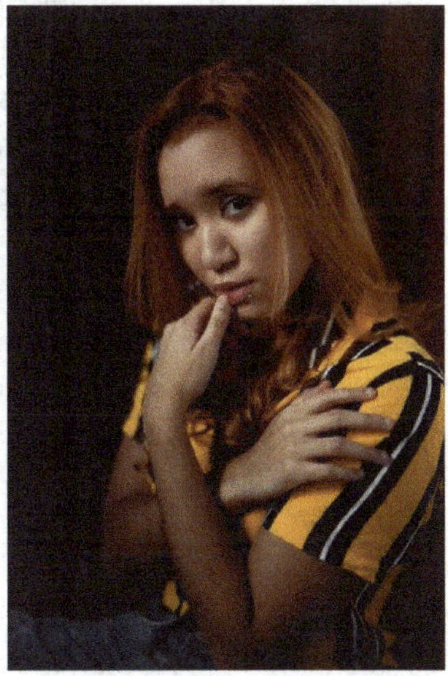

BEHAVIORAL FLIPS

Sometimes unexpectedly swing from social avoidant behavior to aggressive behavior geared to competitively assert the self.

DERIVED DISABILITIES

Tendency for isolation affects all aspects of life. Alcohol can be misused as a self-antidote to social awkwardness.

AWARENESS

Conscious (Neurotic Disorder).

CHARACTEROLOGICAL FILIATION

Egocentric

QG LAYER-PARTITIONS

1 [(-4, -3, -2, -1), (+1, +2, +3, +4)**]**

STATISTICS

The prevalence of Social Anxiety Disorder in adults is 7.1% and higher in females than males. Adolescents have a higher rate than adults.

INSIGHTS

The Quanto-Geometric Norm of Monocentrism that informs normal Layer **1** with its entire suite of partitions is responsible for the observable behaviors associated with *Social Anxiety Disorder*, specifically *Timidity, Solitude, Indifference, and Introversion*, for the retreating forms of behavior, as well as *Conservativeness* and *Competitiveness* in the disinhibited forms of behavior.

It is generally understood that child abuse and emotional abuse expressed mainly as ridiculing may trigger *Social Anxiety Disorder*. However it is only the predisposition to this form of morbidity given in the accrual of the above-mentioned mental fits that ultimately provokes the dysfunctional reactions observable in the morbidity. While there is a higher emphasis on the left-chiral partitions for the morbidity, it is important to note that in the variant of Aggressiveness, the accrual is experienced more on the right-chiral partitions. It is also well worth noting that a swing from morbidity based on the left-chiral partitions to morbidity based on right-chiral partitions where the individual experiences Aggressiveness may become permanent. In many cases the subject executes that flip from very conscious motivations, as it develops in the form of a compensation to the physiological pain or discomfort associated with the retreating behavior.

Adults with extremely low birth weight have been reported with significantly higher shyness, behavioral inhibition, impaired socialization, lower sociability and emotional well-being than their normal birth-weight counterparts in the morbidity.

PATOLOGICAL AFFILIATES

Selective Mutism

Selective Mutism applies to a person's behavior manifesting extended retraction from speaking in particular situations or most, while that person shows no physical condition that impedes speaking. This Disorder most often occurs in children, and is commonly exemplified by a child speaking freely when in the home quarters but not at school. *Selective Mutism* is a psychogenic disorder appearing in children who are very shy or going through a period of social withdrawal or isolation.

Diagnosing selective mutism ordinarily involves a multidisciplinary team of professionals which includes speech language pathologists, pediatricians, psychologists, and psychiatrists. This multiform approach is due to the fact that certain speech language disorders have the same symptomatic effects as *Selective Mutism,* which make a differential diagnosis a requirement in this case. Examples of the former are stuttering, aphasia, apraxia of speech, or dysarthria. We are uniquely concerned here with *Selective Mutism* caused by psychological factors, on account of which it becomes a Disorder in the same nosological class as *Stuttering*.

Despite the rapprochement, *Selective Mutism* does not share the same etiological roots as *Stuttering*. An important feature of *Selective Mutism* is that the subject appears to consciously self-censor himself or herself in producing speech. When the subject feels emotionally safe, i.e. while at home, he or she will freely speak, but not at school where peer pressure or learning pressure under instructors creates enough tension to contribute to a communication blockage. It is important to stress, however, that it is againt a backdrop of predisposed mental conditions that such a blockage occurs. Concordantly, *Selective Mutism* in children is known to be tightly associated with excessive shyness, or plainly Social Anxiety Disorder. The left-chiral palette of partitions on Layer 1 of the Foliate constitutes the pensive engine causing the behavior, namely *Timidity*, *Solitude, Indifference,* and *Introversion*. It is thus clear that, in the condition of a psychogenic dysfunction, *Selective Mutism* is not a disease in its own right, but more genuinely a symptom set of Social Anxiety Disorder.

Intermittent Explosive Disorder

Intermittent Explosive Disorder (IED) is an aggressive behavior well intended to harm in one way or another someone else who does not wish to be victimized. It is referred in the simple term of "committing violence" in its extreme form of physical harm resulting in injury or death. There are two types of aggressions in IED: emotional (impulsive) and instrumental (cognitive). Poor impulse control, substance use, as well as antisocial personality tendency can be at the core of the sadistic aggressiveness expressed in Intermittent Explosive Disorder.

PASSIVE –RESPONSIVE SYMPTOMS

Hearing echoes, experiencing sensations of tingling, head pressure and chest tightness. Suicidal and parasuicidal gestures as well as self-mutilation may occur. Aggressive attacks are preceded by a sense of tension or tight situational stress. Degree of triggering psychosocial precipitants or cause of stress is often squintly proportionate with the much higher intensity of the subsequent aggressive response.

ACTIVE-REACTIVE SYMPTOMS

Experience sudden intense impulses towards physical and emotional aggression prior to committing the act. Outbursts resulting in assault acts to persons or animals, or destruction of property. Heightened verbal tone, yelling, vituperating during episodes of aggression. These attacks typically result in injury to or death of other people. Frequent unwarranted heightened irritability and rage.

KNOWN VARIANTS

Belongs to the family of Impulse-Control Disorders. Emotional type when driven by outright impulsive emotions and Instrumental or cognitive type if attacks are intently planned and executed.

LANGUAGE

Generally loud and disruptive, insults, curses. Individuals describe explosive episodes as "spells" or "attacks".

BEHAVIORAL FLIPS

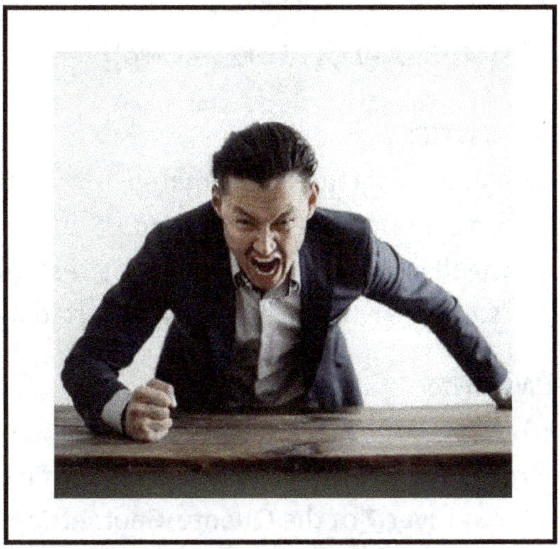

Reports from some individuals indicate that their aggressive episodes are often preceded by such symptoms as sensations of chest tightness, head pressure, and hearing an echo, followed by tingling, tremors and palpitations at which point the spree of violence unleashes as a morbid episode. In some other cases, the same suite of individual states appear to be mixed in their succession. Whether one group of symptoms orderly precedes the other or the individual mental fits within the nosological spectrum are intermixed, it is clear that the excitation of the states of the Mentation body at the same Layer **7** are flipping from one chiral side to the other.

DERIVED DISABILITIES

Severely affects interpersonal relationships, both in family and in the social order. Inability to maintain a job or complete an education. Some subjects reported engaging in 27.8 high-severity aggressive acts during their worst year incurred 2–3 outbursts requiring medical assistance. Across the lifespan, the mean value of property damage due to aggressive outbursts was estimated at $1603.

AWARENESS

Conscious (Neurotic Disorder). Psychotic instead whenever patients hear hallucinative echoes or commit horrific criminal acts such as crimes of human dismemberment.

CHARACTEROLOGICAL FILIATION

Paradoxical

QG LAYER-PARTITIONS

7 [(-4,-3,-2,-1), (+1, +2, +3, +4)]

STATISTICS

Lifetime prevalence is estimated 4-6% of the population in some studies. No broad consensus yet. Of studied US subjects with IED, 67.8% were found to have engaged in direct interpersonal aggression, 20.9% have threatened others with personal aggression, and 11.4% exerted aggression against material objects[26].

INSIGHTS

The suite of sensations or mental fits experienced in *Intermittent Explosive Disorder* clearly relates to violence or conflict as the core Norm subsuming behavior at Layer **7** of the Quanto-Geometric Mentation Foliate. The entire spectrum is involved from Angst, to Anxiety to Fury as the nosological terms of the description are clearly evocative of these states. Note that anxiety, which is oftentimes comorbid in mental disorders, is here a genuine etiological expression of the disorder as a prime root instigating it.

The distinction between impulsiveness and predetermined intent in the expression of aggressiveness in the disorder is a secondary level of categorization that mostly relates to the orthoflows occurring throughout the Foliate. In one case, the impulses (orthoflows) manage to directly reach the conscious instance of the Mental in a raw fashion. While in the other case, they are overtaken by the partitions making up the conscious instance which introduce a level of rationalization in dealing with them.

---

[26] ***"The prevalence and correlates of DSM-IV intermittent explosive disorder in the National Comorbidity Survey Replication"****. Arch. Gen. Psychiatry.* ***63*** *(6): 669–78. doi:10.1001/archpsyc.63.6.669. PMC 1924721. PMID 16754840*

Mythomania

Mythomania or *Pseudologia Fantastica* is the behavior of habitual or compulsive lying. First described in the medical literature in 1891, the characteristics of *Pseudologia Fantastica* are: (1) the stories are not entirely improbable and often have some element of truth; (2) the stories are long lasting; (3) the stories are told for internal psychological reasons rather than external gain, and tend towards fancifully presenting the person (i.e. being fantastically brave, knowing or being related to many famous people); and (4) they are not quite delusional (that is, upon persistent confrontation, the individual can ultimately acknowledge them to be untrue).

PASSIVE –RESPONSIVE SYMPTOMS

Feigning of illnesses either to assume the sick role of victim (Munchausen syndrome) or to obtain secondary gains of capturing attention the subject doesn't have. Feelings of shame and guilt from social experience or interactions, i.e. deficient grades at school, personality lacks from development delays, feelings of inadequacy with respect to siblings, etc. Compensatory enhancing of self-esteem in the face of shame is a common qualitative theme among many of the factious or delusional stories composed by mythomaniacs.

ACTIVE-REACTIVE SYMPTOMS

Constant daydreaming in telling episodic stories made up of both the imaginary and truistic elements of reality. Create a new reality that allows for fulfillment of their own wishes or self-aggrandizing fantasies. The person embellishes his or her own personal story to impress people. Generally considered a compulsive liar in search of grandeur for whom telling fantastic lies becomes a way of life. Moves between conscious deceit and delusion, at times believing his grandiose tales while at others able to acknowledge their mendacity.

KNOWN VARIANTS

Pseudologia Fantastica is part of a spectrum of factious disorders or so-called Personality Disorders. Munchausen syndrome, Malingering, Imposture, Peregrination (frequently moving town or even country, presumably to avoid detection of the lies).

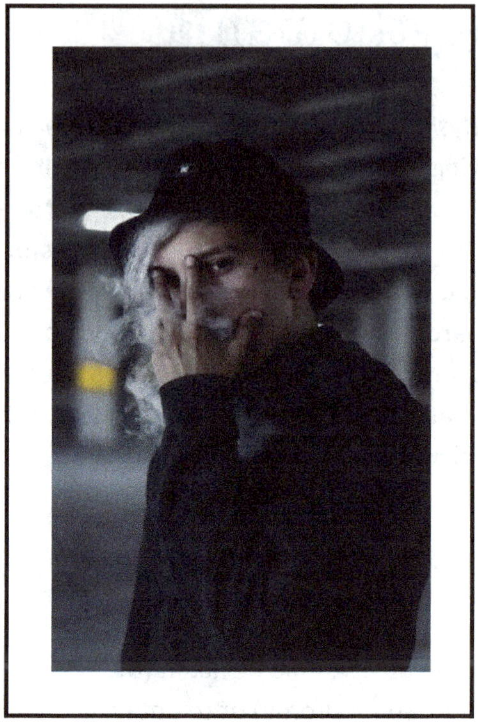

LANGUAGE

Excited, embellished, rants of repetitive statements with tendency to amplify meaning. Superior verbal ability. *"Can I just be depressed and suicidal*?" says one patient when confronted with pressure to explain his fictional narrative (he thought he needed a dramatic reason to receive help for his factitious unwellness).

BEHAVIORAL FLIPS

People with Mythomania may knowingly experience severe mood swings, feel greater instability and insecurity, and are said to lack a stable sense of self.

DERIVED DISABILITIES

The Disorder affects interpersonal relationships, destroys trust and lives.

AWARENESS

Conscious (Neurotic Disorder)

CHARACTEROLOGICAL FILIATION

Hyperbolic

QG LAYER-PARTITIONS

4[(-4,-3,-2,-1) (1, 2, 3, 4)]

STATISTICS

Prevalence in the general population is 1%.

INSIGHTS

In this Disorder, the patient exhibit grandiosity in telling extrapolating stories to augment his self-importance. In many of these fantasies, he plays an utterly heroic role. He may portray himself as stoically enduring extreme hardship and still being well alive, i.e. coping well *"despite having sustained a number of musculoskeletal injuries resulting in chronic pain while playing Division I football in college..."* or despite *"both of his parents, multiple siblings, and cousins having died during his early childhood."* All verified false claims. He will also have the audacity to challenge the very medical professionals that he is seeking help from, i.e *"by requesting placement at an inpatient psychiatric facility for electroconvulsive therapy", so* telling them what his treatment must be. The fabrications can also be very presumptuous, i.e. *"that he had been drafted by the National Football League"* or "that *"he is a tenured mathematics and physics professor at a prestigious university studying time bends in space using some of Einstein's old formulae."* The partitions pertaining to the right chiral group of Layer **4** of the Mental Foliate are all ostensibly in display here.

However much of a perpetual actor who never runs out of masks the Mythomaniac may be, we must be keen in comprehending that his feelings of shame, guilt, regretfulness, low self-esteem are prime drivers of his behavior overall. He clearly experiences those feelings both in their raw expression in reaction to a negative social or family experience and as projections in feigning illnesses either to assume the sick role (Munchausen syndrome) or for capturing attention. From there, it is easy to see how he is flipping from one set of mental fits to the other by compensation.

Lastly, the peculiar mix of realistic elements of their lives with delusional fantasies in their storytelling, for which they will sometimes go to the extra lengths of moving town to keep them plausible to people, and in which they believe despite their being aware that they created them, is a faithful representation of the hybrid traits of the Quadratic Norm of Ambivalence in Quanto-Geometric physics. Despite the fact that compulsive lying is controversially counted among the symptoms of this disorder, we report it in the nosology, being well aware that this symptom more genuinely and principally belongs to Pathological Lying which we alternatively coined Paradoxical Lying.

Kleptomania

Kleptomania (Pathological Stealing) is an impulse control disorder characterized by uncontrollable impulse to steal with reduction in psychic tension and anxiety while the act is in execution. The Kleptomaniac experiences salacious pleasure during the act of stealing. This illness affects the patient's social and occupational life, and may expectedly have deleterious legal consequences.

PASSIVE –RESPONSIVE SYMPTOMS

Experience a significant level of anxiety in the lead up to acts of theft by compulsion. Uncontrollable urges to engage in stealing other's property which are an expression of the increase in tension before the act. Experience naughty pleasure and gratification during the act of theft, but commonly feel depressed and guilty after the fact.

ACTIVE-REACTIVE SYMPTOMS

The Keptomaniac is motivated to steal objects that she can afford, does not need and which hold little monetary value. She does not steal to satisfy covet or for financial gain, and she does not plan or premeditate the acts of theft. The individual is aware of possible legal implications, and, nevertheless, they are overridden by the impulse.

KNOWN VARIANTS

None

LANGUAGE

Patients can find such beautiful excuses for stealing property that they appear to be quite natural to others.

BEHAVIORAL FLIPS

No known flip.

DERIVED DISABILITIES

Comorbid substance use. Unable to maintain good civic behavior in social settings. Consequences of kleptomanic behavior can be very serious, from being fired from work, to being expelled from school, to arrested by law enforcement and convicted for theft.

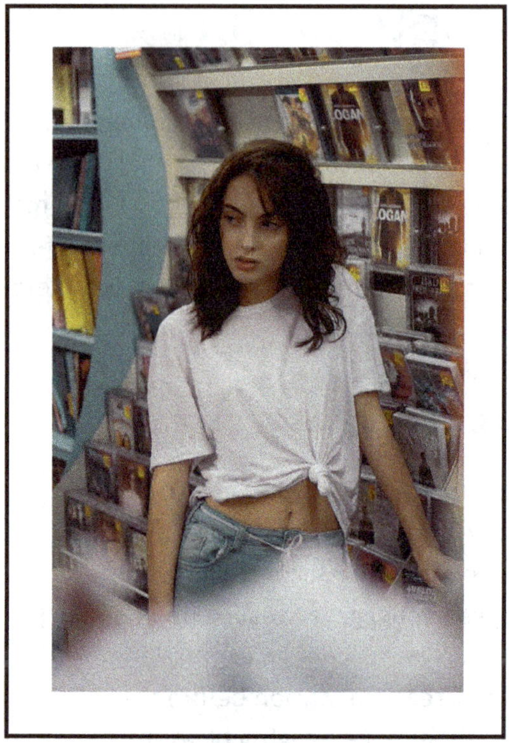

AWARENESS

Conscious (Neurotic Disorder)

CHARACTEROLOGICAL FILIATION

Paradoxical

QG LAYER-PARTITIONS

7[(-4, -3, -2, -1)]

STATISTICS

In the US, it has a prevalence of 0.3 to 0.6% of the population.

INSIGHTS

Psychiatric science has not been able to offer thus far a credible plausible explanation of the cause of Kleptomania. The usual so-called "defense" mechanisms have been unable to produce a rational etiological scenario. Some clinicians view in Kleptomania just another member of the obsessive-compulsive spectrum of disorders. They unjustifiably reason that many individuals experience the impulse to steal as an *alien*, unwanted intrusion into their mental state, which is not much of an interpretative explanation. Other clinicians believe that kleptomania may be a variant of mood disorders akin to depression.

The QG psychophysics perspective offers the endogenous cause of Kleptomania to be in the accrual of essentially the lelf-chiral partitions of Layer **7** in the Mental Foliate, in particular the Anxiety partition. There is no accrual in the right-chiral set of partitions, which is the reason why psychiatry is unable to provide an explanation for the disorder, accustomed as it is to provide explanations based on mood swings, compensation and defense mechanisms, which represent a dynamic that involves transflows occurring between the two sets of chiral partitions on individual Layers of the Foliate.

The Kleptomaniac is strictly moved by the urge of being conflictive in causing disruption to order and rule of law. This is an expression of the Paradoxical Norm procuring the nature of the partitions making up Layer **7**. The paradoxical act of stealing is realized through the apprehension and anxiety states in the prior visualization of the act and joined to the salacious satisfaction procured by the act in breaking the social norms. Why theft? Theft just represents one way for the root apprehension or anxiety to materialize from representations embedded in the partitions themselves as a result of education and social interaction, just as the same root partitions would instead gear a subject to masochistic behavior based on embedded representations favoring this type of rapport.

Fetishism

The concept of a "fetish" evokes an adoration and obsessive fascination with physical objects or natural events. In this context, a "fetish" is an object with the power to elicit sexual arousal in an individual. *Fetishism* is in itself the behavior associated with sexual arousal to inanimate objects or body parts not traditionally viewed as sexual. Distress is generally a component of the nosology as well.

PASSIVE –RESPONSIVE SYMPTOMS

Patients are curious, sensitive and inquisitive about various forms of the fetish objects, as well as their texture and size, i.e. women's high heel shoes. Show no interest in genitalia or sexual characters of the opposite sex. They will hold, rub, smell and taste the fetish object itself. Most do not engage with a sexual partner or, if they do, prefer solitary sexual enjoyment with their fetish, if not asking the partner to wear the fetish during sex. The fetish object makes them feel safe sexually. Fetishists so display a serious level of superficiality in experiencing their sexuality through impersonal objects or non-genital body parts.

ACTIVE-REACTIVE SYMPTOMS

Patients collect inanimate objects and/or focus on body parts for sexual arousal and gratification. Often collect the images of these objects as well. They typically collect shoes, undergarments, lingerie, stockings and focus on thighs, breasts, hands, nape of the neck, feet, etc.

KNOWN VARIANTS

Form fetish and Media fetish. In Form fetish, it is the form of the object that is relevant, i.e. high heels. In Media fetish, it is the material from which the object is made which takes significance, i.e. leather or silk (undergarments).

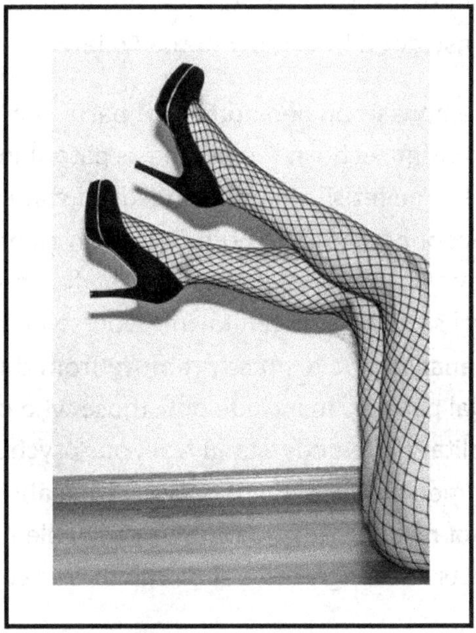

LANGUAGE

Live with their fetish as a "heavy secret". Refer to natural sexual intercourse as "sexual action" being stranger to them.

BEHAVIORAL FLIPS

Unknown/Unreported

DERIVED DISABILITIES

Social and occupational impairment.

AWARENESS

Conscious (Neurotic Disorder)

CHARACTEROLOGICAL FILIATION

Realistic

QG LAYER-PARTITIONS

2[(-4, -3, -2, -1), (+1, +2, + 3, + 4)**]**

STATISTICS

Fetishism is more prevalent in men (almost 3% of the general population) than in women (0.4%).

INSIGHTS

The Quanto-Geometric Binarity norm that informs normal Layer **2** is instrumental in bringing best unequivocal understanding of the etiology of Fetishism. The Fetishistic slant is the tone given by the Binary Layer to sexual activity in the psychosexual context. As such, it is distinct from most other paraphilia, which are instigated by Layer 7 of the Foliate.

The emphasis on perceptivity of particular objects of Reality, including their reverberating echo in the psyche, is patent in the disease as its most crucial character. The fetishist notably needs to stare at or insistently imagine the fetish object or body part in order to obtain an erection and sexual gratification. Furthermore and very significantly, the fetishist person may never engage in an actual sexual act of genital intercourse in the entire course of life as reported. In this analysis, we expressly remove from this group patients who engage with a sexual partner, to include only those who obtain sexual arousal from their fetish in solitary. We understand from our psychophysics that they are so much overwhelmed by the perception and visual absorption of the fetish object that they do not need a sexual partner for sensible human sexual interaction. The fetish objects knowingly bring their minds to a certain level of fixation.

While some level of fetishism is normal in human sexuality, it becomes a qualified dysfunction when it is the only way to achieve sexual gratification while inducing personal distress and negatively affecting other areas of functioning.

The fact that the disorder expressly affects women brings support to our psychophysics perspective in that it is an overaccrual of the left chiral partitions that is responsible for the onset of the disease. The additional fact that in males it creates female-gender-orientated behavior further supports the view that an exacerbation in the perception of objects of Reality is responsible for the disease. Effectively, in many of its variants such as fixation on female legs, high heels, stockings, tape of the neck, breasts, gloves, intimate lingerie, etc., fetishism disorder shows male identification with female gender and behavior.

Another orthodox psychoanalytic hypothesis seeks to put emphasis on such fetish as legs, fingers or gloves bearing a morphological connotation as a substitute penis represented by the fetishist acting on himself. It is unclear whether such fetish hypothetically recalls the horror of castration since apparently they bring reassurance to the subject. If they did in any ways, they would nevertheless put the subject in the role of a female, which rejoins the turn of our interpretation. In all, the clearest analytic interpretation of the disease remains along the line of exacerbated perceptivity of objects of Reality, per thought partitions pertaining to Layer 2 of the Foliate, with an overboard influence on sexual behavior.

Lastly, it is worth stating that the former breakup of fetishism into a so-called *partialism* disease, *"involving sexual arousal by a body part, such as feet, breasts, or buttocks"* had little merits due to the culturally driven connotation associated with these anatomic parts in the normal sociocultural context. That subtype had been justifiably deprecated.

PATHOLOGICAL AFFILIATES

Transvestic Fetishism: Having established that the disease of Fetishism is to be attributed to individuals who do not engage in any form of shared sexual interaction, preferring to remain solitary in sexual enjoyment through their fetish, we are driven to reconsider the category and nomenclature assigned to Transvestic Fetishism.

With that exclusivity criterion being defined, we find that Transvestic Fetishism cannot be affiliated to the main disease of Fetishism, since Transvestic Fetishist patients do engage with partners for sexual enjoyment, to whom they would ask wearing the fetish for their own arousal. Hence the Fetishism label in the name Transvestic Fetishism becomes unwarranted or inappropriate. Again, it is worth insisting, in support of this deprecation, that within the framework of our phsychophysics, the restriction of Fetishism to strictly solitary sexual arousal through the fetish is consistent with the **paroxysmal level of perceptiveness as the cause of the disease**, since in this case the patient would demonstrate lack of the need for sensible human interaction (or Foliate-to-Foliate cisgender pairing as defined for love) for sexual arousal but the strict view of a non genital object.

Voyeuristic Disorder: A morbid behavior involving the act of secretly observing an unsuspecting naked person, whether in the process of disrobing or engaging in sexual activity. Most normal men given the opportunity to observe a woman undressing herself would not avert their eyes. To be morbid, the "peeping" must be recurrent and the urges intense or recurrent. Oftentimes, voyeurs are socially and sexually underdeveloped, thereby accusing a level of *superficiality* in their psychosexual development. They tend to engage in sexual activity later than other groups, and are reportedly less likely to marry than experimental controls and other sex offenders as well (Smith, 1976). There is evidence suggesting that voyeurs may be equally predisposed to other paraphilias (e.g., sadomasochism, zoophilia) (Langevin et al., 1985). They often come from a childhood with good relationship with both parents but with the parents in open discord. Their peeping seems thereby a reaction to parental conflicts and a result of the anxious need to confirm good empathy and harmony between the parents as evidenced in intercourse.

Be that as it may, the only reason why children with that sort of a background would orchestrate a reaction this kind to conflicts between parents, is a predisposed terrain, with a Mental Layer 2 in high paroxysm, per temperament proneness, akin to Fetishism.

Cotard's Syndrome

Cotard's Syndrome, also called *Délire des Négations*, is a mental disorder in which the individual commonly experiences nihilistic delusions concerning the body and reality in general, in terms of their inexistence, as well as delusions of immortality and hypochondrial delusions alike.

PASSIVE –RESPONSIVE SYMPTOMS

Patients believe they are deceased or that they don't exist at all, or that they cannot breathe at all any longer, that their heartbeats have stopped, that they have no more blood in their veins, no more bowels, etc. Might see their body and other people's body become miniscule, same for animals and objects in the environment. Often refuse to eat or keep up personal hygiene. Feel internal organs rotting and being destroyed. The syndrome associates frightful inner anxiety, visual hallucinations and extreme stupor. Self-accusation and even self-mutilation and suicide may ensue.

ACTIVE-REACTIVE SYMPTOMS

A particular patient may pretend that he has been suffering for more than 6000 years, or has 300 worms in his stomach. One may speak of his esophaguses (plural) and his bladders (plural) being fretted by hundreds of worms. They have a grandiose or exaggerated view of their bodies, which they see with twinning, bigger and a higher number of organs than the natural single ones. Some pretend that their belly has been opened up to remove loads of diamonds. Another believes his eyes no longer exist but that he had several pairs in his coffers, which were in fact stars in the sky as he affirms. Delusions of immortality are frequent.

KNOWN VARIANTS

Body Integrity Identity Disorder (BIID). Depersonalization/Derealization Disorder.

LANGUAGE

Very paradoxical nihilistic verbiage about the inexistence or surrealism of their body parts and the natural world.

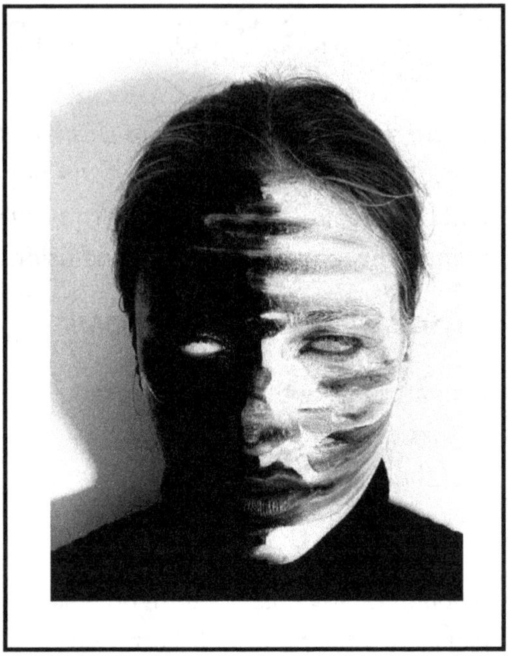

BEHAVIORAL FLIPS

Cotard had identified two clear states in this disorder: a depressive state of delirium (ideas of negations and suicide) and an expansive state (state with a grandiosity wrap on the negation ideas). There is a switching or transitioning according to Cotard between the *depressive* delirium and the *exaggerating* delirium states.

DERIVED DISABILITIES

Inability to maintain proper hygiene, affecting social life. Affected by incurability, they do not seek treatment.

AWARENESS

Unconscious (Psychotic disorder)

CHARACTEROLOGICAL FILIATION

Paradoxical

STATISTICS

Rare disorder with quite unknown distribution in the population. One study suggested about 1% affected. No difference between men and women.

QG LAYER-PARTITIONS

7[(-4, -3, -2, -1) (+1, +2, + 3, + 4)]

INSIGHTS

We assign the etiology of this Disorder to the Mental Foliate's set of partitions pertaining to Layer 7, per the paradoxical norm subsuming them. The nosology of the Disorder is well reflected in the generalized mentation of negation, anxiety and dystopic motivation that subsumes these partitions. The string of negative and self-destructive thoughts explicit in the symptoms is well represented in the negative wing of the suite of partitions on Layer 7. Self-resentment, self-repugnance and neglect infused by partitions **7(+2)** and **7(+3)** orchestrate the main impulses from the right side of the distribution. They are also responsible for fueling the exaggerating state of delirium, much of it through inner projective and compensative mentation within the representational sublayers.

The grandiosity or exaggerating tone of the ideas that make up the state of exaggerating delirium in the nosology must be understood as outright dystopic motivational representations, perhaps with an added compensatory or projective tone. That the subject believes he has no eyes, that he has several pairs in a box, and that they are in fact stars in the sky is a way to disown his two natural eyes, remove them from his body and to chaotically deconstruct and reconstruct the natural world out there with stars that are dystopically human eyes.

The dystopic tones of mentation in the state of exaggerated delirium should not be confused with the hyperbolic tone in root thoughts associated with paranoia, as one might incline to assess. Furthermore, the dystopic representations in Cotard's Syndrome are not delusions as characterized in the current definition of the disorder but hallucinations in their own right.

Perfectionism

A neurotic *Perfectionist* is somebody obsessed with giving an appearance of perfection to others. Perfectionists do not rely on own judgement for the assessment of thoroughness in accomplishments but remain wary of others' favorable opinion in sanctioning their actions. They need other people's approval to feel safe. Asking questions whose answers the person has no real interest in but only to otherwise show personal cleverness, perfectionists are prone to show condescension and to grant themselves inflated self-importance.

PASSIVE –RESPONSIVE SYMPTOMS

Harbor doubts about oneself, self-worth, thereby translating a low self-esteem; doubts about ability to perform and fear of failure. Self-underestimation that leads to setting extremely high standards about personal performance. Failure to deliver on the promise, at times because of procrastination, reinforces the sentiments of doubts about performance capabilities. Own negative thinking tends to lead the individual to mistakenly feel unsuccessful. Inept "all-or-nothing" thinking leading them to believe achievements are either total or inexistent.

ACTIVE-REACTIVE SYMPTOMS

Busy building a façade of personal qualities for constant display to others in the social environment as a way to put forth their putative moral, intellectual and affective superiority. Fond of giving treats to others even when the means to do so clearly falter. Will give away tickets to events at their own expense without even being able to afford one for themselves after the fact. Want to know that others are aware of their largesse and generosity and will slip in conversations the help given to others because they are influential, generous, etc. They constantly seek other people's acknowledgment of their qualities.

KNOWN VARIANTS

Inferiority complex – *Impostor Syndrome* are disorders of the same class - Neurosis of Failure.

LANGUAGE

Very paradoxical nihilistic verbiage about the inexistence or surrealism of their body parts and the natural world.

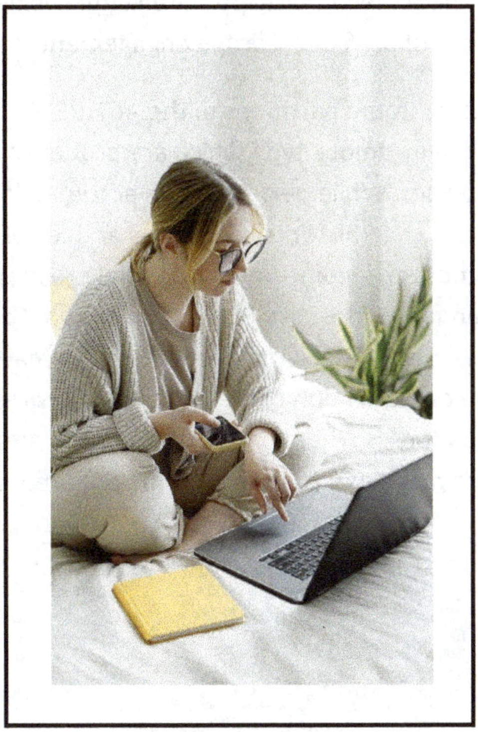

BEHAVIORAL FLIPS

No known swings.

DERIVED DISABILITIES

In professional life, may be slow to produce results due to delays in overperfecting the works.

AWARENESS

Unconscious (Psychotic).

CHARACTEROLOGICAL FILIATION

Intellectual.

QG LAYER-PARTITIONS

3[(-4, -3, -2, -1), (+1, +2, + 3, + 4)]

STATISTICS

Unknown. No consensus on criteria for Perfectionism to be considered maladaptive behavior.

INSIGHTS

We assign the etiology of this Disorder to the Mental Foliate's set of partitions on Layer 3, per the associativity norm subsuming them. The nosology of the Disorder in terms of the report for *PASSIVE-RESPONSIVE* Behavior is well reflected in the set of partitions represented in Doubt, Aberration, Idiocy and Disorientation. They reflect the undercurrent of maladaptation and disability in the analytic paralysis experienced by the Perfectionist. On the other hand, it is clearly the root thoughts of Discernment, Perspicacity, Clairvoyance and Lucidity that animate the impulses for intellectual achievement and overachievement in terms of *perfection-prone* engagement.

It is the same partitions in the *ACTIVE-REACTIVE* set that will fuel achievements of the ingenious type which are proper to the human spirits socially qualified as geniuses. While perfectionism accounts for achievements of many highly accomplished historical figures, examples of extreme, or perhaps abnormal, perfectionism leading important thinkers to withhold their works in an untimely manner i.e. do exist. Such is the case of Carl Friedrich Gauss, who is estimated to have been otherwise able to advance mathematics by 50 years. The embedding and orchestration of life experience representations within the root thought partitions is what is going to make the difference between an authentic genius, with no maladaptation, and the talented hard-work perfectionist.

Psychogenic Stuttering

In general, *Stuttering (a.k.a Stammering)* is characterized by repetition of sounds, syllables and words, prolonging a word or sound, blocking of speech and difficulty with articulation. It may be associated with facial tics, eye blinks, facial flushing, perspiration and eye movements. Psychogenic Stuttering is a category of speech disturbance that most commonly manifest as disturbance in fluency and voluntary control over any component of speech production. Generally, the onset of psychogenic stuttering is sudden and temporarily related to an impacting event.

PASSIVE –RESPONSIVE SYMPTOMS

Speech blocking, increased speech hesitancy. Sentiments of despair and self-pity. Difficulty to articulate words, phrases and sentences. States of despair and sadness will cause facial flushing, blushing and eye blinks. Intentional silences during the act of speaking to control the oncome of speech.

ACTIVE-REACTIVE SYMPTOMS

Lack of fluency, repetition of syllables, words, sounds, prolonging words or sounds, introjecting interjections or sounds of the patient's own make up. Facial tics, eye movements, increased perspiration, lip tremors and head jerks. Fist clenching may also occur.

KNOWN VARIANTS

Developmental and Neurogenic Stuttering.

LANGUAGE

Problems with language constitute principal nosological elements of the disorder as described above for symptoms manifestation.

BEHAVIORAL FLIPS

Symptoms of stuttering largely vary throughout a person's day. Swings are constant between the efector elements of the behavior and the affector elements.

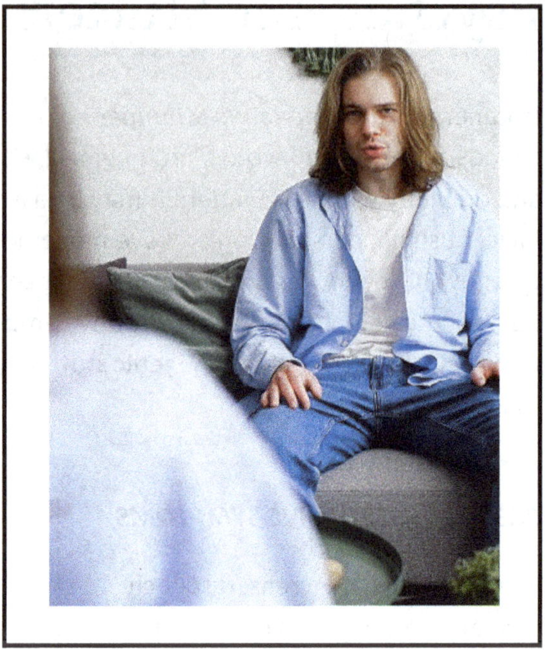

DERIVED DISABILITIES

Patients can lose confidence in social situations due to feeling scrutinized or their patience being put to test. Affects personal relationship and career advancement.

AWARENESS

Conscious (Neurotic Disorder)

CHARACTEROLOGICAL FILIATION

Matrixial

QG LAYER-PARTITIONS

6 [(-4, -3, -2, -1) (+1, +2, +3, +4)]

STATISTICS

1% of the general population, 8% of people experience the onset of stuttering during their lifetime; it is twice more common in boys.

INSIGHTS

Psychogenic Stuttering is generally viewed as a comorbid component of mental dysfunctions. However, in the QG framework of interpretation, the main disorders associated with stuttering are rooted on Layer 6 of the Mental Foliate.

In particular, depressive disorders that come as a result of emotional marital breakdown are principally rooted in the *PASSIVE-RESPONSIVE* partitions pertaining to Layer 6 (Despair, Sadness, etc). Likewise, it is possible to note the close relationship that exists between stuttering as a disturbance in verbiage with the notable alterations occurring in language in Bipolar Disorder, a dysfunction rooted on Layer 6. Bipolar patients are driven to a very notable repetitive mode in speech severally expressed as: clang associations, rhymes and puns, echolalia and word salads. They are also prone to neologisms. Note that stuttering has little or much less to do with inner linguistic structures themselves as it does with locution. In that regard, note that stuttering is almost never accompanied with writing impairments.

The above clearly explains why stuttering knowingly disappears while singing. It so occurs because stuttering appears as a precursor to the act of singing as all of the elements of stuttering are fairly orchestrated in the fine art of singing in different dimensions. This element of artful repetitiveness (or re-producing) is intimately inherent to the partitions of the *ACTIVE-REACTIVE* chiral set of Layer 6. Stutterers can therefore become very talented in fine arts, in particular the art of acting. Let's listen to famous actor Bruce Willis: *"I could hardly talk. It took me three minutes to complete a sentence. It was crushing for anyone who wanted to express themselves, who wanted to be heard and couldn't. It was frightening. Yet, when I became another character, in a play, I lost the stutter. It was phenomenal."*

Approval Compulsion

Approval Compulsion is the compulsive need by a character of personal knowledgement from the social environment. It is traditionally viewed as a fense mechanism against pervasive self-doubt manifested through feelings of unworthiness, weakness and insignificance. Brain imaging has evidenced tion of pleasure in the brain when people get positive feedback concerning their character or reputation. However, the constant or excessive urge for self-approval from others in this disorder bears a morbid character in need of treatment.

PASSIVE –RESPONSIVE SYMPTOMS

These individuals frequently change their minds to prevent being questioned or losing others' acceptance. Compulsion to justify everything and anything they do in offering excessive justifying explanations. They may be innerved or angered by any disagreement coming from other people in their circle. Alternatively, they hide any possible disagreement or discomfort of their own when something of their dislike occurs. Some publish on line an excess of personal photos looking for "likes" of approbation or praise.

ACTIVE-REACTIVE SYMPTOMS

Immediate approval by the subject of the words pronounced by the person of the moment he or she is interacting with, with his own mimics and stereotypes. At times the subject repeats in an echoing manner the words of his/her interlocutor, oftentimes a superior, even to the point of repeating or mimicking the mannerisms of the latter. Behaviour is frequently agitated, with sudden bursts of words.

KNOWN VARIANTS

Perfectionism -- Impostor Syndrome.

LANGUAGE

Mimics and stereotypical words or phrases. Language focuses on seeking praise, approval, flattery in a compulsive manner. The language repeats and mimicks others.

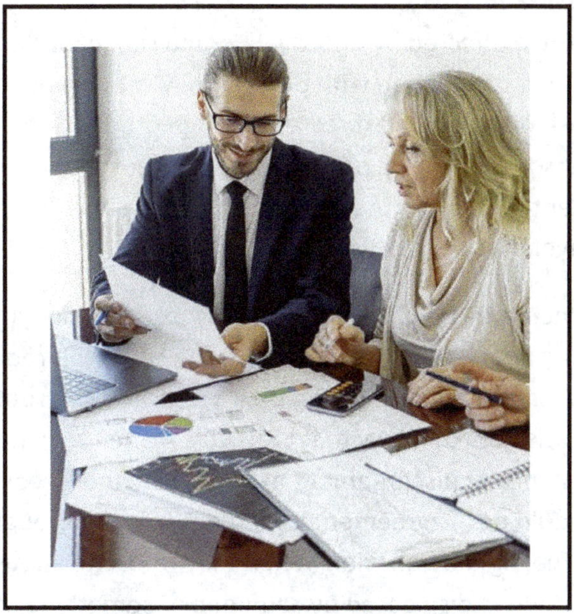

BEHAVIORAL FLIPS

Swings between, on one hand, compulsion to justify anything they do and search for praise and, on the other hand, the offering of their own approbation to the point of mimicking their interlocutor's mannerisms.

DERIVED DISABILITIES

Shallow interpersonal relationships.

AWARENESS

Conscious (Neurotic Disorder)

CHARACTEROLOGICAL FILIATION

Intellectual

QG LAYER-PARTITIONS

3 [(1, 2, 3, 4)], (+1, +2, +3, +4)],

STATISTICS

As part of Obsessive-Compulsive Disorder, its prevalence is 1% of the population on that account.

INSIGHTS

People affected by Approval Compulsion experience strong feelings of association or connection with others. They feel the need for a bijective connection with other peers expressed through other's approval of their actions and their personality, which puts them at the center of a web of connections. This form of mentation and behavior perfectly obeys the Associative norm at the heart of Layer 3 of the Mental Foliate.

When they tend to give too many explanations to justify what they do or opine, they are expressing uncertainty fueled by the root thought of Doubt. When they constantly keep changing their views, it is the root thought of Confusion or the clumsiness of Idiocy that is at work. When they lose their temper at every single instance of disagreement expressed by their peers, as if everyone in the world should be in agreement with them, it is the thought partition of Aberration that is fueling the behavior. When they refuse to show the least amount of discomfort when displeased by someone or something, it is also the partition of Aberration that is at work.

Seen in cognitive psychology as a member of the group of disorders associated with Compulsive-Obsessive Disorders, in QG Mentation analysis, Approval Compulsion represents a dysfunction in its own right, very closely associated with Perfectionism, Impostor Syndrome and Inferiority Complex. The designated group of Compulsive-Obsessive Disorders is not, in QG Mentation analysis, legitimate, since, as we shall see, each of the members develops a dysfunction rooted on a specific Layer that is not always Layer 6, the principal Layer instigating obsessions or mania. Consequently, Approval Compulsion is not per se a risk factor or a so-called defense mechanism.

Neglect Syndrome

Neglect Syndrome, also called *Hemispatial Neglect, Unilateral Neglect, Hemi-inattention, or Hemineglect* is a serious and disabling consequence of brain strokes. It can be defined as a defective ability to explore or attend to stimuli presented on the side contralateral to the brain lesion. This inattention towards one side of space is, by definition, not caused by visual impairments (visual field defects). It usually results from damage to the right parietal area which leads to inattention to the left side of the space. In left parietal lesions, attention is typically maintained on both sides by the right parietal area. This disorder is strictly of neurologic nature. We are listing it here only due to its peculiarity in relation to the chiral architecture of the meta-level structure of human Mentation which subsumes the human brain's biological organization.

PASSIVE –RESPONSIVE SYMPTOMS

Neglect Syndrome is usually associated with other neurological symptoms, i.e. hemiplegia, anosognosia, impaired working memory and reduced attention. Patients fail to be aware of one side of their body, may deny ownership of the limbs on the affected side (somatoparaphrenia). They can ignore one-half of all objects, have failure to recall auditory information on the affected side after distraction (anterograde variant), or unable to recall the contralateral half of a previously known scene (retrograde variant).

ACTIVE-REACTIVE SYMPTOMS

Neglect is hardly ever an isolated syndrome and may involve, in addition to visual, auditory and somatosensory perceptions, proper kinetic symptoms where patients exploration of the environment is biased towards the ipsilateral side. Initiation of motor behavior fails in the contralateral side of the body, they miss half of the space (anosognosia). Some patients will not use the limbs in the counterlesionial side of the body in a behavior known as motor neglect. They can shave half of their face, only eating half of their food on their plate, walking into walls, ignore people on their left, or fail to dress their left side.

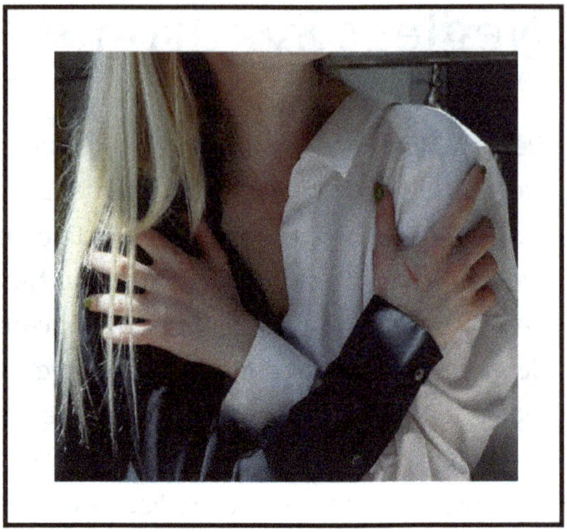

KNOWN VARIANTS

Somatoparaphrenia, Neglect of the extrapersonal space, Representational neglect (anterograde and retrograde), Motor (Intentional neglect). Also tightly related to BIID and Cotard's Syndrome, per associated nosology. Frontotemporal Dementia is a neurological par to this illness.

LANGUAGE

Evolves around unawareness of the deficits. Patient may omit words when reading text on the one side of the page, or misread one side of individual words (neglect dyslexia).

BEHAVIORAL FLIPS

*"Interestingly, an individual patient's degree of neglect can fluctuate strikingly, even within the same day. This depends upon factors such as overall arousal, which is known to be affected by right hemisphere stroke. In addition, although many people show neglect on more than one type of task, some groups of patients show **dissociations**, demonstrating a **lateralised bias** on only one test and normal performance on others; even these characteristics may vary over time."* – See Commented Bibliography.

DERIVED DISABILITIES

Allochiria and *Constructional Apraxia.*

AWARENESS

Absence of conscious awareness (Psychotic).

CHARACTEROLOGICAL FILIATION

Paradoxical

QG LAYER-PARTITIONS

7[(-4, -3, -2, -1), (+1, +2, + 3, + 4)]: Pertains entirely to the full Foliate contained in each of the dual Mental Body. The accrual occurs asymmetrically in one Foliate.

STATISTICS

In USA, the incidence rate for unilateral spatial neglect following a stroke is over 80% in right-sided stroke patients. Right-sided unilateral neglect resulting from left hemisphere damage was found at least to some degree in 43.5% of stroke patients.

INSIGHTS

In this dysfunction, patients experience unawareness of their specific deficits. They remain unaware of the neglect or extinction their cognition and behavior exhibit as much as they are unaware of occurring hemiplegia. They submit to a delusional belief relating to the contralesional limbs or side of the body, such that they do not believe that the limb/side belongs to them. This artifact tightly relates Neglect Syndrome disorder to Cotard's Syndrome and Body Integrity Identity Disorder, all of which are fueled by accrual of the roots thoughts pertaining to Layer 7 of the Mental Foliate. This rapprochement must not obscure the fact that the Mental Foliate does not belong to the biological brain, each being harnessed by a physical metric of a different nature through which they entertain a correspondence and superposition relationship. This rapprochement in fact solidifies that hypothesis, because there is no known brain lesion basis to Cotard's syndrome and BIID.

Inferiority Complex

Inferiority Complex is an abnormal or pathological mental state which leads the individual to self depreciation and undervaluation, to become unduly sensitive, and to be too eager for praise and flattery as well as prone to adopt a derogatory attitude toward others. These feelings of inadequacy affect the individual's activities of daily living. They may ultimately cause social integration failure and maladjustment. The maladjustment will be due to drawing unrealistic views of oneself, self-depreciation and hypersensitivity to rejection. The feelings of inferiority in the Inferiority Complex are postulated to be as conscious as they may be subconscious and afflicted individuals have the tendency to overcompensate for them. Alfred Adler coined the term in 1920.

PASSIVE – RESPONSIVE SYMPTOMS

Feelings of inferiority or insecurity. Discomforting feelings of impotence and fear of incapacities of one kind or another. Inability to adjust to these feelings due to lack of recognition of one's natural or circumstantial limitations. Low self-esteem and frequent avoidant behavior. Underlying feelings of pain due to these inadequacies.

ACTIVE-REACTIVE SYMPTOMS

Conscious sublimation of feelings of impotence and inadequacy into a constant stance of superiority, excessive pride, exaggerated aggressiveness, pathological mistrust, overly boosted self-confidence, despising others, need to humiliate others, etc. Experience urge to be always right, to outclass and command others, to always be the first, to constantly find faults in others

while finding it difficult to admit own mistakes.

KNOWN VARIANTS

Social anxiety disorder, Dependent Personality Disorder, Perfectionism.

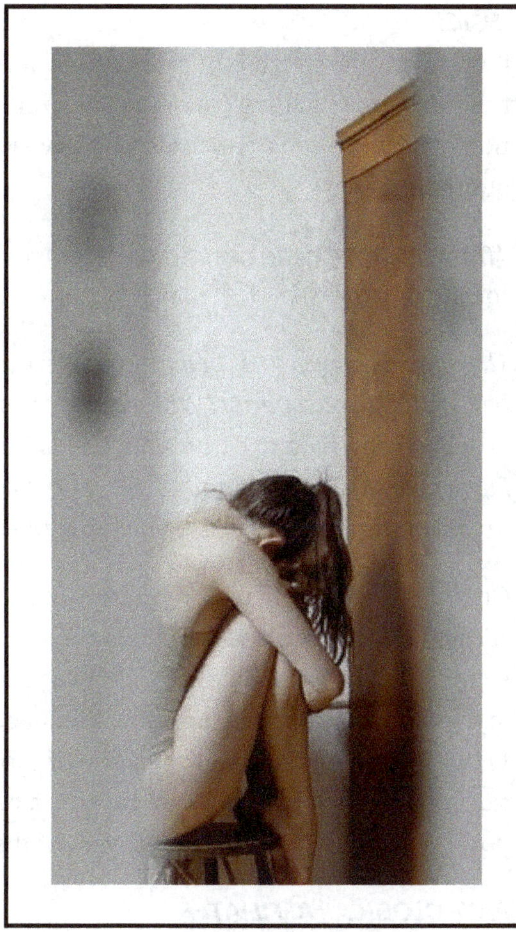

LANGUAGE

Evolves around themes of self-depreciation, vacillations and needing reassurance.

BEHAVIORAL FLIPS

Compensation swings between discomforting feelings of inadequacy and impotence on one side and, on the other side, sublimated feelings of pride, superiority and urges to be always right, etc. They either feel inferior or believe they are superior, going from one to the other.

DERIVED DISABILITIES

Failure to socially adapt and to integrate to professional working teams, not accepting advice, displaying a spirit of contradiction and opposition, demanding submission and imposing stances of superiority.

AWARENESS

Conscious awareness (Neurotic Disorder)

CHARACTEROLOGICAL FILIATION

Intellectual

QG LAYER-PARTITIONS

3[(-4, -3, -2, -1), (+1, +2, + 3, + 4)]

STATISTICS

4.2% in young population.

INSIGHTS

It is important to highlight expressions of the right chiral partitions of Layer **3** in this disorder which are generally analyzed in terms of unconscious compensation mechanisms in analytic psychology, at least partially. A psychologist is quoted to say:

"They experience the need to teach others, to direct and lead, they feel the need to counsel others...

They do not conceive of being "equal" to anyone. They either feel inferior or they believe they are superior. When a "compensating" neurotic patient feels inferior, he will do anything to astonish peers, to be admired for his knowledge, his intelligence, his elevated thoughts, his regards and courtesy towards others, his human warmth, etc... They are obviously thirsty of prestige."

One can see here the direct reflection of the partitions of *Discernment, Perspicacity, Clairvoyance* and *Lucidity,* which the subject thinks he/she is displaying at every moment and every occasion in attitude and opinions. Whether he does so in reaction to strong feelings of inadequacy and inferiority or not, the personality build up on an overintensification of the mental fits germane to that chiral side of the distribution on that Layer is a perfectly conscious act, which has nothing to do with the deeper Layers of the Unconscious.

PATHOLOGICAL AFFILIATES

Intellectual Disability

Intellectual Disability, formerly known as *Mental Retardation*, is characterized by impairment of Intellectual capabilities in relation to an individual's ability to learn, reason, make decisions and solve problems, on the one hand, and on the other, adaptive capabilities, acknowledged to be the skills necessary for day-to-day life, i.e. self care, effective personal communication, and spatial interaction with others.

PASSIVE - RESPONSIVE SYMPTOMS

Lack of curiosity, trouble understanding social rules, difficulty with logical thinking as manifest in deficient problem-solving. Difficulties learning academic skills. Do not understand how to pay for things bought. Trouble regulating emotions and behavior. Immaturity in social interactions compared with peers, with support needed in nearly all daily living tasks.

ACTIVE - REACTIVE SYMPTOMS

In the developmental stage, failure to timely meet intellectual developmental markers, i.e. slow to sit up, crawl, or walk compared to most other children, slow in learning to talk compared to the average children, or show trouble speaking and remembering things. Limited spoken language. Delayed in mastery of practical skills such as feeding oneself, dressing up and the exercise of toilet hygiene. Explosive tantrums possibly resulting from self-realization of these inequities or blockage caused by the same.

KNOWN VARIANTS

Variants have been categorized according to severity level as: Mild, Moderate, Severe and Profound. Down Syndrome is another notable variant with organic (chromosomal) causes instead of psychogenic.

QG LAYER-PARTITIONS

3[(-4, -3, -2, -1), (+1, +2, + 3, + 4)**]**

STATISTICS

Intellectual disability affects about 1 percent of the population, and prevalence for severe intellectual disability is approximately 6 per 1,000 people, according to the DSM-5 report.

INSIGHTS

It is important to stress that deviations in normal adaptive behaviors depend on the severity of the condition. In general, mild intellectual disability is typically associated with academic difficulties and a somewhat inappropriate concrete approach to solving problems. Severe intellectual disability typically results in limited communication and the need for support in nearly all activities of daily living.

It is no less important to stress that any form of interference with normal brain development may knowingly cause *Intellectual Disability* or *Mental Retardation*. Notably, other physiological diseases and physiological accidents or injuries may be causal factors. What's more, among the known causes of Intellectual Disability, physiological accidents or pathological agents play an eminent role. In two-thirds of cases of *Intellectual Disability*, the causal factors are completely unknown, however.

Mental science commonly believes that people affected with *Intellectual Disability* have co-occurring mental, neurodevelopmental, medical, and physical conditions. When a genetic condition has caused the disability, the individual may also exhibit the characteristic physical features of that condition known as *Down Syndrome*. The pensive condition that is always responsible for the disease in its psychological aspect is spurred by the Left-Chiral palette of the partitions on Layer **3**. Note that the symptoms slated to be of an *ACTIVE-REACTIVE* nature are for the most part lexically rendered as failures or lacks instead of straightforward intent or positive motivation. What this means is that they are in fact a result of an over accretion of the opposite pensive partitions. When the pensive partitions of *Aberration, Doubt, Idiocy* or *Disorientation* are constantly spurring the production of thoughts, there are few occasions left for intelligent coordination, insightful intellection, and positive calls to retrieve memories alike, in order to sustain agile learning and skillful coordination. Flips to the Right-Chiral partitions of Layer **3**, which would relieve the situation, do not occur for many different reasons, leaving the individual in the postration of idiocy and disorientation. This also means that, in the psychogenic cases of the Disorder, there is indeed no lack of cleverness per se in the sufferer's mind, contrary to what the frequent IQ diagnostic tests might suggest. At this effect, it is important to realize that sufferers are not oblivious to their inabilities, they are in fact well aware of their inabilities from observation and reflection stimulated by their Right-Chiral intellection faculties. They do have access to the comprehension of these intellection inequities. And that stands for the very reason why they experience these well known tantrums and anger at themselves for these inequities, as well as the proness to suicide duly registered in that population.

Lastly, we will strongly caution against the common association of Intellectual Disability with Autism Disorder. Although the kind of cognitive impairment present in Autism Disorder may have a few remote similarities with Mental Retardation Syndrome in their expression, they originate from two very different pensive normals of the Foliate. It will be at the end very difficult to assimilate the high intellectual exaltation visible in Autism or Schizophrenia in their high fly symbolic artistry with the typical idiocy and disorientation proper to Intellectual Disability, and only pay attention to the notable mental impenetrability in Autism or Schizophrenia that equally results in deficient learning by sufferers. The alleged comorbidity between the two disorders simply does not exist.

Specific Learning Disorder

Specific Learning Disorder (or Learning Disability) affects a significant number of school children in any of the three learning areas: (1) reading, (2) writing and (3) math. At times learning disabilities can affect an individual's understanding of what they read or their understanding of spoken language. There is conventionally frequent association of these disorders and their variants with *Attention-Deficit Hyperactivity Disorder (ADHD)*, albeit unjustifiably so from our psychophysics vantage.

PASSIVE - RESPONSIVE SYMPTOMS

Persistent difficulties in reading as well as arithmetic and mathematical reasoning. Inaccurate, slow or effortful reading. Difficulties remembering number facts.

ACTIVE - REACTIVE SYMPTOMS

Persistent difficulties with writing. Inaccurate, slow or effortful writing. Poor written expression or elaboration that lacks clarity.

KNOWN VARIANTS

Reading Disorder is a variant that is also referred to as *Dyslexia*. *Dyscalculia* is another variant that is a persistent Disorder concerning math understanding. *Dysgraphia* affects a person's ability for handwriting as a fine motor skill.

LANGUAGE

Spoken language is not fluent and written language is characterized by inability to decode words and impaired reading comprehension.

BEHAVIORAL FLIPS

Bolstering self-esteem in overcompensation for the learning deficit; challenging rebellious behavior in reaction to stress caused by stigma.

DERIVED DISABILITIES

Many more subjects of study are affected by the inability to understand written text and calculate. Overall decreased academic achievement and inability to achieve full potential. Negative impact on social and interpersonal relationships.

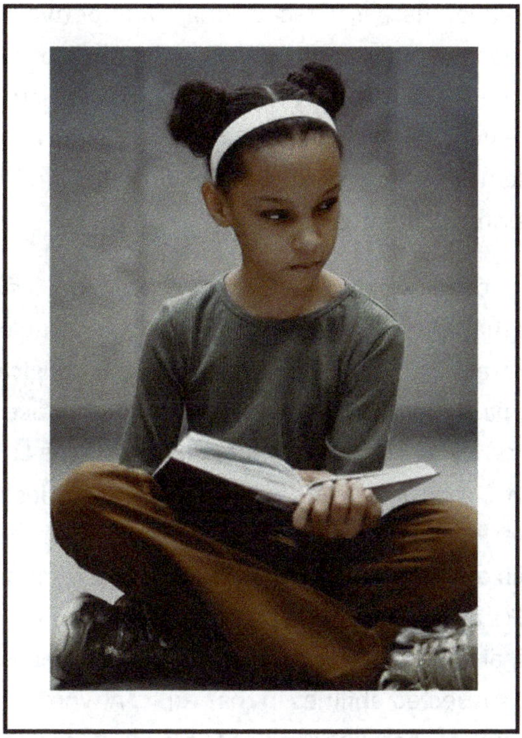

AWARENESS

Conscious (Neurotic Disorder)

CHARACTEROLOGICAL FILIATION

Associative Character

QG LAYER-PARTITIONS

3[(-4, -3, -2, -1)]

INSIGHTS

There are reportedly many myths concerning Learning Disability Disorder. One of them is that smart students cannot accuse this type of Disorder. The pushback against this myth from seasoned professionals in the Learning field is that *"Specific learning disabilities and IQ are not connected, and that many individuals who struggle with reading, writing, or math are bright and successful students."* This assessment rejoins our view that IQ tests does not bear out the important fact that in *Intellectual Disability*, a member of the same family of Disorders, positive intelligent intellection remains unaffected. It is simply masked by the flood of negatively oriented intellection arising fom the pensive primitives at the Left-Chiral side of Layer **3**, which steals the show so to speak. The example of Albert Einstein who was admittedly a poor student positively argues in that direction. IQ tests do not contemplate and evaluate the circumstances in which the Right-Chiral side of the Intellection Layer in affected Minds becomes expressive. It is important to realize that idiocy and brightness belongs to the same mentation normal (or Layer). So therefore, from our psychophysics perspective, there is in fact a connection between the faculties evidenced by IQ measurements and the associative skills of reading, writing and computing. It is not however a direct relationship or assessment because there are structural elements within the mentation framework and internalized psychosocial elements (within the representation sublayers) that such tests ignore in their assessment of intelligence.

Our conclusion is that a *Specific Learning Disability* is not necessarily a Disorder of the psychiatric order, but only at the outset an impairment at the educational or training level resulting from a psychological conflict or problem. The specific impairment may be caused by social practice or taboo, or parenting or educators' influence, majorly internalized at the Left-Chiral side of the impaired Foliate. A father having had himself difficulties with mathematical logic may expressly drive his children in the belief that they too will suffer the impairment and as a result they so become conditioned to fail in that subject. It will only take a diminution or subtraction from his constant debilitating influence in that regard, perhaps in favor of life circumstances, for them to start showing their unsuspected abilities in that topic. A woman, under the influence of social customs emphasizing the unfitness of women for mathematical logic, computation and engineering, may find herself in an unidentified psychological blockage to proficiently use a computer or its broad and deep resources beyond web browsing imagery, or to engage a career in those fields. It is worth making the special mention here about how mathematicians and professionals of the core sciences like physical science have decisively managed to obscure those sciences to the rest of humans all over the globe in their expressions and dissemination, for the benefit of personal pride and ascendency and, historically, for securing a win in the competition to serve Royalty. In these circumstances, most human beings under all latitudes find themselves challenged in those sciences and present with a sure learning disability.

It is also clear that an oppressive climate from parents, educators and a sociopolitical environment will block self-expression and in the making thwart personal positive intellection as well.

In conclusion, *Specific Learning Disability* qualifies only as a circumstantial impairment, no matter how long it perdures. The Left-Chiral Layer 3 paroxysm, which is responsible for the observed symptoms, does not necessarily rise to Level 3 which qualifies a neurosis, as much as it does in the close parent disorder of *Intellectual Disability*.

Guilt Syndrome

Guilt is the feeling resulting from a wrongdoing of the moral order. It is also useful to distinguish guilt, which stems from judgmental self-evaluation of a wrongful behavior with a sanction, from shame, a related emotion stirred by a sentiment of moral wrongdoing alike but in a lesser degree. The feelings of Guilt (and shame as well) are considered self-conscious and moral emotions since they play a crucial role in materializing and guiding moral behavior, the internalized moral norms being socially defined. *Guilt Syndrome* is an emotional complex whereby the individual's mind remains orbiting around those acute feelings of underestimation of self. It should also be well understood that the sentiment of Remorse is duly part of this emotional complex, being the extreme end of this class of mental fits.

PASSIVE –RESPONSIVE SYMPTOMS

Feelings of regret, tension after a regretful behavior such as being deceptive to others. Feelings of insecurity and low self-esteem evidenced in often feeling down on oneself. Tendency to give up easily or start out any effort with the attitude of being already defeated. Feeling frequent need to withdraw in social situations.

ACTIVE-REACTIVE SYMPTOMS

Fear that anybody and everybody is out there persecuting them. Rooted in burst of presumption, the feeling is that "No, I am not untrustworthy, the other person is the one who is the double-dealing snake." Negatively judging self and own behavior with no justifiable reason, a behavior that qualifies as judgementalism.

KNOWN VARIANTS

Survivor's Guilt, Guilty Father syndrome, Mommy Guilt Syndrome, Layoff Survivor's Syndrome, Guilty Vacation Syndrome.

LANGUAGE

Language is expressive of culpa or mea culpa, excessive apologizing, making up for the perceived wrongdoing in practice.

BEHAVIORAL FLIPS

It is well known ever since Shakespeare that guilt entails paranoid behavior (persecution). Effectively, he wrote: "Suspicion always haunts the guilty mind; the thief doth fear each bush an officer." Clear swings between paranoid suspicion and sentiments of guilt.

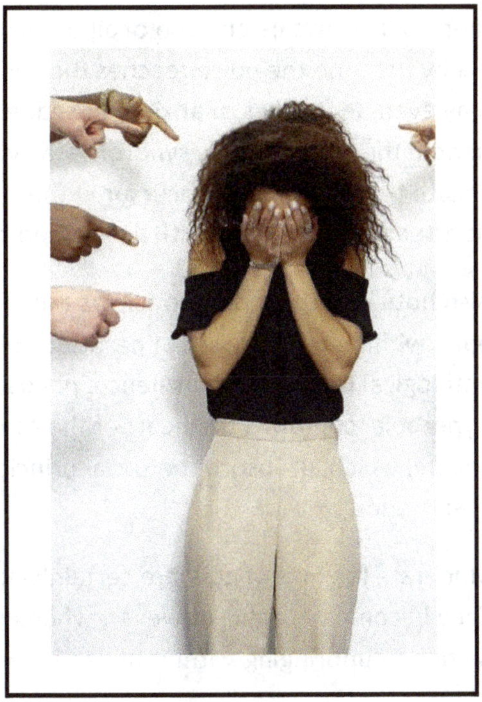

DERIVED DISABILITIES

Inability to reach one's goals and feeling "stuck" as they oftentimes effectively are.

AWARENESS

Conscious self-awareness (Neurotic Disorder).

CHARACTEROLOGICAL FILIATION

Hyperbolic

QG LAYER-PARTITIONS

4 [(-4, -3, -2, -1), (+1, +2, +3, +4)]

STATISTICS

18.5-22.2% prevalence

INSIGHTS

It is often assessed in analytic psychology that lying, cheating or stealing are common examples of acts that may elicit feelings of guilt, towards advancing an etiology for Guilt Syndrome. It bears repeating vehemently here that not because these feelings are present in the nosology of the syndrome they are actually part of its etiology. Worth reminding how the orthoflows develop across the channels cutting through the diverse mental layers. Because the travel impulse crosses partitions on the same channel represented in the orthoflow, there will always be an echo of all the partitions encompassed within the channel by the time the pulse reaches the conscious hypocursor. So therefore, there may even be feelings of anxiety or sadness consciously experienced by the patient in the throes of this syndrome. Nevertheless, the main Layer of the Mental Foliate that fuels the hypocursor in this illness, which requires special therapeutic attention, is Layer **4**, with its accrued partitions in the circumstance.

Also note that the moral principles are of social provenance and become imbued within the entire set of partitions of Layer **4**. The Quanto-Geometric primal ontological Norm of Ambivalence, philosophically equivalent to Manicheic Hyperbola, conforms the heart of the root partitions at Layer **4** of the Mental Foliate, which all absorb the social principles of good v. bad that regulate group coexistence.

Moderate feelings of guilt are certainly adaptive for normal social functioning. They become neurotic, however, when unduly accrued as a result of social interaction or upbringing within the family setting.

Grief Reaction

Grief (Sadness) is the emotional process of coping with a loss or a moral pain experienced as a loss. The process involves many different emotions, actions, and expressions, all of which help a person come to terms with the loss. Such a loss may be in the realization of a loved one's passing or the breakup of an intense enamoring relationship. The intense commotion that follows the loss of a mate as a result of an unexpected breakup has many of the same expressions that accompany the mourning for the loss of a loved one in death. While this reaction is normal, the grief that lingers on and does not diminish in intensity over time, however, is of a morbid nature. The subject is viewed to be unable to "get over" his/her sadness and despair.

PASSIVE –RESPONSIVE SYMPTOMS	***ACTIVE-REACTIVE SYMPTOMS***
Silence or constant reflective mood. Weakening of facial traits, i.e. a shattering of all facial commisurae. A detectable weakening of all vegetative functions. Withdrawal and frequent absence of emotional expression are ostensible. Abundant and persistent tearing, frequent sobbing and sighing. Sudden intense emotions of painful loss fueled by remembrances. Often painful feelings of being abandoned. Ritualistic verbal responses or exclamations. May go as far as to wear an article of the deceased's clothing.	None

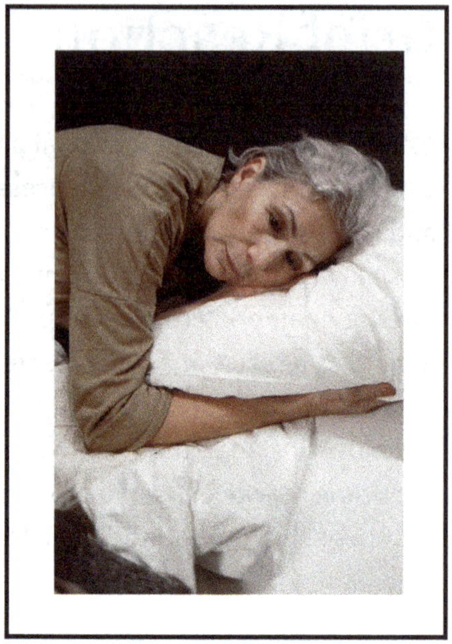

KNOWN VARIANTS
Verbal, Non verbal. Complicated Grief, Prolonged or Unresoldve Grief.

LANGUAGE
Sighing and sobbing. Sudden exclamations or verbal rituals.

BEHAVIORAL FLIPS
No applicable flip because the nosology and etiology of the illness are concentrated on the left-chiral side of the affected Layer of the Mental Foliate.

DERIVED DISABILITIES
Lack of socialization, depression, leading to suicidal thoughts/attempts.

AWARENESS
Conscious awareness (Neurotic Disorder).

CHARACTEROLOGICAL FILIATION
Matrixial

QG LAYER-PARTITIONS
6 [(-4,-3,-2,-1)]

STATISTICS
Unknown but 10% have *Complicated Grief*.

INSIGHTS
The following is to add to the nosology of this Disorder as seen in the so-called *Complicated* or *Unresolved* Grief:

- Continued disbelief in or inability to accept the separation.
- Continued preoccupation with the loved one and the manner of the separation.

- Intense sorrow and emotional pain, sometimes including bitterness or anger.
- Unable to enjoy good memories about the loved one.
- Blaming oneself for the death or separation.
- Wishing to die to be with a deceased loved one with possible suicidal attempts in both the cases of breakup of a passionate relation and passing of a loved one.
- Excessively avoiding reminders of their loss.
- Continuous yearning and longing for the loved one (feeling part of themselves died with the deceased love one).
- Trouble pursuing interests or planning for the future after the separation or feeling that life is meaningless or empty without the loved one.

Clearly the left-chiral side of Layer **6** of the Mental Foliate is responsible for this Disorder in all its forms as the associated thought partitions manifestly represent the mentation engine fueling the symptoms.

Split Personality Disorder

Split Personality Disorder also known as *Multiple Personality Disorder* or *Dissociative Identity Disorder (DID)* is a chronic psychopathological condition which typically manifests after trauma or childhood sexual abuse. It includes disruption in the patient's memory and identity. Patients with DID show different identities and do not remember the event or the other alter egos after coming back to thier original identity. In other words, each personality has its very own life train. DID is also characterized by unexplained loss of personal information from one's memory.

PASSIVE –RESPONSIVE SYMPTOMS

Blurred sense of identity. Feeling detached from self and one's emotions. Perception of people and things around self as distorted and unreal. Sense of detachment expressed as sensation of being outside of oneself and observing one's own actions, feelings and thoughts and the very self from a distance, as though watching a movie. World may feel unreal. Commonly amnesia and blackout: memory loss of certain time periods, events, people and personal information. There is marked discontinuity in sense of self and sense of agency.

ACTIVE-REACTIVE SYMPTOMS

Individual may feel two or more people talking and living inside himself/herself as though possessed by other entities. Identities are discrepant and opposite, each with own name, being well-ingrained with own personal history, behavioral patterns including different voices, gender, mannerisms and even physical/biological qualities such as need for eye glasses. The transition from one personality to another is often sudden and brought about by stress. Notably, sleepwalking and automatic writing.

KNOWN VARIANTS

Depersonalization – Derealization Disorder. Also Sleepwalking Disorder and Conversion or Somatoform Disorder.

LANGUAGE

Patient can speak a different foreign language during *alter* states, language is consistent with each personality and is suggestive of amnestic information. The person refers to himself or herself as "we".

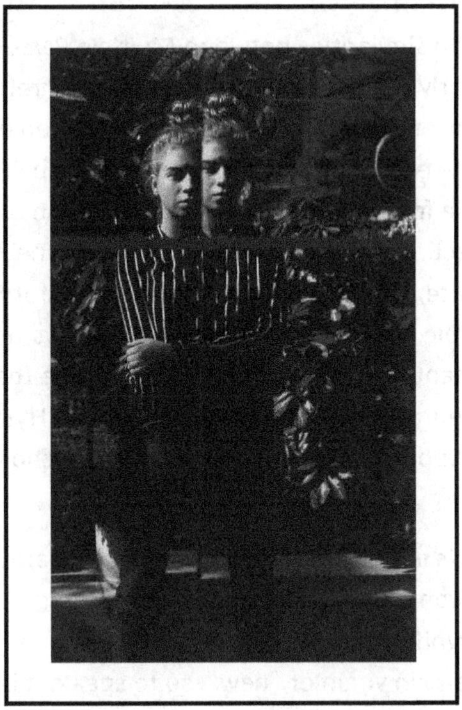

BEHAVIORAL FLIPS

In many cases, flips between sleep-walking in a second state at nightly hours and typical daytime neurotic alter expression.

DERIVED DISABILITIES

Substance abuse. Severe distress and impairment in functioning, the disturbance not being part of normal cultural or religious practices. Problems with sexual adjustment; uncontrollable increased sexual behavior; prostitution.

AWARENESS

Conscious (Each identity is fully aware of self – Neurotic Disorder).

CHARACTEROLOGICAL FILIATION

Metamorphogenic

QG LAYER-PARTITIONS

5 [(-4, -3, -2, -1) (+1, +2, + 3, +4)]

STATISTICS

The estimated DID prevalence around the globe is about 5% among the inpatient psychiatric population, 2%–3% among outpatients, and 1% in the general population.

INSIGHTS

The similarities between *Multiple Personality Disorder* and *Hysteria* had caught early on J. M. Charcot's attention as reflected in his choice of name for the disease: *Hystero-epilepsy.* Babinsky, then enlisted in Charcot's instruction, noticed the exacerbation of suggestive capabilities in the disease which were responsible for the bewildering multiplication of alter personalities in the impaired subject. Indeed the fragmentation engine constituted in Layer **5** of the Mental Foliate, whose norm is Disorder, Transformation or Alter-ation, is majorly responsible for the very modality of this Dysfunction. We have discussed this assignment in *Hysteria* and it is easy to see that *Multiple Personality Disorder* is one neurotic version of the psychosis of Hysteria, both of which have not stopped flabbergasting neurologists and psychologists since the 1800's.

It is important to note that in the characterological version of this Disorder, the Utopian (or Metamorphogenic) Character, newness and its pursuit represent a significant expression which, on the sexual plane, compels these characters to remain virgin or "new", so to speak. It is no surprise that knowingly a traumatic impact, at early age or not, on the sexual life of these subjects, in terms of violating their virgin intimacy as they feel, bears the potential to impair them beyond repair and cause a severe fragmentation or *alter-ization* of their personality. Once the damage has occurred, it can accordingly throw them into dehumanizing compulsive sexual behavior up to the extreme of prostitution, this sort of personality representing the very *alter* to their *pure* primal self-representation.

PATHOLOGICAL AFFILIATES

Dissociative Amnesia

Dissociative Amnesia is a dissociative disorder usually induced by trauma or severe stress whereby the individual suffers memory loss affecting an entire lifestyle. The subject of amnesia can be a specific event or the person's very own identity or personal history.

PASSIVE - RESPONSIVE SYMPTOMS

Feeling confused. Unconscious blockage of a specific trauma or inability to recall autobiographical information, i.e. not recalling family members, friends, coworkers or former plans shared with others.

ACTIVE - REACTIVE SYMPTOMS

May engage into establishing a new identity by relocation.

INSIGHTS

We consider *Dissociative Amnesia* a direct affiliate disease to *Split Personality Disorder*. In many cases a trauma, which the psyche perceives as a highly unexpected and unusual event, triggers the Disorder. It becomes orchestrated by a Foliate's Layer **5** likely already in accretion as the syndrome observed in *Dissociative Amnesia* expressing a personality fragmentation, with *alter(s)* to the *pure* primal self-identity. The severity in the accretion of Layer **5**'s partitions conditions the strength and plurality of the personality split.

Compulsive Gambling Disorder

Pathological Gambling is defined as a pattern of repeated gambling and preoccupation with gambling (per DSM – 1980). Some psychiatrists have proposed to treat this disorder according to the disease model, akin to alcoholism, whereby gambling is viewed as a disease or sickness of the mind. Behaviorists, on the other hand, see pathological gambling as a learned, conditioned response. Due to the reinforcement of intermittently winning one or two jackpots, between losing a few, the gambler is putatively motivated to keep playing until the positive reinforcement is given again (Pavlov's theory). Various research studies have shown that this reinforcement in intermittent schedules is extremely difficult to reduce or stop.

PASSIVE –RESPONSIVE SYMPTOMS

Loss of interest in normal activities. Downplay gambling losses, majority of the time is spent and centered on the few wins. Self-pity, desperation, guilt and shame when losing. Empty promises, not fulfilling commitments, chasing own losses. Not assuming responsibility for losses and deceiving others, inveterate lies to minimize the relevance of financial losses.

ACTIVE-REACTIVE SYMPTOMS

Hightened interest in gambling activities such as gambling odds, hearing about new games to be played, new locations of casinos or lottery stations. While winning, emotional excitement is common. Grandiose thoughts and fantasies (i.e. in false superiority), accompanied with inability to sleep when losing or winning.

KNOWN VARIANTS

Professional, Antisocial, Casual, Serious Social, Relief and Escape, Conservative, and Compulsive Gamblers.

LANGUAGE

Tangential speech (frequently and repeatedly changing conversational topics to others that are hardly related). Pressured speech (rapid, excessive, and frenzied speaking).

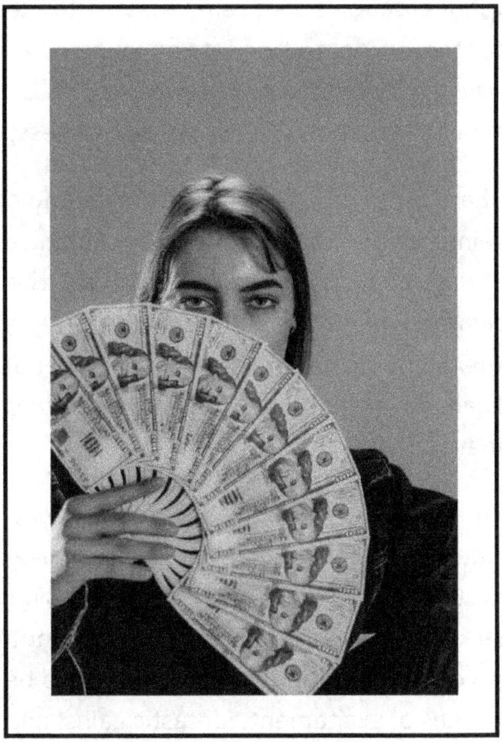

BEHAVIORAL FLIPS

Reported mood swings (See commented Bibliography).

DERIVED DISABILITIES

Associating with shabby characters. Financial difficulties leading to financial ruin. Personal problems possibly deriving from a life of crimes, depression and despair which may lead to suicide.

AWARENESS

Conscious (Neurotic Disorder)

CHARACTEROLOGICAL FILIATION

Utopian

QG LAYER-PARTITIONS

5 [(-4, -3, -2, -1), (+1, +2, + 3, +4)]

STATISTICS

2-3% of the US population suffers from this disorder.

INSIGHTS

The most important driver of this Disorder is the urge for newness and surprise, due to an accrual of the root thoughts germane to Layer 5 of the Mental Foliate. The norm that subsumes this layer is that of Change or Metamorphosis. The Visionary mind fit is the one feeding the grandiose fantasies of riches or big wins and superiority. The Utopic mind fit keeps the individual subject to the thrill of winning huge sums of money. Whereas the inability to stop financial ruins with rationalization about self-behavior, the tendency to dishonor commitments, and for the subject to turn into an inveterate liar (repeated lying to self and others), have everything to do in this case with Daydreamming, the illusion of hallucination and creation of fables (fabulousness).

There is not much to draw, from an etiological standpoint, from the putative reinforcement of intermittently winning one or two jackpots, between losing a few, by compulsive gamblers. It is not the intermittency that creates the positive reinforcement. It is ultimately the underlying mind state of thrill of winning, either chimeric or utopian in nature, that drives and motivates the gambler to keep playing until the spectacular winning transformation is eventually given, if it ever does.

The details about mood swings experienced in the illness are squint in the literature. Per reference in Commented Bibliography, they are de facto reported to occur, albeit in not sufficient details as might be desired. Notwithstanding this lack of details, one may argue that compulsive gambling requires a form of psychic dissociation driven to fluctuate between emotional and behavioral extremes of excitement, fantastic gains, and respectively disappointment or despair at the tune of major losses. Like in Delirium disorder, compulsive gambling represents a form of escapism from reality.

Phobia

Phobia is an intense, persistent and irrational fear directed to anything as a subject. It is usually specific to an object, situation, activity or a person. The fear is oftentimes proportionally greater than the actual danger posed or threat. People with specific phobias are also highly distressed about experiencing the fear itself, and will often go to great lengths to avoid the object or situation in question.

PASSIVE –RESPONSIVE SYMPTOMS

Feeling terrorized by or in intense fear of a perceived threat represented in the presence or proximity to an object, environment or situation, or by anticipation thereof (e.g., flying, heights, animals, receiving an injection, seeing blood). Except at times in children, the person recognizes that the fear is out of proportion to the actual threat posed. Avoids the phobic situation(s) or endures said situation(s) with intense anxiety or distress. Exposure to the feared item or situation almost always leads to an immediate anxiety response, which may take the form of a panic attack (dizziness, nausea, breathlessness, tachycardia). Crying or freezing reaction in children.

ACTIVE –REACTIVE SYMPTOMS

In children, the anxiety may provoke tantrums or clinging behavior. Avoidant behavior consisting in running away from the situations or threats are usually part of the behavior.

KNOWN VARIANTS

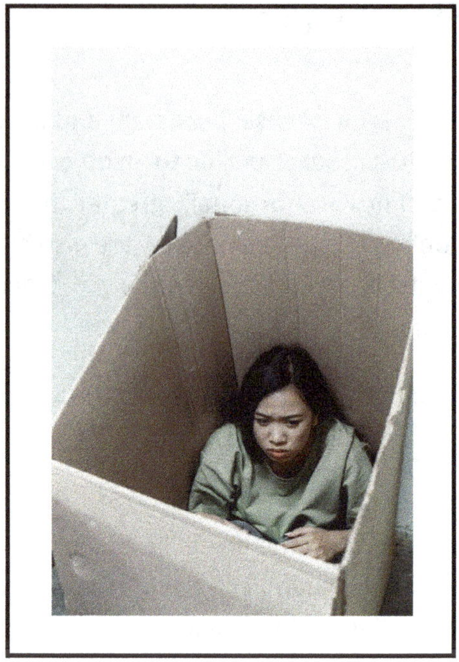

Natural environment: Astraphobia (fear of lightning), Hydrophobia (fear of water), Dendrophobia (fear of trees), Amatophobia (fear of dust), Keraunophobia (fear of thunder), Mysophobia (fear of dirt), Nyctophobia (fear of the dark), Pyrophobia (fear of fire). Hemophobia. Generalized Anxiety Disorder.

Animals: Batrachophobia (fear of reptiles), Cynophobia (fear of dogs), Equinophobia (fear of horses), Ailurophobia (fear of cats), Arachnophobia (fear of spiders), Microphobia (fear of germs), Ornitophobia (fear of birds), Pteronophobia (fear of feathers), Zoophobia (fear of animals), Ophidiophobia (fear of snakes).

Mutilation/Medical Treatment: Trypanophobia (fear of needles), Dentophobia (fear of dentist), Hematophobia (fear of blood), Emetophobia (fear of vomiting), Ereuthophobia (fear of blushing), Genophobia (fear of sex), Pathophobia (fear of disease), Pnigophobia (fear of choking).

Situations: Claustrophobia (fear of closed-in spaces), Agoraphobia (fear of open spaces), Aerophobia (fear of flying), Glossophobia (fear of speaking), Acrophobia (fear of heights), Agoraphobia (fear of public or open space), Claustrophobia (fear of closed space), Ochlophobia (fear of crowds), Triskaedekaphobia (fear of number 13), Xenophobia (fear of strangers), Xenoglossophobia (fear of foreign languages).

LANGUAGE

Language is characterized by increased speech rate, rhythm and volume, screaming during phobia situations. Sometimes, simpy hearing words that depict the specific phobia are sufficient to trigger the symptoms.

BEHAVIORAL FLIPS

From the fear and anxiety caused by a situation to uncontrolled outbursts of anger and frustration, typically in a young child.

DERIVED DISABILITIES

The avoidance, anxious anticipation, or distress during the feared situations interferes significantly with the person's normal routine, work or school functioning, or social activities or relationships, or there is marked distress about having the phobia. Depression can be associated with or derive from persistent phobias.

A teenager with a dog phobia avoids at all costs going to houses of friends and family who own dogs - A businessman with a fear of flying loses out on business opportunities because of his inability for fast travel - A woman with a needle phobia avoids getting blood work her primary care physician deemed necessary for her physical health - A young man with a fear of enclosed spaces takes the stairs each day to his office on the 11th floor to avoid taking the elevator until disabling fatigue sets in.

AWARENESS

Conscious (Neurotic disorder) – Unconscious when hallucinations settle in and the Disorder becomes psychotic.

CHARACTEROLOGICAL FILIATION

Paradoxical

QG LAYER-PARTITIONS

7 [(-4, -3, -2, -1), (+1, +2, + 3, +4)**]**

STATISTICS

The year-long community prevalence estimate for specific phobias is approximately 7%-9%.

INSIGHTS

The Quanto-Geometric norm of contradiction that informs normal Layer **7** duly motorizes this disorder which is centered on the expression of conflict and fear at the heart of the left-chiral set of partitions making up the Layer. In Claustrophobia, one can see the rapprochement with the fear of being locked up in a jail cell, the closed space, i.e. an elevator, being suggestive of a loss of personal freedom. In Agoraphobia, which duly pertains to this family of disorder, the fear of losing one's privacy or self- secrecy by projecting oneself into an open space is quite obvious. Although the right-chiral set of partitions may become active as well, as manifest in children when they take to tantrum, the onus remains on the left-chiral set.

It is important to not confuse this disorder with Social Anxiety Disorder, aka Timidity, and the diverse forms of obsessions or mania, a common analytic flaw. Though one may see a form of obsession in the repetitive or persistent expression of a fear, the nature of these mental fits are quite different, both emanating from different mentation roots. Same holds true for Social Anxiety Disorder, which is not an anxiety disorder at first order, but an ego-centric dysfunction. The presence of anxiety in the nosology of Social Anxiety Disorder is simply a result of secondary orthoflows, due to layer crossing, as the subject becomes keenly aware of the intimidating situation. The primary layer responsible for the morbit accrual imbalance must always remain the principal object of treatment and consideration.

PATHOLOGICAL AFFILIATES

Generalized Anxiety Disorder

Generalized Anxiety Disorder is characterized by a persistent excessive worry regarding a variety of events or activities (e.g., work or school performance) without any reasonable justification in terms of objective impact of events. People with Generalized Anxiety Disorder find it difficult to control their worry, perceive threats in events and situations where there is none. They are also indecisive, nervous and irritable.

Paranoia (Megalomania)

Paranoia or Megalomania is a peculiar thought process that causes one to have a persistent suspicion and mistrust of others. Paranoid individuals feel persecuted or that someone is out to get them. They may also perceive they are in danger while also feeling misunderstood or disbelieved. They have the cy to mentally and physically isolate themselves and may be unable to work with others, thus leading to dysfunctional interpersonal relationships. Paranoid thinking is for certain a common human characteristic, particularly in display in the sphere of sociopolitical regulation and organization. Lack of insight is common in both acute and chronic paranoid states.

PASSIVE –RESPONSIVE SYMPTOMS

Pervasive mistrust of others, a belief that harm will occur, an attribution that others intend to harm. Preoccupied with unjustified doubts about the loyalty of friends and associates. Reluctance to confide in others due to fear that the information will be used maliciously against them. Bear compulsive grudges which they may hold for a long time. Read hidden meanings in benign remarks.

ACTIVE-REACTIVE SYMPTOMS

Perceived persecutors are either unspecified or relatives, the police, neighbors, medical personnel, the government, etc. Paranoid delusions of conspiracy-driven thinking is self-focused. Estranged behavior, isolating from others, strained relationships. Virtuoso of absurd logic and reasoning. Prone to endless lies. Cleverly Insinuate situations where they play a prominent role, with factitious relationships with the famous. Refusal to submit to norms.

KNOWN VARIANTS

Religious, Erotic, Persecutory, Reformatory, Hypochondriacal, Litigious, Jealous paranoia, and Delusions of grandeur. Paranoid Personality Disorder.

LANGUAGE

With the paranoid, others constantly walk on egg-shells in language, since they tend to read hidden meanings leading to persecution in otherwise benign remarks. Language develops along the line of straight logic invoking absurd and factitious circumstances and situations.

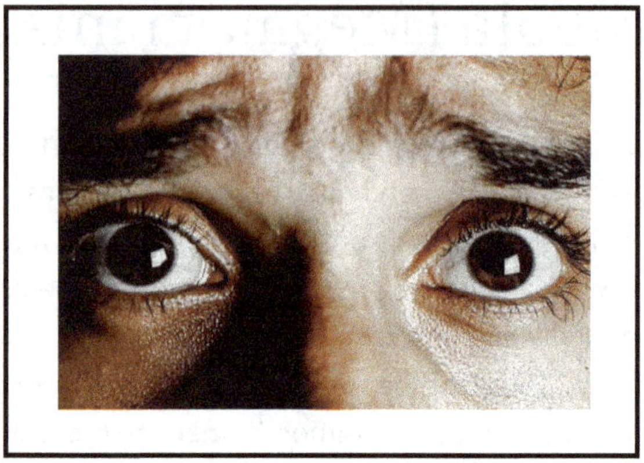

BEHAVIORAL FLIPS

Constantly flipping between sentiments of victimization causing i.e. isolating and barricading in own bedroom to avoid family members and sentiments of superiority and stoicism: *"he oftentimes believes that he is being persecuted because his remarkable intelligence and lucidity turn him into a dangerous person, reason why he is pushed aside."* In factitiously braving oneself against continuous perceived or imaginary threats, the mind is in constant chiral swing.

DERIVED DISABILITIES

Paranoia is associated with low social cohesion, stated of worry, sleep deprivation, substance use, victimization, abuse, trauma and certain cognitive biases. Its flares are common in other psychoses such as dementia and epilepsy as well as certain brain injuries.

AWARENESS

Semi-Conscious

CHARACTEROLOGICAL FILIATION

Hyperbolic

QG LAYER-PARTITIONS

4 [(-4, -3, -2, -1) (+1, +2, +3, +4)]

STATISTICS

Prevalence of *Paranoid Disorder* is 1%.

INSIGHTS

The paranoids' notable refusal to submit to social or family norms is due to their core belief that they are the embodiment of Norms themselves, and thus inaccessible to externally imposed principles or norms. It is a remarkable fact that those entrusted with the social mission to provide social norms of coexistence, that is to say politicians as law makers and executive enforcers, knowingly exhibit this famous behavior of being subject to relentless persecution on the part of other players in the conduct of their professional political activities. The other is always out there to get them and to counter their actions. The belief that paranoid attributions increase when, in experimental settings, participants interact with opponents, making the social context influential, holds as a tangential analytic view, since the core motives for this behavior are the root Mentation fits composing Layer 4 of the universal mental Foliate. Remorse, guilt, shame, indignity as well as presumption, audacity, stoicism, and heroism are manifestly the main ideation basis for the core symptoms exhibited in the illness as described.

Worth noting that paranoia knowingly emerges in adolescence and peaks during adulthood and late age.

Hypochondria (Illness Anxiety Disorder)

Hypochondria, renamed *Illness Anxiety Disorder,* is defined as a preoccupation with the fear of having a serious illness or being in danger of developing one, despite appropriate medical examination dismissing the fact or possibility. The most conspicuous feature of this disorder is seeking excessive reassurance from physicians, medical references, or self-inspection. Many patients, however, also fear they will receive upsetting information if evaluated and thus avoid consultations and remain preoccupied with physiologic events, believing they are physically ill. In certain cases, true malfunction of kidneys, constipation, genital and endocrine problems may be observed.

PASSIVE –RESPONSIVE SYMPTOMS

History of going indiscriminately to incessant medical checkups with fables about having certain specific pathological conditions. Obliviousness to doctor's reassurance of good health, with excessive and persistent doubt of well-being that only increases the presumed physical symptoms. Falsely assumes or imagines that hurt is harm. Continuous and irrational monitoring of symptoms. High level of anxiety, nervousness. Depression may follow.

ACTIVE-REACTIVE SYMPTOMS

Continuous unjustified urges to seek medical consultation. Daring presumption that good health is symptom free and that any symptom is equivalent to illness. Construe or visualize innocuous symptoms as syndromic health threats. Maintain a utopian vision about health care habits stipulating i.e. that "one should not never hesitate visiting the doctor on anything unusual or it will be too late." The preoccupation may be symptom based, with a focus on bodily functions (eg, heartbeat, sweating, peristalsis), minor physical abnormalities (eg, a small sore or an occasional cough), or vague and ambiguous physical sensations (eg, "tired heart," "aching veins"), all chimerically imagined by the subject.

KNOWN VARIANTS

None

LANGUAGE

It focuses on specific symptoms related to the patient's factitious unwellness. Common verbiage: *"Cancer runs in my family."-- "My father died when he was my age."—"I have a weak heart."*

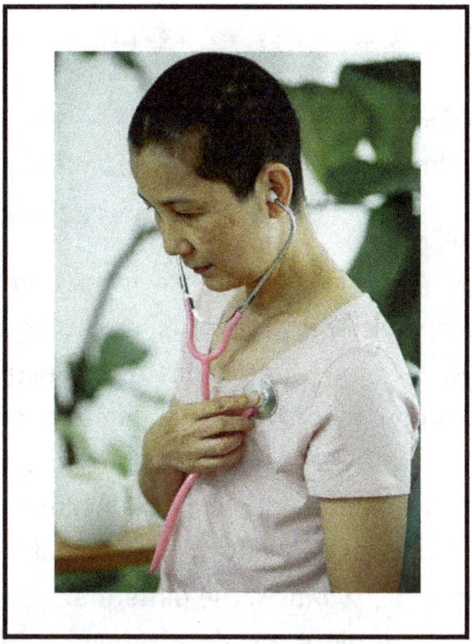

BEHAVIORAL FLIPS

The changing mood of Hypochondriacs, between what seems to be sadness and an ego-centric attitude is well known clinically. However these mind fits are co-morbid affect, the disease finding its most authentic swing expression in: Excessive, irrational fear and fabulation of organic disorders, on one side, and, on the other side, continuous intent monitoring of disorder symptoms with urges to continually seek medical consultation.

The *"doctor shopping"* behavior is a further product of the patient's distrust in the doctor's information as long as they do not correspond to his/her fables.

DERIVED DISABILITIES

In most patients, the unwellness conviction is functionally disabling and persists despite appropriate evaluation and reassurance of good health. In addition, patients have difficulty maintaining a job, performing daily activities, maintaining relationships.

AWARENESS

Conscious (neurotic) and Unconscious (psychotic)

CHARACTEROLOGICAL FILIATION

Utopian

QG LAYER-PARTITIONS

5 [(-4, -3, -2, -1)(+1, +2, +3, +4)]

STATISTICS

Lifetime prevalence rate estimates vary widely and range from 0.8% to 8.5%.

INSIGHTS

The driver of Hypochondria is the urge for biological alterations per the reformism and visionary mind fits, due to an accrual of the root thoughts pertaining to Layer **5** of the Mental Foliate. For instance, exposure to illness-related information in the media likely influences onset of severe illness anxiety disorder in these patients. The constant preoccupation with illness is identifiable as a representation in delirium, hallucination, fabulousness, and daydreaming making up the partitioning at the left side of the Foliate. When the disease reaches the level of a psychosis, the patient exhibits very clear episodes of hallucinations, and an absolute certainty of being affected by imaginary disorders.

Hypochondria can begin at any age, but most commonly occurs in early adulthood. Symptoms often arise during periods of increased stress but may be more directly triggered or influenced by recovery from a serious illness, diagnosis of an illness in a loved one, or the death of a close friend or relative.

Schizophrenia

Schizophrenia was initially designated "dementia precox" by Emil Kraepelin. Subsequently, Bleuler recognized that dementia was not a characteristic of "dementia precox" and suggested the term "schizophrenia" or splitting of the mind. Schizophrenia is a chronic disorder which typically manifests as withdrawals and a total loss of contact with reality (environment, persons and events), so reflecting a profoundly impaired cognition. Competing models for conceptualizing schizophrenia have ultimately concorded in that it meets the criteria for an authentic disease.

PASSIVE –RESPONSIVE SYMPTOMS

Subject appears mentally to be totally cuto ff from reality. Seems to live in a perpetual dream of his/her own. Indifference to others is total as the patient appears totally centered on self, hence the alternative nomer of *autism* for the disease. Various hallucinations of different senses (touch, smell, taste, vision) with the auditory ones being the most common. Somatic or religious delusions with a grandiose character. Manifest loss of motivation, social withdrawal and neglect, emotional blunting. Notable poverty of speech. May indefinitely keep the most uncomfortable positions that they are set to take. Frequent unexpected impulses or prolonged repetition of uncommon weird gestures. Often staring stuporously into space with total loss of reactions.

ACTIVE-REACTIVE SYMPTOMS

The hallucinative voices may speak directly to the patient, whether in the form of comments or received commands. They may criticize the patient's behavior or discuss among themselves the patient's condition. Agitation and yelling are common. Strange behavior of whispering or avoiding use of the telephone, television or computers. Grimaces, mimics, claps, rhythmic motion of a peculiar nature. The feeling that thoughts, actions and body are externally controlled leads to the specificities of the delusional behaviors (delusions of persecutions or control). Oncome of violent impulses are common as well. Thought disorder manifests as tangential and circumstantial, with illogical speech. Poor hygiene due to self-neglect.

KNOWN VARIANTS

Paranoid, Catatonic, Disorganized (Hebephrenic), Undifferentiated and Residual. Schizophreniform Disorder, Autism.

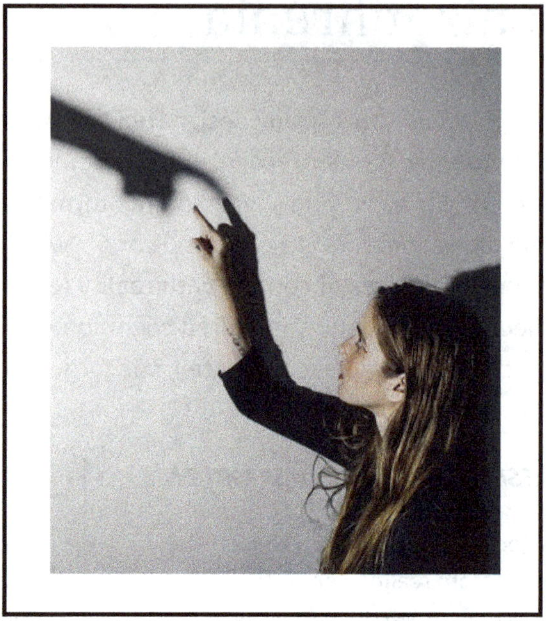

LANGUAGE

Language in Schizophrenia can be nonsensical, concrete with a literal flavor in some way, and unintelligible. Disorganized speech manifests as word salad, punning, perseverance, incoherence, echolalia (repetition of other's words). In terms of content, schizophreniac use fewer words, more objects per subject, fewer qualifiers per verb, more negative words. The syntax, diction, and words use give it a characteristic contour which is very unique to the disease. Example: *"A growing pattern had climbed on me".* The rate, rhythm and volume of speech are also affected.

BEHAVIORAL FLIPS

In catatonic schizophrenia patients maintain rigid postures for prolonged periods of time (i.e. mimicking others' movements), if not stereotypic repetitive movements such as nail biting and rocking, grimaces, posturing, etc. And then all of a sudden, he/she flips and bursts into a violent impulse that is in nature gratuitous, blind and absurd. For instance, he jumps on the clinician to strangle him or her. The most interesting flip in this disease of great relevance to our swing concern occur when certain patients go from withdrawal and stupor to an intellectual activity that discloses in symbolic artforms a highly elevated intellectual exaltation. They are able to deliver extraordinary artistic works when riding on this positive wing of the partition set of their thoughts distribution, on the concerned layer.

DERIVED DISABILITIES
Psychosocial disabilities affecting a range of faculties, behavior patterns and social bonding: emotional functioning, cognitive ability, energy and drive, psychomotor function, pain, relationships with others, employment, education, self-care, communication, domestic and leisure activities, quality of life, skills and vocations as well as treatment compliance.

AWARENESS
Mostly unconscious (Predominantly psychotic Disorder)

CHARACTEROLOGICAL FILIATION
Symbolic

QG LAYER-PARTITIONS

8 [(-4, -3, -2, -1) (+1, +2, +3, +4)]

STATISTICS
Prevalence of Schizophrenia worldwide is rated at just under 1%. There is variation of the disease within populations and risk factors such as season of birth, parental age, birth complications, infections, autoimmune diseases, cannabis use, ethnicity, and urban residence.

INSIGHTS
The Quanto-Geometric norm of Selflessness (Universalism - Perfection) that informs normal layer **8** of the Mental Foliate is the key to the analytic understanding of Schizophrenia. Patients with schizophrenia do not usually attain their full psychosocial potential within human societies as known. Canonical QG analysis may afford a better understanding of the nosology and etiology associated with the disease.

The consecrated view that the schizophrenic is cut off from reality is a misleading interpretation of what is truly happening in the disease and only caters to the behavioral appearance exhibited by the patient. The fact that the schizophrenic is not responsive to others does not make his/her psyche an *autistic* psyche in terms of an egocentric stir. In fact the patient's mind is wide open to reality in an utterly ostensible manner, well demonstrated in the inability to focus on single objects or individualities (loss of personal contacts) and the broad overture on symbolic expressions further possibly portrayed in artistic works. All attributable to the loss of the sense of self replaced by a sense of universalism which finds its full expression in the metaphoric or symbolic language.

It would be more proper to state that the patient is not only cut off from external reality as it appears but the internal sense of self seems to vanish as well, given the frequent state of stupor and the absence of self hygiene (attention to self) that equally characterize the disease.

The full set of thought partitions associated with Layer **8** offers the required grounds for the etiology of the disease.

PATHOLOGICAL AFFILIATES

Schizoid Personality Disorder
Schizotypal Personality Disorder

Schizoid Personality Disorder is characterized by avoidance of social presence and interaction with peers and other members of the social environment. Sufferers also show a limited range of emotional expression, appear to be dismissive of others and lack the desire or skill to form close personal relationships, including sexual relations. They may appear to lack humor and emotions altogether as they don't react to praise or criticism.

One can easily see here the specter of Autism and avoid confusing the isolation behavior with that which is expressed in *Social Anxiety Disorder* in particular.

The aforedescribed traits for Schizoid Personality Disorder are even more pronounced in *Schizotypal Personality Disorder*, which adds to the prevalent autism trait of the disease unsual beliefs and maneurisms whereby the individual senses presence of absent people, dresses in peculiar unmatching clothes, pronounces odd vagueries and rambling during conversations. These departures and others are clear neurotic harbingers of full-fledged Schizophrenia.

Exhibitionistic Disorder

Exhibitionistic Disorder is the paraphilia in which a person experiences recurrent and intense sexual fantasies, sexual urges or behaviors, all involving the exposure of genitals to an unsuspecting and non-consenting stranger. It is accompanied with significant distress or impairment in social, occupational and/or other important areas of psychological behavior. Very broadly, flashing one's totally nude body or partially nude body parts (exposing one's genitals: breasts, penis, or vagina) in a public place is considered exhibitionistic morbidity.

PASSIVE –RESPONSIVE SYMPTOMS

Motivation for self-harm by affected females demonstrated in the nervous thrill of being reported for indecent exposure.

ACTIVE-REACTIVE SYMPTOMS

Experience sexual urges resulting in distress. Online dissemination of nude photographs involving one's genitals to anyone. Or under the influence of alcohol intoxication. Sexual fantasies, and behaviors involving exhibiting one's genitals to unsuspecting individuals or animals. Executing on sexual impulses for a non consenting person. Excessive masturbation and preoccupation with sex and chasing non consenting victims.

KNOWN VARIANTS

- Seek sexual arousal by exposing genitals to pre-pubertal children.
- Seek sexual arousal by exposing genitals to physically mature individuals
- Seek sexual arousal by exposing genitals to both prepubertal children <u>and</u> to physically mature individuals.

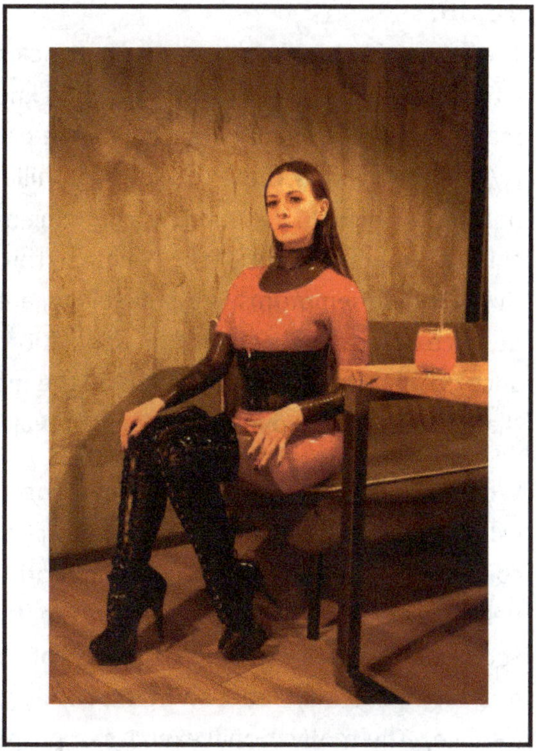

This Disorder belongs to the same family of Sadistic morbidity.

LANGUAGE
Language may exhibit anxious prosody and specific sexual verbiage to produce shock. Most expressions in Exhibitionistic Disorder are nonverbal.

BEHAVIORAL FLIPS
Unknown

DERIVED DISABILITIES
Possibly an unrelenting obsession with sexual intercourse or activity, and hypersexuality (having extremely frequent or suddenly increased sexual urges or sexual activity). Pedophilic sexual tendencies. Those sorts of disabilities deriving from the impairment of Exhibitionism as a consequence have only been hypothesized and not systematically proven. Forensic implications are real however.

AWARENESS
Conscious (Neurotic Disorder)

CHARACTEROLOGICAL FILIATION
Paradoxical

QG LAYER-PARTITIONS
7[(+1, +2, +3, +4)]

STATISTICS
Much less common in females; in males has a prevalence of 2-4%.

INSIGHTS

The onset of Exhibitionistic disorder typically occurs sometime in late adolescence or early adulthood and knowingly prevails largely among the male population. In accordance with the principle of a gender identity/expression crisis at the root of paraphilic disorders, we stipulate an exacerbating paroxysm in the dynamics defining male gender taking place at the right-chiral or Animus Sector of the Foliate in this case. Given the exacerbation of Active-Reactive symptoms in the nosology, and given that this very chiral preponderance defines male gender (in opposition to passive-responsive preponderance defining female gender), it is all the more congruent and understandable that this disorder is overwhelmingly prevalent in males.

When it comes to females, we must recognize that the repetitive and aggressive exhibition of breasts and vagina to attract or compel a male to sexual intercourse represents an Active-Reactive motivational behavior emanating from the right-chiral side of the Mentation Foliate. It suggests an accrual of the Animus Sector of the Foliate which, in the case of a female, can most plausibly occur as a result of disparity between Mental Body gender (male) and biological gender (female). The motivational exercise of purposeful sexual attraction is of course part of natural female sexuality. However, the analyst is in good stead to inquest and invoke gender determination disparity when the motivation becomes morbidly paroxysmal.

For this qualification, the woman exhibitionist must preferably give other signs of non sexual male behavior, such as the desire of being in control of peers, males in particular, in daily living. Even the explicit desire to be in control of males through sexual exhibition is a valid confirmation. Such an admission would elicit the competitive drive that is natural to male gender.

In all cases, whether patient is male or female, when the intention of instigating fear or disgust, causing an aggravation of any kind is part of the exhibitionism, even when the patient is secretly hoping of being reported or somehow castigated for the exhibitionistic behavior, the intervention of the Layer 7's palette of mentation partitions is clearly there fueling the disorder as well.

The Quanto-Geometric norm of Paradox or Antagonism that informs normal Layer **7** of the Foliate is key to the etiological comprehension of the second nosologic stream of Exhibitionistic disorder. In particular, the right-chiral side partitions of the Layer prevalently protagonize those symptoms as they become overly or morbidly paroxysmal (beyond level 2).

Exhibitionists are inarguably motivated by the impulse to create a **shock** to their chosen victims, to use their sexual attributes (genitalia in particular) as a means to unleash shocking appearance or portrait of self to the target person. In the case of males, the shock consists in the threat of causing harm with their penis as a sort of heuristic sword. As they perceive their victims' shocked response to their outrageous behavior, sexual arousal ensues or obtains enhancement. Therefore, by showing up his naked body and penis, the exhibitionist exerts a threat of aggravation in forced sexual penetration in order to elicit terror or shock from their victims. As a paraphilic disorder, exhibitionistic behavior, per DSM-5, must otherwise cause or involve personal harm or risk of harm to others to qualify as such. The latter condition is clearly given in exhibitionism in the agency of psychological shock towards experiencing sexual satisfaction.

PATHOLOGICAL AFFILIATES

Frotteuristic Disorder

Frotteuristic Disorder pertains to the same strain of disorders as Exhibitionistic Disorder and is characterized by the presence of recurrent and intense sexual arousal from touching or rubbing against a non-consenting person, generally a woman in a crowded area, as manifested by fantasies, urges or behaviors.

ACTIVE-REACTIVE SYMPTOMS

The frotteur usually touches, rubs against or gropes the victim’s breasts, legs, buttocks or genitals or else rubs his own pelvic area or erect penis against the victim’s body, generally from behind.

The frotteur is active in public places and crowded areas such as subways, buses, elevators or dance halls which can protect his anonymity.

"Evidence indicates that the courtship disorders [such as Frotteurism] are associated with a preference for eliciting an alarmed reaction from an unfamiliar target."[27] Here again, the frotteur manifestly attempts to scandalize the victim in order to obtain sexual gratification or enhancement thereof. They know full well that touching intimate parts of a stranger will scandalize the person because everyone protects their intimate parts and nobody summarily engages in intimacy with someone they don't know or feel stranger to. On their part, it is a highly audacious, malicious and offensive act.

STATISTICS

Prevalence of Frotteuristic disorder may be as high as 35%. There is currently no consensus on the percentage.

---

[27] See Commented Bibliography.

Sexual Sadism Disorder

Marquis de Sade, 18th century author and aristocrat, was the first to describe, among others, *Sexual Sadism* from a clinical perspective, in his book *"The 120 Days of Sodom"*. In his thesis, von Krafft-Ebing defined sadism as the experience of sexual, pleasurable sensations (including orgasm) in producing acts of cruelty, bodily punishment afflicting a person or even when witnessing it, be the victim animals or human beings. The diagnosis of *Sexual Sadism Disorder* requires prolonged intense sexual arousal from inducing physical or psychological suffering in either a non-consenting or consenting person, as manifested by imaginary fantasies and behaviors. Clinically, the entity must cause significant impairment in important areas of life as a diagnosis requirement.

PASSIVE –RESPONSIVE SYMPTOMS

Intense feelings of sexual excitement when fantasizing about or witnessing another individual undergoing physical or psychological pain. Depressed mood.

ACTIVE-REACTIVE SYMPTOMS

Use of cutting, burning metal devices to induce pain as well as mutilation and strangulation. Angry behavior and emotional detachment. Most often experienced by males who have erotic fantasies by inflicting pain to others earlier in life. Extreme forms of pornography may enhance it. Infliction of psychological suffering, i.e. verbal abuse, physical suffering, assault or bondage. Frequent rehearsal of sadistic acts.

KNOWN VARIANTS

(B&D) Bondage and Discipline, (D&S) Domination and Submission, (S&M) Sadism and Masochism. Also Minor Sadism (mostly illustrated in the works of Marquis de Sade) and Major Sadism which can lead to such profoundly violent sexual acts as rape-murders.

LANGUAGE

Language depicts excitement at the infliction of pain, emotional emptiness and aloofness.

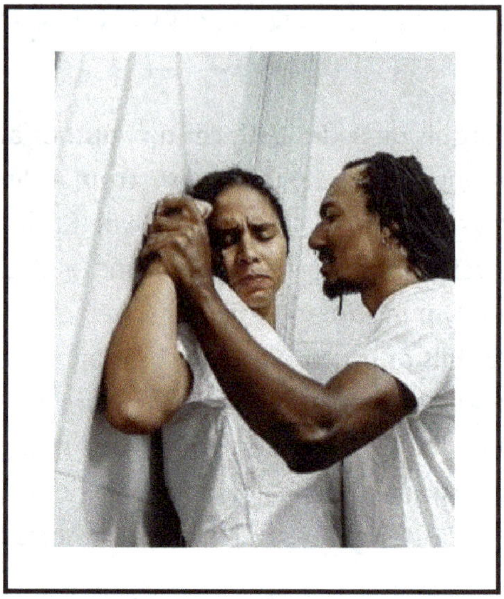

BEHAVIORAL FLIPS

It is well known and acknowledged that often an affected individual obtains sexual excitement from both sadistic and masochistic activities, in what are clearly behavioral sadomasochistic swings. The flip resides in the movement between perceptive sensation of pain to the motivation of inflicting it.

"No clear lines divide sexual sadism and sexual masochism, and the predispositions are often interchangeable. The conditions may coexist in the same individual... This relationship is supported by the finding that those who entertain masochistic fantasies also engage in sadistic fantasies."

DERIVED DISABILITIES

Prone to commit acts of criminality entailing many legal consequences.

AWARENESS

Conscious in the minor (Neurotic Disorder). Unconscious in the major (Psychotic Disorder – at the height of sadistic acts the Sadist is in a second state).

CHARACTEROLOGICAL FILIATION

Paradoxical

QG LAYER-PARTITIONS

7[(-4, -3, -2, -1) (+1, +2, +3, +4)]

STATISTICS

Among criminal offenders, *Sexual Sadism Disorder* has a prevalence of less than 10%. In the general population, its prevalence is unknown.

INSIGHTS

The Quanto-Geometric norm of Paradox/Antagonism that informs normal Layer **7** is instrumental to the etiological understanding of *Sexual Sadism Disorder*. Layer **7** includes on the positive chiral side the psychic states of *Resentment, Repugnance, Wickedness and Fury*, which are manifestly at the heart of the sadistic behavior. Note that sadism and masochism generally coexist in a variable degree. They both partner with pain as a common denominator in the biological expression of the phenomenological normal of Conflict or Antagonism. It is quite straightforward to relate *Sexual Sadism Disorder* to the specific states making up Layer 7 of the Mental Foliate. The Left-Chiral side which showcases such mental fits as *Terror, Fear, Anxiety* and *Perplexity* inarguably provides the root mentation activity for the psychosis of Masochism in general, counterpart of Sadism. Those states understandably also inform sexual behavior experienced by the subject in *Sexual Sadism Disorder*, stirring it to the enjoyment of pain (or conflict), since those mentation roots are the birthplace of the very mental experience of pain. Further, pain can either be purely psychogenic or the echo of a biological condition or event.

Sadism and Masochism knowingly work together, including in their sexual expressions, by virtue of the accrual of Layer 7 partitions in their fullness in the Mental Foliate, from our psychophysics perspective. In Sadism there is a prominence of the Right-Chiral set of partitions over the Left-chiral one within the accretion, and vice versa in Masochism.

PATHOLOGICAL AFFILIATES

Narcomania

Narcomania or *Drug Addiction* is an uncontrollable desire for narcotics. Its expression is a clear attempt or complacency to self-destruction, since the affected are duly cognizant of the physical and physiological damage they may or are in effect causing to themselves. Its onset by pure psychogenic implses directly relates it to Sadism and Masochism (or Sadomasochism) in their condition of top-level expression of this class of disorders. The insistent urge in Narcomania for self-harm, or pleasure from self-harm, is a typical attribute of Layer 7 overaccrual.

Gender Identity Disorder

Magnus Hirschfeld coined the term *transvestite* in 1910 to refer to patent interest in crossdressing in general. He used the term to describe individuals who are in the habit of intently wearing clothes of the opposite sex. The group of transvestites identified by M. Hirschfeld consisted of both male and female individuals, in the whole spectrum of sexual orientation, namely heterosexuals, homosexuals, bisexuals and asexuals. Formerly denoted transvestism, this disorder became labeled *Gender Identity Disorder* and lastly *Gender Dysphoria*. Male transvestites or crossdressers are men who wear female clothing and often both admire and imitate women, but do not self-identify as gay men or transsexuals. They further generally deny having fetishistic urges or intentions, in the sense that they are not interested in female dresses and do not wear female dresses to the aims of eliciting sexual arousal.

PASSIVE –RESPONSIVE BEHAVIOR

Overwhelming and persistent feeling that they belong to the gender other than their biologically determined gender. Transvestite men imitate women's mannerisms. Transvestite women imitate men's mannerisms. In children adoption, men would like to be and behave like mothers and women would like to be and behave like fathers. Strong conviction that feelings experienced are like those of the other gender.

ACTIVE-REACTIVE BEHAVIOR

Actively and permanently wear dresses of the other sex in lieu of those of their biological sex. Feelings of empathy and appreciation for persons of the other sex, i.e. transvestite men experience empathy for women, would espouse their cause (appreciation). Desire to get rid of secondary sexual characteristics or prevent their development. Desire for those characteristics to be like the other gender's.

KNOWN VARIANTS

Formerly known as Transvestism and now Gender Dysphoria.

LANGUAGE

Language and voice are colorful, the pitch is borrowed from the sex of impersonification.

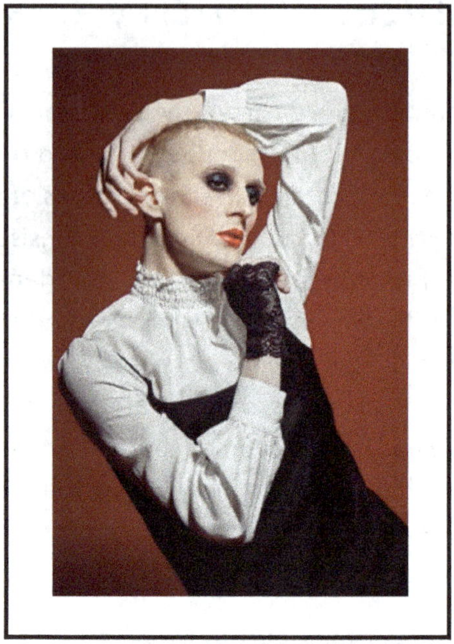

BEHAVIORAL FLIPS

Unknown

DERIVED DISABILITIES

Relationship conflict, inability to keep a functioning marriage resulting in separations or divorce. Performance at school or work may be impaired. Very high rate of suicide attempts.

AWARENESS

Conscious (Neurotic Disorder)

CHARACTEROLOGICAL FILIATION

N/A

QG LAYER-PARTITIONS

Entire Left-Chiral Side of the Foliate
or Entire Right-Chiral side of the Foliate
in cross contrast to biologically-determined Gender

STATISTICS

From 0.5% to to 1.2% of the population with about the same percentage in men as women.

INSIGHTS

This disorder is a very peculiar form of dysunction, almost unique in its kind. It must not be confused with any of the other forms of sexual transvestism where interactive sexuality or sexual arousal is central to the individual's motives. We have indulged the use of the label Transvestite for the disorder because it was the term coined early on by Hirschfeld for this specific nosology. From our perspective, Gender Identity Disorder is the most appropriate denomination, because the disorder showcases a blatant self-identity disparity between the Mental Body and the Biological body.

The peculiarity of this disorder resides in the fact that it etiologically involves the entire mentation Foliate which is in gender disparity with the actual biologically-determined elements of gender in the individual's body, as discussed in Chapter 2. The gender produced by the prevailing chiral side in the Mentation Foliate is in disparity with the gender determined in the biological body.

Notice that we have changed the labels for the Symptoms block in that we have substituted the word BEHAVIOR to SYMPTOMS. Effectively those sentiments and desires experienced by the patient have not the tone of any extreme or morbid excess that could not be felt at the same level by otherwise healthy or normal individuals. Transvestite individuals, in their full consciousness, do not consider that they are mentally sick and have expressly objected early on to the Transvestism label in favor of crossdresser, a habit of their full cognizance. However, the impairment does exist, and it resides in the fact of the disparity that we have discussed and the inner workings of what constitutes gender at the Mental level. Nevertheless, it remains an open question which way is best appropriate to resolve the disparity. Is it best resolved by readjusting the biological gender through biological *transgenderism in* clinical procedures as currently practiced in medical science, or by readjusting the Mentally-determined gender? The most legitimate answer may lie in the understanding of and perhaps abilty to manipulate the mechanism that correlates the biological body to the Mental body. We do not address this question in this treatise.

Transvestic Disorder

In *Transvestic Disorder*, the individual experiences intense sexual arousal from crossdressing, as manifested by fantasies and urges. The peculiarity of these fantasies, urges and atypical crossdressing acts are acknowledged by the individual and cause clinically significant distress or impairment in important areas of life.

PASSIVE –RESPONSIVE SYMPTOMS

Feel conflicted about the desire to behave like a woman, being a man, or to behave live a man, being a woman. Distressed by the resulting inability to function in various areas of life. Fully taking the role of the other sex when crossdressing. Patients with this disorder will have sex during or following the crossdressing, resulting in feelings of sadness, distress, humiliation and self-condemnation due to crossdressing urges and acts. May be further distressed by a partner's negative reaction to the behavior. Also worries about rejection in the social and professional environments.

ACTIVE-REACTIVE SYMPTOMS

Persistent and intense sexual arousal from fantasizing about wearing clothing of the opposite sex, frequently wear one or more pieces of garments of the opposite sex. May wear either a partial garment of the opposite sex or a complete outfit, along with women's wigs and makeup. Under continuous urges to cross-dress, else their desire may fluctuate or occur in a series of episodes. Behavioral pattern of purchasing clothing with the intent of crossdressing, proceeding to wear them in crossdressing displays, and then throwing them away in hopes of quitting. Tend to collect clothing for the strict purpose of crossdressing. Frequently unable to quit per their wish.

KNOWN VARIANTS

Dual-role transvestism. With fetishism: the individual is sexually aroused by fabrics and materials.

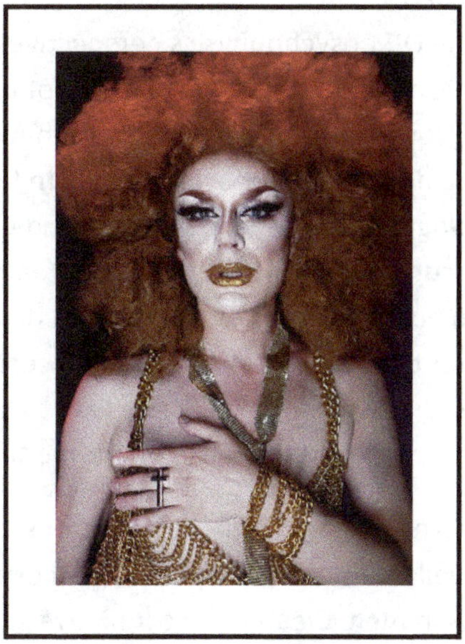

With autogynephilia: the individual is also aroused by thoughts or images of self as female – Autogynephilia is also known as eonism, sexo-aesthetic inversion, or automonosexuality.

LANGUAGE

Language and voice are colorful, the pitch is borrowed from the sex of impersonification.

BEHAVIORAL FLIPS

Constantly flipping between the desire for sexual arousal from cross-dressing and the distress and self-condemnation that leads them to extemporaneously throw away the crossdressing articles.

DERIVED DISABILITIES

Relationship conflict, separations or divorces.

AWARENESS

Conscious (Neurotic Disorder)

CHARACTEROLOGICAL FILIATION

Paradoxical

QG LAYER-PARTITIONS

7[(-4, -3, -2, -1), (+1, +2, +3, +4)]

STATISTICS

The prevalence of Transvestic Disorder is still unknown and likely to remain so, since most affected individuals are reluctant to report their sexual fantasies and behaviors.

INSIGHTS

In the QGT psychophysics perspective, we assign a paroxysmic Layer **7** to Transvestic disorder. The keyword to spot in the nosology of this disorder is Conflict, the Norm of this Layer. Also note that the distress experienced in this disorder is not a derived or comorbid symptom but a direct innate one pertaining to the etiology. In fact, it is because the individual is feeling paroxysmic distress that he crossdresses. In that regard, note that individuals with Gender Identity Disorder who equally crossdress do not feel distraught about it but instead feel good about their crossdressing. In Transvestic Disorder, the individual is driven to crossdressing specifically as a way to behave like a woman (in the case of man) as his particular response to intervening societal or parental pressures.

A stern and harsh father, even prone to chastisements, or a masculine mother, as well as abusive same-sex sexual experiences, may be the triggers of this neurosis in men. Clearly, the conflictive situations arising from parental interactions as known in analytic orthodoxy which drive the young person to heuristic castration represent legitimate etiological drivers in the onset of this disorder. However, the analyst always has to consider that all this negative background may have been present in other people's lives and nevertheless never brought them to this acute disequilibrium level. It is only because of a predisposed mental terrain, which our psychophysics recognizes as paroxysmal Layer 7 of their Mental Foliate, that the aforementioned factors bring these patients to the pathological level of the paroxysm.

Lastly, it is important to recognize that the sexual arousal Transvestites experience is felt in the condition that they are sexually impersonating. In other words, female Transvestites impersonating men feel projective sexual arousal, while male Transvestites impersonating female feel sexual arousal in terms of expectant passive penetration.

PATHOLOGICAL AFFILIATES

Transvestic Fetishism

In this disease, the patient both crossdresses and engages in a form of fetishism consisting in asking sexual partners to wear the fetish objects in order to visually stimulate their sexual arousal. In contrast to Fetishists, these patients do find meaning in human interaction for sexual activity and do not just seek sexual arousal from the strict observation of a non genital object in a solitary act.

The nature of the sexual desire itself is an important factor to best understanding of these paraphilia. The literature available on the subject unfortunately does not bring that aspect of the disorder under sufficient light, if at all. Reports on the nature of the sexual desire in those cases falter altogether. One important question: Is the partner a man or a woman? If the partner is a man, the individual ought to be considered a crossdresser that feels he is a woman, and looks for a male partner. That would make his Transvestic Fetishism an affiliate of Transvestic Disorder, and rejoins the aforedescribed characterization. Were the partner a female, it would probably mean that the individual is essentially a Fetishist which does not really feel the need for the female partner and that a marital obligation probably imposes the partner. He will be asking the female partner, as reported, to wear or do strange things that she feels uncomfortable with and will not do. In that case, he could as well have used a mannequin, and he would have still obtained an arousal to his satisfaction. Very tellingly, a Fetishist man reveals, in his own words "that he would have practiced the heterosexual act of intercourse if only a woman would have consented to wear his female shoes", of which he kept an extensive collection through the course of a life in which he never had sex with any woman.

Therefore, decisively conclusive analysis is not yet possible and requires more clinical data.

Hoarding Disorder

Hoarding Disorder is characterized by the compulsion to accumulate and store material belongings at all costs, including those with no value such as junk mail, old newspapers that most people would discard. This accumulation leads to cluttering hoarders' living space which may pose health hazards. Clutter may cover any surface in the home, from floors to furniture, leaving the hoarder barely with walking path through the living space. Hoarders feel emotionally attached to these items with a sense that they will need them in the future. This behavior is alarming to the people around the individual and usually leads to complaints from family members, neighbors and even local law enforcement.

PASSIVE –RESPONSIVE SYMPTOMS

Emotional attachment to collected items with fear of losing them. Feelings of insecurity and that others are emotionally indifferent to the hoarder. Often self-neglect ensues. Pervasive tendency to low self-esteem. Reclusiveness and unfriendliness are common personality traits found in hoarders. Generally remain in house-bound seclusion and come across as quite eccentric. Display a significant level of indifference to others, though they think others have no interest and affection for them.

ACTIVE-REACTIVE SYMPTOMS

Obsessively accumulates material items or possessions which result in persistent difficulty discarding or parting from them, regardless of their value or lack thereof. Emotionally attached to the items they compulsively preserve or collect. Consequently feel distressed about discarding any of their possessions. See no problem with their compulsion to accumulate and reason that they might need these items in the future. Compulsion to accumulate possessions leads to clutter of living spaces and compromise use of living spaces. Sometimes engage in excessive acquisition of unneeded items or for which there is no available space.

KNOWN VARIANTS

Animal Hoarder, Paper Hoarder (newspapers, magazines, mail, etc.), Photograph Hoarder, Clothing Hoarder, Container Hoarder, Food Hoarder, Garbabe and Human Waste Product Hoarder.

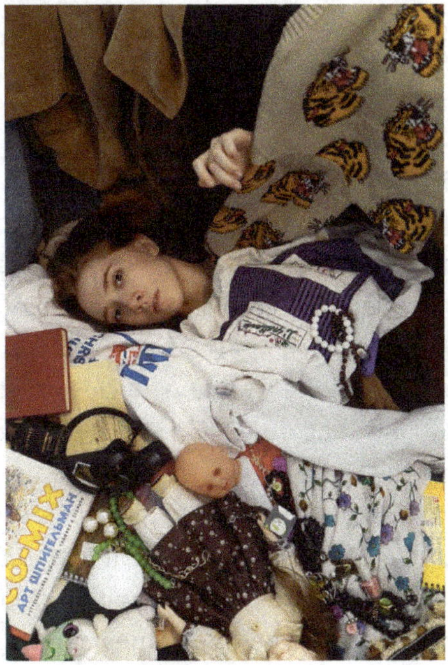

LANGUAGE

Language reflects deep stubbornness: *"I keep good stuff, you hoard junk."*

BEHAVIORAL FLIPS

Indifference is in hoarders intertwined with stubbornness and tendency to argue for self-justification. They would swing from one type of behavior to the other.

DERIVED DISABILITIES

Inability to maintain a safe place. According to the Fair Housing Act, hoarding is a mental disability that may pose health hazards by animal or flea infestation, falls or fire.

AWARENESS

Conscious (Neurotic Disorder)

CHARACTEROLOGICAL FILIATION

Egocentric

QG LAYER-PARTITIONS

1[(-4, -3, -2, -1) (+1, +2, +3, +4)]

STATISTICS

An estimated 2 to 5% of people in the US population are affected with hoarding disorder. The National Alliance on Mental Illness (NAMI) Massachusetts estimates that up to 5 percent of the world's population exhibit clinical symptoms of hoarding.

INSIGHTS

Under the Unary Norm of Egocentrism, hoarders show paroxysmal behavior responding to the whole array of mentation partitions pertaining to the referred Layer in their mental Foliate. The passive-responsive partitions of Normal Layer **1**, namely *Timidity, Indifference, Solitude and Introversion* fuel the pervasive tendency to low self-esteem. Reclusiveness, which is a common personality traits found in hoarders, is to be attributed to a working of the left-chiral partitions of the Layer as well, in particular the Solitude pensive partition. On average, hoarders are knowingly social loners who live alone. It is through their mental states of timidity and solitude that hoarders tend to give themselves to seclusion in a house-bound condition. That also speaks to the fact that hoarders reportedly tend to be three times more obese than the average person. Indifference leads them to eccentric displays as they show little care for what others may think of them and their behavior. Their manifest stubbornness, tendency to argue for being right vis-à-vis others, and compulsion to accumulate or collect are engenders of the palette of right-chiral partitions of the Layer, namely *Conservativeness*, *Possessiveness*, *Competitiveness* and *Cupidity*.

Psychoanalytically, various defense mechanisms have been linked to hoarding, such as denial, regression, reaction formation, justification and sublimation. However, the pensive results of these mechanisms are best accounted for as impulses surfacing into the Conscious Cognos via orthoflows from their Layer 7 sources. The true direct drivers of the compulsions manifest in Hoarding are offsprings of the partitions belonging to Layer 1 of these individuals' Mentation Foliate, which directly spell out their pensive quality or nature. It is only when the entire Layer becomes overly paroxysmal that the compulsion becomes manifest as a dysfunctional syndrome.

Furthermore, it is worth noting that in order for the mentioned psychoanalytic exegesis to hold, it would have to eloquently explain why similar parent-related developmental dynamics result in hoarding dysfunction in one individual and not another. We have not seen an exposition of this sort of formalism for this case.

Hoarders' urge for self-appropriation and attachment to collected objects is so profound that in the case of animal hoarders i.e., they often have trouble giving the animals up, even when the well-being of the animals is clearly at stake and the animals, like dogs and cats, are sick and in unquestionable disarray under their watch.

Pedophilia Disorder

Pedophilia is a disorder characterized by arousing fantasies about or sexual urges for prepubescent children. The affected individual has either acted upon these sexual desires, or is under stress due to these desires. The lower age threshold generally considered for this disorder is 16 years old, and an age gap between the pedophile and the child of at least 5 years. When the individual has not risen to the point of acting materially on these sexual urges for children, or is loath to or preoccupied about causing damage to these young lives, the ease is considered by many clinicians to be more of a compulsive disorder type.

PASSIVE –RESPONSIVE SYMPTOMS

Intense, repetitive sexual arousal from fantasies, urges, or behaviors involving one child or more (usually aged 13 or under). Generally show depressed mood and low self-esteem.

ACTIVE-REACTIVE SYMPTOMS

Attempt to lure and attract children by filling their own homes with toys, games, bikes and swimming pools as baits. Maintenance of collections of child pornography. Salacious exposure of children to nudity through pictures, videos, language or shared activities. Types of activities may be as simple as just looking at a child or undressing and touching a child. Acts often involve oral sex or touching of genitals of the child or the offender. Aggressive compulsion by many to materially abduct their coveted young sex partners. May tragically progress to commission of material rapes of young children. These sexual impulses are generally accompanied with Impulsive behavior.

KNOWN VARIANTS

- Exclusive type: sexual attraction to children only.
- Non exclusive type: sexual attraction to adults and children.
- Attraction to boys.
- Attraction to girls.
- Incestuous only: boys or girls in the pedophile's own family.
- Virtuous Pedophelia (Pedophilia Obsessive Compulsive Disorder)
- Hebephelia
- Hephebophelia

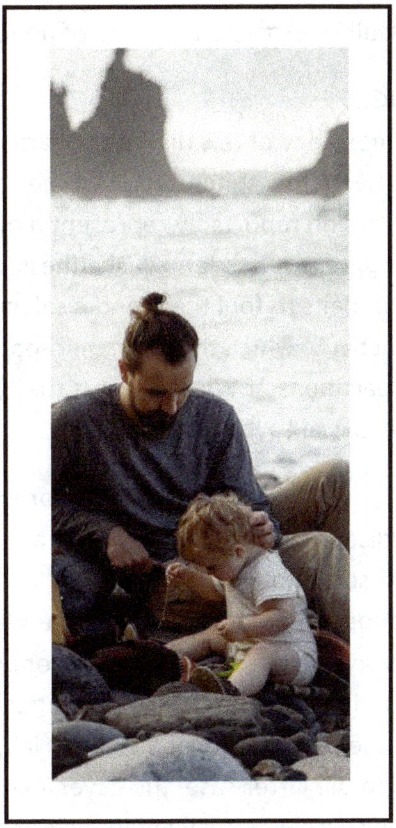

LANGUAGE

A pedophile talks the talk *"I am just like you"*. Language may be persuasive, flirtatious.

BEHAVIORAL FLIPS

Unknown

DERIVED DISABILITIES

Criminal sexual offenses, child abuse. A pedophile may be a professional who works with children. Often, the pedophile is a single male over 30 years of age. The internet provides ideal disguise for such sexual predators searching for potential victims.

AWARENESS

Conscious (Neurotic Disorder)

CHARACTEROLOGICAL FILIATION

Paradoxical

QG LAYER-PARTITIONS

[Left-Chiral Sector] of Foliate

7[(-4, -3, -2, -1)(+1, +2, +3, +4)]

STATISTICS

In adult men, the prevalence of pedophilia is below 5%.

INSIGHTS

The nosology of this disorder clearly shows the imprint of an intense dynamic regime on the Anima sector of the Foliate, in as much as low-down mood and depression reportedly represent a major part of its symptom set. Additionally, the aggressiveness and wickedness in active abduction of innocent children, the use of baits to foul them and a salacious introduction of young children to sexual activity, which they are unprepared and inapt for, bears the clear imprint of the partitions of Wickedness (Cruelty) and Fury at the right-chiral side of the Paradoxical Layer of the Foliate.

For the analyst, these two components should hold for the etiological basis of the disease, given that there are a number of challenges with the diagnostic of the disorder on account of so-called multimorbidity. For that matter, incisive diagnosis of pedophilic disorder endeavors to specify whether the individual is exclusively attracted to children or not, the gender that the individual is attracted to, whether the sexual urges are limited to incest or not as well as whether the individual has materially acted on these sexual urges for children or not. In the latter case, the Layer 7 component does not apply to the etiology. The disease essentially manifests as a dysfunction with the Anima sector of the individual's Mental Manifold arising from a gender disparity between Mental Body and biological body, as discussed in Chapter 2. The Anima Sector of the subject's Mental Manifold bears the accrual that stamps gender in lieu of the Animus Sector. The individual subsequently finds himself distressed by a flurry of sensations aroused in his body to which his unbeknownst female Mental Foliate feels estranged. Following is the corresponding observable nosology:

- Unwelcome spontaneous thoughts and images of sexual acts with a child.
- Unwelcome spontaneous thoughts and images of a naked child.
- Experiencing undesired arousal sensations even with mere thoughts of a child's company.
- Fictional thoughts of having sexually molested a child.

- Fictional thoughts of having blacked out or erased from own memory sexual abuse or molestation of a child in the past.
- Eluding normal situations that involve even the most common and simplest physical contact with a child.
- Eluding normal activities or duties towards children such as bathing, changing clothes or diapers, as well as other routine care-giving activities.
- Constant reviewing for subtle indicators or past events and encounters which may accuse pedophilic behavior of some kind on their part.
- Eluding articles or shows that depict pedophilia, either explicitly or allusively.
- Constantly looking for advice and reassurance from trusted loved ones regarding their feelings of self-doubt and guilt.

One of the most salient traits of these symptoms is the now understandable estrangement that embroils the individual's thought processes vis-à-vis his attraction for children. To complete the etiological tableau of the aforementioned nosology, one may psychoanalytically invoke the special nurture that females feel for babies and little children, which is very present in the estranged female Foliate, to be chiefly responsible for this particular strain of the disorder. It would account for a contribution of the group of representational sublayers involved in the impairment. The aforedescribed nosology pertains to the so-called *Virtuous Pedophilia* or *Pedophilia Obsessive Compulsive Disorder*.

Female Sexual Interest-Arousal Disorder (FSIAD)

Female Sexual Interest-Arousal Disorder is characterized by either a lack or a significant reduction in sexual interest on one hand, or, on the other hand, a lack of sexual arousal during sexual activity. Formerly known under the term frigidity, the disease used to cover inability to experience orgasm in sexual interaction as well. Official psychiatry has come to segregate the orgasmic deficiency symptom from the disorder and assign the label *Female Orgasmic Disorder (FOD)* to the last as a disorder in its own right. Female sexual response is however known to be one, with the following 5-phase cycle: desire, arousal, plateau, orgasm, and resolution.

PASSIVE –RESPONSIVE SYMPTOMS

Low libido and/or unresponsiveness to sexual stimulation. Discomfort or emotional pain during intercourse. Incapacity to demonstrate complete feminine let go or yield, or trust and confidence in a sexual male partner. Inability to self-abandon to masculine interaction in the expression of their sexuality. Possible persistent feelings of low self-esteem and poor body image, constant stress or feelings of depression. Lack of any pleasure of sorts during sexual encounters and inability to reach orgasm with absence of genital lubricating secretions. Discomforting flashbacks of possible past sexual abuse.

ACTIVE-REACTIVE SYMPTOMS

Aversion of sexual activity. Rejection or repugnance of the natural feminine sexual role of passiveness. Lack of sexual fantasy or sexual musing leading to sexual desires. Hence marked decrease in sexual activity and desires for sexual intercourse. Feigned fatigue to avoid engaging in sexual activity with partner.

KNOWN VARIANTS

Life-long type – Acquired type – Generalized type – Situational type.

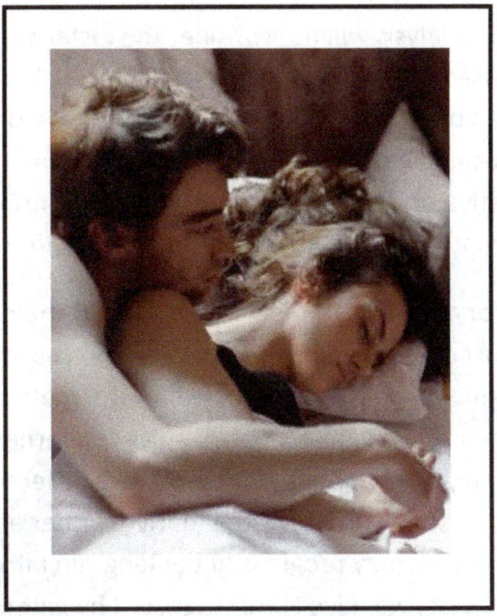

LANGUAGE

Avoidance of conversations or exchanges about sex.

BEHAVIORAL FLIPS

Extemporaneously switching intimate conversations during sex from erotic to casual.

DERIVED DISABILITIES

Overeating, resorting to alcohol or drugs use to compensate for the inability to have sex. Avoiding or delaying sex and shared intimacy, may incur masturbation as well. Partner relation issues. Libidinal deficiency may have been caused by religious or cultural beliefs.

AWARENESS

Conscious (Neurotic disorder)

CHARACTEROLOGICAL FILIATION

Paradoxical

QG LAYER-PARTITIONS

[Left-Chiral Side] of Foliate overaccrued.

7[(-4, -3, -2, -1) (+1, +2, +3, +4)**]**

STATISTICS

Overall, the disorder can affect 22-43% of women up to age 59. As a breakdown, the prevalence of women who have desire difficulties is 64%, arousal difficulties 31%, orgasm difficulties 35%, and sexual pain 26%.

INSIGHTS

This analysis will not consider the instances of the disorder that are purely caused by physiological dysregulations, but only its psychogenic cadre and the possible psychosomatic projections thereof. One ought to consider that the specific phase that is affected may be due to a quantitative trend but not a qualitative one. It is therefore all the more fitting to consider altogether the entire symptomatic spectrum of the disorder in the behavioral order.

Strong feelings of resentment against their partners, or the hatred in jealousy caused by partner's behaviors or choices, are among the first factors of female frigidity in marital or couple life. The male partner's attitude during copulation, when showing inability to display tenderness and rocking love but instead rough, careless, self-centered and unaffectionate physical interaction with the female partner, is a prime motive for her ensuing rejection of sexual interaction. The latter may progress in the long run into full-fledged, distressing FSIAD. In this case, we have FSIAD triggered by external causes.

These factors are of the same nature as sexual abuse whether by a stranger or a family member in settling the disorder in the female patient. In both cases we are dealing with mistreatments instigating a resentment or repugnance response to sexual activity.

It is clear that the main nosological expression of FSIAD concerns the ability to yield and assume a passive role in psychological expression as relates to love, per dictate of the predominant Anima side of the female Foliate. To that extent, and in the context of a paradoxical character, the implicated components of the Passive-Responsive psyche at the left-chiral side of Layer 7 of the Foliate may become preponderant in the sexual response, and galvanize morbid behavior as their dynamics reach over accrual. It is the *Anxiety, Angst, Anguish* and, in the case of intervening rape, the *Terror* in the manifestation of experienced sexual activity, that, in the disorder, fuel much of the female patient's aggravating inner sensations with respect to sex. It is by virtue of a counter-reaction to those sensations from the partitions at the right-chiral side of the Layer that compensation by way of frigidity will ensue, which may be not only psychological but entail physiological projections as well (absence of orgasmic pelvic and vaginal responses).

It is important to raise another plausible etiological dimension of the Disorder. Very significantly, other female patients with FSIAD confide that they are only able to have sexual relations with their husbands if and only if *"they feel sorry for them or when their husbands are momentarily in a low-down mood".* This may be interpreted either as the result of empathy or a shadow desire to dominate instead. When the patient will admit that she can only reach satisfaction in sexual intercourse if *"she outright dominates her partner in the act",* the analyst must outrightly consider a pathological basis of sheer disparity between gender identity in the Mental Foliate and that of the biological body. Other reported tendentious language that dictates this diagnostic is i.e. *"I will never accept to be the puppet of a man"* or *"I am a woman by accident, I could never submit to this inferior role considered vacuous."* Some women will not even accept to wear a female bathing suit at the beach. In these cases, we are dealing with not only masculine motives of an Animus-driven Foliate but, very particularly, with the right-chiral partitions of *Resentment, Repugnance, Wickedness and Fury* of a paroxysmal Layer 7.

From an etiological perspective, we must understand all of the above citations to have come from patients who experience the disorder as a result of internal autogenic impairments as opposed to external factors. Again, only on account of the internal psychophysical dynamics, can the analyst understand why somebody who may have experienced all the trauma in the qualified external causes of the disorder or more does not actually get to succumb to it while another who actually was spared does succumb to it.

Should the psychosocial pressure of male dominance wherever it exists become overboard, and the natural empathy between daughter and father reach an extremum level within the representational sublayers of the young female Foliate, both factors are going to create a perfect storm of gender identity crisis therein, causing a chiral paroxysm switch between the two sectors of the Foliate in the determination of gender identity. The Animus sector of the young female Foliate takes over causing a psychosomatic disjunction between gender in the mental Manifold and the physiological elements of gender. The severe sexual intercourse dysfunctions exhibited in the nosology of the Disorder are all assuredly borne out of this disparity. This is the psychophysics background on which the psychosocial and familial elements of development generally invoked in orthodox psychoanalysis by virtue of pure logic truly materially play out in these cases.

Understanding the entire etiological background in the diagnostic analysis is evidently paramount to successful therapy. The specifics of adequate genital stimulation, application of lubricants of one or the other kind, physiological treatment of vaginal pain, etc., are all important elements to achieve momentary relief. These measures are however contingent upon the specific primal psychogenic causes of the Disorder. Only by addressing those root causes can a treatment of any class break down the morbid barrier to an entirely pleasurable female's sexual experience, as noted in the introduction.

PATHOLOGICAL AFFILIATES

Female Orgasmic Disorder (Frigidity)

As previously mentioned, the specific fringe of the disorder that only shows lack of orgasm, or so-called anorgasmia, as the symptom has been labeled *Female Orgasmic Disorder*. Both the typical altered state of consciousness and the corresponding pelvic, uterine and vaginal responses do not show up. That is the case even despite preliminary sexual excitement evidenced in desire and arousal. In other cases, there may be instead markedly diminished intensity of orgasmic sensations or marked delay of orgasm from any kind of stimulation, leading to female distress.

KNOWN VARIANTS

Anorgasmia can be either Primary, in which a woman has never experienced orgasm through any means of stimulation, or Secondary, in which a woman is anorgasmic after having been orgasmic. Secondary anorgasmia can be classified as situational (e.g., when a woman can experience orgasm via masturbation but not with a partner) or generalized.

INSIGHTS

Most of the variants above mentioned, if not all, likely fall under the case of psychogenic causes to the disorder. It is clear that an inquest of possible physiological causes to the disorder is in order as a precondition to engaging a psychogenic etiological analysis. All the analytic elements invoked in the case of FSIAD apply. We have abstained from including the sub label "orgasm" in the FSIAD nomer for the Disorder in order to keep the current nomenclature conveniently unaltered.

It is worth mentioning that sleep deprivation and stress are important contributing factors to anorgasmia. Existing treatments of any kind with antidepressants or antipsychotics, as well as many blood pressure pharmacological agents, may seriously affect or provoke the condition. Various hormonal states such as pregnancy, breastfeeding, and postmenopausal state can be equally associated with decreased libido. Certain chronic medical conditions, including hypothyroidism, may contribute as well. In women of reproductive age, contraception may become the culprit.

Erectile Disorder

Erectile Disorder (ED) may be rightly viewed as the correspondent in men to the female arousal and orgasmic disorders. Formerly known as Male Erectile Disorder, ED is characterized by the inability to achieve or maintain an erection sufficient for satisfactory sexual performance, or a noticeable decrease in erectile rigidity during partnered sexual activity. Cases where it is associated by medical diagnosis with chronic medical illnesses such as sedentary lifestyle, diabetes mellitus, hyperlipidemia, obesity, hypertension, testosterone deficiency or prostate treatment, drug and alcohol use, and various types of medications are of no interest for this study and are not considered here. We retain only the psychological cases to the effect of this study. Note that age or the later phases of the lifecycle should never be underestimated and represent an important contributor (or risk factor) to the dysfunction.

PASSIVE –RESPONSIVE SYMPTOMS

Trouble getting an erection or not every time the person is sexually engaged. Or else trouble maintaining an erection for normal sexual activity. Reduced sexual desire. Fatigue. Sexual performance anxiety or generalized anxiety, depressed mood.

ACTIVE-REACTIVE SYMPTOMS

Poor confidence about maintaining an erection. Find no satisfaction in sexual intercourse. Infrequent ejaculation during sex. Decrease in sexual desire concomitant with depressed mood.

KNOWN VARIANTS

- Lifelong type
- Acquired type
- Generalized
- Situational
- Due to Psychological factors
- Due to Combined factors

LANGUAGE

In Erectile Disorder, the male speech may sound depressive and anxious, express frustration during sexual intercourse or undergoes periods of silence. May be less charged with affection and emotion.

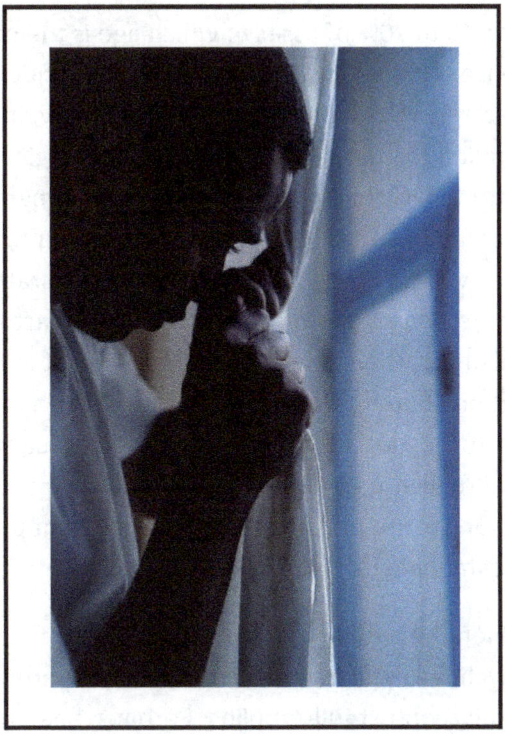

BEHAVIORAL FLIPS

From anxiety, fear of sexual failure, and stress about sexual performance to active sex avoidance and anger.

DERIVED DISABILITIES

Smoking, drinking alcohol or using drugs. Interpersonal difficulty and communication problems. Inability to maintain a healthy relationship with risks of separation or divorce.

AWARENESS

Conscious (Neurotic disorder)

CHARACTEROLOGICAL FILIATION

Paradoxical

QG LAYER-PARTITIONS

[Left-Chiral Side] of Foliate overaccrued.

7[(-4, -3, -2, -1) (+1, +2, +3, +4)**]**

STATISTICS

The prevalence of ED increases with age at a range of 40-70% as men age between 40 to 70 years old.

INSIGHTS

The 40 to 70% of cases in which age is the main factor causing erectile impotence or sexual disability cannot be considered psychopathology but a natural decline in the vitality of the Human body. In this regard, in Chapter 2 we have studied the tight relation between biological vitality and libido. Second, the very natural fact that arousal and orgasm in men occur very quickly, in any case much more quickly than they do in women, seem to suggest that men are naturally vulnerable to a shortening in the duration and weakening in the strength of arousal and orgasm caused by adverse factors of either biological or psychological order. Therefore the psychotherapist is well advised to highly consider education about managing sexual interaction for affected patients and refrain from hasty diagnosis of deficiency. It is also clear that healthy living, good nutrition and regular physical exercise that are able to maintain or restore vitality of the organism are prime remedy or significant palliative to the disorder worth recommending.

When the pathology is clearly there per the described symptom set, the known psychoanalytic exegesis that bears on parental negative influence within the family context fully applies. Perhaps, heeding to both patient's and parents' language in those cases may help elucidate the roots of the disorder even further for the purpose of this analysis. The following are common remarks by sexually impotent men in analysis:

- *My mother is the only woman I have ever loved and admired.*
- *It's a reflex with me, I compare every woman with my mother. None outlives the comparison.*
- *I have married my wife because her eyes look the same as my mother's...*

But others say:

- *I have been so torn by my mother's authority that when I talk to my wife it looks like my mother is standing right in front of me.*
- *My mother used to say: after all I've done for you I hope that you will stay with me for as long as possible. A boy ought to stay with his mother.*

- *I have been raised and spoiled by my mother like sugar. She considered every girl that approached me her personal enemy and used to warn me about "the girls that take away the boys from their mothers".*

These remarks put in evidence the deep mutual attachment between boy and mother. The Oedipus situation evoked in orthodox analysis is clear therein. It is also clear in some of these remarks that the attachment on the mother's part is morbidly excessive, which creates the grounds for an internal conflict for the boy, as commonly viewed in psychoanalysis. The neurosis in the young mind in development, in terms of unconscious compensation mechanisms or defense mechanisms, is inevitable. The logic gives us that the boy is doomed to become "girly", sexually impotent in his male attributions, aka loss of masculinity or virility.

In attempting to render a clear representation of the psychophysics of these pensive interactions, one ought to consider the deep affectionate empathy that exists between the boy and his mother. Normally these transactions will remain seated in the representational sublayers of the young boy's Foliate. However, when these empathetic transactions involving the mother become too intensely accrued in the course of the boy's development, their impact in his Mental Foliate engenders an identity crisis that swings the gender-defining accrual of root partitions from the Right-Chiral sector of his Foliate to the Left-Chiral sector. This chiral swing of an entire sector of the Foliate creates a disparity between the natural gender imprinted in the biological body and the new inverted one in the Foliate. This new psychophysics landscape constitutes indeed the basis for best understanding of the language aforequoted from sexually impotent men in analysis.

PATHOLOGICAL AFFILIATES

Male Hypoactive Sexual Desire Disorder

Male Hypoactive Sexual Desire Disorder is defined as persistent or recurrent lack of erotic thoughts, fantasies, and desire for sexual activity. These symptoms must clinically cause significant distress about the condition to the patient in order to arise to morbidity status. Often, men with MHSDD present with erectile dysfunction as well. Because the latter appears to be a more significant symptom, it may eclipse the existence of MHSDD as part of the symptom set that is manifest in a particular patient. Analysis that seeks to granularly detect deficiencies across five individual components of sexual intercourse activity should pay discriminate attention to this caveat.

Premature Ejaculation Disorder

The **International Society of Sexual Medicine** has determined the following symptom set in Premature Ejaculation:

- Ejaculation always or nearly always occurs prior to or within about 1 minute of vaginal penetration in newly initiated sexual experiences.
- Clinically bothersome reduction in latency time, often to about 3 minutes or less.
- Inability to delay ejaculation on all or nearly all vaginal penetrations.

It is also known as rapid ejaculation or early ejaculation. We consider the psychophysics etiological profile of these affiliate disorders to be the same or nearly the same as that of the main Erectile dysfunction disorder.

Delayed Ejaculation Disorder

Delayed ejaculation (DE), formerly known as Male orgasmic disorder is the persistent or recurrent difficulty, protraction, or inability to obtain orgasm and ejaculation after sufficient sexual stimulation. In men, both orgasm and ejaculation occur simultaneously even though they represent two different phenomena. Other synonymous names are: retarded ejaculation, inhibited ejaculation, inadequate ejaculation, idiopathic anejaculation, primary impotentia ejaculationis, or psychogenic anejaculation.

PASSIVE –RESPONSIVE SYMPTOMS	***ACTIVE-REACTIVE SYMPTOMS***
Necessity of long protracted stimulation from partner to achieve an orgasm/ejaculation and at times the latter is completely defaulting at end of exercise. Often engage in very peculiar patterns of self-stimulation or masturbation to reach orgasm/ejaculation.	Patient may ejaculate and in small amount only with manual or oral stimulation or one specific form of stimulation. Often requires a special form in speed and pressure of penis stimulation only attainable in solo masturbation for ejaculation to occur. Erotic stimulation may require different modalities some of which may be overtly paraphilic in nature. Experiences dry orgasm (aspermia), delayed orgasm, retrograde ejaculation. Dissatisfaction with sexual intercourse in general.

STATISTICS

Jern et al. and Bancroft et al. demonstrated that men with homosexual orientations had a significantly higher frequency of DE than heterosexual men.

INSIGHTS

A number of psychosexual scenarios have been invoked in orthodox psychoanalysis to explain the oncome of *Delayed Ejaculation* in the psychological landscape, namely: fears of pregnancy and fertility issues, defiling the partner, fears of castration, rejection, fear of loss of control, fears of intimacy etc. In the word of Juza Chen, however: *"Although some of these factors may contribute to the etiologies of individual men with DE, no well controlled studies have provided comprehensive support for any of the various hypotheses."*

Towards a sensible etiology of the disease the analyst must heed two important known facts:

- Erotic stimulation required by the affected male may be overtly paraphilic in nature.
- An overwhelming majority of affected men exhibit homosexual orientations.

Both suggest a projective incapacity resulting from a misplaced paroxysm at the Left-chiral Sector of the Foliate which should be naturally dwelling instead on the Right-chiral Sector, for one, and, for the other, a paroxysmal Layer 7 in the Layer hierarchy. All concordant with the etiology reported above for the main disease in the group.

Nymphomania

The term *Nymphomania*, frequently used in popular language to denigrate women sexually, is not quite welcome currently in formal science of the mental despite its use in nomenclature. It was initially coined in Europe during the Victorian era to describe women who were willing to have sex with any man they encountered. The male version of the behavior was coined *"Don Juanism"* or *"Satyriasis"*. Those two terms have been abandoned and the label *Nymphomania* now applies to males exhibiting the behavior as well. Also known nowadays as *Erotomania, Hypersexuality* or *Compulsive Sexual Behavior*, the disorder is defined by increased libido, intrusive and distressing sexual thoughts and urges with promiscuous behaviors.

PASSIVE –RESPONSIVE SYMPTOMS

Intrusive, distressing sexual thoughts. Feelings of guilt, shame and inadequacy. Repeated uncontrollable thoughts about having sex. In women and homosexual men, compulsion to be sexually penetrated or to be subject to sexual interaction. Manifest no preference or partners, thereby exhibiting promiscuity. Spill into compulsive masturbation when partners become sparse or difficult, and compulsive use of pornography alike.

ACTIVE-REACTIVE SYMPTOMS

In heterosexual men, repeated uncontrollable urges and behaviors of engaging in sexual penetration.

KNOWN VARIANTS

None

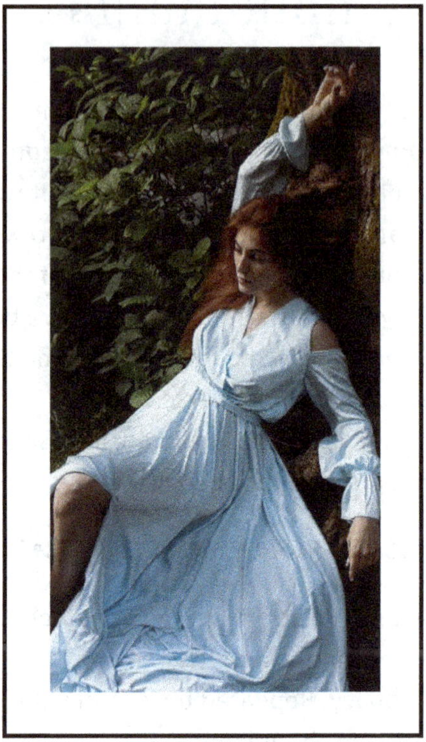

LANGUAGE

The language is characteristically rich in sexual lexicon.

BEHAVIORAL FLIPS

Unknown

DERIVED DISABILITIES

Substance use, increased risk for STDs, proneness to high-risk sexual behaviors. Frequent relationship failures.

AWARENESS

Conscious (Neurotic Disorder)

CHARACTEROLOGICAL FILIATION

Paradoxical

QG LAYER-PARTITIONS

In women and homosexual men:

[Left-Chiral Side] of Foliate overaccrued

7[(-1, -2, -3, -4)]

In men and lesbian women:

[Right-Chiral Side] of Foliate overaccrued

7[(+1, +2, +3, +4)]

STATISTICS

Known to be likely more common in women and homosexual men. Apparent prevalence of 3-6% in the population.

INSIGHTS

It is well known that stress and recent traumatic life event predispose to this disorder or act as triggers. It is well understood that these conditions (stress and trauma) respond to specific activity of the left-chiral side of the Mental Foliate. In addition, the prevalence of both women and homosexual men in exhibiting this disorder strongly advocates for a congruence of the statistics with an active role of the Anima side of the female gender Foliate in the disorder. It remits to an overactive left-chiral side of the Foliate in the case of affected women and, in the case of homosexual men, a disparity that dysfunctionally construes a female Mental Foliate for the individual instead of a male Foliate that matches the male gender identity in his biological body.

Here also, the additional imprint of a paroxysmal QG Layer **7** is ostensible in the psychophysical background of the disorder. It is important to note that we do not discard the possibility of a Layer **6** accompaniment instead of a Layer **7** in the etiology of the Disorder. It will be up to the analyst to make that determination through the psychometric tests proposed at the end of this study. Since there can never be two different individual Layers in paroxysm in a subject's Mentation Foliate, the Layer overaccrual that coparticipates in the disorder will be the same one that already accrued to determine the individual's character, in this case Layer **6**.

Sexual Masochism Disorder

Sexual Masochism Disorder (SMD) is an intense sexual arousal when the fected individual is set to experience suffering which might involve humiliation, submission to battery or bondage, whether the inflicted aggravation is real or simulated. To rise to the level of a disorder the fantasies and actions must cause prolonged or significant distress, and/or impairment in important areas of life. SMD belongs to the class of so-called algolagnic disorders which are rized by infliction of pain and suffering for sexual gratification.

PASSIVE –RESPONSIVE SYMPTOMS

Sexual arousal from being beaten, bound, or otherwise subject to pain and suffering. The sexual masochistic individual is at the receiving end of spanking, cutting, burning, whipping, binding, strangulating by a partner in the sadistic role, and for ecstatic sexual pleasure. Use of cloths, leather, metal chains, handcuffs in bondage are common for stimulation.

ACTIVE-REACTIVE SYMPTOMS

Their Individual partners are sadistically aroused by fantasies of pain infliction in others, images of distressed faces of women or semi-nude women in bondage.

KNOWN VARIANTS

Asphyxiophilia, which is when the individual restricts his or her breathing in order to achieve desired arousal.

LANGUAGE

Language depicts excitement and pain, failure, emptiness, despair.

BEHAVIORAL FLIPS

Unknown

DERIVED DISABILITIES

May rise to behavior decried or punishable by the Law, i.e. accidental asphyxia, mutilation. Scarring may result from inflicted masochistic wounds, trauma, depression.

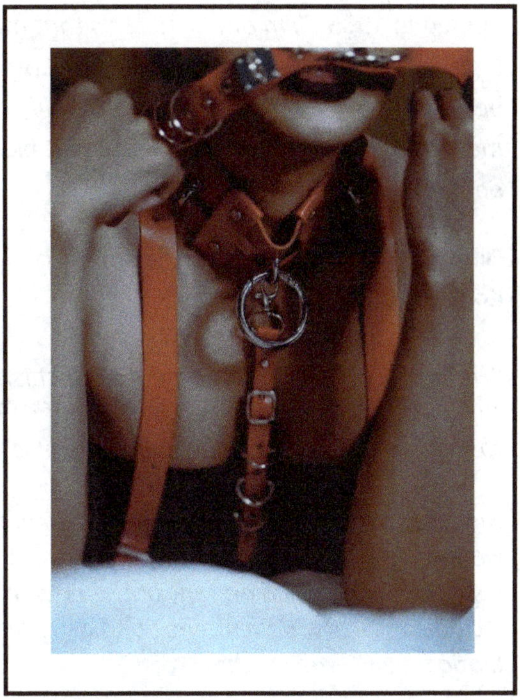

AWARENESS

Conscious (Neurotic disorder)

CHARACTEROLOGICAL FILIATION

Paradoxical

QG LAYER-PARTITIONS

[Left-Chiral set] of Foliate

7[(-4, -3, -2, -1)]

STATISTICS

The prevalence in the population is unknown, essentially because there is no agreement on the defining elements of the Disorder among practitioners.

INSIGHTS

Paroxysmal exacerbation of the Left-chiral set of the entire Foliate is chiefly responsible for the disorder. To this background, is adjoined an extra level of exacerbation of the partition set pertaining to Layer 7 of the Mental Foliate. The Left-chiral block of the Foliate accounts for the expression of sexuality as the main theme in the dysfunctional behavior: it is all around sexuality. The particular participation of Layer 7 as an independent superimposed current accounts for the self-victimizing characterizing the disorder. In this case, participation of Layer 7 is limited to its left-chiral partition group.

There is a huge controversy in psychology and psychiatry about the gender prevalence of masochism in general, and thus sexual masochism as well. Dr Eleanor Galenson, a member psychoanalyst of the New York Psychoanalytic Institute, opined in 1985: *"I'm one who feels that masochism is more prevalent among women than men."* Arnold Cooper at Cornell University Medical College instead believed that *"Masochism is not sexually differentiated. Masochism is present in men as well as women. Its cause is not biological, but rather, an aspect of development."*

Glenn Collins in the New York Times article **Women and Masochism: Debate Continues**[28] further writes:

"For women," Dr. Caplan said, "masochism has come to mean the presence of suffering rather than the enjoyment of it. This is a distortion that does damage to women because they believe the evil is within."

However, Dr. Natalie Shainess, a psychiatrist and psychoanalyst who practices in New York, defined masochism as "a group of personality traits based on self-contempt and based on fear of the power of others." She added: "These traits include passivity, dependence and usually the insufficient dissolution of the symbiotic tie with the mother."

Our psychophysics framework makes the firm prediction that women are more likely to suffer from this disorder because of the natural exacerbation of the passive left-chiral side of their Mental Foliates which at the same time defines their female gender or sexuation.

---

[28] The New York Times, Glenn Collins, December 2, 1985, Section B, Page 12

Voyeuristic Disorder

Voyeuristic Disorder (Peeping Tom) is a paraphilic disorder that involves intense and recurrent sexual arousal from observing unsuspecting and non-consenting naked individuals, while in the process of disrobing themselves or engaging in their own sexual activity. Voyeurs experience arousal from urges, fantasies, and impulses resulting from these activities. Official psychiatry requires VD to induce marked distress and social or occupational impairment and the patient to be at least 18 years of age. Voyeuristic activity under 18 years of age is considered normal and not criminalized in the law. *Voyeur* is a French word that means "seer", "watcher" or observer.

PASSIVE –RESPONSIVE SYMPTOMS

Intense sexual arousal from observing unsuspecting naked individuals in the process of getting undressed or engaged in sexual activity or sexually-explicit behavior. Accompanied with shyness, low self-esteem, loneliness, guilt or shame, subjective distress.

ACTIVE-REACTIVE SYMPTOMS

Memorialize and spy on unsuspecting individuals in private areas such as dressing rooms, locker rooms, bedrooms, bathrooms with the use of cameras and drones. Upskirting a woman without her consent by male voyeur. May be driven to other forms of similar sexual assault for arousal by observation. Onset of sexual fantasies and urges triggered by low-mood phases.

KNOWN VARIANTS

Frotteurism-Voyeurism: disorder which presents with both symptom sets.

LANGUAGE

Most expression in Voyeuristic Disorder is nonverbal, but language may exhibit depressive, anxious, or cyclothymic overtones.

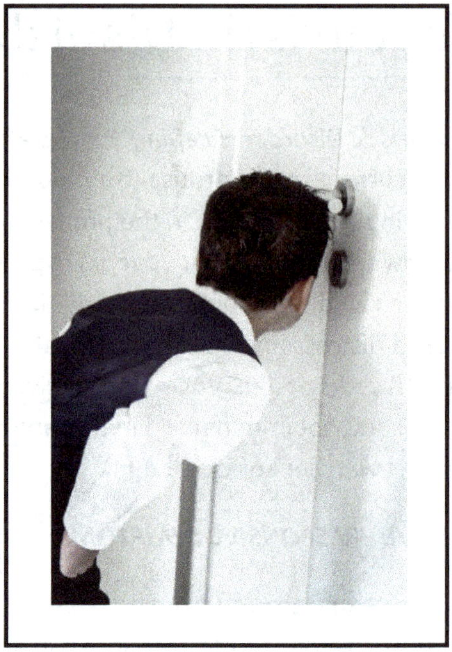

BEHAVIORAL FLIPS

Only in the variant *Frotteurism-Voyeurism* where the individual can flip between one dimension of the disease and the other.

DERIVED DISABILITIES

Substance misuse, sexual preoccupation, hypersexuality, criminal behavior associated with certain personality profiles. Internet pornography addiction (internet sexual addiction may pose a risk in vulnerable individuals with abusive trauma).

AWARENESS

Conscious (Neurotic disorder).

CHARACTEROLOGICAL FILIATION

N/A

QG LAYER-PARTITIONS

[Left-Chiral Side] overaccrued

2[(-4,-3,-2,-1)] or 7[(-4,-3,-2,-1)]

STATISTICS

13% men and 4% of women may be voyeurs.

INSIGHTS

The *Voyeur* must be considered to be someone who is so utterly passive psychogenically that in sexuality he has gone beyond the point of feeling pleasure from being acted upon but will be aroused by mere identification with someone he observes being sexually acted upon. Note that children who manifest curiosity by peep-holing their parents' bedroom to watch sexual activity do not qualify for voyeurism. We will also note that elder men who may engage in forthright private watch of live sex by compensation of age-related impotency do not qualify for voyeurism either, no more than anyone who circumstantially watches pornographic movies does.

This assessment is equally valid for voyeurism that involves simple observation of nudity for self-arousal. It invokes a marked preference for passiveness in the exercise of sexuality.

Analytically, the male voyeur suffers from gender identity disparity between the Mental Body and the biological body. Whereas in the case of a female voyeur, we are facing an exacerbation of the Anima Sector of the Foliate. When the symptom set of the disorder points to voyeurism as the one single dysfunction confronting the patient, whether male or female, Layer paroxysm, which is an inevitable, may well lie with Layer 2 of the Foliate which is canonically observational or perceptive. In the case of a nosology accusing *Frotteurism-Voyeurism*, Layer paroxysm most likely lies with Layer 7 of the individual's Foliate. From here, one can readily see why a masochistic component, originating from the left-chiral partition set of Layer 7, may be part of the disease as well, making for a pretty multi-faceted symptom set for these disorders. As a reminder, Layer paroxysm for morbidity is superimposed by 2 or 3 gradients over gender determination accrual. This framework sets the basis for clear analytic insight into another important stream of the intricate comorbidity predicaments so very much disparaging to analysts.

It is understood that, as some reports indicate, *Voyeuristic Disorder* may originate from an accidental sighting of someone who is naked, disrobing, or participating in sexual activity, and that repeated viewing may drive the subject to the point of pathological behavior. Psychogenically, all of this plays out on the representational substrata laid over the root pensive partitions which ultimately condition the normal and pathological responses of the Mental Foliate as prime factors.

Pseudocyesis (False Pregnancy, Phantom Pregnancy)

Pseudocyesis is a psychiatric condition in which a female displays a false belief of being pregnant. The belief is deemed false because she is clinically not pregnant with a fetus, even though signs of pregnancy may show up, such as back pain, breast changes, nausea and vomiting, interruption of menstrual periods, swollen belly, etc. A normal person that experiences these signs and is fully cognizant that no justifying act of sexual intercourse or artificial insemination has occurred will outrightly dismiss them as signs of an ongoing pregnancy. When in those conditions the belief of a pregnancy persists in the woman's mind, those beliefs qualify as delusional making her a mentally ill person. Several historical figures, such as Mary Tudor, struggled with this form of morbidity.

PASSIVE –RESPONSIVE BEHAVIOR

Weight gain or swollen belly. Nausea. Interruption of the menstrual period. Feeling of fetal movements. At times labor pains.

ACTIVE-REACTIVE BEHAVIOR

Irregular periods, breast changes, vomiting, constipation, appetite changes. Enlarged and tender breasts with changes in the nipples, and possibly milk production. Strong or persistent desire to have a child.

KNOWN VARIANTS

Non medical Amenorrhea.

LANGUAGE

The language is uncharacteristically rich in pregnancy themes.

BEHAVIORAL FLIPS

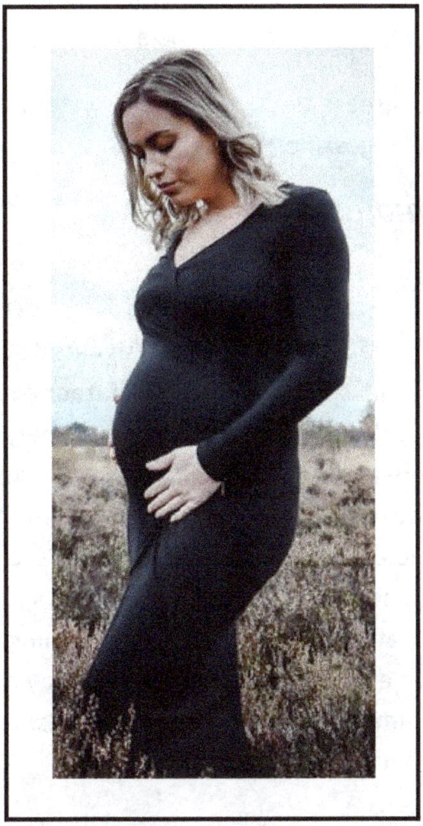

Mood swings from depressed to euphoric (same as those known in real pregnancy).

DERIVED DISABILITIES

Judgement may be so clouded that patient may demand an Emergency C section to deliver a non existent fetus.

AWARENESS

Unconscious (Neurotic disorder)

CHARACTEROLOGICAL FILIATION

Metamorphogenic

QG LAYER-PARTITIONS

5[(-1, -2, -3, -4) (+1, +2, +3, +4)]

STATISTICS

Pseudocyesis is very rare and affects women between 20 to 39 years of age. It can be found in both pre-menarchal and postmenopausal women, as well as in multiparous women.

INSIGHTS

In general, there is a preexisting psychological landscape in which Pseudocyesis develops. As a woman feels an intense desire to become pregnant, possibly owing to infertility, repeat miscarriages, an impending menopause, or a desire to get married, a Layer 5 already in accretion by character within the Mental Foliate may become so overaccrued that it psychosomatically potentialize the endocrine system to release the set of hormones that initiates the peculiar body alterations for pregnancy. Her body will then produce such pregnancy signs as a swollen belly, enlarged breasts, and even these sensations of pelvic fetal movement. The release of hormones (such as estrogen and prolactin) in that circumstance leads to the actual pregnancy symptoms.

This disease tightly relates to hysteria in its etiology. More details in our etiological exegesis for Hysteria.

PATHOLOGICAL AFFILIATE

Couvade Syndrome

Couvade Syndrome, also designated sympathetic pregnancy, is a proposed condition in which an expectant father experiences some of the same symptoms and behavior as the pregnant mother, his wife. Again, one has to discard cases where a real pregnancy of the wife exists, and the husband is reacting by sympathy to the wife's pregnancy experience or presenting with the symptoms due to biological exchange of secretions as regards to hormone-induced changes. In genuine cases, Couvade syndrome's symptoms most often include major weight gain, altered hormone levels, morning nausea, and disturbed sleep patterns. In more extreme cases, symptoms may come to include labor pains, fatigue, postpartum depression, and nosebleeds. The labor pain symptom is commonly known as sympathy pain.

It worth noting that there is a very large spectrum of symptoms that affected male individuals may exhibit, namely: stomach pain, back pain, indigestion, changes in appetite, weight gain, acne, diarrhea, constipation, headache, toothache, cravings, nausea, breast augmentation, breast growth, dry navel, hardening of the nipple, excessive earwax, and insomnia.

Etiologically, a Layer **5** in excessive accretion is prevalently the culprit. In cases where labor pains, cravings, and postpartum depression are sympathetically present, overaccretion at Layer **6** of the individual's Mental Manifold is likely to be the culprit, possibly owing to preexisting accretion by character at that Layer. The very heavy **Matrixial** characteristics of pregnancy in the loved one (wife), once internalized by the patient, would decisively contribute by sympathy (or identification) to the onset of symptoms of the kind in that affected husband.

Histrionic Personality Disorder

Histrionic Personality Disorder is characterized by constant attention-seeking, emotional overreaction or dramatization, and seductive behavior. People affected by this condition tend to overdramatize situations of life, at the risk of impairing their relationships in general, which frequently ends up leading them to depression. Flaunting exaggerated emotional displays as a matter of course, they lead others to believe that their acquaintances or relationships are more intimate than they really are. They are also highly suggestible in the sense of susceptibility to easy influence by others.

PASSIVE –RESPONSIVE SYMPTOMS

Exhibit excessive emotionality—a tendency to regard everything in life in an emotional manner. Constant attention seekers who feel uncomfortable or unappreciated when they are not the center of attention. Constant seeking of approval. Excessive sensitiveness to criticism, easily influenced by others. Habitual flirtatious and sexually provocative behavior. Rapidly shifting emotional states bearing the likes of shallow to others; Indisposed and discomforted when their attention- and attraction-seeking efforts meet indifference. Prone to depression when relationships fail.

ACTIVE-REACTIVE SYMPTOMS

Self-dramatization, and theatricality. Acting or looking overly seductive. Always want to be "the life of the party." Excessive concerns about their looks. Believe their relationships are more intimate than they actually are. Excess of showing in emotions, manners and physical appearance may come to embarrass others.

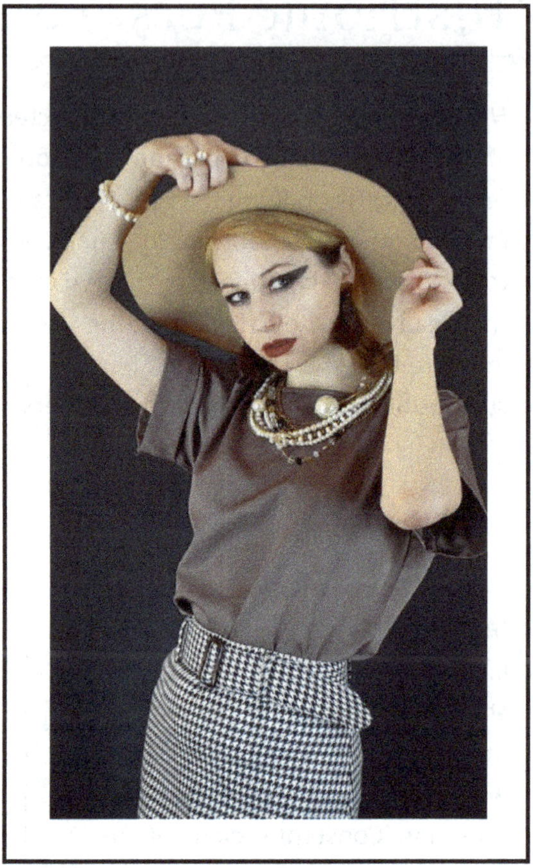

KNOWN VARIANTS

Millon identified the following subtypes: Appeasing, Vivacious, Tempestuous, Disingenuous, Theatrical, and Infantile.

LANGUAGE

Speech is dramatic, colorful, and impressionistic.

BEHAVIORAL FLIPS

Unknown

DERIVED DISABILITIES

Unable to properly handle relationships: Excessive public displays of emotion, such as embracing casual acquaintances with passion, sobbing uncontrollably over minor setbacks, or having temper tantrums.

AWARENESS

Conscious (Neurotic Disorder).

CHARACTEROLOGICAL FILIATION

None.

QG LAYER-PARTITIONS

[Left-chiral Sector] of Foliate

1 [(-1, -2, -3, -4)]

STATISTICS

The prevalence of Histrionic PD in the general population is 2-3%. Overwhelming in females within that segment of the population.

INSIGHTS

A notable overaccretion in the dynamics of the Left-Chiral Sector of the Foliate which normally determines female gender with one gradient of accrual is responsible for the Disorder. The attention-seeking, the incessant seductive behavior, the flirtatiousness are all female characteristics pertaining to the Left-chiral Sector of the Foliate. To the same account of the overly heightened Anima Sector go sufferers' high suggestibility and susceptibility to the influence of others, as well as their own seeking of treatment for depression upon relationship failures.

The self-centrism that has been noted in the nosology of this disorder is not a first-order quality but a result of the constant feminine attention-seeking and desire to attract. However, a legitimate Layer **1** contribution accounting for this trait is entirely plausible, since morbid single Layer overaccretion may also contribute to the patient's dysfunction.

The high prevalence of females in the population being affected by this disorder strongly advocates for our QG psychophysics attribution to an overaccrued Anima Sector of the Mental Foliate.

Narcissistic Personality Disorder

Narcissistic Personality Disorder (NPD) is characterized by a need and demand for attention, admiration and extreme praise, as well as a belief that the affected deserves special treatment above and beyond others. Often he/she holds an exploitative view of relationships. The condition also shows an inflated and unjustified self-regard, focus on being successful and powerful, a belief in one's superiority and an expectation of adulation. There is oftentimes a failure to understand the feelings or needs of others, and a display of arrogance in interpersonal interaction.

PASSIVE –RESPONSIVE SYMPTOMS

Infatuation with oneself about one's attributes. Entertain belief that they are more attractive and intelligent than everyone else. Identity issues, inflated self-esteem, focus on power and success. Need for attention, praise and admiration accompanied with lack of empathy.

ACTIVE-REACTIVE SYMPTOMS

Marked and unending interest in charming the other sex. Entertain charming strategies they exert time and time again with a propensity to manipulate. Tendency to exploit relationships and partner with others for the purpose of conquering the other sex. Arrogance in interpersonal relationships. Envious of others or belief that others are envious of them. Enraged when told they aren't beautiful or brilliant but indifference when told they are jerks. Bragging, refocusing the topic of conversation, making exaggerated hand movements, talking loudly, and showing disinterest by "glazing over" when others speak.

KNOWN VARIANTS

Grandiose (Overt) and Vulnerable (Covert). In the Grandiose subtype of NPD there is displays of self-importance, entitlement, fantasies of admiration. The vulnerable subtype tends more toward hypersensitivity to insult, self-criticism, feelings of shame, helplessness, and social withdrawal.

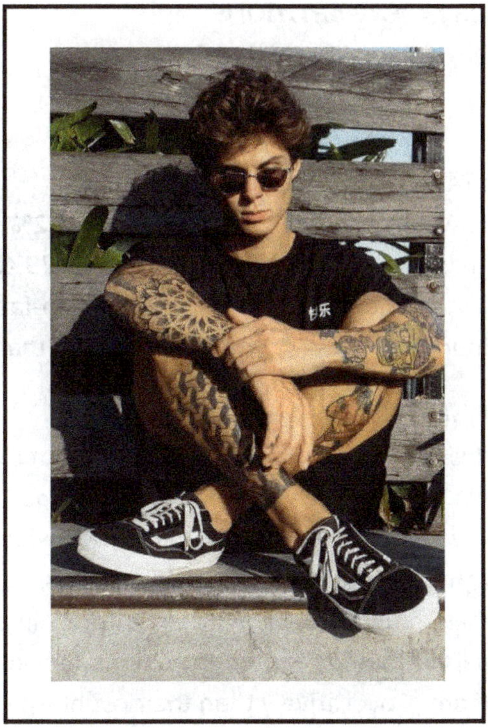

LANGUAGE

Men: talk loudly. Express disinterest in the mate of the moment to keep her hooked: *"Every three weeks or so I remind her that I continue to have options, and continue to choose her."* Women express their volatility and capriciousness: "*Not so fast! It's too early in the relationship for you to touch me like that,*" after a "*You have interesting eyes*".

BEHAVIORAL FLIPS

Unknown

DERIVED DISABILITIES

Inability to handle criticism, poor interpersonal relationships. Inability to handle long-term relationships, leaning toward short-term hookups and promiscuity.

AWARENESS

Conscious (Neurotic Disorder)

CHARACTEROLOGICAL FILIATION

None

QG LAYER-PARTITIONS

[Right-chiral Sector] of Foliate

6 [(+1, +2, +3, +4)]

STATISTICS

Prevalence varies between 1% and 6.2% of the population; it is more common among male in the proportion of 50-75%. Further, psychologist Frederick Stinson and colleagues conducted face-to-face interviews with 34,653 adults and found that men are more narcissistic than women across the lifespan.

INSIGHTS

It is important to note the high level of similarity between the nosology reported for *Histronic Personality Disorder* and that of *Narcissistic Personality Disorder*. The sexual orientation of behaviors in both disorders take common highlight in both repertories of symptoms. As reported in the nosology of NPD, both males and females take keen interest in charming the other sex as an unending part of their daily preoccupations. While female narcissists consistently dress more provocatively than their counterparts, male narcissists resort to displays of wit and braggadocio towards females — in other words, both narcissistic men and women engage at long last in time-tested sexual strategies. This sexual inclination is so strong in NPD that some psychologists, including Jonason and then graduate student Nicholas Holtzman of Washington University in St. Louis went so far to argue, in the evolutionism vein, that narcissism may have evolved as a strategy to secure short-term sexual partners.

The above leads us to several conclusions:

1. The plausibility that NPD symptoms in women are better reported to *Histrionic Personality Disorder* on account of the incessant and unmitigated trend to charming the other sex that make up Histionists' daily living, at the very least as a variant of HPD.
2. *Narcissistic Personality Disorder* may justifiably be considered the male version of *Histrionic Personality Disorder* on account of the high prevalence of Men over women in the distribution of the Disorder in the population.

3. The etiology of *Narcissistic Personality Disorder* strongly rests on an overaccretion of the Animus Sector of the Mental Manifold as the original male gender determinant of that Body and so deemed to register the over accrual triggering the dysfunction.

Note that while Histrionistic women may become anxious when their charms meet indifference or resistance, narcissistic men care little about being taxed jerks and take it as part of their quarry. An understandable distinction on account of the specific Sector of the Foliate that is hyperactive in each case. Again here in NPD, it is entirely plausible that an overaccrual by one of the nine Layers plays a role of second-order causal factor of the Disorder, in particular Layer 6, due to the high level of seduction trend demonstrated in the dysfunction.

Sadistic Personality Disorder

Sadistic or *Antisocial Personality Disorder* is nothing but sadistic behavior tered on the perpetration of cruelty from a deep propensity to harm others. In addition, sadists ordinarily exhibit habitual lying, use of different aliases to foul others and conning for personal profit. The subject is often totally indifferent to having hurt or mistreated others, or stolen someone else's property. This pairment is oftentimes accompanied with a total lack of remorse, and a complete inability to distinguish between good and bad. It is naturally difficult to apply this set of conditions to children due to the fact that they are still in velopment and have not reached the self-determination maturity required for this exhibit to fully apply. More in the ***INSIGHTS*** block.

PASSIVE –RESPONSIVE SYMPTOMS

ACTIVE-REACTIVE SYMPTOMS

Persistent lying or deceit to exploit others. Deep cynicism and open disrespect to others. Luring others through charm or wit strictly for personal gain or pleasure. Frequently violating the rights of others through intimidation and dishonesty. Frequent law-breaking criminal behavior. Hostility, significant irritability, agitation, aggression or cruelty towards people and animals demonstrated in killings and physical destruction. Unnecessary risk-taking or dangerous behavior that is inconsiderate of safety of self or others. Irresponsible habit of failing to meet financial or work-related obligations.

KNOWN VARIANTS
Pure Pyromania

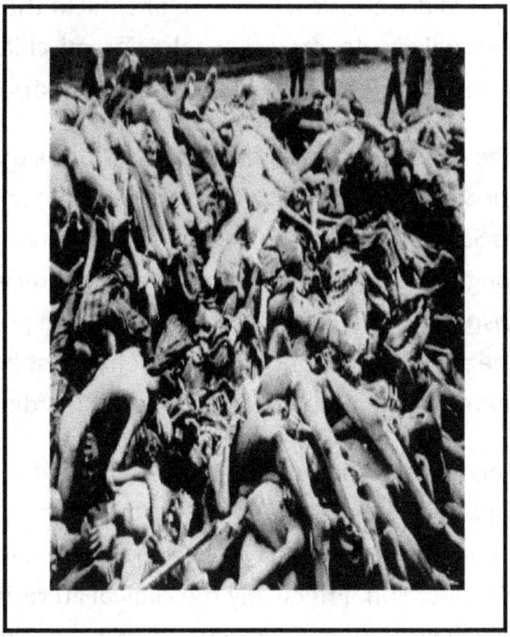

LANGUAGE
Use of slurs, negative and cursive statements, emotionally intense or charged vocabulary. Also inability to express love or intimacy.

BEHAVIORAL FLIPS
None

DERIVED DISABILITIES
Notable higher rates of suicide or homicide in this population. These patients become a burden to their families owing to frequent collateral substance abuse and unemployment.

AWARENESS
Unconscious (Psychotic Disorder)

CHARACTEROLOGICAL FILIATION
Paradoxical

QG LAYER-PARTITIONS
7 [(+1, +2, +3, +4)]

STATISTICS
Overwhelming in men (arsonists, serial killers, genocide executioners, etc.)

INSIGHTS
It must be noted that often the law traumatically seeks a difficult line of demarcation amidst responsibility criteria for applicable punishment to the affected youngsters. Responsibility criteria become in this case quite an equivocal ques-

tion to discern since children are still in the phase of internalizing social norms. Certainly acute impulsive behavior, mischievousness, excessive irritability and unjustified aggressiveness are forerunners of the disorder in young age.

The Quanto-Geometric norm of paradox that informs normal Layer **7** is the basis for *Sadistic/Antisocial Personality Disorder*. We have chosen to list this disorder as *Sadistic/Antisocial*, even though the term *Sadistic Personality Disorder* has long been deprecated in psychiatric medicine in favor of *Antisocial Personality Disorder*, because we recognize that the prevalent symptom of this disorder is the perpetration of Cruelty. Cruelty must be considered to be the axis that nucleates all the other directly related disorders as pathological affiliates.

This disorder has inarguably been one of the most controversial in psychiatry and psychology, because the slippery line between what appears to be one nosological set and another has left the science unable to establish proper lines of classification. Effectively the clinical literature offers a flourished line of labels which include, *Antisocial Personality Disorder, Sadistic Personality Disorder, Malignant narcissism, Psychopathy, Sociopathy,* etc. Several have been officially deprecated as previously mentioned but continue to be used by many professionals in practice and clinical literature[29], i.e. *Sociopathy, Psychopathy, Sadistic Personality Disorder,* etc.

In our sense, those discrepancies in classification are firstly due to a misunderstanding of the intimate pathological nature of the Disorder. The spectrum of exhibited symptoms very notably match the pensive states of *resentment, repugnance, wickedness,* and *fury* which form the right-chiral side of Layer **7** in our psychophysics framework. From our vantage, *Sadistic/Antisocial Personality Disorder* must be preeminently understood as a psychosis. Two key points to sustain this view are shortly discussed.

Most analysts agree that a psychopath does not have what they call *"a conscience".* He steals with no moral qualms whatsoever, only able to mimic or

---

[29]**Epidemiology, Comorbidity, and Behavioral Genetics of Antisocial Personality Disorder and Psychopathy**, Kimberly B. Werner1, Lauren R. Few2, and Kathleen K. Bucholz2, Psychiatr Ann. 2015 April ; 45(4): 195–199. doi:10.3928/00485713-20150401-08

feign being conscientious to avoid being identified or singled out. The sociopath knowingly has little of it. The cruelty that a sadistic person will display, such as that perpetrated by a cannibal or a body ripper assassin, undoubtedly shows this lack of conscience of sorts. It is in fact not so much a lack of conscience as it is an inability relating to the same kind of inflexibility ostensible in the expression of psychosis in general. At the height of these acts of violence or aggression, the individual is definitely in a second state that qualifies as outright hallucination.

The hallucination element constitutes the very reason why affected individuals are not able to see other human beings for what they are, kindred that is, and knowingly consider them as objects they can operate on or manipulate. Their coldness and inability to empathize spell out as a detachment resulting from the artifact of hallucinating. Those who have engaged in violent passionate crimes, such as dismemberment of loved ones, would argue in their defense that at the moment of the act they had *"lost their mind"*. We shall take them at their words. It is another way to speak of hallucination, or to express that they had lost contact with reality. These elements, who have engaged in high acts of murder, reportedly display *"disorganized thinking, hallucinations"*. It is important to understand that the hallucinatory component is always there even when what is visible is *"rage, resentment, envy, impulsivity and lability"* as reported, because the Modus Operandi is always a dystopic mental departure from reality. Lewis and Yarnell (1950) report these telling nosological details of pyromaniacs in their well-known study ***Pathological Firesetting***: *"The [psychological] reasons for the fires are unknown; ... These offenders are able to give a classical description of the* ***irresistible impulse****. They describe the mounting tension; the restlessness; the urge for motion; the conversion symptoms such as headaches, palpitations, ringing in the ears, and the* ***gradual merging of their identity into a state of unreality****; then the fires are set... Once they have started the fires, thrown the neighborhood into confusion, and are assured the fire engines are working, the tension subsides, and they can go home and drop into a peaceful sleep."*

Perhaps, one of the best ways to represent this pathological state is to picture a deeply inebriated person that hypothetically has not succumbed to psychomotor disequilibrium. He would be as such engaging cold headedly in all sorts of verbal and physical aggression towards others, loved ones and others, while hallucinating (seeing or hearing things that are unreal or projected – or unable to see physical reality for what it is) as known of the state of deep inebriation. In many cases, Sadists would denature reality and choose to believe – and attempt to lead others to believe – in what they originally knew as patently untrue, a behavior otherwise known as bigotry as well. And they end up believing in their own lies or their own fabrications. The operation of constructing a lie and ending up believing in it is a deconstruction or fictitious transformation of reality and represents an inner working of hallucination.

The level of paroxysm in the committed act of violence constitutes the barometer to gauge whether or not the individual has reached the point of hallucinating in his/her dysfunction. An arsonist responsible for burning down multiple neighborhood buildings is probably at a higher paroxysmal level in the disease than a so-called psychopath who has spent a lifetime "backstabbing" coworkers at the office, as vernacular language has it.

The different aforementioned labels that had been put forth thus far in the science for this class of disorder are not based on this significant underlying distinction, the distinction between neurosis and psychosis, that is. What official psychiatric science has done is identify a *personality* component in the disease which it believes has been perverted into *antisocial* behavior. From our psychophysics standpoint however, personality impairment is an active component of all mental disorders as previously discussed. No more so in sadistic impairment flares than it is, say, in Hoarding disorder. The litter resulting from the compulsion to keep everything and never trash anything is certainly a mark of personality that would make the social agent called the landlord loath to rent his properties to any such temper: clearly a personality disorder with inconvenient social consequences, which makes Hoarding no less of an *antisocial personality disorder* as well.

Once one understands the central role played by Cruelty in this sort of pathology, it is easy to aggregate the other nosological sets to the Sadistic root, primarily along the line of intensity of visualization and perpetration of cruelty as reflected in the distinction between neurosis and psychosis. The other level of distinction between those different forms of manifestation of the disease essentially relates to representations resulting from the individual's mental orchestration of parental and social interaction during the developmental phase of life. The state of Mind of an arsonist setting fire to acres and acres of wild life with clear intent to scathingly damage society is probably just plainly comparable to that of a heinous individual kidnapping minority ethnic people to hang them off tree branches. Hence, the distinction between one form of the impairment and the other in this case is not fundamental but secondary. Should one make this distinction a fundamental one, it will probably remain blind to the fact that the overwhelming majority of Sadists belong to the male gender, leaving the analyst unable to ever explicate or unravel the underlying reason. Our analytic line automatically elucidates this important statistical fact in identifying the disease as a paroxysm of the pensive states pertaining to the right-chiral side of Layer **7** of the Foliate, consistent with our definition of male gender.

We discuss the elements of a possible new nomenclature for this tree of disorders below.

PATHOLOGICAL AFFILIATES

Following is a comparative analysis between symptoms experienced by the group labeled Psychopath and the parallel group labeled Sociopath, in an attempt to elicit a new possible nomenclature.

PSYCHOPATHIC SYMPTOMS

Inability to form emotional attachments. Experience joy from aggressive and predatory acts. Ability to deceive people through charm and polished language. Skilled at gaining the eventual victim's trust. Display coolness and calmness with ability to carefully plan their crimes. Complete lack of conscience.

SOCIOPATHIC SYMPTOMS

Hot-headedness actively engaging in the exercise of violent acts. Show squint level of conscience and empathy. Less able to play along with ruse and treachery. Make it plain they're not interested in anyone but themselves. Often blame others and have excuses for their own behaviors and lacks.

While these differences may bear forensic significance, they are not fundamental from the psychological standpoint. Further, the two titles do not reflect the actual nature of the difference. A sociopath should be understood to commit crimes or acts of violence within the social order, such as a serial killer or a genocide executioner. A psychopath should be understood to commit crimes or acts of violence within the personal or family setting, a characteristic that is not reflected in the label. If somebody, unrelated by blood to a family, sets fire to an inhabited home with the intention of killing all the members of that family, that act should qualify as a social crime and fittingly the perpetrator a sociopath. If somebody within the same family should set the family home on fire in order to kill the other members of the family, the act should qualify as a private-setting crime and the perpetrator described with a qualifier for a compartmentalized setting (Sociopath Minor perhaps), not the psychopath label. The term psychopath is linguistically a descriptor for an impaired psyche incline to commit acts of cruelty. In order for anyone to qualify as a sociopath, you must be first a psychopath. Therefore, on that account alone, the parallel use of these two labels, justifiably deprecated officially since the advent of the replacement term *Antisocial Personality Disorder*, should also be clinically abandoned altogether.

Furthermore, it is quite difficult to establish a hierarchy line between Psychopathy and Sociopathy that is consistent with nosology. Because psychopaths are generally considered to lack all conscience, and even experiencing joy from aggression and dishonesty, one would tend to flag their impairment to be deeper than that of sociopaths. However, sociopaths are knowingly the ones who experience propensity to commit acts of high cruelty such as murders, which cannot stand second to psychopaths' lack of conscience and mischievous joy. Lastly we find no value whatsoever in the Malignant Narcissism label and summarily dismiss it.

In this context of classificatory impropriety, it becomes all the more sensible to review the known forensic categories and establish the psychological basis that leads to their specificities, given that the visualization and perpetration of Cruelty constitutes the true axis of this aggregate of impairments. We distinguish the following three classes of impairments based on reported nosologies for killers essentially.

Mass Destruction Sadist: Arsonist (pyromaniacs), Murderer of more than one individual at any one time, Member of a terrorist organization or unlawful militia, Executioner of a terrorist act, Genocide intellectual author, Genocide executioner, Head practitioner of death cults, Accessory to death cults. Means of killing or destruction are immaterial to the qualifier. Whether the offender has expectation to be killed in the acts, participates in the act by executing suicide, or not is irrelevant.

Some of the acts of cruelty or destruction perpetrated under this category of Sadism are familicide-suicide, suicide bombing, gang violence, classroom retaliation (against teacher or other pupils), disgruntled employee retaliation, and pseudo commando.

Spree Sadist: Executes a string of sadistic acts of the same kind or of different kinds at various different geographical locations without any cooling off period between the interventions, or execute successive sadistic acts of a different nature involving the same geographical location and the same victim. An illustration of the first case is a spree killer who murders a string of people in various locations without any cooling off period. An example of the second case is a rape murderer who rapes the female victim and then executes her by suffocation, gunshot, laceration or dismemberment, or a rape murderer who kills the female victim and then proceeds to rape her dead body.

Serial Sadist: Executes two or more sadistic acts of same or different nature one after another at different locations, and observing a time lapse between the interventions. An individual who repeatedly drowns his cars in the ponds around town in order to fraudulently collect vehicle insurance compensation most certainly belongs to this group. An arson occurring in a domestic violence case with the purpose of hiding another crime including murder and for financial gain is indeed an act or series of acts perpetrated by a serial Sadist.

Pyromania

Of pyromaniacs, Lewis and Yarnell further write:

"The majority of pyromaniacs, incidentally, start fires in their own neighborhood. With some the impulse asserts itself episodically with extended periods of "normality" intervening; with others, it controls them night after night; in either instance they almost always have to set a fire when the impulse appears. Such offenders will continue, each fire being a facsimile of the first, until a more powerful force, usually embodied in the "arm of the law," steps in and commands them to stop.

These are the mysterious "firebugs" who terrorize neighborhoods by going on solitary fire-setting sprees, often nocturnal, during which they torch off trash fires in one building after another without regard to property or life."

These pyromaniacs well fit our category of serial Sadists. Note that an important distinction between pyromaniacs and arsonists is that arsonists start fires for the purpose of revenge or vengeance, whereas pyromaniacs start fires for personal gratification. Pyromania is defined to be the madness with fire under an irresistible impulse or fascination with the same leading the subject to set damaging fires time and time again.

Epilepsy

Epilepsy is a neuropsychic disease mainly characterized by both seizures or loss of conscious awareness and muscular dysregulations such as convulsions. Some institutions have attempted to redefine the disease in order to reach a better working definition for clinicians. Said definition not enjoying universal consensus, it is best to simply consider that two unprovoked seizures are required for a diagnosis of an epilepsy syndrome. From our perspective, it is perhaps more significant to ensure that the purely psychic or psychogenic aspect of the ease is reflected in the definition, since it directly connects to our psychophysics etiological vantage of the syndrome. Further, there has been an inflation of types of the disease traditionally, which regrettably does not obey a clear rarchy principle, even though they may be factual manifestations of the disease. Such is the division of old distinguishing *petit mal* epilepsy and *grand mal* epilepsy. It is worth mentioning the intervention of EEG measurements as a support to specifc diagnoses since the reformist definition calls for an *"abnormal* (uncommon) *and excessive* (paroxysmal)" electrical discharge in the brain, as to whether *focalized* or *synchronously* spread throughout.

PASSIVE –RESPONSIVE SYMPTOMS

Odd feelings, perception of factitious smells and tastes, feelings of "out-of-body" separation, feeling detached, with people or situations looking strange. Transient seizures. Feeling oneself spacey, fuzzy. Absence: stopping of all activity and staring into space for a few seconds. Mental confusion and forgetfulness or memory lapses. Numbness, weakness, sleepiness, daydreaming episodes.

ACTIVE-REACTIVE SYMPTOMS

Jerking or convulsive movements of arm and leg pertaining to one side of the body. Tongue biting during convulsions. Incessant eye blinking and lip smacking. Feeling of electricity in part of the body. Tingling, falling. Sudden urination or defecation, and even ejaculation in male subjects during convulsions. At times, furious anger that may lead to unmotivated murder. Mouth foaming. Juvenile runaways.

KNOWN VARIANTS

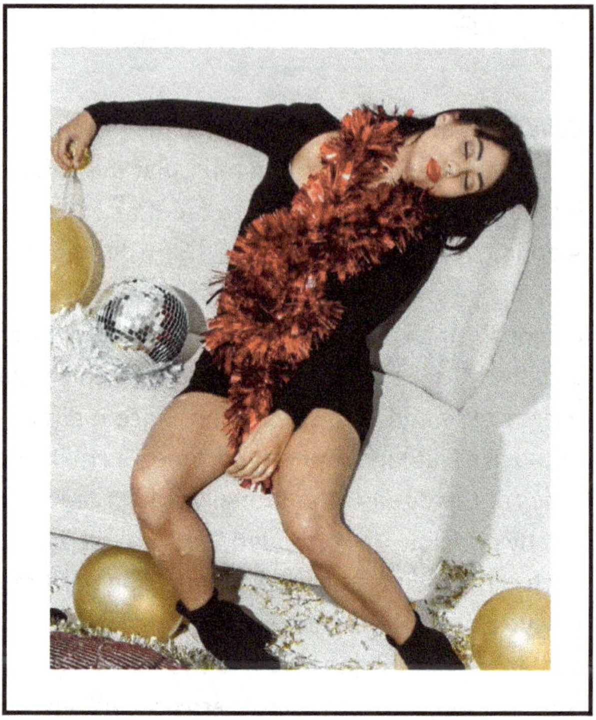

In reference to the Seizure type, the following variants have been identified: *Absence, Myoclonic, Atonic, Tonic,* and *Tonic-Clonic.*

In reference to the electric brain response, the following variants have been identified: *Focal, Generalized, Combined Generalized/Focal, Unknown.*

LANGUAGE
Language disturbance varies with seizure type, localization and severity. Difficulty in producing words, aphasia, comprehension issues.

BEHAVIORAL FLIPS
Alternations between seizure crises showing stare spells (absence seizures) and convulsive crises.

DERIVED DISABILITIES
At risk of physical injury, drowning, vehicular accidents, pregnancy complications. Bone breaking and head injury resulting from uncontrollable falls. Risks of reduced lifespan by sudden death. Psychosocial effects by reduction in employment opportunities and possibility of marriage.

AWARENESS
Unconscious (Psychotic Disorder)

CHARACTEROLOGICAL FILIATION
Asymptotic

QG LAYER-PARTITIONS

[Left-chiral Sector][Right-chiral Sector]
of Foliate at Ground 0
9 [(-1, -2, -3, -4) (+1, +2, +3, +4)]

STATISTICS

In the US, 1.2% of the population suffers from active *Epilepsy*.

INSIGHTS

Amidst the huge diversity of facts making up the general nosologic cadre of Epilepsy, singling out two important symptomatic trends of the disease will help us assertively probe its root causes. The developmental phases in which epilepsy mostly tends to occur is one such pointer, which we shortly address.

1.- Asexuation Causal Factor

The onset of epilepsy is knowingly most common in children (age 10 and younger) and older adults (age 60 and older). Therefore, it is fair to note that the disease tends to occur in an asexual developmental context, because in those two age brackets sexual life is naturally moot. For women, for instance, it tends to occur in a phase of life well removed from the reproductive cycle or well into menopause. At age 60, most men naturally experience significant reduction in sexual vigor both psychologically (libido) and physiologically (erection / ejaculation); those trends are further accentuated in the 70's in most cases. This takes us back to the mechanism of sexuation discussed in Chapter 2, in particular the consideration given to the quality of an asexual Mentation Foliate. Analytically, a man or woman age 75 i.e., by virtue of severe reduction of libido, has become identifiable or comparable to a little boy or girl who is completely devoid of sexual thoughts, despite the recognition of their belonging to a distinct sex group per body anatomy. Recent studies reveal the following astounding facts about male fertility in Epilepsy not only in the age-60 and over bracket but including males in their reproductive cycle:

"Epilepsy does have an impact on reproductive function and fertility. Statistically, men with epilepsy (MWE) have a disproportionately high risk of reproductive dysfunction, which manifests as diminished potency and abnormal sperm cha-

racteristics and can decrease fertility. Specific findings regarding reproduction and fertility among men with epilepsy include the following:

One study found that MWE were only 36 percent as likely as their male siblings without epilepsy to father a pregnancy.

In a study comparing sperm in healthy males to sperm in epileptic men, researchers found that all MWE—regardless of whether they were taking antiepileptic medications (AEDs)—exhibit abnormalities in the structure and function of their sperm far more frequently than do healthy males."

It is also a well known fact among epileptologists that Temporal Lobe epilepsy is linked to testicular endocrine dysfunction, libidinal dysfunction, affecting even the male epileptic's ability to recognize subtle cues from the sexual partner that are integral to establishing intimacy. The latter two are clearly symptoms of a psychological nature. However, overall these are deep correlational dysfunctions at the biological level that cannot be accounted for by psychosocial factors generally invoked in orthodox psychoanalysis or analytic psychology in general. They can only be elucidated in the psychophysics framework that we have postulated with the specific modus operandi of establishment of sexuation in the Mental Foliate. What we are seeing here is clearly a failure to establish, reach or maintain the Ground 1 level paroxysm at one chiral Sector of the Foliate, which is the expression of accomplished sexuation. The Foliate remains in a condition closer to the Ground 0 level, without a clearly defined chiral paroxysm of any binary Sector, a condition that expresses asexuality. It is a profound dysfunction of the psyche or Mentation Foliate.

This etiological proposition is further corroborated by the fact that in the maturation phase of sexuation kicked off by puberty, there is a trend to lesser onset of the disease in the population. Effectively, sexuation maturation with the development and exercise of secondary sexual characteristics (phase between adolescence and age 60) represents an added layer of intensity of sexual characteristics slated to palliate sexual hypoexpression or asexuation in the Mental Foliate. At this effect, note that the disease may optionally disappear entirely in affected children as soon as their pubertal development commences.

To the end, a statement like *"Epilepsy does have an impact on reproductive function and fertility."* is as inappropriate as inaccurate from our viewpoint. It is instead sexual dysfunction created within the Mental Body or Foliate that galvanizes the dysfunctional cadre observable in Epileptic disorder. Because it is so, we are deemed to see dysfunctional expressions specifically related to one or the other chiral group of pensive partitions of the Foliate, in particular a fast switching between one group and the other. On that account, the symptoms of Mental Confusion, which the left-chiral partitions of Layer 3 are responsible for, are part of the symptom set of epilepsy. Statistical studies reveal that the suicide rate among people with epilepsy is 5 times greater than that of the general population. Suicide is a masochistic act attributable to the left-chiral side of Layer 7, but it may be the consequence of a Layer 6 Depression alike through the Distress channel orthoflows. Since the epileptic syndrome covers that entire chiral side of the Foliate, suicide then becomes one of its manifestations. Unmotivated utter fear and anxiety, left-chiral partitions of Layer 7, equally join the palette of symptomatic manifestations of Epilepsy as precursors of every crisis. Daydreaming, a left-chiral Layer 5 pensive partition, reportedly participates in the syndrome as well.

At the right-chiral Sector, we have seen the exacerbation of the Partitions of Wickedness and Fury at Layer 7, when the epileptic furiously and impulsively attacks and kills somebody with no justification. The very characteristic convulsions are no more than the expression of Agitation as a generic response of the entire Animus Sector of the Foliate projected at the biological level. Muscular rigidness without convulsions, biting of the tongue, spontaneous orinating (Layer 7), defecating (Layer 7) and ejaculating (Layer 6) ought to be added to the same account of a generalized motivational commotion at the right-chiral side of the Foliate. The sensation of strangeness of self (alter-self), with people and situations feeling different, that is part of the aura preceding the crises, is a right-chiral Layer 5 production emanating from the partition of Reformism.

Before addressing the second major etiological stream of Epilepsy, it is important to highlight the fact that the same trend of depotentialization of male sexual and reproductive faculties and abilities has its counterpart in females as well. There is evidence that epilepsy may shorten the reproductive cycle of women in a particular strain of the disease, as an asexual push, forcing their menopausal phase to occur a decade earlier. This trend is particularly visible in women with catamenial epilepsy, those who experience a worsening of the seizures near the time of menstruation, that is. Furthermore, the very fact of symptom worsening during the reproductive period must be understood in terms of a diminishment of reproductive capacity, since those symptoms in their nature are slated to undermine any pregnancy. Concordantly, it is interesting to note that women who had a pattern of catamenial epilepsy were more likely to have fewer seizures after menopause, whilst showing more seizures during the period of changes just before menopause (perimenopause).

The asexual trend to depotentialize the epileptic female's reproductive faculties takes place in one of 3 different modus operandi:

1. In some women, seizures occur most frequently just before menstruation or during the first few days of menstrual bleeding, owing possibly to the fast drop in progesterone that occurs before menstruation in this instance. A reversal by intake of natural progesterone may even help with seizure control.
2. Other women experience seizures most frequently in the middle of their cycle, at time of ovulation, which is when there is a natural rapid increase in estrogen to stimulate ovulation at this time.
3. Some women have more seizures during the entire second half of their menstrual cycle, from mid cycle to the onset of menstrual bleeding. The seizures stop at the act of menstrual bleeding, the latter being a confirmation that the eminently female act of procreation will not occur. This pattern is usually seen in women with the potential to not ovulate at all and not produce, as they effectively don't, enough progesterone.

In conclusion, the asexual trend in the disease is indisputable. The fact that in its early onset, convulsions involve only one chiral side of the body is further indirect indication of the chiral character of the disease. In this case it shows an incipient sexual mark of the disease which will disappear in asexuation as the disease progresses and imposes the asexual trend.

2.- Important Causal Factor of Layer 9 Overaccretion

A brief visit to the necrology chapter in medicine is necessary in order to understand the nature of a subset of symptoms in epileptic syndrome. First, a recount of these particular symptoms.

1. Feelings of detachment or out-of-body separation
2. Feeling oneself spacey and fuzzy
3. Alterations of the sense of smell such as perception of factitious smells
4. Absence consisting in sudden stillness while staring vaguely into open space
5. Irregular loud breathing
6. Mouth foaming
7. Irregular muscle contractions, some resulting in convulsions
8. Irregular muscle distensions, resulting in downfalls and numbness
9. Temporary confusion and loss of consciousness
10. Non breathing after return of conscious awareness

There is some level of evidence that alteration of the sense of smell or perceptions of factitious smells may be a sign of imminent death. Dr. Jayant Pinto, associate professor of surgery at the University of Chicago, writes that the *"loss of the sense of smell does not directly cause death, but it's a harbinger, an early sign that something has gone wrong."* Dr. Pinto conducted a study involving 3000 patients from age 57 to 85 who were asked to identify 5 distinct scents in the primary class of odors (fish, leather, peppermint, oranges and roses), which led to the above conclusion while rejoining anecdotal reports on the subject. Symptomatic presence of alteration of the sense of smell with no known organic basis in epileptic syndrome is firmly indicative of a connection between epilepsy and clinical death. Now, let's follow through with a brief description of the process of agony, as commonly known in necrologic medicine.

The dying subject remains in a quiet flat laid down position whenever possible. There is a weakening of consciousness, with limbs getting colder and pale, while breathing becomes irregular. A state of confusion may occur preceding somnolence. Pharynx secretions lead to loud breathing, which may also be due to an atoning of the throat muscles. This sort of breathing causes the characteristic "rale de la mort", which an intervening change in position may diminish. The "rale de la mort" only continually occurs when the person is no longer able to acknowledge it. It may last hours and represents an indication that death is imminent. The pharynx secretions may become visible as mouth foaming off the lips.

When the agony happens to last longer, i.e days, the state of somnolence along with the accompanying mental confusion may vary in depth. It may alternate with moments of clearer wake or presence.

The very moment of death is accompanied with muscle contractions which may lift up the thorax, similar to breathing. After breathing has stopped altogether, it is possible that the heart may still beat for a few seconds. Some convulsions may equally appear thereafter. In some cases, a stare spell occurs at the moment of death, in particular if the person was keeping an interaction with someone at the bedside. The stare spell remains after the moment of death, requiring someone to close the deceased's eyelids.

One of the very sine qua non conditions of agony is immobility in a flat laid down position. It is of utmost import to recognize that what the muscular conditions within epileptic seizures are attempting to realize or mimic is the muscular condition that materialize the flat laid down condition of immobility in the process of agony. Muscular conditions in seizures are as follows:

1. Tonic seizures – Tonic seizures cause stiffening of the muscles. These seizures usually affect muscles in the back, arms and legs and may cause downfalls.
2. Atonic seizures – Atonic seizures, also known as drop seizures, cause a loss of muscle control, possibly resulting in sudden collapse or downfalls as well.
3. Clonic seizures – Clonic seizures are associated with repeated or rhythmic, jerking muscle movements, usually affecting neck, face and arms.
4. Myoclonic seizures – Myoclonic seizures usually appear as sudden brief jerks or twitches of arms and legs.

While the distinction in the set of muscles that affects body control in epilepsy may be useful to establish, the overarching insight must be that such muscular reactions are only a means to a pursued goal, which is agony posture adoption and necrological activity. We will let the reader compare and establish the similarity between our necrological description with the aforementioned subset of epileptic symptoms and the elements inherent to the process of dying. From the QG psychophysics perspective, the Transcendental Norm imbued in Layer **9** along with a paroxysmal level by the palette of partitions comprising that Layer are to be held responsible for the necrologic set of symptoms in the disease of Epilepsy. *Inanity, Cluelessness, Austerity*, and *Patience* indeed inform any of the epileptic phases. In particular, the partitions of *Inanition* and *Cluelessness* play a key role in developing the characteristic symptom subset of death. Everyone knows that the state of inanition may indeed ultimately lead to death. It is also the chief orchestrator of generalized immobility observable in the disease. The stare spells and the confusion in certain types of epileptic seizures are directly enacted by the partition of *Cluelessness*. During agony, the right-chiral partitions of *Temperance*, *Endurance*, *Resilience* and *Tenacity* are what guide the entire Mental Body through the process of Transcendentalization which we call Death. A discussion of these features would take us into the realm of Religious Traditions, which lay outside the original motivation for this publication. However, a brief evocation of a known fact from the annals of allopathic medicine may make the point.

During the infamous bloody period of the French Revolution, many of the condemned to the guillotine were asked to blink for as long as possible after decapitation, for medical investigative purposes. Some found the means to comply with the request as best they could, for as long as thirty seconds following the lethal strike, and one may wonder out of what resource or courage. Others went much beyond this call and cooperated with observers to implement specific reactions to stimuli following beheading. Dr. Beaurieux was one such observer in the case of a convicted murderer by the name of Languille, who was sent to the guillotine. Dr. Beaurieux interacted with him (or his head) after his execution at 5:30 AM on June 28th, 1905. From the ***Archives d'Anthropologie Criminelle***, here are Dr Beaurieux's observations:

Here, then, is what I was able to note immediately after the decapitation: the eyelids and lips of the guillotined man worked in irregularly rhythmic contractions for about five or six seconds ... I waited for several seconds. The spasmodic movements ceased. The face relaxed, the lids half closed on the eyeballs, leaving only the white of the conjunctiva visible, exactly as in the dying whom we have occasion to see every day in the exercise of our profession, or as in those just dead. It was then that I called in a strong, sharp voice: 'Languille!' I saw the eyelids slowly lift up, without any spasmodic contractions ... Next Languille's eyes very definitely fixed themselves on mine and the pupils focused themselves ... After several seconds, the eyelids closed again, slowly and evenly, and the head took on the same appearance as it had had before I called out. It was at that point that I called out again and, once more, without any spasm, slowly, the eyelids lifted and undeniably living eyes fixed themselves on mine with perhaps even more penetration than the first time. Then there was a further closing of the eyelids, but now less complete. I attempted the effect of a third call; there was no further movement and the eyes took on the glazed look which they have in the dead.

I have just recounted to you with rigorous exactness what I was able to observe. The whole thing had lasted twenty-five to thirty seconds."

Talk about courage, resilience and perseverance. It is important to keep in mind that death is not a prime act of destruction but a prime act of Transcendence as far as the Mental Foliate is concerned. Destruction of the biological body as a QG Phenotype is an after-runner of the successive major events taking place during the process of Death. Despite the fact that death in real life may occur accidentally, Death is not an accident of Life but a function of Life. At this effect, it is opportune to remember the following fact which many practitioners well know. The terminal phase of many illnesses may be punctuated by episodes of severely increased gravity. These episodes are oftentimes followed by a period of improvement. In general, and very importantly so, death will occur as the end stage of a worsening stretch following a duly developed improvement or stability period. In other words, the body and the Foliate prepare themselves for the event or function of Death, the event of Transcendentalization that will be taking place, that is. The Mental Body or Foliate orchestrates it through the resources of the Asymptotic Mentation Layer (Layer 9).

Yet one may wonder whether what occurs in Epileptic Disorder is an enactment or simulation of the process of Death or Agony, or a real implementation of the process without reaching the point of culmination or complete departure of the Foliate Body. Two possible outcomes of the syndrome unequivocally answer this question. For one, the condition known as *Status Epilepticus*, a state of continuous seizure activity lasting more than five minutes, or frequent recurrent seizures without regaining full consciousness in between, creates the real risk of permanent brain damage and clinical Death. On another count, Epileptic dysfunctions also create the risk of so-called *SUDEP (Sudden Death in Epilepsy)*, whose cause remains totally unknown. The specialists believe that patients with frequent tonic-clonic seizures may be at higher risk of *SUDEP*. It is estimated that overall about 1 percent of all people with epilepsy die of *SUDEP*.

We shall also remind the reader that what causes the death-oriented Epileptic syndrome is an exacerbation of the paroxysm at Layer 9 bringing it to the psychotic level.

Our psychophysics etiological perspective calls for a rekindling of the taxonomic order hitherto adopted for the many variants of Epilepsy. The classification must be inspired by the two major etiological trends above discussed for the syndrome.

One last but not least important remark. From a strict psyschophysics perspective, a dimension of intra-layer analysis, which in this treatise we do not engage, would bear the fact that the course of epileptic disease responds to the mathematical derivative of the Life Function *V(r)* (Fig. 2.1) expressed as *d(V)/dr*. Very specifically, the disease tends to occur in lifecyle phases where the derivative *d(V)/dr* is at a very low gradient, which , per the graph, corresponds to infancy and elderly phases of life as characterized along the *r-axis*. This mathematical characterization applies to intralayer dynamics, and puts our etiological analysis on an even more rigorous basis.

Alzheimer's Disease

Alzheimer's Disease is one of the most common causes of so-called Dementia, amounting to up to 70% of the cases of disorder under this label. The term Dementia is from the French word *"Démence"* for Demented which is an inauspicious term in disuse in francophone psychology. As applied to *Alzheimer's Disease*, the term has been restricted to mean both a neurodegenerative disorder and a psychological clinical syndrome characterized by progressive deterioration of the cognitive function. The decline in cognition significantly affects patients' personal daily activities (driving, shopping, housekeeping, cooking, managing finances, and personal care) and interactive social functioning alike.

PASSIVE –RESPONSIVE SYMPTOMS

Severe memory impairment, difficulty recalling date, events, time and place (i.e. inability to recognize where they are and how they got there), personal information, especially newly acquired information. Aphasia (difficulty finding words or making sentences). Deficits in visuospatial functioning (inability to recognize objects and faces). Confusion, disorientation, mood changes. Unfounded suspicions about family, friends and professional caregivers. Delusions. Behavior may elicit fear, anxiety and signs of being depressed. Cortical brain cell inactivity and degeneration, with neural circuit inhibits.

ACTIVE-REACTIVE SYMPTOMS

Endlessly repeat statements and questions. Difficulty speaking, swallowing and walking. Executive functioning impairment (planning, decision making, reasoning). Decreased ability in praxis or purposeful movements. Endless wanders in open spaces and getting lost in familiar places.

KNOWN VARIANTS

Lewy Body Disease, Fronto-temporal Dementia, Dementia due to Parkinson's Disease, Dementia due to hippocampal sclerosis. Dementia due to Cerebrovascular disease.

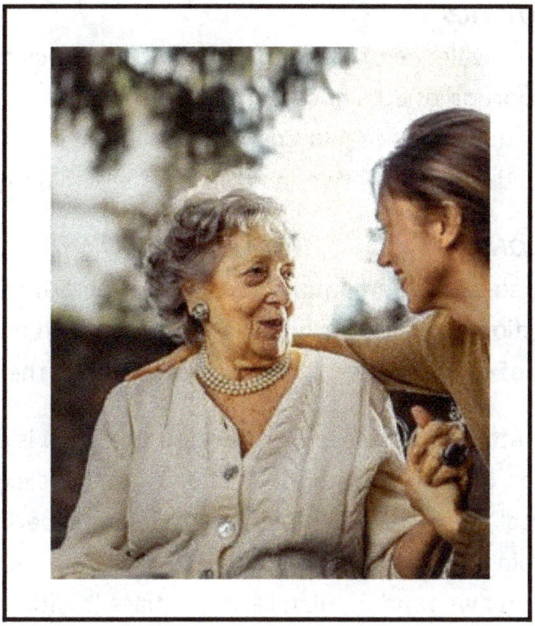

LANGUAGE

Aphasia, difficulty with structured sentences. Repetition of words or sentences. People who are bilingual show signs of Alzheimer's later by 4.5 years in comparison to people who speak only one language.

BEHAVIORAL FLIPS

Reported changes in mood fits, presumably implicating one par to the other.

DERIVED DISABILITIES

Balance issues, slow movement, shakiness, stiffness, difficulty attending to activities of daily living such as toileting, eating, coughing, choking, propensity for infections, death.

AWARENESS

Unconscious (Psychotic Disorder): Most do not acknowledge own intellection disability.

CHARACTEROLOGICAL FILIATION

Archetypical

QG LAYER-PARTITIONS

[Left-Chiral Sector] of Foliate

9 [(-1, -2, -3, -4) (+1, +2, +3, +4)]

STATISTICS

The prevalence of Alzheimer's disease is much higher among females in the proportion of 80% of cases. Only in the US there are 5 million Americans living with this disease. Mild Cognitive Impairment (MCI), a syndrome which is situated clinically between normal aging and dementia has a prevalence of 3-24%.

INSIGHTS

This so-called dementia disorder must be primarily understood as an attempt to functionally freeze or hibernate the brain, on one hand, and on the other, a result of overaccretion of the Anima Sector of the Foliate.

The attempt to freeze or hibernate the brain is a Layer **9** determinant at first order, consistent with the trait of asymptotic expansion subsumed in the typological nature of the Layer. The notion of Hibernation is our common way of describing the process of "end without end", although, as an end, in culture in general we tend to mistakenly conflate it with the state of Death or disintegration. We have amply discussed Death in the analysis of the epileptic syndrome and stated that it is in fact a process of transcendentalization essentially. Hibernation is a close parent, if not the same process under a different lens. Perhaps the state of Lethargy may make for the common denominator between the two concepts. Far from a casual fact, statistical psychopathology reveals that a vast majority of patients affected with Alzheimer's syndrome are in the elderly phase of their lives, the serial or infinitesimal ending phase of life. It is an overaccretion in the dynamics of the Layer **9**'s pensive partitions eliciting the above qualities that is going to plunge the Mind into this expansive and expctant storm, as one major etiological component of Alzheimer's disease.

On that account, the quality of mentation itself becomes infinitesimal, taking the likes of a freeze or sclerosis, leaving the content of Mind with something expressible as no more than a behavioral-pensive vector, so to speak. In other words, there is not a lot of "thoughtfulness" or thoughtful content in the pensive partitions of *Inanity* or *Austerity* for instance, when stretched out in excessive accretion. In general, this expectant aspect of the Norm at Layer **9**, in all cases of the disease, becomes intimately responsible for the very difficulty in eliciting thoughts and language expressing thoughts as a major symptom of Alzheimer's disease. The hibernating freeze of mentation is also expressed in a thinning of the very mnemonic faculty, which appears as another striking symptom of the disease. One must understand, however, that memory as a whole in its distribution throughout the psychic Foliate, in all of its capacities – storage, registration, recall, etc. – remains unchanged. It is the overall thinning of intellection that impairs the mnenomic faculties at an accrued Layer 9 in the disease. One might simply say that memory there and then hibernates.

The expectant tendency to freeze or hibernate subsumed in the Layer 9 Norm of the Foliate is even expressed at the neurological level. Effectively, in Alzheimer's Disease cortical and neocortical neurons fill up with Lewy bodies and beta-amyloid molecules forming detectable plaques, while tangles build up within the interstitial neural medium. Tangles and plaques are all assumed to block communication between contiguous neurons, effectively freezing the neural circuits. Neurologists tend to believe of late, as more research develops, that inhibition of interneuron communication stands for a major causal factor of the disease. In our sense, the partition of *Inanity* is to be held chiefly responsible for the orchestration of the indicated neural developments, either by projection onto the biological map or correlatively with the latter.

In the same analytic vein, one may observe that the Left-Chiral partitions of Layer 9 accuse an expectant state of the Mind more than the Right-Chiral ones do, i.e. *Resilience* or *Tenacity* vs. *Inanity*. But because this tendency is more accused at the chiral Anima side of the Foliate as a passive-responsive quality, it gives women more extensive longevity over men, per the psychopathological statistics related to the disease. This outcome is easy to understand when we remember the accretion role played by the Left-Chiral partitions in female sex determination. What's more, the entire Left-Chiral Sector of the Foliate plays an eminent role in the disease as well, which we will shortly address.

Overaccretion of the Anima Sector of the Foliate is visible in many symptoms that are rooted on many different mentation Layers at that chiral side. Notably, confusion, disorientation, mood flashes, paranoid suspicions about family, friends and professional caregivers, in addition to behaviors that elicit fear, anxiety and signs of being depressed, as reported in the nosology section. This etiological aspect of the disease, as indicated earlier, readily explains why women are so overwhelming prone to be affected by this disorder in comparison to men, evidently on account of a Foliate that is already in accretion in its Anima Sector. Some clever researchers have found that the reason why more women are tabulated affected with the disorder than men is due to their longer longevity with respect to men. Granted them this conclusion, they would then have to explain in turn the possible reasons why women live longer than men. Matter-of-factly, it is the intersection of two clear etiological factors that lead to this outcome, from our analytic perspective: accrued *Asymptotization* from the Layer 9 Norm leading to hibernation processes and agency of the Anima Sector of the Foliate.

Finally, the impairment that stirs *Alzheimer's* patients to repeat acts of life or redo things over and over again goes on account of the trend to extensiveness or prolongation that is notable in the Layer **9** Norm of Asymptotization and keenly transpires in the right-chiral partitions of the Layer, namely *Temperance, Endurance, Resilience,* and *Tenacity*. Their forever wandering in open space through city streets, which is usually construed as being geographically lost and not knowing where they are, obeys the same subjacent instigating motivation.

Suicidal Obsession

Suicidal Obsessions are underrepresented and are generally classified as an Obsessive-Compulsive Disorder. They are ego-dystonic in nature and bear an sive character. The patient finds himself or herself with these recurrent and ending thoughts of death or self-harm, occurring time and again throughout the day. Whilst some individuals visualize outright suicidal acts, others experience recurrent thoughts involving self-injury or self-mutilation. These obsessions may occur spontaneously, seemingly out of nowhere, or may be triggered by unpleasant activities. Even pleasant activities may lead the patient to this slant of morbid thinking.

PASSIVE –RESPONSIVE SYMPTOMS

Fear of committing suicide (i.e. fear of slitting one's wrists, hanging oneself, or overdosing on medications). Fear of jumping off of a building or another high place. Fear of stepping out into oncoming traffic and being hit by a car. Fear of jumping in front of an oncoming train or subway. Fear of grabbing hot pans or stove burners. Fear of driving off bridges or intentionally crashing head on into other vehicles. Fear of intentionally disfiguring one's face with a curling iron. Fear of intentionally crushing one's car or oneself under the garage. Even fear of becoming depressed and then feeling compelled to commit suicide.

ACTIVE-REACTIVE SYMPTOMS

People with suicidal obsessions do not actually want to act or make good on their thoughts. Else they may be unsure about whether they "really" want to act on their thoughts. Projective thoughts such as "what if I pickup that knife and slit my throats" may show up as well.

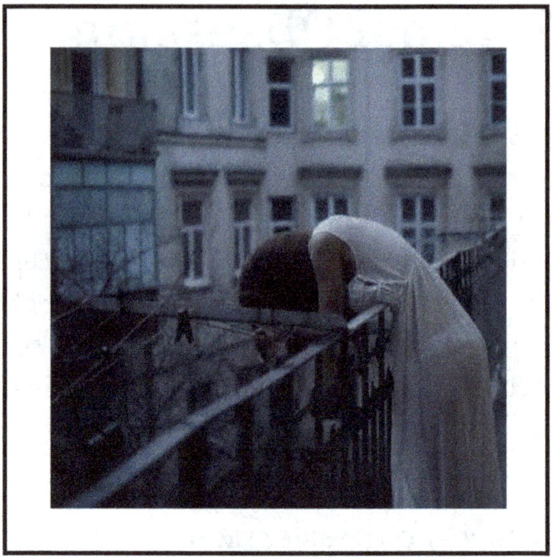

KNOWN VARIANTS
N/A

LANGUAGE
Language mainly bears anxious prosody.

BEHAVIORAL FLIPS
Unknown

DERIVED DISABILITIES
At risk of ultimately committing suicide.

AWARENESS
Conscious (Neurotic Disorder)

CHARACTEROLOGICAL FILIATION
Paradoxical

QG LAYER-PARTITIONS
7 **[(-1, -2, -3, -4)** (+1, +2, +3, +4)**]**

STATISTICS
No specific data allegedly due to comorbidity with other disorders.

INSIGHTS
The Quanto-Geometric Destruction norm that informs normal layer **7** is the basis for *Suicidal Obsession* Disorder. There is an amalgam of terror, fear, anxiety and perplexity imbued in the suicidal obsessive ideation spurred by the Left-Chiral side of the Foliate. The Right-Chiral partitions participate in the morbidity in terms of eliciting 1) an avoidance of lethal objects and 2) projective thoughts about harming oneself.

While some individuals may truly fear acting on the self-occurring suicidal thoughts (i.e., actually killing or harming oneself), others fear the moral or spiritual implications of simply having these unwanted thoughts calling for suicide or self-harm. For instance, some people feel disturbed by thoughts that qualify them as "bad," "evil," or "sinful" people. Others fear that thoughts of committing suicide may signal something in the works that is dangerous to their good health, such as the onset of depression, schizophrenia, or other types of terrible mental illness.

Suicidal obsessions may become explicit as projective thoughts of harming oneself. They manifest in such thoughts as "What if I lose control, pick up that knife, and kill myself" or images such as mental scenarios focusing on self-harming behaviors like cutting, shooting, hanging, or medicine overdosing. Regardless of the form, in many cases, suicide and self-harm obsessions are accompanied with pseudo-analytic cogitations, the likes of "What if I secretly want to follow through on these thoughts?"

It is important to make a distinction between suicidal obsession as a disorder in its own right and other forms of morbidity in which suicidal thoughts are present, i.e. the depressive phase of Bipolar Disorder. Except for masochism, the instigation to the suicide act is a function call originating from other Layers of the Mentation Foliate to right-chiral Layer **7**. In Bipolar Disorder i.e. it is the intense feelings of misery and despair at Layer **6** that trigger such calls through the conscious rationale that life is consequentially no longer worth living. In those cases the determination to execution of the act is pretty straightforward, which may drive the subject to repeated attempts of suicide should they factually fail for one reason or another. Also note that in those instances the motivation for self-mutilation is not there either, as it generally is in Layer-**7**-triggered impulses, thereby demonstrating that the visualization of suicide is directed to solely putting an end to the unbearable enduring of sufferings (Left-Chiral Layer **6**).

In other cases where the call to suicide is impulsed by Layer **7**, such as Masochism or Sado-Masochism, the compulsion to self-destruction is pugnant, and further consciously experienced as an inner irresistible drive to commit the act for itself, and thrillingly so. In this case, the function call directly originates from Layer **7**.

In Suicidal Obsession Disorder, the right-chiral call to commission of the act is at its lowest level, being at the level of a projective figuration. It is thus fair to conclude that the compulsive aspect is weak in this Disorder, or missing altogether, whereas the obsessive aspect is highly prominent. We understand that compulsion is Active-Reactive in nature whereas obsession is Passive-Responsive in nature.

Body Dysmorphic Disorder

Body Dysmorphic Disorder or *Dysmorphophobia* is a psychiatric disorder described by Morselli in the late 1800's and in which the preoccupation with an imagined or slight real physical defect causes significant distress. The preoccupation with the appearance is judged excessive since the defect may not even be noticeable to other people. Despite the alternative label of Dysmorphophobia, the disease is not an authentic phobia.

PASSIVE –RESPONSIVE BEHAVIOR

Hours agonizing about their looks in what appears to be an obsession with their appearance. Some realize they look worse to themselves than to others and that their view of their appearance problem is exaggerated and distorted. Others are convinced of the accuracy of their view of that physical "defect" in their body. Mistaken feeling that other people are taking special notice of their "defect" by staring at it, making fun of it or laughing about it subreptitiously. Feelings of shame and fear of being rejected by others due to their supposed "defect".

ACTIVE-REACTIVE BEHAVIOR

Constant lengthy appearance checking in the mirror for an "imagined" or minor physiognomic defect. Frequent gauging of their appearance against others or images in magazines or billboards. Hours of "grooming" themselves by applying make-up, changing clothes or re-arranging their hair to "correct" or cover up the "problem". Camouflaging or hiding their supposed defect by wearing a hat, a wig or sunglasses. In extreme cases, some wear a mask or hood over their head, or acting or standing in a certain way in public to mitigate the "defect". Others weigh or measure themselves continually or wear big and baggy clothing to hide perceived "huge" hips or large breasts. Habit of wearing many layers of clothing to appear larger or more muscular. Some men (especially those who suffer from "muscle dysmorphia") lift weights or exercise excessively to bulk up. Mistakenly seek cosmetic surgeons or dermatologists for surgery or medical treatments to do away with their body problem.

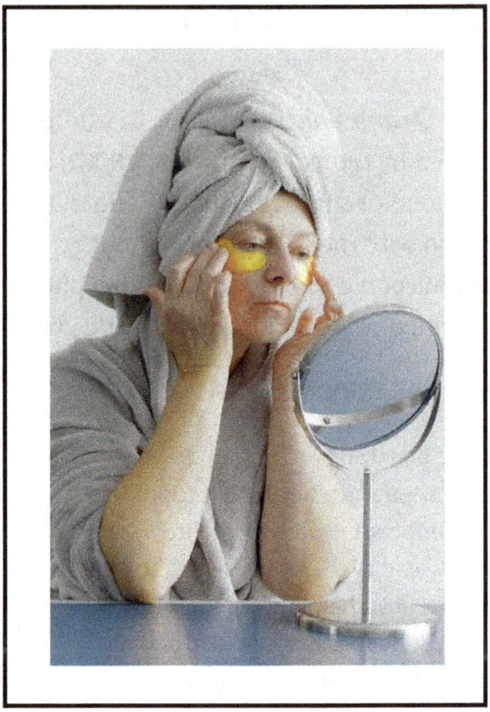

KNOWN VARIANTS

Muscle Dysmorphia, Body Dysmorphic Disorder by Proxy.

LANGUAGE

Language focuses on magnifying the perceived body "flaw" and elicits anxiety.

BEHAVIORAL FLIPS

From Despair and Self-Pity about their perceived "flaw" to seeking others' Sympathy by attempting to convince them of the ugliness of the perceived "flaw" or obtaining from them a graceful acknowledgement of their "flaw".

DERIVED DISABILITIES

Social isolation due to fear of embarrassment by going to school or work. May become depressed with suicidal thoughts due to desperation about their "defect". Dysfunctional dating and avoidance thereof. May bear multiple scarring due to repeated or multiple cosmetic and other surgical procedures.

AWARENESS

Conscious (Neurotic Disorder)

CHARACTEROLOGICAL FILIATION

Matrixial

QG LAYER-PARTITIONS

6 [(-1, -2, -3, -4) (+1, +2, +3, +4)]

STATISTICS

Body Dysmorphic Disorder has a general population prevalence of 1.7-2.9%.

INSIGHTS

The Quanto-Geometric Norm of Harmony that informs normal Layer **6** is the basis for Body Dysmorphic Disorder. There is a clear quest for beauty, attractiveness and seduction in that preoccupation about a small or imaginary defect, as pertains to the right chiral partitions of Layer **6**. The frenzy of special diets and unnecessary procedures are nothing else but a constant attempt at garnering admiration and an unwavering desire to trigger passion.

It would also appear that a small or innocuous body defect functions as a pretense or alibi for the unleashing of autogenic and excessively intense feelings of despair, self-pity and sadness that equally characterize the morbidity in Body Dysmorphic mentation. Such feelings unmistakably originate from the Left-chiral partitions of Layer **6**.

Dependent Personality Disorder

Dependent Personality Disorder (DPD) is a life prevalent disorder characterized by a specific form of distortion of interpersonal relationships. Dependency is a naturally occurring experience in society by virtue of the universal need to seek guidance, approval and support, in particular during times of weakness. Anytime such a need is accompanied with high levels of persistent distress or negatively affects one's ability to function as expected by most others in interpersonal relations, an underlying psychopathology is likely to present requiring a diagnostic probe.

PASSIVE –RESPONSIVE SYMPTOMS

Preoccupation with relationships, fear of abandonment and rejection. Feelings of powerlessness. Constantly seeking closeness and intimacy. Preoccupations with attachment resulting in feeling uncomfortable alone. Lack of self-confidence causing difficulty starting projects. Tendency to belittle their own abilities. Witholding or refraining from expressing disagreements with others by reason of need of empathy. Given to rely on others for self-care. Unrealistic expectation of being left alone to take care of themselves while being presumably unable to.

ACTIVE-REACTIVE SYMPTOMS

Difficulty managing interpersonal boundaries. Tendency to develop relationship ties. Search for empathy resulting in difficulty making decisions without advice and reassurance from others. Abdicate own responsibility for the satisfaction and discharge of their personal needs and flip it to others. Willingness to go to great lengths to obtain support, empathy or admiration by others (i.e. discharge unpleasant tasks, tolerating abuses, etc.).

KNOWN VARIANTS

Passive-aggressive and Counter-dependent.

LANGUAGE
Difficulty expressing disagreement, anxious prosody.

BEHAVIORAL FLIPS
Unknown

DERIVED DISABILITIES
Passivity, docility, relationship problem. Proneness to abuse tolerance.

AWARENESS
Conscious (Neurotic Disorder)

CHARACTEROLOGICAL FILIATION
Matrixial

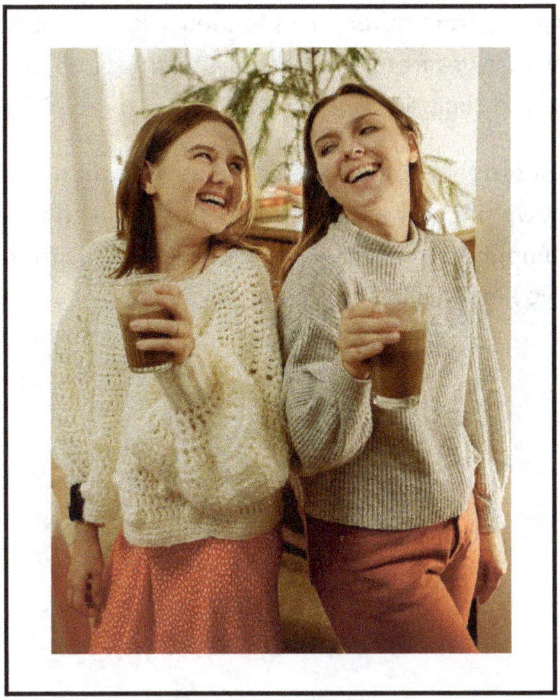

QG LAYER-PARTITIONS
6 **[(-4, -3, -2, -1) (+1, +2, +3, +4)]**

STATISTICS
Prevalence of DPD is less than 1% in the population. Diagnosed more often in women, but in some studies, prevalence figure is the same for both sexes.

INSIGHTS
The Quanto-Geometric Norm of Harmony that informs normal Layer **6** of the Foliate is instrumental in developing the behavior seen in DPD symptoms. There is a certain prevalence of the symptoms rooted in the Left-Chiral partitions over the Right-Chiral ones. It is also notable that the most active partitions are located center-left and center-right of the distribution on the Layer. These pensive partitions overall percolate into behaviors that somewhat indirectly express the mentation primitives innate to the former, instead of an outright visible expression of the primitive. There is a great need to *fit* or *couple with* manifest in the search for empathy, sympathy and admiration to some extent, as well as inspir-

ing pity from others. This tendency is evidenced in their inability to extricate themselves from doomed partnerships and prefer malingering in them as observed clinically.

Consequently, the nosological demarcation of this disease is clear from the viewpoint of the Mentation Foliate Map and shall not yield to comorbidity assumptions. In particular, the association with the so-called Obsessive Compulsive Personality Disorder should be avoided.

Authoritarianism

Authoritarianism is primarily viewed as a syndrome in which a person displays behaviors stirred by tyrannical impulses. The subject is obsessed with control of others, imposes personal rules and might even willfully cooperate with authorities to enforce social rules and norms. He/she exercises aggression toward those who violate the imposed norms, shows an ostensible lack of compassion, while holding stereotypic or superstitious beliefs in general in relation to those norms and rules. These subjects might even go to the extra lengths of using firearms to keep their spouses under control with threats or punish other loved ones for ever showing weakness to others.

PASSIVE –RESPONSIVE BEHAVIOR	***ACTIVE-REACTIVE BEHAVIOR***
	Power craving, urge for domination, discrimination and offensive behaviors. Intolerance for members of other social or ethnic groups. Urge for surpassing in competition everyone else. Aggressive tendency for leadership, yet with simplistic reasoning. Use scare tactics to dominate and subdue people. Promote a culture of fear, prejudice, and rigid thinking. Prone to impose rules on other people which they do not abide by. Always alert for an opportunity to punish someone, especially family members.

KNOWN VARIANTS

Non coercive forms of Domination or Disguised Domination: use of drama and excessive affection and care to cover up the compulsion for control.

LANGUAGE
Language displays cynicism, explodes and strikes out in abusive bursts. Insults and threats telling people "they would never amount to nothing" or "be anything".

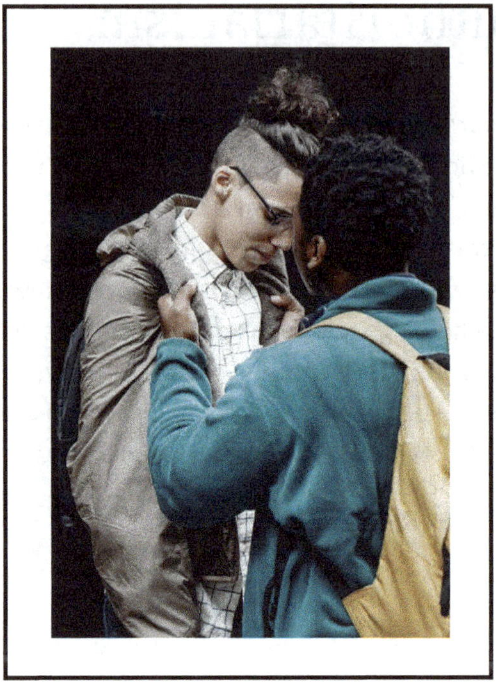

BEHAVIORAL FLIPS
Unknown

DERIVED DISABILITIES
Risk of becoming a threat to partners. Tense relationships that become unviable over time. Inability to raise children in a healthy manner with frequent state custody interventions. Civic dysfunction: at risk of problems with the law due to hostile behaviors edging criminality.

AWARENESS
Conscious (Neurotic Disorder)

CHARACTEROLOGICAL FILIATION
Hyper-Egocentric

QG LAYER-PARTITIONS
Right-Chiral Layer 1 compendium (Hyper-Quantum Operator)

STATISTICS
Insufficient data to establish prevalence.

INSIGHTS
The QG Hyper-Quantum Operator is key to these patients' morbid tendency for

Authoritarian behavior. It is important to understand that the aspiration to domination is the main morbid driver in the disorder. The patient consciously organizes a psychological cadre to serve this compulsion. At this effect, all the hatred and wickedness that present with the domination symptoms are secondary to the latter and represent the individual calling on these intellection resources to build his dominion.

Therefore, a clear distinction must be made between a morbid antisocial bigot or a morbid ruler instigating genocides to consolidate or remain in power, in which cases Layer **7** is hyperactive, and a family or close-circle bound individual obsessed with controlling relatives and friends through hostile behavior as a means but not the motivation. The distinction may not be easy to delineate, however scrutinizing the full spectrum of symptoms may unequivocally bear out the difference. In Authoritarianism, the Hyper-Quantum operator materializes an utter exaggeration in the expression of Layer 1 pensive partitions (expressly the right-chiral ones), the premises of which we have seen at the Charaterological level as the Hyper-Egocentric character type.

It is important to highlight the noncoercive form of Authoritarianism as a variant whereby the compulsion for domination is camouflaged under a barrage of apparent goodwill, affection and love, especially in the context of parenting (i.e. a grandmother or an aunt raising a child). In those cases, the morbid behavior of false love and care becomes so hoarding, oppressive and intoxicating that it may in turn induce neurotic behavior in the cherished young person.

Lastly, note that if Authoritarianism appears to be of mild or benign morbidity as a disorder, or an exaggeration of normal character traits, it is a false impression primarily due to the fact that the dysfunction in order originates from the Conscious Cognos. To that extent, the patient will never lose touch with logic and reason, and will never be delusional, akin to i.e. Perfectionism or ADHD, and all the other disorders rooted in Layer 1, 2 and 3. Authoritarianism is subject to the same paroxysm metric that rules all Disorders and elicited by the paroxysm level that characterizes a neurosis.

Separation Anxiety Disorder

Separation Anxiety Disorder (SAD) is characterized by excessive anxiety directly caused by physical separation from familiar individuals and home. Children with this disorder avoid or refuse anxiety-inducing situations. Beyond the normal velopmental phase of 6 to 12 months, SAD is considered an abnormal extension of anxiety from motherly weaning. Both genetic and psychosocial factors seem to play a role in the disorder.

PASSIVE –RESPONSIVE SYMPTOMS

Intense distress with crying when separating from a parent or close caring person, or from home. Excessive worry about losing the attachment figure to injury, sickness or death. Excessive preoccupation that something disastrous will happen to separate them from the attachment figure. Persistent fear of being alone, i.e. that a parent will leave and never return.

ACTIVE-REACTIVE SYMPTOMS

Temper tantrums. Refusal to engage in activities that require any separation at all. Refusal to sleep away from home.

KNOWN VARIANTS

None

LANGUAGE

Restrictive, receptive and expressive vocabulary; content and use of words can be affected.

BEHAVIORAL FLIPS

Unknown

DERIVED DISABILITIES

Restriction in social communication. Clinging behaviors. School refusal which will hamper progress in education and success in learning processes.

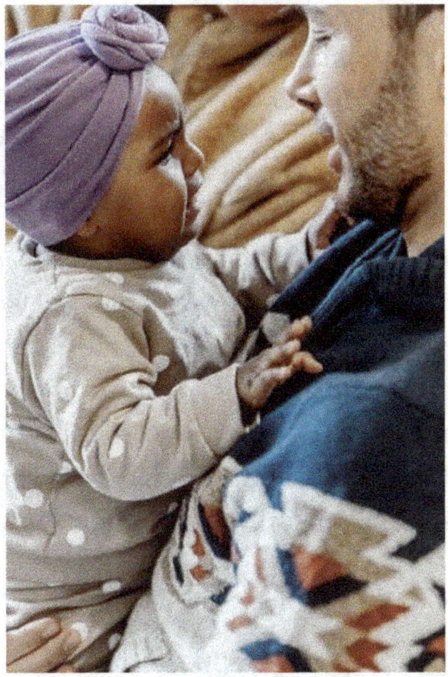

AWARENESS

Conscious (Neurotic Disorder)

CHARACTEROLOGICAL FILIATION

Matrixial

QG LAYER-PARTITIONS

6 **[(-1, -2, -3, -4) (+1, +2, +3, +4)]**

STATISTICS

Approximately 4.1% of children will exhibit a clinical level of separation anxiety, while one-third persist into adulthood if left untreated.

INSIGHTS

Jill T. Ehrenreich et al expressed the following etiological viewpoints[30] in relation to the disorder: *"Twin studies have shown that overprotective and over involved parenting behaviors are central to the development and maintenance of childhood anxiety. Furthermore, parental intrusiveness appears to be a specific risk factor for SAD among children with anxiety disorder diagnoses (Wood, 2006). In this context, intrusive parenting is characterized by disproportionate regulation of the child's emotions and behavior as well as autocratic decision making. Parental intrusiveness is often enacted by providing excessive assistance in the child's daily activities, such as dressing or bedtime routine, thus preventing the child from engaging in and mastering age-appropriate behaviors and activities.*

---

[30] Separation Anxiety Disorder in Youth: Phenomenology, Assessment, and Treatment – *NIH Psicol Conductual. 2008 January 1; 16(3): 389–412. doi:10.1901/jaba.2008.16-389*

These intrusive parental behaviors, aimed at reducing or preventing the child's distress, may instead encourage the child's dependence on parents, thus impacting the child's perceptions of mastery over his or her environment."

The above described psychosocial experience comes to be majorly internalized in the representational sublayer of the Foliate in development at the level of Layer **6**. It is only when they find a set of Left-Chiral partitions on that Layer already in accretion that a morbid tide will ensue jeopardizing the overall dynamics of the Foliate. The above etiological language ultimately requires a psychophysics translation to explain how all of that occurs in the Mind of individual patients. Only the Harmonic Norm inherent to normal Layer **6** is able to construe a response to an event of separation from a loved one or decoupling, because Layer 6 is the intrapsychic region or crucible that crystallizes coupling, matching and empathy phenomenologically.

PATHOLOGICAL AFFILIATES

Infantile Neglect Disorder

Infantile Neglect Disorder (IND) is our newly proposed label for the integration of *Reactive Attachment Disorder (RAD)* and *Disinhibited Social Engagement Disorder (DSED)*. In *Infantile Neglect Disorder* there is a syndromal variant with over accrual prevalence of the Left-Chiral pensive Partitions of Layer **6** accountable for the expression of the Disorder as *Reactive Attachment Disorder*. In parallel with this variant, there is another with over accrual prevalence of the Right-Chiral pensive partitions of Layer **6** accountable for the expression of IND as *Disinhibited Social Enagement Disorder*.

In addition, the representational sublayers pertaining to Layer **6** of the Foliate have internalized a history of psychosocial neglect from parents and caregivers which not only spurs the over accrual of the root partitions therein, but influences by their specificities the expression of the particular morbid impairment either as a DSED or RAD syndrome.

Infantile Neglect Disorder

Under the new label *Infantile Neglect Disorder (IND)*, we are joining together *Reactive Attachment Disorder (RAD)* and *Disinhibited Social Engagement Disorder (SSED)* following the categorization formerly offered in DSM-IV in which *Disinhibited Social Engagement Disorder* was proposed as a subtype of *Reactive Attachment Disorder*. In order to avoid introducing a disruption in the classificatory code for the formerly known entities, we are not calling for deprecating their labels. However, the analysis that follows will forcefully show that their integration under one single entity serves better the etiological understanding of these two Disorders, hence assuredly clinical treatment measures as well.

COMMON CORE

PASSIVE - RESPONSIVE SYMPTOMS	***ACTIVE - REACTIVE SYMPTOMS***
Persistent insatisfaction of basic emotional needs for comfort, stimulation, and affection by caregiving adults as a result of social neglect. Few or no stable attachments to parents, relatives and otherwise closed ones possibly deriving from repeated changes of primary caregivers. Absence of selective attachments possibly caused by rearing in unusual settings that limited the opportunities for such preferential bounds (e.g. an institution with high child-to-caregiver ratios).	None

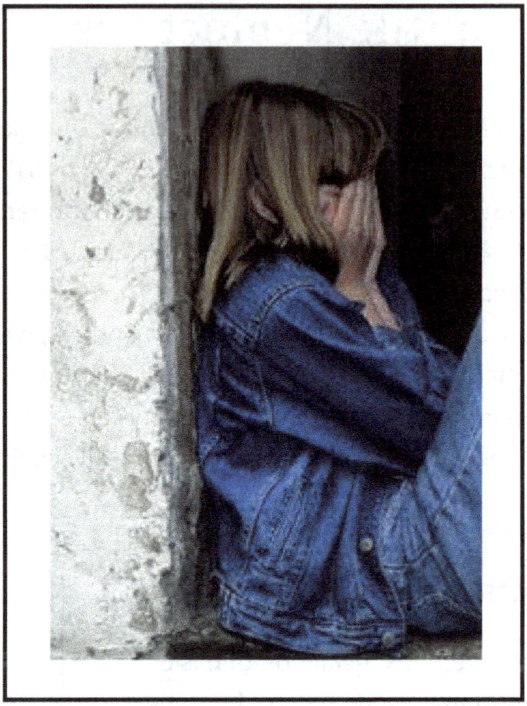

These symptoms are clearly duced by objective social neglect negatively perceived and disparagingly internalized by the affected child. They are knowingly present in both syndromes. The DSM explicitly requires this history of social neglect to be additionally satisfied for a qualified diagnosis of *Disinhibited Social Engagement Disorder* from behavior. However, social neglect must become a subjective internalized experience in order to produce any psychological impact whatsoever on a child's Mental Body. We have thus appropriately reformulated syntactically the DSM requirement in the above nosologic report. Furthermore, in *Reactive Attachment Disorder* it is also clear that the same kind of parental neglect and abandonment the child's emotional development has to confront in order to produce the reverse attachement reaction evidenced in its label.

It is judicious to consider *Disinhibited Social Engagement Disorder, Reactive Attachment Disorder* as well *Separation Anxiety Disorder* to be part of the same cluster of mental impairments or so-called attachment impairments. While parenting in *Separation Anxiety Disorder* is for the most part overbearing in intrusion in the child's life, in the other two cases, or simply *Infantile Neglect Disorder*, it is parental neglect and abandonment that the child's emotional development has to face and cope with. In both cases, the deep emotional hurt experienced by the child spurs an emotional reaction of empathetic (or harmonic) nature common to both syndromes.

Disinhibited Social Engagement Disorder

Children with disinhibited social engagement disorder show an ostensible, exaggerated and unjustified friendliness to strangers. They feel so comfortable around unknown and unfamiliar people that they would climb into their cars or accept an invitation to a stranger's home without hesitation. This uninhibited friendliness toward strangers puts affected children frequently at great risk of social harm that can be life threatening or dangerous to their safety, should the disorder be left untreated.

DSED PASSIVE - RESPONSIVE SYMPTOMS

Inability to make judgments about whether a stranger looks kind or mean based on an individual's face or psysiognomic appearance like most kids do.

DSED ACTIVE - REACTIVE SYMPTOMS

Open trust of strangers inconsistent with culturally sanctioned rules and customs, and social boundaries. Willingness to talk to, engage or go away with an unfamiliar adult with little or no hesitation. Venturing away with no concerns, even in unfamiliar settings, with no check back with the adult caregiver. Reaching out to a complete stranger for emotional support when in need (i.e. after fall and hurt at the park or playground). Or Telling random passerby of a hurt or even siting on a stranger's lap on a park bench to cry. Indiscriminately seek physical affection (i.e. sit on stranger's lap in waiting room or hug passerby at the grocery store or sit with another family at the park as if invited to their picnic).

KNOWN VARIANTS

None

LANGUAGE

Very naïve. May strike up a highly personal conversation with an unfamiliar adult at the playground. Older children: *"I want to go to your house"* when meeting a new classmate for the first time.

BEHAVIORAL FLIPS

Flips between kindness cravings and empathy, and intently making loud noises and otherwise noticeable behavior to capture attention and sympathy.

DERIVED DISABILITIES

Confuse and ennerve caregivers with incomprehensible indiscriminate openness. Adolescent sufferers are likely to develop problematic relations with peers, parents, teachers, and coaches. They knowingly tend to develop superficial relationships with others, struggle with these conflicts, and continually demonstrate indiscriminate behaviors toward adults.

AWARENESS

Conscious (Neurotic Disorder)

CHARACTEROLOGICAL FILIATION

Matrixial

QG LAYER-PARTITIONS

6 [(-1, -2, -3, -4) (+1, +2, +3, +4)]

STATISTICS

Fairly rare disorder affecting 20% of children in high-risk populations (children raised in orphanages or through placement in multiple foster care homes).

INSIGHTS

It is very clear that the lack of attention, care and affection from closed ones, parents and relatives, who might be absent altogether in the child's immediate environment, is what prompts this indiscriminate openness to and trust of perfect strangers. By middle childhood, affected children often show verbal and physical overfamiliarity as well as inauthentic expression of emotions. For instance a preteen may laugh when others laugh, all to cozzily feel that she belongs, to empathize or incite empathy. They may instead show sadness just to better manipulate a social situation, in lieu of the expression of a genuine emotion.

Inarguably the pensive partitions of an overtiding Layer **6** of the Foliate, with concentration at the Left-Chiral side of the Layer, are fueling these reactions. Neglect during infancy has been spotted to be the major cause of this Disorder. However, there is often misunderstanding about what constitutes neglect and what in general contributes to the development of so-called attachment disorders in children. Most importantly, contrary to common myths, the disorder is admittedly not caused by placing a child in daycare, nor will a child necessarily develop *DSED* by being routinely placed in the crib when crying. Most certainly, not all neglected children will develop DSED and many will grow up with healthy relationships exempt of lasting attachment impairments. Again this is another instance worth the reminder that it is the predisposed terrain of an already tidal Layer which will allow the overbearing resonance with internalized psychosocial factors to unleash the pathological condition.

Reactive Attachment Disorder

Reactive Attachment Disorder (RAD) is considered a rare but serious condition in which an infant or young child fails to establish healthy emotional bonds with parents or caregivers. The Disorder may develop if the child's basic needs for comfort, affection and nurturing are left unmet. Typically, these children are either fostered in special children's homes or other institutions that sort and endure frequent changes of foster homes or caregivers, or live with parents who have severe mental health problems, show criminal behavior or engage in narcotic substance abuse impairing their parenting. Other triggers may be prolonged separation from parents or other caregivers due to hospitalization. This Disorder ordinarily onsets in early childhood before age 5 is reached.

RAD PASSIVE - RESPONSIVE SYMPTOMS

Sadness and listless appearance. Not seeking comfort or showing no response when comfort is given. Watching others closely but not engaging in social interaction. Unexplained withdrawal. Fail to ask for support or assistance or to reach out when picked up. Unexplained withdrawal, fear, and failure to smile. No interest in playing interactive games.

RAD ACTIVE - REACTIVE SYMPTOMS

Children may react violently when held or comforted; their behavior consists in being difficult to console, and difficult to discipline. Failure to smile. Irritability. Attempts to elicit temper outbursts or self-injurious behavior. Frequenly inhibited academically.

KNOWN VARIANTS
None

LANGUAGE
--

BEHAVIORAL FLIPS
None

DERIVED DISABILITIES
Research suggests that some children and teenagers with RAD may display callous, unemotional traits that can include cruelty toward people or animals. However more research is needed to demonstrate the direct relationship of these behavioral traits with RAD.

CHARACTEROLOGICAL FILIATION
Matrixial

AWARENESS
Conscious (Neurotic Disorder)

QG LAYER-PARTITIONS

6 [(-1, -2, -3, -4) (+1, +2, +3, +4)]

STATISTICS

Estimated is 1% prevalence rate in all children under 5 years old, 35% of maltreated toddlers in a foster care.

INSIGHTS

While in DSED children are indiscriminately forthcoming and open to other people, in RAD they are rather withdrawn, distrust people and the world, and in general carry a low mood. The deep emotional hurt experienced by the child in the absence of affection and emotional parental neglect spur in each case a different emotional reaction.

In DSED, the Right-Chiral pensive partitions of Layer 6, in particular *Sympathy* and *Admiration*, fuel the behavior in a compensatory manner, while in RAD the Left-Chiral partitions of the same Layer are the ones directly in control of the behavior, essentially the partitions of *Sadness*, *Sorrow* and *Pity*, outrightly emanating from the situation of parental lack of love. In the severe cases, *Despair* is also involved. Therefore, the fullness of the conditions necessary for a visualization of these two syndromes in one is unquestionably satisfied, each subsyndromal set qualifying as a variant of the main Disorder which we designated *Infantile Neglect Disorder.*

One must not lose sight however that a predisposed terrain in the embodiment of a preexistent accrued Layer **6** is ultimately accountable for the over accrual which constitutes the pathology in both cases. It is clinically well understood that most children who are severely neglected do not get to experience neither one nor the other syndrome, consistent with the empathetic predisposition that must exist at Layer **6** of the psyche for the psychosocial factors to resonate internally, producing the specific observable syndromes. Clearly, the difference in the pathological emotional orchestration resulting in a specific facet or variant of the Disorder is mainly a dependency of the kind of faulty parental/caregiver interventions endured by the child.

That the two sets of impairments are tighly related to one another in nosology and etiology and better understood as counterparts of one another under the common label of *Infantile Neglect Disorder*, as previously argued, is to us a fact in plain sight. Further, despite the uncertainty about whether or not RAD occurs in children older than 5 years of age, akin to DSED which extends into adolescence, it remains clear that they are both the consequences of parental neglect creating a child's morbid attachment predicament. More research is needed in order to precisely situate DSED within the prodromal course of RAD, a conclusion we have been driven to from the reviewed research literature. In all, their common symptomatic core pertaining to emotional neglect history of the sufferers definitely speaks to the affine traits and onset conditions characterizing the two syndromes and validating their reunion in one Disorder.

Post Traumatic Stress Disorder

Post Traumatic Stress Disorder (PTSD) is an intense mentation commotion that follows the witnessing or experiencing an unusual, extraordinary or exceptionally impacting event by the affected individual. The mentation paroxysmal bance may be immediate following the event or more or less delayed in the succession of events making up daily living, even within the succession of mental phases of the lifecycle.

PASSIVE –RESPONSIVE SYMPTOMS

Emotional distressful commotion or numbing resulting from observing or experiencing , in the act and after the fact, devastation or death typically from raging fires, seismic or cyclonic destruction, war mayhems, torture or torturous deaths, violent deaths by wounds or dismemberments or live cremation, genocides, dehumanizing treatments, belliquous or sexual assault, vehicular accidents, sudden death of a loved one, or even receiving a life-threatening diagnosis. Discomforting flashbacks, nightmares or intrusive memories evocative of the original stressful event(s) on a backdrop of feelings of horror or fright. Inability to henceforth experience positive emotions naturally. Hyperarousal such as anxiety and sleep disturbances. Possible distorted blame of self or others.

ACTIVE-REACTIVE SYMPTOMS

Commotional active remembrance of the event possibly causing dissociation. Irritability and difficulty concentrating. Intent avoidance of reminders of the traumatic event(s) such as particular situations, places, and people.

KNOWN VARIANTS

Acute Stress Reaction Disorder.

LANGUAGE

The language can traumatically express the anxiety and shock related to the stressful event mixed with profuse tears.

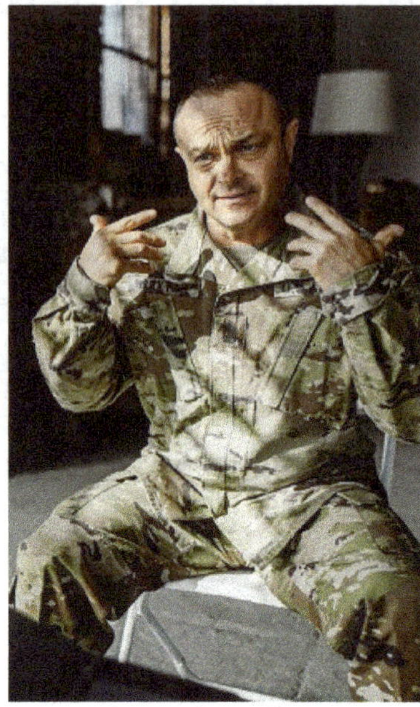

BEHAVIORAL FLIPS

People who experience PTSD may have persistent frightening thoughts embroiled in memories of the stressful event(s) and feel detached and/or numb, or may be easily startled. Possible dystonic flips between the numbness of deep fright and the disquiet of being startled. A peculiar flip between left-chiral partitions in overtone and right-chiral ones in due tone.

DERIVED DISABILITIES

In its very severe forms, PTSD will significantly impair an individual's ability to function properly at work, at home, and in social settings.

AWARENESS

Unconscious: Inability to discern between reality, past events and circumstances provoking the symptoms makes it a psychotic Disorder. The person incidentally thinks he is brought back or still lives a time and circumstance that are past and exist no more. Such a form of mentation qualifies as hallucination.

CHARACTEROLOGICAL FILIATION

Paradoxical

QG LAYER-PARTITIONS

7 [(-1, -2, -3, -4) (+1, +2, +3, +4)**]**

STATISTICS

Lifetime prevalence of PTSD in general population is 6.8%. In adolescents, the prevalence is higher in females than males. The prevalence of PTSD among certain populations exposed to high rates of traumatic events, including physical injury, military combat, peacekeeping, disaster, and rape, have demonstrated much higher rates of PTSD than the general population (prevalence estimates range between 10% and 40%).

INSIGHTS

Currently, official psychiatry requires the symptoms to last for more than one month and a 6-month delay for the first manifestation of symptoms. Subthreshold traumatic responses in the first 6-month period after occurrence of the stressful event officially qualifies as "delayed expression". Typically, the severity of the symptoms diminish over time, however 25% of PTSD patients with delayed onset knowingly experience a monotonic increase in the severity of symptoms over time

Because of the incidence of wars and interethnic hatred in the history of mankind, and the spread of violence in the contemporaneous world alike, traumatic mentation disorders, of which Post Traumatic Stress Disorder is the maximum expression, has become a prevalent disease in the human population. About one half of all U.S. adults will experience at least one traumatic event in their lives. However, it is important to stress, from the clinical vantage, that most of those individuals do not develop PTSD, at least in the aftermath immediately following the mental shock incidentally caused by the stressful event, including a reasonable period thereafter.

People presenting with PTSD symptoms are known to have often been exposed to multiple traumatic events. Therefore, it is important to stress that the nosology of the disorder is likely to show an onset consequential to a previous succession or an accumulation of exposures to multiple traumatic events of more or less acute severity. Therefore, one is safe to conclude that:

- The onset of the Disorder seemingly requires an intrapsychic predisposition to this type of dysfunction.

- Once a trauma history has been registered in the psyche and reaches a certain severity threshold, the next traumatic event will unleash the commotional tide and bursts that destabilize the psyche in the peculiar manner known to PTSD.

As frequently mentioned previously, the psychosocial conditions of living and facts of life become registered in the psyche at the representational sublayer level all throughout the Mentation Foliate. Where the traumatic conditions and events (raging fires, killings, rapes, etc.) find resonance is at Paradoxical Layer **7**, evidently by virtue of the phenotypic nature of pensive partitions at the left-chiral side of the Layer *(Terror, Fear, Angst, Anxiety).* Note that the perpetrators and their acts bear a phenotypic nature that matches the partitions at the right-chiral side of the Layer *(Resentment, Repugnance, Wickedness, Fury).* When a casual neighborhood electricity outage triggers in someone hyperarousal acts such as running and hiding in deep distress, looking frenziedly for cover, in uncontrolled and uncontrollable maelstrom, and terrified like hell, you may be witnessing i.e. PTSD expression in the exiled son of a President whose brutal and lethal ouster from power in an overnight military coup scarred for life (without treatment, that is).

It is worth noting that the common view that sees a high rate of PTSD comorbidity with other mental disorders, such as major depressive disorders, alcohol abuse and/or dependence, anxiety disorders, panic disorder, borderline personality disorder and antisocial personality disorder, is not exactly correct from our psychophysics perspective. We have amply discussed the dimensions of normal layer partitioning and orthogonal channels or anti-symmetric threads with the binary Sector partitioning which all conform the mentation Foliate Map and subtend the psychopathological dynamics of a dysfunctional Mental Foliate. This foundational canvas provides the critical psychopathological elements that are common to all mental disorders. It is only in the absence of a broad understanding of this foundation that mental impairments can be viewed as comorbidity agglutinating mental disorders or sets thereof in an unfortunate amalgam defying unified and effective diagnosis (See Commented Bibliography for PTSD).

As we have seen, notwithstanding the fact that one same Layer may elicit differing disorders, there are multiple different ways for a normal Layer to participate in and characterize a specific disorder. The element of shock that is omnipresent in the paroxysmally stressful event causing PTSD symptoms, ultimately embodied in the representational substratrum at Layer 7, has for certain a special tidal impact on the associated root partitions making up the Layer. Further, the representations are also responsible for intensity modulations among the partitions in accretion. Detailed psychometric probing of all the partitions participating in a particular disorder will bear out those distinctions, although in this study we have not addressed the details of transflow currents circulating longitudinally across a pensive Layer that would disclose those partition tides. Very particularly, individual partition responses condition such mechanisms as the compensation and defense mechanism as studied in Chapter 4, as well as the eponymous behavioral flips or swings that we have listed for a number of disorders. In PTSD we can see the peculiar form taken by this swing at Layer 7 which is in accretion mainly at one chiral side.

PATHOLOGICAL AFFILIATES

Panic Disorder

In many ways, *Panic Disorder* is similar to PTSD to a significant degree. It is a sudden onset of intense fear or discomfort which peaks within minutes. The PASSIVE-RESPONSIVE symptoms consist of fear of "going crazy", fear of dying, derealization and depersonalization, tingling or numbness, chest and abdominal pain, nausea, chills and hot flashes. On the ACTIVE-REACTIVE side, the following symptoms are common: palpitations, shaking, sweating, shortness of breath, sensation of choking and dizziness. Also common in the disease is a constant conscious worry about having more panic attacks, which supports a diagnosis of neurosis for Panic Disorder. Overall, it may be viewed as a mild version of PTSD.

Anxiety Syndrome

496 is described as an anticipation of a future threat in response to an intense and overwhelming sensation of fear. The latter manifests in an excessive worry

associated with emotional or physical expression. The most common PASSIVE-RESPONSIVE symptoms are: feeling tense, feeling of dread, anticipating the worst, headaches, insomnia, and fatigue. To keep in line with the same QG layer manifestation, for the ACTIVE-REACTIVE side, one may note: feeling jumpy, restlessness or irritability, racing heart, shortness of breath, tremors, sweating, frequent urination or bowel movements, and upset stomach. This syndrome is also a neurosis.

Oppositional Defiant Disorder

Oppositional Defiant Disorder (ODD) is characterized by repetitive defiant and hostile behavior, and lack of cooperation toward persons in authority. It affects both children and adults. This abnormal behavior seriously interferes with the child's functioning and psychosocial development. In adults, it seriously hampers their familial and social interactions. Many uncertainties still exist about ODD as a legitimate morbid disorder, given that it is rarely examined as a distinct psychiatric disorder, despite its dubious distinction of leading cause of referrals to youth mental health services.

PASSIVE –RESPONSIVE SYMPTOMS

N/A

ACTIVE-REACTIVE SYMPTOMS

In children, temper tantrums, arguing with adults, questioning rules, annoying people, not admitting own mistakes, refusal to comply with adults' requests, anger issues, harboring grudges, spitefulness, seeking revenge. Affected adults often lose temper and argue with family members and coworkers. They actively defy or refuse to comply with rules and laws. Deliberately annoying people as much as they are easily annoyed by others. Angry and resentful, spiteful or vindictive. Blame others for their own mistakes or misbehavior.

KNOWN VARIANTS

Disruptive Mood Dysregulation

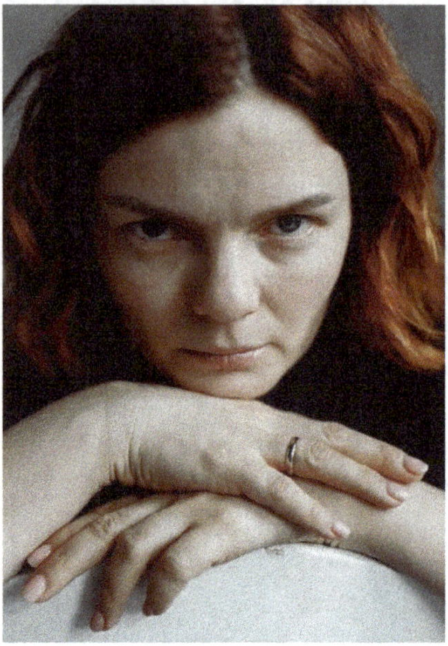

LANGUAGE

The language has mean and hateful vocabulary when subject is upset.

BEHAVIORAL FLIPS

Unknown

DERIVED DISABILITIES

Inability to discern between reality and symptoms, impairment of functioning in various areas.

AWARENESS

Conscious (Neurotic Disorder)

CHARACTEROLOGICAL FILIATION

Paradoxical

QG LAYER-PARTITIONS

7[(-1, -2, -3, -4) **(+1, +2, +3, +4)]**

STATISTICS

Lifetime prevalence in the population is 10.2% with preeminence among males.

INSIGHTS

A 10-year long study[31] of subjects' lifetime diagnostic status of ADHD, ODD and Conduct Disorder (CD) has found the following outcome:

"**Results:** *ODD persisted in a substantial minority of subjects at the 10-year follow-up. Independent of co-morbid CD, ODD was associated with major depression in the interval between the 4-year and the 10-year follow-up. Although ODD significantly increased the risk for CD and antisocial personality disorder, CD con-*

---

[31] **The Long-Term Longitudinal Course of Oppositional Defiant Disorder and Conduct Disorder in ADHD boys**: findings from a controlled 10-year prospective longitudinal follow-up study – J Biederman et al - 2008 Jul;38(7):1027-36. doi: 10.1017/S0033291707002668. Epub 2008 Jan 21.

ferred a much larger risk for these outcomes. Furthermore, only CD was associated with significantly increased risk for psychoactive substance use disorders, smoking, and bipolar disorder.

Conclusions: *These longitudinal findings support and extend previously reported findings from this sample at the 4-year follow-up indicating that ODD and CD follow a divergent course. They also support previous findings that ODD heralds a compromised outcome for ADHD youth grown up independently of the comorbidity with CD."*

The vision implicit in the abovementioned study and the exegesis of the study findings is a typical example of how the notion of comorbidity may muddy visibility in the intricacies of mental disorders, due to the ignorance of the subjacent psychophysics factors that control symptoms of disorders. First, the categorization of Conduct Disorder is problematic by virtue of the principled fact that if behavior is a broadly cast expression of Mind, then conduct becomes an epithet for all forms of disorders in their condition of troublesome expression of behavior. Second, in the ignorance of the matrix arrangement of the Mentation Map of which orthogonal threads with dynamical flows (orthoflows) become a consequential derivative, it is not possible to delineate the significant underlying differences between symptomatic elements that might appear to participate in different types of disorders. Therefore, the rapprochement between ODD and ADHD, albeit ultimately justified in our vision as expressions of disorders equally rooted on the right-chiral side of the Mentation Foliate, cannot ascertain (1) their etiological belonging to two distinct root Layers of the Foliate and (2) that their relationship between one another is carried out via orthogonal flows.

Effectively, overaccretion at QG Layer **7** is the etiological hallmark for ODD in which the pensive partitions of *Resentment*, *Repugnance*, *Wickedness*, and *Fury* fuel the morbid stubborn and rebellious conduct as observed. In the event that inciting psychosocial factors are significantly registered at that stratum of the Psyche, a preexisting accretion level per character determination will result in a push to over tidal accretion. The event of a neural accident or shock caused by psychotropic drugs or alcohol ingestion may be the trigger to the morbid tide, whether the latter is permanent or circumstantial.

From our perspective, ODD is most fruitfully scrutinized by studying its relationship with other disorders from the same etiological spectral root and chiral partition set than through the perspective of a remote relationship with other disorders via orthoflows pertaining to the underlying normal dynamics of the Foliate. Orthoflows represent a natural mechanism that would account for much of what has been quite erratically termed in psychopathology comorbidity or multimorbidity.

Juvenile Conduct Disorder

We gather under this Label the legal qualifier *Juvenile Delinquency* and the DSM psychiatric disorder named *Conduct Disorder*. Both notions concern children and adolescents on the one hand, and, on the other, societal interaction through individual personal conduct. In that way, under the Label *Juvenile Conduct order*, we parsimoniously restrict the very general notion of conduct to the dimension of personal conduct and to the specific juvenile group targeted by the pathological categorization. The affected display early conflictive social tions requiring the pressing intervention of law enforcement beyond parental control.

PASSIVE –RESPONSIVE SYMPTOMS

ACTIVE-REACTIVE SYMPTOMS

Aggressiveness in the form of intimidation or bullying others, causing purposeful physical harm to animals or persons and committing rape or using a weapon. Deceiptful behavior such as brazen lying, forgery, trespass breaking and stealing. Destructive behavior such as arson or vandalizing property. Violation of rules that may include skipping school, running away from home, drug and alcohol use and premature sexual activity.

KNOWN VARIANTS

- Prone to Status offenses: runaway, underage drinking, illegal purchases.
- Prone to Property crimes: larceny, burglary, theft ,and arson.

- Prone to Violent crimes: robbery, rape, murder, and aggravated assault.

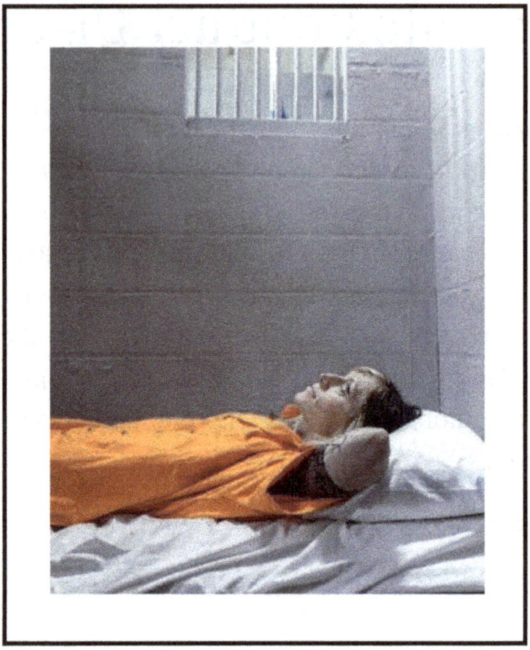

LANGUAGE
Use of slurs, ruthless vocabulary. Inability to express love or intimacy, depressive prosody.

BEHAVIORAL FLIPS
Unknown

DERIVED DISABILITIES
Poor performance in school, community and at home. Perverted social agent engaging in illegal substance abuse, homicide, criminal intolerance of others due to origin, ethnicity or religion, subject to arrests, suicide, etc.

AWARENESS
Conscious (Neurotic Disorder)

CHARACTEROLOGICAL FILIATION
Paradoxical

QG LAYER-PARTITIONS
7[(+1, +2, +3, +4)]

STATISTICS
9% of juvenile arrests are among children below age 13. Boys with *Juvenile Conduct Disorder* are more likely than girls to display aggressive and destructive conduct, girls being more prone to deceitful and rule-violating conduct.

INSIGHTS
QG layer **7** is the birthplace of *Juvenile Conduct Disorder* as the Right-Chiral pa-

lette of partitions of *Resentment, Repugnance, Wickedness,* and *Fury* become prominently hyperactive in the syndrome.

Currently, some adolescents who are in trouble with the law will be labeled juvenile delinquents but will not meet criteria for so-called *Conduct Disorder* due to the limited scope of their conduct transgressions. We feel that the two criteria should be much more in line with one another, and that ultimately the psychiatric definitions should be accurate enough to constrain and inform the legal definition of this Disorder. Our label change for the Disorder is an attempt to arrive at such a unity while we firmly believe that the new pathological metric based on intensity of pensive primitives bears the potential to provide the objective basis for the sought-after reconciliation. At the very least this approach does away with the arbitrary number of symptoms (or violations) required for a qualified diagnosis as it currently stands, which is in mismatch with what warrants arrest and reformation in jurisprudence. That all said, the least that, for its own, an equanimous justice system can do is to be fair and forthright to the diverse citizenry at large in its applicable delinquency qualifiers and tightly peg to the science of psychiatry for its punishment and remediation measures, which does not appear to always be the case.

Bulimia – Anorexia Nervosa

Bulimia Nervosa is characterized by recurrent episodes of binge eating followed each by voluntarily induced vomiting, indiscriminate laxative use, and even fasting between binges, whereas *Anorexia Nervosa* is considered an eating disorder characterized by extreme and prolonged fasting, an intense fear of gaining weight, and a distorted perception of the person's body physiognomy. In official psychiatry, those two diseases have traditionally been treated as one, as evidenced in DSM-IV. We have chosen to retain this categorization of one same disease, under the joint label *Bulimia-Anorexia Nervosa,* due to the solid support that our etiological framework preferentially brings to this analytic visualization, as amply discussed in what follows.

PASSIVE –RESPONSIVE SYMPTOMS

BULIMIC

Being preoccupied with or insistently complaining about body shape and weight. Living in fear of gaining weight. Negative views of oneself, obsession with body image or physiognomic appearance. Avoidance of eating in public. Intense fear of gaining weight. Use of unneeded laxatives, diuretics or enemas after regular eating in the purging subtype. Sadness.

ANOREXIC

Keep the body in chronic if not constant starvation through fasting or dieting. Denial of hunger calls or making excuses for not eating. Avoid eating in public. Prepare elaborate meals for others but not eating them. Ritualistically spitting food out after chewing them. Excessive complaints about body fats. Frequent mirror checking for imagined body flaws. Misuse of laxatives, diet aids, diuretics or enemas to eliminate waste. Sadness. Fatigue, dizziness or fainting. Extremely low libido. Flat inexpressive mood. Social withdrawal.

ACTIVE-REACTIVE SYMPTOMS

BULIMIC

Binging even when not hungry and eating food not of the person's normal taste. Feeling a loss of control during binging, i.e. unable to stop eating or cannot control what to ingest. Fasting, restricting calories or avoiding certain foods between binges. Use of fasting or excessive exercise in the non purging subtype to keep from gaining weight after bingeing. Self-induced vomiting to eliminate ingested food. Going to the bathroom right after eating, during meals or for long periods of time. Excessive use of dietary supplements or herbal products for weight loss. Suppressed anger at oneself.

ANOREXIC

Extreme weight loss, or not making expected developmental weight gains, causing an extremely thin personal appearance. Lying about how much food had been eaten. Suppressed anger.

KNOWN VARIANTS

There are 2 classified subtypes for Bulimia: purging and non purging. Destructive Binge Eating. Avoidant/Restrictive Food Intake Disorder.

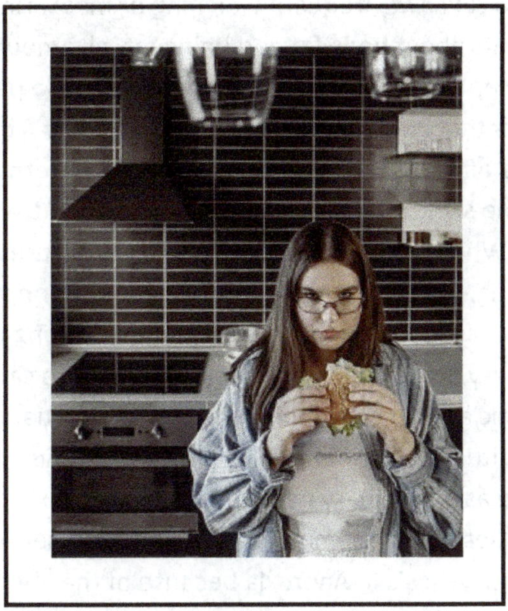

LANGUAGE

Language focuses more on non fat-related words, can be depressive in prosody.

BEHAVIORAL FLIPS

Binary flips between bulimic food binging (right-chiral) and anorexic food depravation (left-chiral) in both crescents of the disease (Bulimia and Anorexia).

DERIVED DISABILITIES

Having sores, scars or calluses on the knuckles or hands. Various medical complications can occur: flatulence, constipation and abdominal pain, delayed gastric emptying, Mallory-Weiss esophageal tears, rectal prolapse, amenorrhea due to low body fat, cardiac toxicity from ipecac (an emetic drug), damaged teeth and gums, enamel erosion from gastric acid, calluses on middle phalanges from using fingers to induce vomiting (Russell's sign), sialadenosis. In patients with anorexia nervosa as the major, a reduction in bone mineral density is also evident. Intolerance of cold. Irregular heart rhythms. Low blood pressure. Dehydration. Swelling of arms or legs. Abnormal blood counts. Irregular heart rhythms. Low blood pressure. Dehydration. Soft, downy hair covering the body. Dry or yellowish skin in light complexion people. Insomnia. Absence of menstruation. Submitting the body to excessive exercise. Changing or unstable body weight.

AWARENESS

Drastic reduction in interest for sex advocates against the quest for attractiveness, particularly in Anorexia. The frequent checking in the mirror for imagined physical flaws, frequent weighing or measuring the body and incessant complaints about body fat and being fat, all amount to a degradation in the patient's perception of reality. Some of these female patients would fast and observe diets that put their waist line at about 3 or 4 in. wide under the constant pressure of a large belt, causing alarming concerns to both strangers and loved ones at the sight of what is clearly a high risk to their physical or physiognomic integrity. While bulimics' behavior seems to accuse a loss of control over their binge eating, which takes the likes of a compulsion, anorexic patients seem to have lost sound contact with reality when denying to themselves and others they are hungry and make excuses for not eating to satiate hunger, refusing to eat in public as if an act of sinning, lying about quantity of ingested food, adopting eating rituals, etc. Analytically, it is fully justified to view the bulimic side of the disease as an ordinary neurosis and its anorexic side trending to delusional neurosis. Despite the somewhat compromised sense of what's real, there is no qualified psychosis in Anorexia because of the absence of unmitigated hallucinations. Hence in both cases the patient's awareness remains conscious.

CHARACTEROLOGICAL FILIATION

Matrixial

QG LAYER-PARTITIONS

7 [(-1, -2, -3, -4) (+1, +2, +3, +4)]

STATISTICS

Bulimia Nervosa has a prevalence of 2% to 3%, while Anorexia has a prevalence of 0.5% to 1%. Both affect mostly females and in an even higher proportion those who are college educated. Males are affected by eating disorders at a rate one tenth of that of females.

INSIGHTS

The most important identifiable trend in this joint disorder of Bulimia-Anorexia Nervosa is an obsession with activity of the digestive system, a biological element that conforms to the universal Norm of Destruction from a QG perspective of the organization of the living. The patient's ailment specifically manifests in the form of either an overstimulation of the digestive system or a hypostimulation of the same. In either case, the behavior primarily seeks to realize the infamous act of self-destruction. This attempt centers on the biological element of destruction par excellence in the living body, the digestive system, that is. The biology of digestion and the digestive system directly relates to the Paradoxical Mentation Layer of the Foliate which embodies the Norm of Destruction on the mental plane.

Analysts have traditionally, and erroneously so, emphasized the concern for body appearance in the expression of the disorder, in particular in the case of Anorexia Nervosa. This preoccupation is in fact rather secondary and simply represents a conscious rationalization of the disorder symptoms by the patient, which are in fact unconsciously orchestrated by Layer **7** of the Mental Manifold. What we face here is a disease that manifests in two different crescents: one that compels the patient to self-harm by passive refrain of food intake or starvation, and another that instead actively compels the patient to self-harm by a gross hypertrophic intake of food. The bulimic may go through significant periods of fasting steadfastly motivated by this quest for self-harm. Some analysts believe that the fast is to stimulate binging. In fact, the binge may occur with the patient not feeling hungry at all. In any event, what the patient is doing is instigating a dystopic mayhem throughout his/her body by using the capabilities of the digestive system. The binge in itself is an act of stimulation of the digestive system. But because it naturally takes too long for the overabundant amount of ingested food to be fully digested and excreted as anal waste, the patient turns to vomiting, employing all kinds of methods to induce vomiting as an act of buccal digestion or waste purge. The behavior is all about the experience of destruction and self-destruction or self-harm. So therefore, the difference between the purging and non purging type in Bulimia is of little significance.

Bulimia nervosa was described as an ominous variant of anorexia nervosa by Russell since 1979. More research effected since then has erroneously led official psychiatry to the recognition of bulimia nervosa and anorexia nervosa as two distinct syndromes. It is well established, however, that many patients who suffer from anorexia nervosa do exhibit clear bulimic features. They understandably have more difficulty reaching normal body weight and tend to be and stay at lower body weights (even after treatment). These anorexic patients do binge and purge, similar to individuals with Bulimia. Clinically, anorexics are known to be prone to developing binge eating after treatment as well. A 1997 study reported that 30% of treated anorexics developed binge-eating behavior in the 5-year period following hospitalization. The following interdisciplinary assessment between general Medicine and Psychiatry about Bulimia has been issued since 2003 in the publication **Primary Care Companion to the Journal of Association of Medicine and Psychiatry**: *"When assessing a normal or overweight patient with bulimia nervosa, it is important to gather historical information about the presence and duration of past anorexia nervosa. Anorexia nervosa complicated by bulimic symptoms is associated with higher mortality rates than those from bulimia nervosa alone."* The connection between anorexic food starvation and bulimic food binging is clear and not difficult to spot and highlight in the prodromal course of the dysfunction, from a formal analytic viewpoint. Most tellingly, the binary swings between food binging of bulimic nature (right-chiral) experienced by Anorexics and food depravation or fasts of anorexic nature (left-chiral) experienced by Bulimics is a clear and unequivocal indication that this is a single two-crescent Disorder where a subset of the symptoms may play the role of either a minor or a major in a disease to be viewed as one *(Bulimia-Anorexia).* Therefore, to establish a rigid line of separation between the two disorders resulting in two staunchly differentiated pathologies is unequivocally unjustified.

Furthermore, the intent for outright self-harm is a pathological feature that is omnipresent in all forms of Bulimia and Anorexia. Self-injury is flagged to be a serious clinical concern for patients with Bulimia Nervosa. In one study, 34% of bulimic patients reported having intentionally injured themselves at some point in their lives, while 21.3% reported having injured themselves in the 5 months prior to the study. These patients most often injure themselves by lacerating or scratching their arms, hands, legs, or face, with many of these injuries resulting in profuse bleeding and posterior scarring. Anorexic patients, for their own, are known to engage in the following deleterious activities: alcohol and psychotropic substance misuse or abuse, self-injury to their body and suicide attempts following persistent suicidal ideation. Consequently, self-mutilation or self-harm is not reportedly an isolated trait among the dysfunctions, but a major symptom that reveals the true overall sado-masochistic nature of the disease, consistent with its optional rooting on the right-chiral or left-chiral pensive set of partitions of Layer **7** of the Foliate (at the right-chiral side compulsion to harm not others but the self amidst repugnance for self).

It is fair to conclude that, when all symptoms are taken into consideration, *Bulimia Nervosa and Anorexia Nervosa* are best etiologically understood as the same Disorder *Bulimia-Anorexia Nervosa* with two variants characterized by a minor and a major role, both to be appropriately applied to the two chiral subsets of the spectrum of common symptoms. This longitudinal spectrum is that of Layer **7** of the Mentation Foliate. When it comes to the *Destructive Binge Eating* variant, it only becomes legitimate as such if its symptom set is strictly limited to the Right-Chiral side of Layer **7**, with no minor represented in the Left-Chiral side of that normal.

Lastly, note that the chiral categorization of this family of Disorders is very similar to the demarcation taking place in Bipolar Disorder previously studied.

PATHOLOGICAL AFFILIATES

Rumination Disorder

Rumination Disorder is characterized by recurrent food regurgitation, whereby the patient may re-chew, re-swallow or spit out the food. These regurgitations must neither be accompanied by other gastric symptoms such as nausea or vomiting, nor occur in the context of a medical condition, for them to qualify as *Rumination Disorder*. They shall instead be considered part of *Anorexia - Bulimia Nervosa*, *Binge Eating Disorder*, or *Avoidant/Restrictive Food Intake Disorder*, should they occur as part of the larger individual syndromes of these Disorders.

PASSIVE - RESPONSIVE SYMPTOMS

Feeling of pressure, belching, nausea, bloating, heartburn, abdominal pain, headaches, dizziness, or sleeping difficulties; constipation.

ACTIVE - REACTIVE SYMPTOMS

Regurgitation, rechewing or expulsion of food which begins soon after eating and does not occur during sleep; diarrhea.

DERIVED DISABILITIES

Hygiene of neglect reflected in poor breath and damaged teeth. Malnutrition is a common complication as well resulting from the marked inability to maintain healthy nutrition habits.

INSIGHTS

Rumination Disorder is part of the cluster of Food-related mental disorders orchestrated by over accretion of Layer **7** of the Foliate.

Trichotillomania - Dermatillomania

Trichotillomania or *Hair Pulling Disorder* is a compulsion to continually pull out one's hair resulting in factual hair loss. This hair pulling mania is generally followed by unsuccessful attempts to decrease or stop the hair pulling. It is a morbid tic with organic consequences that are more than cosmetic. In catering to the discussion about Obsessive Compulsive Disorders in Chapter 4, we classify *Trichlotillomania* as a mental disease in the class of normal Layer over accretion, independent of the Obsessive Compulsive Disorder and Related categories. We tightly associate it instead with *Dermatillomania* and propose the both as two distinct facets of the same Disorder. We abstain from proposing a new label in order to avoid departing from the taxonomic structure already in place. The discussion that follows will extol the reason for this integration.

PASSIVE - RESPONSIVE SYMPTOMS

An increasing tension before pulling, or when resisting the hair pulling. Enjoyment of sensations of hair thickness on fingers and pulling from scalp. A sense of pleasure or relief after hair is pulled. Repetitive attempts to stop hair pulling perceived as a bad tic or do it less often but without success. Avoidance of social events or close relationships, use of scarves, wigs, or makeup to cover up areas of the body with noticeable hair loss. Significant distress, anxiety, shame, and embarrassment about hair pulling activity itself.

ACTIVE - REACTIVE SYMPTOMS

Compulsively pulling hair out, typically from scalp, eyebrows, eyelashes, beard, pelvis, etc., with sites varying over time. Preference for specific types of hair, with pulling rituals or patterns of hair pulling. Biting, chewing or eating pulled-out hair. Playing with pulled-out hair or rubbing it on lips or face. Many also pick their skin, bite their nails or chew their lips. Sometimes pulling hairs from pets or dolls or from materials such as clothes or blankets.

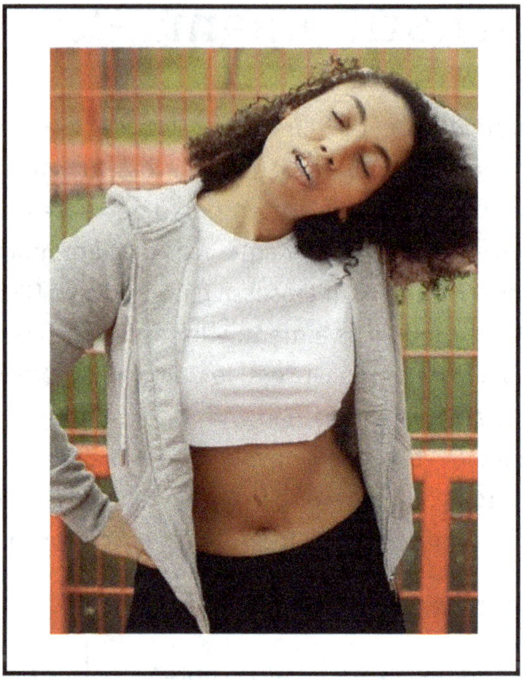

KNOWN VARIANTS

Trichotillomania with minor Excoriation. Minor Trichotillomania with hair pulling symptom alone.

LANGUAGE

"I scratched an itch" or *"I pulled out a hair that didn't belong."*

BEHAVIORAL FLIPS

When patients go from boredom, anxiety and anger to active hair pulling, we are observing an anti-symmetric flip or swing between the two chiral sides of the Foliate (the sensation of satisfaction and enjoyment resulting from the hair pull is masochistic).

DERIVED DISABILITIES

Problems at work, school or in social situations related to pulling out hair. Sores, scars or calluses, skin irritations. Noticeable hair loss, such as shortened or thinned hair, or bald areas on the scalp or other areas of the body, including sparse or missing eyelashes and eyebrows altogether. Chewed hair swabs making it to the bowels may cause serious medical complications. Impaired social interaction as most people with *Trichotillomania* pull hair in private and generally try to hide the disorder from others.

AWARENESS

Conscious (Neurotic Disorder). Note that in Mild Hair Pulling alone, the dysfunction might not arise to the level of a qualified tidal Neurotic Disorder, but only a persistent tic dysregulation controllable by the individual. This would occur when the characterological filiation is not in line with the tidal Layer (Layer **7**).

CHARACTEROLOGICAL FILIATION

Paradoxical

QG LAYER-PARTITIONS

7 **[(-1, -2, -3, -4)** (+1, +2, +3, +4)**]**

STATISTICS

Between 0.6% and 4.0% of the overall population, and 1% in the United States. Because denial of the disorder by the affected is frequent, and many do not seek professional help, the prevalence numbers many not be factually inaccurate. It is however estimated that females are highly more likely than men to develop trichotillomania, some estimates putting the gender-gap ratio as high as 10 females for every 1 male.

INSIGHTS

In *Trichotillomia*, analytic focus has been traditionally set on hair pulling in the Disorder, given that unrelated stress, anger, anxiety and boredom may knowingly trigger hair pulling activity. However, in *Trichotillomia* the intent to self harm is patent as a principle. It is by virture of this principled intent that many affected subjects engage as well in other clearly destructive behaviors such as picking their skin, bite their nails or chew and disfigure their lips. The latter symptoms are genuinely shared with *Dermatillomania* or *Skin Picking Disorder*, and in this case represent a minor in the nosology of the Disorder.

Furthermore, there is a tension inherent to the act of hair pulling experienced as an irresistible need to incur in self-deconstruction, which is followed by relief or pleasure after accomplishing the act of self-harm. These features make *Trichotillomania* an unequivocal expression of Sado-Masochism, much beyond the *obsessive compulsion* qualifier still conferred to the disease in official psychiatry. The unconscious nature of these urges and sensations undoubtedly emanate from the paradoxical Norm and pensive partitions pertaining to Layer **7** of the Mental Foliate, with a noticeable tidal exacerbation on the side of PASSIVE-RESPONSIVE symptoms. The stress, anxiety and anger experienced by the subject are genuinely germane to the roots of the Disorder while the feelings of shame and embarrassment are subsequent conscious reactions to the very potent and irresistible unconscious self-destructive spurs.

It is interesting to note in the language *"I have pulled out a hair that did not belong"* a striking similarity with the sort of language held by patients affected with disorders in the family of *Cotard's Syndrome* (Layer-**7** induced class) who hold that their limbs or organs do not belong to them!

Although the terms Sadism, Masochism and Sadomasochism have been officially deprecated in psychiatry, this is one other case where these qualifiers would justly apply, all exempt of any sexual context as the implicated acts are. Thefore, in Trichotillomania there is a major syndrome in the representation of the PASSIVE-RESPONSIVE side of the normal and a minor in the ACTIVE-REACTIVE side of the normal.

There is for sure any number of psychosocial factors that will drive patients to this particular manner of self-harm or sadomasochistic hair pulling activity. Whatever that external internalized factor is, it can only provoke pathological dysfunction through resonance with the pensive normal of Layer **7** of the individual's Mentation Foliate. The analyst may view in the peculiarity of the dysfunction (pulling hair and skin picking) an attempt to recover primal nakedness and probe the patient's psyche along that line. One can see that this would take us back to intrauterine or fetal state of unborn or not yet existent. Translate a desire to not be or not exist, which is again a Layer **7** paradoxical motivation spurred at the Right-Chiral side of the normal. Yet, the analyst may alternatively probe the psyche for uncovered or suppressed anger toward domineering parents, as has been said. That again takes us back to Layer **7**, Left-Chiral pensive partitions, in the exegetical invocation of a chiral swing from one side of the Layer (- /Anger) to the other (+ /self-Repugnance). Here we opportunely invite the reader to revisit the section regarding psychic equilibration through longitudinal layer transflows and the paradoxical normal nature of defense mechanisms in the disease model discussion undertaken in Chapter 4.

Dermatillomania

Dermatillomania or *Skin Picking* is also alternatively labeled *Excoriation*. Individuals with *Dermatillomania* feel a compulsion to pick the skin throughout their body. They often target face, hands, fingers, arms, legs and scalp, and may spend hours a day on their picking mania, which can last for months or even years. It is generally a chronic condition, although sporadic at times. Official clinical diagnosis requires symptoms to be purely psychogenic, even though organic consequences of this morbid tic may be very serious and transcend cosmetics.

PASSIVE - RESPONSIVE SYMPTOMS

Individuals with this condition spend hours obsessively thinking about picking their skin and trying to resist the urge before giving in. Unrelated stress, anger, anxiety and boredom may trigger skin picking activity. Anxiety, depression, shame, fear of exposure, and embarrassment over the condition.

ACTIVE - REACTIVE SYMPTOMS

Compulsive skin picking extending to pulling, squeezing, scraping, lancing, and even biting both healthy and damaged skin from various parts of the body, including the scalp. May use either own fingers or an instrument, i.e. tweezers or pins. Expectation and wishes for skin spots to appear for more opportunities to skin pick. Compulsion to skin pick on skin spots accumulating pus. Compulsion to dig into or further disturb the irritated skin spots becoming lesions. Compulsion to skin pick on others and even animals. Discomfort about the condition usually leads to attempts at covering up own skin with makeup, clothing, or otherwise.

KNOWN VARIANTS

Minor Excoriation within major Trichotillomania

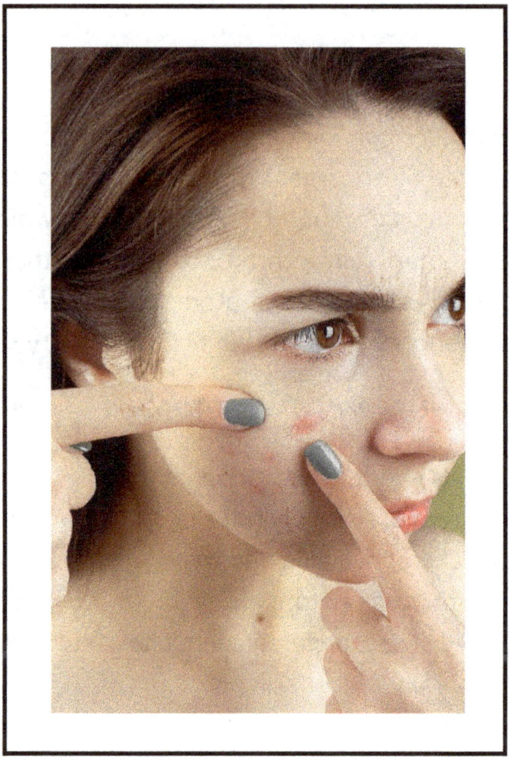

LANGUAGE

"My dog had a bug bite on her neck and I picked it (she can't argue with me). I felt so bad afterwards, but I couldn't stand seeing it..." or *"My partner has mild adult acne so he often gets blackheads and whiteheads I just soooo want to squeeze and pick. I don't but I can't help pointing them out and occasionally asking if I can pick them for him. It's so gross but I hate seeing them."* or *"I pick and pick at my scalp in a nervous fit and do it until it bleeds or becomes raw and sore. Then it scabs and I want to pick the scab. I often do and look at the red scab trying to figure out more... One time I had to go to the nurse because my head was bleeding too badly."*

BEHAVIORAL FLIPS

Swings from Anxiety, Anguish or Angst to Compulsively Furious Skin Picking.

DERIVED DISABILITIES

The disease may interfere with normal social interactions, resulting in patient's uncomfortable relationships with family and friends. *Dermatillomania* often results in visible skin damage and disfigurement from lesions, discoloration, open wounds, scars, and infections.

AWARENESS

Conscious (Neurotic Disorder). Skin picking activity can be automatic, i.e. occuring while watching television or reading a book. It can be focused, with the full awareness of the subject spotted on the pulling activity. This is typical of a tic. In both cases the subject is well aware of the activity in the context of his/her behavior as well as its dysfunctional nature. That is why he or she attempts to react against it.

CHARACTEROLOGICAL FILIATION

Paradoxical

QG LAYER-PARTITIONS

7 [(-1, -2, -3, -4) **(+1, +2, +3, +4)**]

STATISTICS

An estimated 2–5% of the population. Most common among kids between the ages of 13–15 years old but can also affect younger children and adults age 30–45. Estimated to be more present in females than males. Again, the notable embarrassment around the disorder is doomed to skew statistical prevalence numbers.

INSIGHTS

The etiological exegesis that we have advanced for *Trichotillomania* also entirely holds for *Dermatillomania*. We even see that the scalp can also be involved in Skin picking, as much as exacerbation of the pensive partitions of Anxiety and Anguish whose autonomous activity can trigger flips to Skin Picking activity. In addition, the morbid activity in both disorders may extend to other objects, other people or even animals beyond strictly the self. Unlike *Trichotillomania* however, the symptom set accuses higher over accrual on the ACTIVE-REACTIVE side of normal Layer **7** which appears as a major with respect to the lesser number of symptoms on the PASSIVE-RESPONSIVE side as indicated in the nosological block. Therefore, the two Disorders exhibit a complementary major-minor spectrum over the two chiral sets making up Layer **7**. In other words, in one disorder the Left-Chiral set is the major with the Right-Chiral being the minor, whereas in the other, the reverse is true.

The following are some of the psychoanalytic etiological hypotheses that have been advanced to explain *Dermatillomania*:

- It can be understood as a way to decrease one's physical attractiveness due to disfavoring personal attitudes concerning sex.
- It may be a way to discharge uncovered suppressed anger toward domineering parents.
- It may be a mechanism to avoid stressful events or releasing tension that builds up as a result of negative emotions, i.e. impatience, frustration, dissatisfaction, and even boredom.

The latter is wilfully expressed by the sufferers themselves. They are all defense mechanisms and as such they all cycle back to Layer **7** hyperactivity. Some of the language we report show that it is not only limited to a self-harm motive but an endogenous Repugnance trigger with clear intent to find the disgusting or horrendous where there is none or not that much, and not just concerning the self but others as well, including animals. Some of the symptoms reported in the ACTIVE-REACTIVE chiral set further show that it can become quite of a dirty repugnant affair for the seeking.

We lastly note for the record that skin picking can also occur with dermatological conditions, autoimmune disorders, opiate withdrawal, and so-called developmental disorders, such as autism. In the latter, which is the only case of interest to us, it is part of a much larger constellation of somatic symptoms which the subject engages in without any underlying sadomasochistic motive of self-harm or self-disgust, i.e. recurrent hitting of the fists causing a coarse hardening of the phalanxes. Further, it is not a tic in that case, since the subject is unaware of its dysfunctional nature and does not react against it. Therefore, the association is to be dismissed.

In conclusion, the clearly known intersection between the syndromes of the two Disorders demand a mutual definition or at least an integration in their definitions, if we do not want to fall into the caveats of calling for never-ending and intrinsically meaningless comorbidity of disparate disorders. This integration is of a complex order and we believe that the above etiological exegesis has intimately ascertained its correct dimension.

PATHOLOGICAL AFFILIATES

Stereotypic Movement Disorder (SMD)

Stereotypic Movement Disorder is a multiple tic impairment that constrains sufferers to such dysfunctionalities as body rocking, nodding, hand shaking or waving, self-bitting, head-banging, mouthing of objects, hitting self, teeth clenching or grinding. The repetitive hand movements consist of quick, rhythmic, small hand rotations, or repetitive voluntary movements that typically involve the fingers or arms.

There is heavy emphasis in psychiatry in distinguishing SMD tic-like dysfunctionalities from legitimate tics, under the allegation that they consist of voluntary movements and not spasmodic ones. Stereotypies are more fixed, rhythmic, and prolonged in duration than tics are, which generally exhibit brief, rapid, random, and fluctuating motion. However, these so-called stereotypies are as repetitive in their modality as tics are, and both stereotypies and tics cease or tend to be reduced with distraction. In fact, stereotypies are even more repetitive than tics since they are consistent and fixed in their pattern or topography compared with tics, which are variable in their presentation. Therefore, if the distinction between stereotypies and tics is meaningful from a semiological standpoint, it is for certain not fundamental from an impairment viewpoint. We will further see that the difference does not bear out etiologically either.

The most important aspect of SMD nosology is its inherent self-injury component. Aside from body rocking, nodding and hand shaking, the rest of the syndrome is totally self-injurious or self-harming. Bodily injury with this syndrome may go from mild bruising or erythema to hitting hand against body, to lacerations or amputation of digits, to retinal detachment from head banging. What is even more important is that SMD sufferers are not at all distressed by their symptoms and may even appear to derive enjoyment from their repetitive and self-harming stereotypies.

The underlying impulse of this entire syndrome is a sadomasochistic drive from an over tidal Layer-**7** palette of partitions, just as seen in *Trichotillomania-Dermatillomania*. Although there are instances where the syndrome appears to be concurrent with other mental disorders, autism in particular, SMD has been observed as a stand-alone syndrome. It is important to reexamine the evoked comorbitity cases in order to weight whether the three non-injurious symptoms are the ones spotted in comorbid Disorders or not. In that eventuality, the co-morbid qualification should be summarily dropped. We have not seen enough clinical practice cases or enough granular nosologic reports to make that call in our review of the research literature.

We make *Stereotypic Movement Disorder* a pathological affiliate to *Trichotillo-mania-Dermatillomania*.

AWARENESS

Conscious (Neurotic Disorder)

CHARACTEROLOGICAL FILIATION

Paradoxical

QG LAYER-PARTITIONS

7 [(-1, -2, -3, -4) **(+1, +2, +3, +4)]**

Developmental Coordination Disorder

Developmental Coordination Disorder (DCD) also labeled *Clumsy Child Syndrome* is a disorder in which children or adult sufferers demonstrate substantial difficulty in coordinating movements such as those needed to climb the playground, catch balls, complete handwriting tasks or dress up. These movement difficulties interfere with the sufferer's ability to perform everyday tasks and impact their academic performance alike. Although the course of the disease starts in childhood, it should not be considered an infant-related disorder since it will continue into adulthood if left untreated. In addition, the appearance of the disorder may lead others to believe that the sufferer is affected with some form of mental retardation or intellection impairment, a complete misappreciation owing to the very fact that affected people generally demonstrate at least a normal level of intelligence. Differential diagnosis must be keen in discarding other forms of motor dysfunctions that cannot be reduced to this specific type in the diagnosis determination per the presenting clinical nosology of the case at hand.

PASSIVE - RESPONSIVE SYMPTOMS [LEFT CHIRALITY]

Difficulty planning physical movements into a controlled sequence to complete a task, or difficulty remembering the next movement in a sequence despite being instructed how to proceed. Difficulty with activities requiring constant changes (e.g. games like baseball, tennis, etc). Reduced balance and postural control (e.g. unsteady when stepping over a height or when standing while dressing). Difficulty with printing or handwriting, resulting in deficiency in academic subjects such as mathematics, spelling or written language which typically require accurate handwriting or good page organization. Difficulties with organization of school desk, school bag, homework or even the space on a page. Poor sense of medium-related body awareness or self-localization: trouble determining the distance between themselves and objects, and hence bumping into objects or knocking things over and unknowingly invading other people's personal space. Easily distracted. Reduced self-esteem. Frustrated easily when completing tasks. Anxiety when asked to participate in difficult activities.

ACTIVE - REACTIVE SYMPTOMS [RIGHT CHIRALITY]

Difficulty with or delayed in developing gross motor (physical) skills (e.g. running, jumping, hopping, catching balls, climbing), as well as fine motor skills (e.g. handwriting, doing up buttons, threading beads, tying shoe laces), or both. As a consequence, may avoid socializing with peers in physical games (e.g. on the playground) for fear of failure or due to experience with repeated failure. Motor skills not at par with intellection skills., i.e. intellectual and language skills may be quite strong while motor skills are delayed or deficient. Intellection skills only comes to be somehow affected when motor activity is involved in tasks. Demonstrable average or higher than average intellectual abilities.

PASSIVE – RESPONSIVE + ACTIVE – REACTIVE SYMPTOMS [LEFT + RIGHT CHIRALITY]

Difficulty with activities requiring coordinated use of both sides of the body (e.g. cutting with scissors, running, swinging a bat, etc.). Frequent tripping, unsteady walk, fumbling objects and running into others. Difficulty with physiognomic balance. Appears clumsy or awkward in movements compared to friends of similar age (e.g. running awkwardly or holding scissors awkwardly).***KNOWN VARIANTS***

None

LANGUAGE

May complain that *'this is too hard'* or *'I can't do it'* when presented with motor activities.

BEHAVIORAL FLIPS

Choosing to rush through tasks in reaction to poor control or balance that occurs when completing them at a normal or slow rate, as an intent to avoid intolerable completion difficulties. Or very intently extrapolating in taking lots of extra time in performing tasks in order to avoid inaccuracy and incompleteness in their execution.

DERIVED DISABILITIES

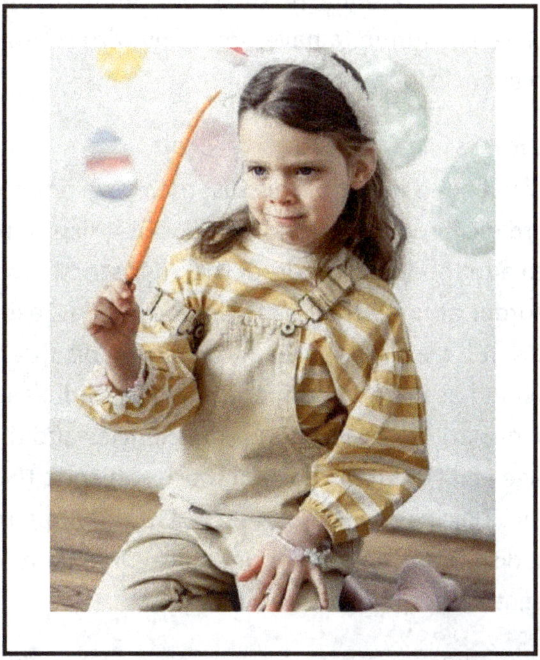

Adults with developmental coordination disorder experience significant troubles in social aspects of their daily lives caused by their motor coordination disabilities. Deficient fine motor skills associated with the disorder causes difficulty with self-care, cooking, housework, and shopping. Weak gross motor skills affect ability to engage in physical activity since their balance and posture are significantly compromised. Also experience difficulties in non-motor domains in the area of executive functioning. Known to impact their inhibition abilities, working memory, and execution attention. In general, motor coordination difficulties will impact academic progress, social integration and emotional development.

AWARENESS

Conscious (Neurotic Disorder)

CHARACTEROLOGICAL FILIATION

Intellectual

QG LAYER-PARTITIONS

3 [(-1, -2, -3, -4) (+1, +2, +3, +4)]

[Left-Chiral Sector] and [Right-Chiral Sector] at par

STATISTICS

Developmental Coordination Disorder is considered a motor skills disorder that affects 5 to 6% of all school-aged children. The ratio of boys to girls varies from

2:1 to 5:1, depending on the group studied. A percentage of 50 to 70 percent of children continue to have problems with coordinated movement through adolescence despite treatment.

INSIGHTS

Several key aspects of this Disorder have not received deserved attention toward elicitation of its etiological roots. First, if the Disorder naturally continues into adulthood if not cured, then it is strictly speaking not a 'developmental' disorder at first order, as the name implies, expressed in retardation of motor skills. It is thus more broadly an all-age disorder. Second, there is a high emphasis that has been put on motor activity deficiencies in the disorder, disregarding the disparity between those deficiencies and the normally average or above average level of intelligence of these subjects. Third, there is never a medical or neurologic basis for the observed motor impairments, strongly suggesting that the disorder is not of a neurological origin but plausibly a conversion or psychosomatic disorder.

The specific motor problems to be witnessed here are not i.e. agitation or incontrolable repetitive impulse dysfunction, but very particularly a coordination dysfunction. Coordination or interrelation is the very Norm inherent to QG Normal Layer **3**. Typically, DCD sufferers not only experience difficulty learning new movement skills but once learned in one environment (e.g. school), they may continue showing difficulties performing the task in another environment (e.g. home); thus requiring to be taught the same task anew in every other environment. This specific symptom exhibits the higher relational aspect of the motor impairment in its pure psychogenic nature, which clearly otherwise involves coordination in its neurobiologic expression.

The palette of pensive partitions pertaining to Layer **3**, from *Aberration* to *Lucidity* answers at once the question as to how can someone showing higher intelligence and insightfulness of clairvoyance be at the same time aberrantly idiotic in anything else, given the broad connectedness of elements of the natural world. The concept of a tide in the expression of the full set of those partitions wonderfully elucidates a syndrome such as *Perfectionism*, in which a de facto high achiever with superb intelligence yet harbors idiotic and morbid doubts about his/her capacities and achievements which everybody else around is keen to acknowledge. Should we leave for a moment the biological motor plan, still in full display here in DCD is the same lack of capacity for interrelatedness that we call *Disorientation*. Said lack will also cause a DCD sufferer to have to re-learn the task set in question at every new environmental setting while being highly proficient intellectually otherwise. The entire motor symptomatic spectrum observable in *Developmental Coordination Disorder* must be peremptorily understood in terms of a conversion of the latter intellection disposition onto the neurological plane to give it the tenure of a psychosomatic Disorder. The overall characteristic 'clumsiness' and 'ackwardness' is created by the Intellection Layer (or Layer **3**) of the Mental Foliate, in an overtidal level of activity, and projected onto the central nervous system. That is the fundamental reason why there is no diagnosable neurological dysfunction subtending this motor-driven Disorder.

Coordinating both sides of the body (e.g., cutting with scissors, or tying shoe laces) is an important element of consideration in the Disorder. In effect, beyond the general coordination problem, there is a specific difficulty with handedness in the disease, notable in the following impairments: problems handling scissors as noted as well as tying shoe laces, but also in other common activities such as walking and handling objects with two hands resulting in frequent tripping, unsteady walk, running into others, on one hand, and, on the other, fumbling objects and poor physical balance. It is important to recognize these apparent coordination problems in terms of being the consequences of a significant handedness impairment. The background landscape subtending this important deficit is a problem with the formation of the ground levels of the Foliate, in terms of Ground-level Accrual 0 of the Foliate experiencing difficulties developing into Ground-level Accrual 1 in order to produce adequate gender determination[32]. As a reminder, ground level 0 is that of a Mentation Foliate

[32] We are somewhat over simplifying the organization of handedness in the analysis here since it implies in fact two composite Foliates as it naturally presents in human ontology. Suffice it to say that in handedness one gains prevalence over the other in phenomenology. For the purpose of this analysis, it is unnecessary to delve into this ultrastructural level of human ontological organization.

with two Chiral Sectors at par in weight, whereas ground level 1 is that of a Mentation Foliate with one Chiral Sector being prevalent over the other. In this case, it is the Right-Chiral Sector (male-determinant) that fails to reach the fullness of natural prevalence, since motorization is what is at stake. This analysis is keenly supported by the known epidemiologic statistical facts about the disease which put males at a marked proportion ranging from 2:1 to 5:1 over females in experiencing the Disorder in the population! Our analytic exegesis is also supported by the fact that the severity of the condition does not worsen over time but the dysfunction simply continues unabated into adulthood, thereby proving to manifest as an underlying permanent condition of the Mental Body once it had settled in, consistent with a one-time accrual shift that failed to occur.

In that sense, one may justifiably further invoke a disparity between a biologically determined male gender identity for the physical body and an asexuated Mentation Foliate borne out by sufferers of *Developmental Coordination Disorder*.

In conclusion, the above etiological advances have made it clear that while the causes of DCD are admittedly not well-understood, the belief among researchers hitherto that it is the result of delayed brain development is simply astray. Likewise, in the light of the above, the appreciation that the ‘motor milestones’ in the dysfunction oftentimes are not exactly delayed but only the ‘acquisition’ of such skills, albeit a judicious observation, does not go far enough etiologically either.

SLEEP & SLEEP-RELATED DISORDERS

Insomnia

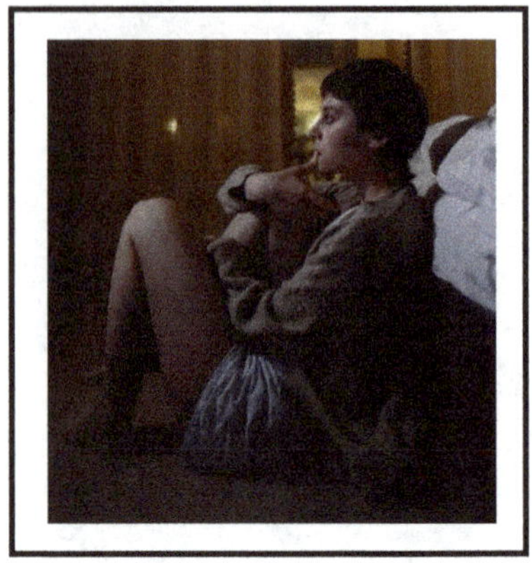

Insomnia is a disorder characterized by a difficulty in initiating sleep and staying asleep for a continued 7-hour period or slightly more as well as a tendency to wake up early in the morning with inability to get back to sleep thereafter.

SYMPTOMS

Affected individuals cannot fall or stay asleep long enough for physiological restoration. Do not feel well rested after sleep. Long periods of overnight wake and difficulty returning to sleep result in a relatively short period of nightly sleep time. Consequently, often experience fatigue or sleepiness during daytime, along with related irritability and inattention.

KNOWN VARIANTS

Two subtypes identified: short-term insomnia (officially symptoms must last less than three months) and chronic insomnia.

DERIVED DISABILITIES

Trouble concentrating on tasks, sometimes to an extreme that severely degrades work performance or social life.

STATISTICS

The US Center for Disease Control (CDC) reports the following: *"In 2014, short sleep duration (less than 7 hours in a 24-hour period) was less common among respondents aged ≥65 years (26.3%) compared with other age groups. The age-adjusted prevalence of short sleep duration was higher among Native Hawaiians/Pacific Islanders (46.3%), non-Hispanic blacks (45.8%), multiracial non-Hispanics (44.3%), and American Indians/Alaska Natives (40.4%) compared with non-Hispanic whites (33.4%), Hispanics (34.5%), and Asians (37.5%). Short sleep prevalence did not differ between men and women...*

Adults who were short sleepers (less than 7 hours per 24-hour period) were more likely to report 10 chronic health conditions compared to those who got enough sleep (7 or more hours per 24-hour period)."

QG LAYER-PARTITIONS

Layer 1 or 2 or 3 over accrued.

MENTATION CURSOR

Hypocursor over accrued.

INSIGHTS

From our QG psychophysics perspective, the primary direct cause of insomnia is a mentation Cursor in Hypocursor mode with a morbid tidal gradient and stalling dynamics as defined in the disease model in Chapter 4. Insomnia is well known to be frequently comorbid to a large number of neuroses. Very understandably, the Hyper-Egocentric character is particularly vulnerable to this type of impairment since it is naturally endowed with a tidal Cursor already. It is important to distinguish between insomnia that manifests in neuroses and that which manifests in psychoses, such as the Manic phase of Bipolar Disorder. In the latter, it is the constant state of intense agitation and sensory stimulation which prevent the realization of the state of hyposensorial stimulation required for sleep. Obviously, all of the disorders driven by extreme agitation or hyperactivity will experience a sleep impairment of the kind.

In a sense, in the case of psychoses with insomnia, we are not really dealing with insomnia per se, since the Cursor is already in a Hypercursor mode with a tidal gradient, but matter-of-factly a state of awaken sleep. Psychotic insomnia is much closer in nature to the expression of somnambulism as awaken sleep, which is in itself a psychosis, than it is to ordinary insomnia. From that very standpoint, the hallucinations that are present in many psychoses may be understood as awaken sleep caused by a highly tidal Hypercursor.

It is not at all improper to take insomnia in any form as a sign of more significant problems from the standpoint of both psychological and physiological health, given the impact of sleep on and the influence it receives from the individual's general state of health. Cultural pressures and customs are for sure important drivers to this impairment, all of which are of utmost significance from a public health perspective in the assessment and prevention of disorders in general.

PATHOLOGICAL AFFILIATES

Insufficient Sleep Syndrome

Insufficient Sleep Syndrome, otherwise called *Sleep Deprivation*, is a sleep disorder that occurs whenever there is no organic or psychological cause to the lack of sleep. It is purely driven by external forcible conditions or personal choices that reduce the necessary amount of time dedicated to sleep for restoration to take place. People with this Disorder tend to ignore its obvious cause. The person routinely spends less than 7 hours in bed at night and typically manifests somewhat slow responses and lack of agility in daily activities, which they oftentimes seek to supplement.

SYMPTOMS

Concentration and attention problems, lowered energy level, reduced alertness. Distractibility, irritability and/or fatigue, frequent consumption of tonics to compensate.

INSIGHTS

Organizing a lifestyle around deprivation of sleep under sociocultural pressures appears to be one of the major contributing factors to this disorder. Despite the fact that no direct medical or psychological causes are responsible for this disorder, it is important to realize that temperamental predisposition may constitute a major driver in this case. People taxed "workaholic" in popular culture are especially vulnerable to this disorder by volition and intent, as they compulsively work hard and long hours into their sleep time.

In general, the three Tempers based on preeminence of the Conscious Cognos, including the Hyper-Egocentric Temper constitute a so-called risk factor for Sleep Deprivation, given the strong appeal of reality on those characters and the tight tendency to transact or manipulate environmental elements in the same. Population statistics for this disorder strongly support this view. The prevalent age group for the sufferers has been measured to be the mid-to-late 30's and it often goes undetected by affected adults until their 40's after the long term effects have added up. Furthermore, it affects a slightly greater number of men than women. And lastly, the voluntary choice of a late-shift work schedule is knowingly not for the "faint of heart" since most are aware of the consequences of those choices as much as the superior benefits of nighttime sleep over daytime sleep to which they renounce.

What's more, the onset of this disorder, apparently benign to the affected, is generally precursory to much more severe syndromes such as Burnout Syndrome, a depletion of the Mental causing one of the most painful and disparaging mental disorders. Medical professionals themselves are knowingly at a high risk[33].

---

[33] The American Medical Association and the Stanford University School of Medicine jointly publish an annual study of burnout symptoms among US physicians, finding in 2017 an average of 44% of 5000 surveyed physicians exhibited at least one burnout symptom.

Hypersomnia

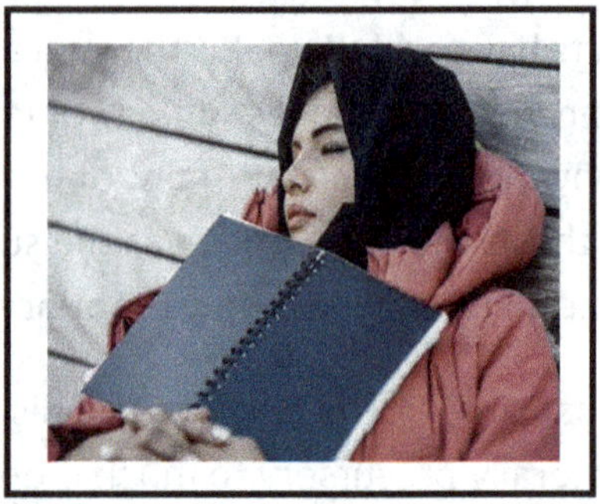

Hypersomnia or Hypersomnolence is a disorder in which the patient experiences significant episodes of sleepiness, even after having had 7 hours or more of deep or quality sleep. It is also less formally designated Excessive Sleepiness, manifest as daytime sleepiness with daily episodes of irrepressible need to sleep, which is not caused by another form of sleep disorder.

SYMPTOMS

Falling asleep several times during the day. Taking naps to combat the sleepiness but not waking up refreshed, or sleeping more than 7 hours but not feeling rested. Presenting difficulty waking up from sleep such as feeling confused or engaging in a struggle to wake up. Patients have difficulty staying awake during the day and fall asleep while at work or school, or even while talking or driving. May show anxiety, low energy, and loss of appetite as well as increased annoyance and impatience.

KNOWN VARIANTS

Subtypes: Idiopathic Hypersomnia, Hypersomnia due to organic/psychiatric condition/medication.

DERIVED DISABILITIES

Memory problems, slow or otherwise impaired thinking, slow to communicate.

STATISTICS

The National Sleep Foundation estimates that up to 40% of individuals present periodic symptoms of hypersomnia and 4-6% of the general population suffer from outright permanent hypersomnia.

QG LAYER-PARTITIONS

Layer 9 over accrued.

MENTATION CURSOR

Hypercursor over accrued.

INSIGHTS

Let us first note, in attending to the naming label for the disease, that Idiopathic Hypersomnia refers to somnolence whose cause is unknown, whereas organic Hypersomnia, the other type referred to in the VARIANTS section is one that is knowingly linked to a deficiency in hypocretin, the hormone responsible for the wake state along with orexin. Therefore it is a fair characterization to qualify Idiopathic Hypersomnia to be of psychogenic origin, whereas organic Hypersomnia is of neurologic nature, possibly originating from medication or neural damage of some kind. It is necessary to make the clarification that in organic Hypersomnia, the hormonal condition does not define sleep, as the monist perspective is quick to conclude, but is only responsible for setting the physiology and physiognomic necessary for the oncome of sleep and the successive development of its internal content. Hypocretin or orexin does not create the contents or dream content of sleep.The fact that Hypersomnia may occur without hormonal dysfunction whatsoever, as it is in so-called Idiopathic Hypersomnia, strongly supports this view.

A critical factor in the determination of Hypersomia and its types are REM readings in order to primarily establish their frequency. For instance, the differentiating feature between Narcolepsy Type 2, which we discuss below as an Affiliate Disorder, and Idiopathic Hypersomnia is the number of sleep-onset REM periods or SOREMP. The Hypersomnia Foundation estimates that *"The diagnosis of Narcolepsy Type 2 requires the presence of two or more SOREMPs on the MSLT (Multiple Sleep Latency Test) or one SOREMP on polysomnography and one on the MSLT. The diagnosis of IH can only be made if the person has one or no SOREMPs on polysomnography and MSLT combined."* SOREMPs are REM sleep periods that abnormally occur within 15 minutes of onset of sleep, while in normal sleep they occur within about 1 hour to 90 mn of sleep onset.

The medical research literature offers profuse reports of REM's in Hypersomnia, which firmly confirm both the existence and the wandering of the Hypercursor throughout the Unconscious Cognos in all forms of the disease since REM sleep is firmly associated with dreams. It is also clear that the disease is essentially due to a dysfunction of the Hypercursor in its dynamics which we attribute to an overaccrual in its intensity, since this mode of the Cursor may untimely occur from wake in the middle of such activities as talking or driving, very inconveniently pulling the self-awareness from Conscious to Unconscious. Another consequence of the overaccrued intensity of the Hypercuror is its abnormal stagnation within the Unconscious Cognos, since the Somnolence is almost endless. Further, one cannot discard that even circumstantial instances of absence of REM dreams in the course of the disease might well be an indication of a stagnation of the Mentation cursor over the left-chiral partitions of Layer **9**, causing the state of awareness to remain in a prolonged or recurrent dormant (hibernating) mode.

Patent is the participation of tidal left-chiral partitions of Layer **9** of the Foliate in this Disorder, notably the partitions of *Inanition* and *Cluelessness*, symptomatically revealed in the confusion accompanying wakeup and necessity for the affected to fight their way to wake from the state of sleep. Furthermore, we have long previously discussed how sleep is a phenomenology attributable to Transcendent Layer **9** of the Foliate, and very intimately to the two aforementioned pensive partitions. The pervasiveness of sleep in this Disorder is only commensurate with a super accretion in the expression of these partitions and the Layer in general, in the condition of their neural projections.

All of the above implicates that the Asymptotic Temperament as much as the Hyper-Asymptotic Temperament stand for sheer precursors or so-called risk factors for Hypersomnia.

PATHOLOGICAL AFFILIATES

Kleine-Levin Syndrome

The Kleine-Levin Syndrome Foundation reports the *Kleine-Levin Syndrome (KLS)* or *Sleeping Beauty Syndrome* to be *"a rare and complex neurological disorder characterized by recurring periods of excessive amounts of sleep [over more than 10 years], altered behavior, and a reduced understanding of the world... In between episodes, those with KLS appear to be in perfect health with no evidence of behavioral or physical dysfunction."*

SYMPTOMS

The Kleine-Levin Syndrome Foundation describes the symptoms of the Disorder as follows:

"In addition to excessive sleep, a Kleine-Levin Syndrome (KLS) patient's whole demeanor is changed, often appearing "spacey" or childlike. When awake the patient experiences confusion, disorientation, complete lack of energy (lethargy), and lack of emotions (apathy). Most patients report that everything seems out of focus, and that they are hypersensitive to noise and light. In some cases, food cravings (compulsive hyperphagia) are exhibited. Instances of uninhibited hypersexuality during an episode have also been reported.

Kleine-Levin Syndrome (KLS) episodes are cyclical. When present, KLS symptoms persist for days, weeks or even months, during which time all normal daily activities stop. Individuals are not able to attend school, work or care for themselves. Most are bedridden, tired and uncommunicative even when awake. Not everyone affected by KLS exhibits all of the symptoms described above.

Affected individuals may go for a period of weeks, months or even years without experiencing any symptoms, and then symptoms reappear with little warning. In between episodes, those diagnosed with KLS appear to be in perfect health with no evidence of behavioral or physical dysfunction. However they function daily with the frightful reality that they could become sick again at any moment. KLS episodes may continue to reoccur for a decade or longer with devastating effects on the adolescent's life and family. KLS robs children and young adults of big pieces of their lives, one agonizing episode at a time.

The mean diagnostic delay for proper Kleine-Levin Syndrome (KLS) diagnosis is four years. This means that it takes the average KLS patient four years before receiving an accurate diagnosis causing undue suffering to patients and families."

We were not the ones to use in this description the words "lethargy", "lack of emotions" (or in fact expressiveness), "apathy", a derivate of *Inanity*, or "reduced understanding of the world", an expression of *Cluelessness*, which we have largely discussed again in this compendium of Disorders and elsewhere in this treatise as ideation or attributes of Layer **9** Mentation.

Last paragraph in the citation underscores the urgent necessity to surpass time-based etiological assessments in psychiatry and psychology in favor of foundational root mentation in their configuration and psychophysics dynamics. The current official diagnostic code requires *"2 to 31 days of recurrent episodes of severe hypersomnia plus at least one of the following:*

1. *Cognitive abnormalities such as feeling of unreality, confusion, hallucinations.*
2. *Abnormal behavior such as irritability, aggression, odd behavior*
3. *Binge eating*
4. *Hyper-sexuality"*

One has to wonder what *"odd behavior"* exactly refers to in this diagnosis, while questioning the rather arbitrary 2-31 day timeframe criterion. It is also important to not confuse the fact of *"sometimes waking only to eat or go to the bathroom"* within Hypersomnolence with the legitimate Binge Eating disease immersed in the very particular symptomatic aura surrounding it, which we already amply discussed. It is understandable that if the body is propelled to remain apathetic for long periods of time as if hibernating, abundant ingestion and digestion of food with subsequent elimination of waste may be a strategy to preserve the thread of life which may become very thin in those circumstances, if it does not opt i.e. for coma which is an even deeper lethargic state. As to hypersexuality in Hypersomnia, it is opportune to highlight that in many biological species copulation is the final act before entering hibernation, with the sperm remaining dormant in the hibernating female. It is thus more likely that in Hypersomnia, hyperactive sexual behavior responds to an emulation of the act of hibernation instigated by the accrued dynamics in Layer **9** of the Foliate. It should not at all be confused with hyperactive sexual behavior in Bipolar Disorder for instance. By the same token, these remarks demonstrate why an etiological assessment stating that hyperactive sexuality is *comorbid* to many different Disorders is a completely erratic visualization.

Narcolepsy Type 1 and 2

Narcolepsy is a condition characterized by excessive fatigue and an extreme tendency to fall asleep whenever in relaxing surroundings. Known Variants are Narcolepsy Type 1 and Narcolepsy Type 2. Narcolepsy Type 1 adds to Hypersomnolence cataplexy (sudden drop of muscle tone) while awake or hypocretin-1 deficiency (neuropeptide controlling awakening). Narcolepsy Type 2 represents Hypersomnia in its strict definition, or Narcolepsy Type 1 without cataplexy or CSF hypocretin deficiency, that is. The differential diagnosis of Narcolepsy Type 2 requires however the presence of two or more SOREMPs on the Multiple Sleep Latency Test (MSLT) or one SOREMP on polysomnography and one on the MSLT. Only one or no SOREMP on polysomnography and MSLT combined takes the Disorder back to Idiopathic Hypersomnia.

SYMPTOMS

An incident of cataplexy in Narcolepsy Type 1 can last anywhere from a few seconds to several minutes and is oftentimes initiated by strong positive emotions, such as laughter and enthusiasm. Sufferers will suddenly lose the ability to control their muscles, resulting in slurring, falling, or being too incapacitated to move, all without falling asleep or losing conscious awareness. Also, sleep paralysis, change in REM sleep, hypnagogic and hypnogogic hallucinations.

INSIGHTS

The etiological exegesis applied to Idiopathic Hypersomnia fully applies here. In addition, one may notice among the reported symptoms the portrayal of swings primarily in the neurologic order with associated behavorial drivers. Cataplexy, as a loss of muscle tone and control of the same, intiated by laughter or sudden enthusiasm, definitely comes across as a neural flip between opposite or anti-symmetric neural nodes or currents, in accordance and correspondence with the binary distribution of the Mentation Foliate as posited in our psychophysics approach.

Restless Leg Syndrome

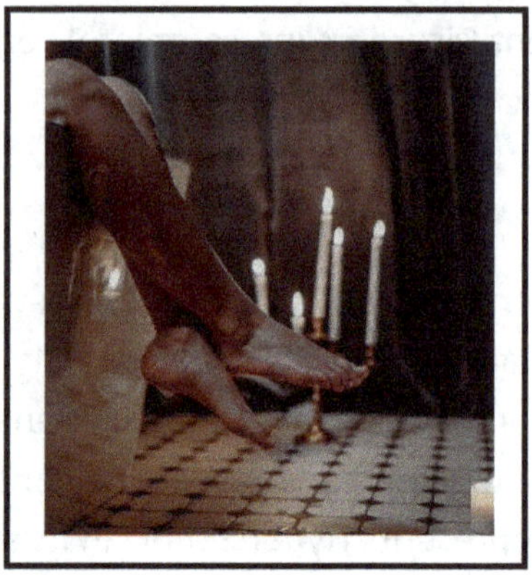

Restless Leg Syndrome (RLS) is a wake disorder with sleep-related elements whereby the affected individual experiences discomforting sleep-ladden sensations of motion requiring actual voluntary motion of limbs to appease them.

PASSIVE –RESPONSIVE SYMPTOMS

Surrogated sensations of aching, itching and electricity flowing in the limb(s). Factitious Limb creeping, crawling, pulling and throbbing experienced as inner limb sensations. May experience difficulty falling asleep and staying asleep.

ACTIVE-REACTIVE SYMPTOMS

Constant actual legs motion to minimize or prevent the discomforting sensations. Pacing the floor, or constantly moving legs while sitting. Tossing and turning in bed constantly. Symptoms worsening at bedtime and symptom-free early morning allowing for more refreshing sleep. Urge to move legs worsening during rest or inactivity.

KNOWN VARIANTS

None

DERIVED DISABILITIES

Resulting exhaustion, along with daytime sleepiness occasionally inherent to the condition can strongly affect mood, concentration, job and school performance, and personal relationships. Inability to concentrate, impaired memory, or failure to accomplish daily tasks. Traveling may become difficult.

STATISTICS

The National Sleep Foundation estimates that up to 7-10 percent of the U.S. population may be suffering from RLS, as it occurs in both men and women, although more prevalently in women. It knows no age, but symptoms typically become more frequent and last longer with age. The severely affected individuals tend to be middle-aged or older.

QG LAYER-PARTITIONS

4[**(-4, -3, -2, -1)** (1, 2, 3, 4)]

MENTATION CURSOR

Quadracursor over accrued.

INSIGHTS

Nobody spends the entire sleep cycle of one night from beginning to end in complete immobility, which a time-lapse video of a night sleep may easily reveal. There is continual visible physiognomic activity of the body during sleep, although the intervals may be quite extended. Yet this activity is restricted to the limited space of the resting bed or whatever other medium upon which sleep occurs. Therefore there is an affect-effector condition and scope that the body administers in order to develop and maintain the state of sleep ata particular location. Hence, it is safe to state that within the perception thresholds and the restrictive motional thresholds set for sleep, the body is aware and maintains awareness of the medium of sleep and the body interaction with that medium. In that context, there exists a specific domain of sensations and reactions that shall be understood as a necessary background for sleep development and preservation across its nighttime cycle.

These typical forms of sensations are not the ones we commonly experience in usual diurnal activity, and they are notably not sensations of cramp or numbness of limbs, or skin sensations. A description of these sensations and reactions, difficult though they are to explain, comes to us from people with *Restless Legs Syndrome*, which they unsurprisingly find abnormal and unpleasant, and mainly locate in their legs and feet, but less commonly in the arms, and more rarely chest and head. Those artifacts are mainly concentrated on the sensation aspect and usually happen on both sides of the body, although they can affect only one lateral side, ranging from uncomfortable to irritating to painful. As described in the *SYMPTOMS* block, thesee sensations mainly are:

- Crawling
- Creeping
- Pulling
- Throbbing
- Aching
- Itchy
- Electric

It is important to emphasize that the first four are strictly inner body sensations, although the lexicon is of a motional nature. There is no actual limb crawling, creeping or pulling which would be motional or effector acts. They are inner sensations that ultimately qualify as projections and that is the main reason why sufferers have difficulties to explain them. In the normal state of sleep, this compendium of sensations and reactions are what is registered under the label Periodic Limb Movement During Sleep, which we discuss thereafter as a sleep syndrome when it becomes excessively frequent.

The Hypercursor is experientially the sole administrator of this stimulus-respone domain in the outright state of developing nightly sleep. What we are seeing in *Restless Legs Syndrome* is a projective evocation of this domain within the very awake state, through a Mentation Cursor that has both the characteristics of the Hypercursor and the Hypocursor modes. It is indeed the **Quadracursor**, grown to the level of over accretion, thereby causing a morbid syndrome.

Whether Layer 4 itself may be over accrued in RLS is a distinct possibility worth probing for a full diagnosis, and constitutes more likely than not a plausibility. In that instance there would be emphasis of the Left-Chiral side over the Right-Chiral side as noted.

Consistent with our analysis of accrued Quadracursor dynamics in the disease model proposition, another exegetic view of this type of dysfunction relates to what normally occurs during the transitioning from wake to sleep. Headbutts and legbutts are ostensible occurences when people are normally transitioning into sleep, headbutts being particularly visible when the medium of sleep is a chair offering no firm back support to the head. It is not difficult to observe the recurrent or periodic limb and head motion occurring when someone else in our company happens to be falling asleep. One may legitimately view the RLS condition as eliciting all the body reactions that normally accompany the state of transition into sleep and causing them to present permanently because the Cursor is stuck. What the condition does is simply to give them constancy. Therefore, it is further very likely that the daytime somnolence infrequently associated with RLS may be light sleepiness following this pattern.

Lastly, the Hyper-Hyperbolic characterological stamp stands for a precursor or high risk factor for this Disorder.

PATHOLOGICAL AFFILIATES

Periodic Limb Movement Disorder

Periodic Limb Movement Disorder (PLMD) is repetitive cramping or jerking of the legs as sleep develops. It is a movement disorder that only occurs during sleep, reason why it is sometimes called Periodic Leg (or limb) Movement During Sleep. The term "Periodic" here refers not to time intervals specifically but the repetitive and rhythmic movements occurring approximately every 20-40 seconds. PLMD is considered a legitimate sleep disorder, since the movements often end up disrupting sleep and consequently lead to persistent daytime sleepiness.

PLMD movements primarily involve the legs, and less commonly the arms. These twitching and jerking movements may occur throughout the entire sleeping night. Though they are a visible expression of the Disorder, they do not constitute the primary symptom of the Disorder as previously discussed. The imperceptible compendium of sensations that precede those limb movements represent the actual charging triggers. Their overaccrual is what ultimately provokes the morbid movements.

PASSIVE –RESPONSIVE SYMPTOMS	*ACTIVE-REACTIVE SYMPTOMS*
None	Movements vary from slight to strenuous wild kicking and thrashing. Typical bending of the knee, ankle, and big toe joints as part of the movement. Last about 2 seconds, manifest as rhythmic and repetitive, occurring every 20-40 seconds. Movements tend to cluster in episodes that last a few minutes to several hours. Severity of movements may change from one night to the next.

KNOWN VARIANTS

Two types are known: (1) Primary PLMD which may be chronic (permanent) and (2) Secondary PLMD which is due to underlying medical cause, subject to disappear if the underlying medical condition is treated.

DERIVED DISABILITIES

Inconvenient urge to sleep during waking hours due to insufficient resting during nightly sleep qualifying as poor sleep.

QG LAYER-PARTITIONS

None

MENTATION CURSOR

Hypercursor over accrued

INSIGHTS

PLMD may admittedly well occur with other sleep disorders and is often particularly linked with *Restless Legs Syndrome* above studied. At least 80% of people with Restless Legs Syndrome also manifest *Periodic Limb Movement Disorder*, which is not a surprise, and as an occurrence when they have transitioned into the full state of sleep, but the reverse is not true. In other words, having *Periodic Limb Movement Disorder* does not imply that *Restless Leg Syndrome* is also in course. It is important to bear clear in mind the distinction between the two disorders, one being a state of compromised or semi-wake (Quadracursor driven Self-Awareness), and the other a state of complete sleep (Hypercursor driver Self-Awareness).

People with PLMD are unaware of the symptoms because the Self-Awareness is unconscious at time of occurrence. They only become cognizant of poor sleep and daytime sleepiness which are the health complaints they raise. They remain unaware of their nightly leg movements unless their partners make a mention.

It is as interesting as important to note that the symptoms of PLMD are mainly ACTIVE-REACTIVE, in contrast with RLS symptoms which are principally PASSIVE-RESPONSIVE. In this case, the association between the two disorders in their similar or parallel traits is not based on Layer dynamics but strictly on Cursor dynamics. The commonality between the Quadracursor and the Hypercursor is based on the semi incorporation of the Hyper mode within the Quadracursor as a hybrid entity.

It is equally judicious to conclude that all disorders based on Agitation as a Right-Chiral-Sector prevalent dysfunction are at risk to see PLMD show up as an authentic and legitimate comorbid partner.

Sleepwalking

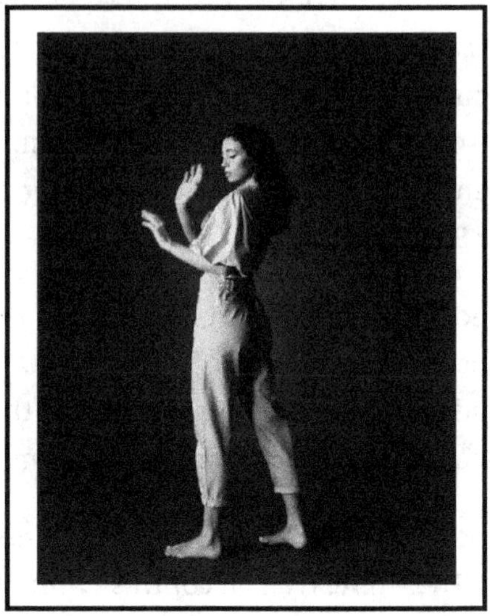

Sleepwalking (or Somnambulism) is said to be an arousal Disorder whereby a person appears to be awake but is actually asleep. The closest natural sleep-like state to *Sleepwalking* endowed with living faculties akin to the conscious seems to develop under the blanket and profiling of the thread of dreams, or REM sleep. However, the body during REM sleep is essentially motionless from the viewpoint of voluntary motion, and functionally engaged in rest, restoration and actualization (or updating). None of this appears to be part of *Sleepwalking*, however. In fact, there is so much lack of true sleep in Sleepwalking that it can lead to excessive daytime sleepiness and learning difficulties.

PASSIVE –RESPONSIVE SYMPTOMS

Sitting up in bed with wide open eyes. Showing a glazed, glassy-eyed expression during episodes. Do not respond or communicate with others. Disorientation and confusion for short period of time after being awakened. Difficult to wake up during an episode unlike normal sleep. Very characteristically, do not remember the episode in the morning when awake, unlike dreams in normal sleep. May also experience sleep terrors.

ACTIVE-REACTIVE SYMPTOMS

Getting out of bed and walking around in slow ambulation. Engaging unconsciously in routine conscious-like activities, such as getting dressed, talking, preparing food or eating. May leave the house and drive a car. Exhibit unusual behavior, such as urinating in a closet, engaging in sexual activity without awareness or jumping out of a window. May become violent during the period of brief confusion immediately after waking or, occasionally, during the act of sleepwalking.

KNOWN VARIANTS

Unknown

DERIVED DISABILITIES

May suffer injuries due to risky behavior, i.e. jumping out of a window or falling down the stairs or leaving the house during winter nights. May cause significant disruption to household members including disturbing their own sleep. Problems functioning during daytime because of disturbed or insufficient sleep.

QG LAYER-PARTITIONS

5[(-4, -3, -2, -1) (+1, +2, +3, +4)]

MENTATION CURSOR

Hypercursor over accrued.

STATISTICS

More common in children than adults and adolescents with 15% of all children between 5 and 12 years of age having sleepwalked.

INSIGHTS

It is important to ascertain the real nature of Sleepwalking Disorder. The disease is otherwise called Somnambulism in order to relate it to the artificial state of Sleep designated Somanmbulism, which was in vogue among 19th Century experimentalists, who were engaged in opposing factions of Mesmerism and Hypnotism advocates. Though there are clear similarities, it is important to avoid conflating Sleepwalking with the artificial sleep state of Somnambulism of paranormal nature. Granular analysis shows that Sleepwalking is not a regular state of sleep. This is clearly borne out by our Symptom presentation in binary wings. That in the awake state, sufferers present with deficiencies typically due to absence of alertness resulting from lack of sleep, such as dragging sleepiness, slow responses and learning inaptitudes, is a clear indication that Sleepwalking is not sleep, neither natural nor artificial. There is no apparent reason why Sleepwalking would not be an expression of REM sleep if it was indeed a sleep state, since the thread of life and awareness that subsumes Sleepwalking activities are exactly comparable to the fine threading evidenced in dreams taking place in REM sleep. However, Sleepwalking occurs during N3 sleep, the deepest stage of non-rapid eye movement (NREM) sleep.

Sleepwalking is in fact a Layer 5 psychosis in which hallucination has completely overtaken the affected individual's mind, because it is doubled with a high accretion of the Hypercursor which for the most part sojourns stagnantly on Layer 5 of the Foliate. What Sleepwalking activities clearly exhibit is the expression of the Alter Self, which we have studied in detail in *Split Personality Disorder*. That is the reason why when awake or back to conscious the conscious person holds no memory whatsoever of what occurred during the episodes. What's more, it is admittedly not easy to take somebody out of this state just like it is to shake somebody out of the hallucinations of a psychotic episode. To a certain point, this metamorphogenic Layer **5** disease is feigning sleep, very much akin to the bewildering sleighs of Hysteria, a Layer **5** psychosis as well.

Lastly, the Metamorphogenic character type is a precursor or so-called risk factor for this Disorder.

Catatonia

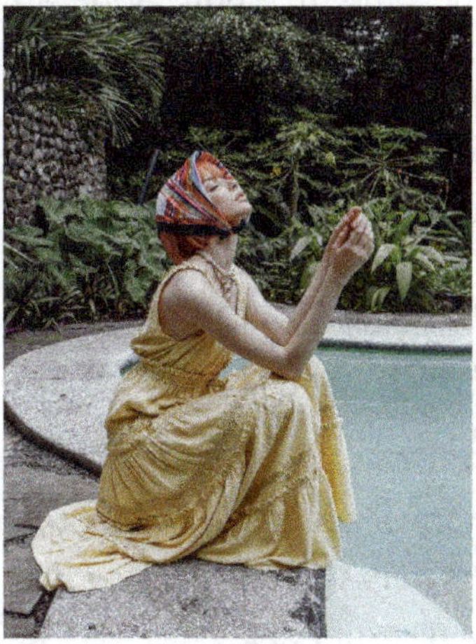

Catatonia, first described in neurology by Karl Kahlbaum in 1874 simply as specific disturbances in motor and behavioral functioning, had to wait for Emil Kraepelin to become a clinical expression of the newly created Dementia Praecox entity, with a chronic course and poor prognosis. Nosological and diagnostic definitions of the Disorder are still argued by clinicians and researchers of this day. We hereby propose a reexamination and redefinition of the Disorder by placing it in its broader historical context and from our particular psychophysics perspective.

PASSIVE –RESPONSIVE SYMPTOMS

Stupor: decreased response to external stimuli and hypoactive behavior. Immobility: akinetic behavior, resistance to being moved. Mutism: verbally unresponsive, refusal to speak. Daze: staring eyes fixed and open for long periods of time. Catalepsy: passive adoption of a posture.

ACTIVE-REACTIVE SYMPTOMS

Waxy flexibility: slight resistance to being moved. Posturing: intently maintaining a single position for a long period of time. Excitement : frantic, stereotyped or purposeless activity. Echolalia: senseless repetition of the words of others. Echopraxia : mimicking the movements of others.

KNOWN VARIANTS

Malignant Catatonia (Catatonia with severe metabolic decompensation) – Stupor (total unresponsiveness to stimuli except for the very intense such as deep pain, bright light or high level of noise or shock).

DERIVED DISABILITIES

May become markedly inoperative and experience extreme difficulty completing daily tasks. For example, the simple act of sitting up in bed may take hours.

QG LAYER-PARTITIONS

6[(-4, -3, -2, -1) (+1, +2, +3, +4)]

MENTATION CURSOR

Hypercursor over accrued and *motionless.*

STATISTICS

In a non-selective cohort of psychiatric inpatients, catatonia was observed in 7% to 17% of cases, and very commonly in those with so-called mood or substance abuse disorders.

INSIGHTS

In the same early period that Kraepelin attempted his nosologic revision of the disease, mesmerism and hypnotism became fashionable in Europe, as experimentalists were able to provoke the so-called *Catalepsy* form of sleep. The etymology of the *Catatonia* label shows its *Catalepsy* origin in the *cata* prefix and the *tonia* suffix to mean muscular tone. *Catatonia* as a clinical mental disorder is a genuine sleep or sleep-related impairment – albeit unknowingly so – with direct connection with the artificial form of sleep historically known as Catalepsy. Although in neurology and psychiatry the term catalepsy has come to mean, as reported in the nosology block, the passive adoption of a somatic posture, the precursor of this condition is forthrightly the continued and indefinite adoption by the dormant subject of a posture under the operator's instruction. If the operator lifts the subject's arm, he or she will remain indefinitely in that posture for the duration of the provoked sleep state. Also note that in that form of artificial sleep, the subject's eyes are open. Hence, clinical *Catatonia* is unquestionably a derivate of Cataleptic sleep. The peculiar wake feature of the Catatonic sleep disorder puts it close to Somnambulism which is more familiar to most, and represents the second of the three prominent forms of artificial or provoked sleep by an operator. The 3rd is Lethargic sleep.

In QG-inspired etiology and visualization, *Catatonia* develops as this uncommon form of awaken sleep, quite akin to Somnambulism in that feature, in which the Hypercursor is not only held captive by a single Mentation Layer, in this case Layer **6** of the Foliate, but constrained to remain indefinitely within the boundaries of one single pensive partition of the Layer as a tendency. This condition accounts for the indefinite posture adoption the individual exhibits in behavior, which in fact is not an inability to move or resistance to motion as believed, but matter-of-factly a persistent single action or act. Should the Cursor land on a Left-Chiral partition, we will see the subject exhibit i.e. fixed staring of the eyes for long periods of time as noted. This fit is described as stupor in the nosology. The main feature in the etiological exegesis of *Catatonia* is the static condition of the Hypercursor, which has lost autodynamism and remains motionless in its superposition over one single partition of the captive Layer.

The senseless repetition of others' words and the mimicking of others' movements known to the Disorder pertain to the Harmonic Norm of the Matrixial Layer, and represent features that are precisely present in Bipolar Disorder, which we know is a Layer-**6** tidal impairment. There is ample consensus that many catatonic symptoms are especially paralled in Bipolar Disorder. Taylor and Abrams demonstrated that there was higher prevalence of Catatonia in patients with Bipolar Disorder compared to those with Schizophrenia. Those particular features are also present in the artificially provoked Cataleptic form of sleep, in which the subject may even attempt to echo in all its forms of expression a simple gestural evocation of an emotional state. For instance, if the individual's fingers are brought onto his or her lips by the operator as if mimicking a kiss, his or her face will proceed to sketch a smile.

Catatonia has long been wrongly associated with Schizophrenia, likely owing to the presence of unusual movements and postures exhibited by sufferers. However, insofar as Schizophrenia is triggered by Layer 8 hyperactivity, the intimate nature of these two Disorders differs from one another. N Bartolommei et al write: *"At present, debate on the nosographic placement of catatonic symptoms lies around the possibility to definitively separate the link between catatonia and schizophrenia, and reclassify catatonic syndrome as an independent diagnostic entity. In the last edition of the DSM [DSM-IV], even if Kraepelin's vision of catatonia is pre-dominant, catatonia is recognized not only as a diagnostic subtype of schizophrenia, but also as an organic mental disorder and as a specific characteristic of major depression or mania within mood disorder. In redefining catatonia as an independent diagnostic category, Taylor and Fink highlighted that the disorder is amply diffuse among psychiatric patients, manifests with a typical symptomatic pattern and a relatively constant clinical course and responds to specific treatment. Thus, it has a clinical picture that can be subjected to diagnostic assessment and reliable prognosis."*

Encephalopathy	Acute onset, bizarre behaviour, altered mental state
Stroke	Acute onset, can present with immobility, mutism and/or altered mental state
Stiff man syndrome	Immobility, fixed posture
Parkinson's disease	Immobility, altered mental state, comorbid mood disorder
Locked-in syndrome	Immobility, mutism
Malignant hyperthermia	Immobility, mutism, altered mental state, instability of autonomic nervous system
Epileptic state	Immobility, mutism, altered mental state, bizarre behaviours
Autism	Mutism, immobility, echolalia, echopraxia
Obsessive-compulsive disorder (Severe forms)	Echolalia/repeated echopraxia, comorbid mood disorder
Elective mutism	Mutism

Fig. 5.2 A tabular report by N. Bartolommei et al of psychiatric conditions that present with putative catatonic expression

It cannot be overstressed that the singlemost important feature of Catatonia is the severe akinetic impairment of an over accrued Hypercursor. The question of what makes possible this akinetic condition of the Hypercursor cannot be answered unless the necessary rapprochement with parapsychological experimentalists' Catalepsy is properly made.

In the West, 19th Century France emerged as the world capital of neurology under the impulse of famed Dr. J. M. Charcot. At the same time, early neurology was immersed in a public debate with metaphysical experimentalists, over the nature of Hypnotic sleep which then was viewed to include so-called human magnetism or Mesmerism. The quest for grander Enlightenment curbed the balance towards an Aristotelian approach to those fundamental questions of human ontology to give us the science of neurology and psychiatry, as known today, in segregation of its implicated metaphysics. The concerns and methods brought about by said metaphysics came to be today orchestrated in the second order science of Parapsychology.

There is no question that in the United States it is that trend which impulsed the unseating of Psychoanalysis in mainstream psychiatry in favor of an empirical pharmacotherapeutic approach to psychopathology since the advent of the DSM-IV. It is understandable that in the absence of the necessary support in fundamental theoretical physics to harness the metric inherent to the metaphysics of the physical realm, western Enlightenment finds itself at an impasse as regards to that paradigmatic question and conservatively settles for knowledge acquisition from the purely observable as it currently stands. It is our profound belief that overcoming the limits of today's psychiatric science dwells in the resolution of questions in the order of the metaphysical metric of matter which only physical science is in the proper position to tackle. This firm determination is to a large extent what has brought us to both the psychophysics approach to human mentation in psychology and psychiatry and the staunch monist perspective that we have by and large developed in this Treatise. We remain convinced that without a fully constructed formalism to elicit human mentation in its very native dimension, the bioneurologic dimension of human mentation embodied in the central nervous system will never be properly and thoroughly mapped, and thus appropriately understood.

Clinical literature about Catatonia is quite prolific as a disorder that has for long posed an enormous challenge to neurology and psychiatry. Yet it is one of the oldest known mental disorders, but also one of the rare lethal ones. It has been characterized as one of the most comorbid mental disorders, defying any form of stringent classification. Marco Solmi et al write in the Schizophrenia Bulletin[34]: *"Catatonia is a complex psychopathological and clinical condition. The difficulties in the clinical diagnosis, conceptualization, and management of catatonia have been described as "the catatonic dilemma." Clinical manifestations of catatonia are extremely heterogeneous and at least 40 separate signs of catatonia have been described, making recognition challenging with frequent misdiagnoses."* Our QG psychophysics scrutiny finds to this Disorder three markedly different dimensions whose specificities most certainly explain the long running etiological trouble psychiatry has endured with it. We shortly address them below.

As previously mentioned, the most striking visible feature of Catatonia is the extraordinary akinetic condition of the body in its physiognomic expression which appears comparable to a frozen photograph in "real time". We have attributed this condition to the Mental Cursor, which we estimate remains stagnant on one single partition of Layer 6 of the Foliate. This stagnant condition is not a Layer property but a Cursor property and as such may be exhibited on any Layer of the Foliate, per our very definition of the Cursor entity. There lies one of the significant reasons why *Catatonia* has been heterogeneously spotted in so many different syndromes in a large variety of Disorders, among them those displayed in the Table in Fig 5.2. They include both psychiatric and medical conditions.

Further, the high level lethality associated with *Catatonia* is a function of the stillness of the Mentation Cursor which is to be comprehended as an extraordinary event in the context of the overall dynamics of the human psyche. The fullness of this realization will easily crystallize should we invoke the quite violent means employed by early 19th century Hypnotists and debuting neurologists contemporaneous to Charcot in order to unknowingly produce this state of the Cursor in already highly psychotic patients. They used to stun the psyche so to speak by submitting it to sudden and extremely high levels of sound, extremely

---

[34] **Schizophrenia Bulletin, The Journal of Psychoses and Related Disorders**, Marco Solmi et al, Volume 44, Issue 5, September 2018.

bright light, as well as potent chemical agents flooding the olfactory sense. Unsurprisingly, modern-day epidemiologic statistics reveal that catatonic stillness is very common among in-patients with substance abuse disorders. Effectively, it requires that much in the level of perceptive stimuli to uncharacteristically bring the Hypercursor to standstill. It also means that the fundamental binary affect-effector core which motorizes the dynamics of the psyche is in jeopardy, affecting even homeostatic mechanisms (we have good reasons to believe that the Hypercursor mediates the brunt of homeostatic regulation occurring during sleep – and these patients are indeed in a dormant state). Concordantly, it is clinically known that catatonic patients unresponsive to treatment invariably progress to lethal metabolic conditions. Work published as late as 1966 firmly demonstrated a high mortality rate for catatonia, even when modern day treatments were applied[35].

Furthermore, despite the fact that both the DSM and ICD have eliminated *Catatonic Depression* as a first-order entity in their taxonomy of mental disorders, and DSM having relegated it to the status of a specifier or subset of symptoms within other major disorders *(Bipolar, Depression, PTSD, Obsessive-Compulsive, etc.)*, we find its imperative clinical nosology consistent with our characterization of Depression as an impairment that involves an entire chiral Sector of the Mental Foliate, specifically and majorly the Left-Chiral Sector. The following is the official list of the known symptoms under so-called *Catatonic Depression* to which we have added Layer assignment:

- Feelings of sadness occurring nearly every day (Layer 6)
- Loss of interest in most activities (Layer 1)
- Sudden weight gain or loss
- Change in appetite (Layer 6)
- Trouble falling asleep (Cursor impairment)
- Trouble getting out of bed
- Feelings of worthlessness (Layer 1 – 3)

---

[35] **The Syndrome of Catatonia**, Behavioral Sciences, ISSN 2076 328X, James Allen Wilcox and Pam Reid Duff.

- Feelings of guilt (Layer 4)
- Fatigue (Layer 8 – Layer 1)
- Difficulty concentrating (Dysthymia)
- Difficulty thinking (Dysthymia)
- Difficulty making decisions (Dysthymia)
- Thoughts of suicide or death (Layer 6 - 7)
- A suicide attempt (Layer 6 -7)
- Irritability (Layer 7 - Agitation)
- Feelings of restlessness (Layer 2 - Agitation)

There is obviously nothing catatonic in the above symptoms, leaving us to surmise that their established putative relationship with *Catatonia* stems from clinically observed prosomal switching of a qualified Catatonic patient to that noted set of depressive symptoms, or perhaps a mix of typical catatonic symptoms with those depressive symptoms. The clinician, however, must be keen in understanding, in the light of granular analysis from our perspective, the distinction in these two different dimensions of the impairments.

In concluding this piece, we intently advance that despite the lethality surrounding the pathological condition of akinesis of the Mentation Cursor, it is not quite an unnatural condition. In fact, both the akinetic Hypercursor and Hypocursor represent a significant pathway to a cluster of special **Paranormal** phenomena. Human Enlightenment, having access to the higher canon of **Norms** regimenting the metric of the physical in its full spectrum, must finally confront and aspire to master those empirical phenomena in order to materialize the next momentous step in the technological, and yes, dare we say spiritual evolution of mankind.

Sleep-Wake Disorder

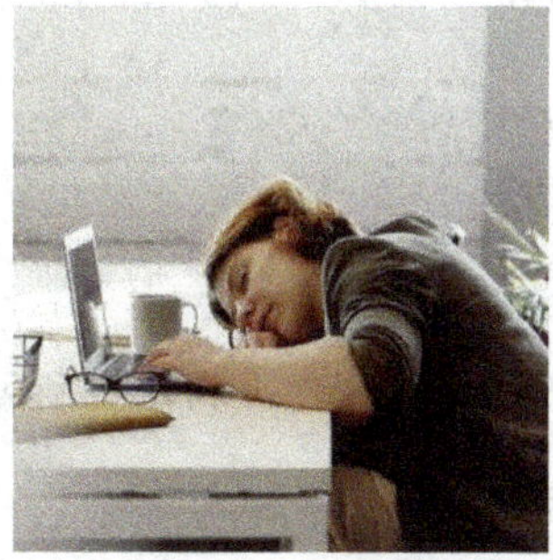

Sleep-Wake Disorder or *Circadian Rhythm Sleep Disorder* occurs when the circadian rhythm, which repeats approximately every 24 hours, is out of sync with natural cosmic alternation between our Sun star and planet Earth that produces day and night. The disease may either result from a dysfunction in the internal psychobiologic mechanism that galvanizes the circadian alternation, or submission to a physical travel course that significant alters the perceived cosmic day/night alternation away from its usual periodicity. This Disorder manifests in several different types and entails problems either falling asleep or staying awake at desired or socially appropriate times.

PASSIVE –RESPONSIVE BEHAVIOR

Problems falling asleep and once asleep to stay asleep. Waking up too early and not being able to resume sleep. Complaints of insomnia and/or excessive sleepiness. Getting sleep but not feeling refreshed after wake. Fatigue, indecisiveness. Frustration and feelings of guilt as relates to perceived inability to restore a daily energy balance.

ACTIVE-REACTIVE BEHAVIOR

Hyperactive, agitated, tossing and turning, doing too much at one time. Poor concentration.

KNOWN VARIANTS

Jet Lag disorder, Shift Work Sleep Disorder, Delayed Sleep-Wake Phase Disorder, Advanced Sleep-Wake Phase Disorder, Non-24 hour Sleep-Wake Rhythm Disorder, Irregular Sleep-Wake Rhythm Disorder.

LANGUAGE
Disinhibited due to sleep deprivation, erratic, curses.

BEHAVIORAL FLIPS
None

DERIVED DISABILITIES
Poor concentration, decreased attention and difficulties with tasks completion.

AWARENESS
Semi-Conscious (Neuro-psychotic Disorder).

CHARACTEROLOGICAL FILIATION
Hyperbolic

QG LAYER-PARTITIONS

4[(-4, -3, -2, -1) (+1, +2, +3, +4)]

MENTATION CURSOR
Quadracursor over accrued.

STATISTICS
Lifetime prevalence: 20 to 40% of US adults report difficulties sleeping at some point in life.

INSIGHTS
Light exposure through the pineal gland and the Suprachiasmatic Nucleus affects the alternation frequency of the psychobiologic circadian rythym, via release of melatonin, an action that keeps the sleep-wake cycle pegged to the indicated natural cosmic alternation producing day and night. In one type of sleep-wake Disorder, the dysfunction is characterized by abnormalities of the circadian system itself.

The most common type of Sleep-Wake Disorder is the one caused by travel through so-called different time zones (time zone being a false and reductionist definition of cosmic spatial phases). They are typically Jet Lag Sleep Disorder and Shift Work Disorder. Jet Lag Disorder involves excessive sleepiness or difficulty falling asleep due to quickly crossing multiple time zones or different space spread phases. Shift work disorder entails problems with alertness (or sleepiness) related to an irregular or untraditional work schedule.

Obviously, when the neurobiologic mechanism that sustains the sleep-wake cycle is impaired, the syndrome typical of the Disorder will be unleashed as well. Various hormones have been implicated in the circadian rhythm: melatonin, cortisol, thyroid stimulating hormone (TSH), and prolactin, thus affecting the sleep architecture. In addition, fluctuations in sex steroid hormones during the luteal phase in women underscore the *Premenstrual Dysphoric Disorder*, in which sleep disruption is common.

In consideration to the elements of the syndrome, it is important to differentiate insomnia in a circadian rhythm sleep syndrome from its manifestation as a standalone Disorder. In the former, insomnia is not a basis inability to sleep but a shift in the necessary sleep phase in the thread of life. It is then almost always concurrent with sleepiness which is the fact of falling asleep in socially inappropriate moments, precisely as a result of the entire shift of the sleep-wake cycle itself.

On the pure psychological plane, it is paramount to underscore that, whatever the nature of the remote or indirect cause of circadian rhythm sleep dysfunction, it only becomes manifest in a syndrome through captivity of the Mentation Quadracursor. The latter stands for the primary mediator between the state of Sleep and that of Wake. The province of the Disorder is Layer 4 of the Mental Foliate because it is the province of the Quadracursor. To assess and elucidate the difference between Insomnia as a Disorder in its own right and insomnia related to a circadian rhythm sleep syndrome, it is paramount to lay bare the mode of the Mentation Cursor in each type of dysfunction. The Hypocursor and accretion of the Conscious Cognos are responsible for the dysfunction in the first case, as previously discussed, whereas in the second case it is the Quadracursor and accretion in the Hyperbolic Layer that must be held accountable.

QG Layer 4 of the Foliate and primarily the Quadracursor hold purview of the primary synchronizing agents of the circadian rhythm which are the light/dark cycle and melatonin. It is interesting to note that the natural endogenous periodicity of the sleep-wake cycle extends beyond 24 hours. Therefore there is a constraint exerted by cosmic day/night alternation and subsequent pineal melatonin over the naturally emerging periodicity of the the sleep-wake cycle that the Quadracursor must endeavor to marshall as a monolith. The critical observation of this disparity which is generally overlooked underscores the idea that the endogenous circadian rhythm is not a "real time clock" or a time duration clock as it has frequently been termed. Instead it genuinely presents as a phase repetition rate ultimately of spatial dimension and involving human wake entropy with associated metabolic activity, reproductive activity and rest or homeostasis.

One other important distinction that is generally ignored in the diagnosis of sleep-wake disorders is the one between sleep and sleepiness. Sleepiness is **not** Sleep. Sleepiness is feeling sleepy while one remains in the wake state or fluctuating therein. The most accurate characterization for that mental fit is semi-sleep/semi-wake, which is a match with our very definition of the Quadracursor. To remain in that hybrid mental fit with the frequency of a chronic condition or as a long-lasting one means that the Quadracursor is held captive within the boundary of Layer 4 of the Foliate and over accrued. This condition of the Quadracursor is also consistent witht the nosologic report of insomnia and/or sleepiness in the many variants of the Disorder. This sort of insomnia is not your typical hard-core insomnia where the sufferer is unable to sleep at all, since she/he does experience sleepiness either during daytime or nighttime. Pure insomnia – whereby the patient is unable to close eyes and sink into any form of sleep all night (or large portion of the night), not even dragging sleepiness – is caused by a stagnant Hypocursor within the Conscious Cognos. Beyond the peculiarities that lead to the classification distinguishing the several indicated variants of Sleep-Wake Disorders, the afore-discussed distinctions must be laid as bare as possible in clinical inquests and reports for a clear understanding of the etiological roots of sleep pathologies from this new psychiatric perspective.

PATHOLOGICAL AFFILIATES

Sleep Paralysis Disorder

The Cursor architecture that we have drafted in this psychophysics analytic theory had allowed us to forthrightly predict a condition of the Quadracursor in which it becomes completely akinetic, akin at the end to the akinetic state of the Hypercursor in *Catatonia*. A catatonic or akinetic condition of the Quadracursor would unleash a behavior in which the mind would manifest a sort of frozen state of a semi-wake/semi-sleep nature.

Effectively, the peculiar but quite common Disorder of *Sleep Paralysis* does exist. It is a state occurring very characteristically either during the wake up slip or the slip into sleep, in which a person is aware or consciously aware but unable to move or speak. Episodes generally last only a few minutes and may occur as a one-off single episode or in a recurrent manner. It is not known to be a harmful impairment or condition, neither physiologically nor psychologically, despite the very real dread it inspires patients. We attribute to the natural brevity of the episodes the main cause for their non-lethality, such brevity being the remote result in phenomenology of the very nature of the Quadracursor as a transition entity.

Etiologically, when the Quadracursor becomes akinetic within the Right-Chiral side of Layer 4, the individual experiences a paralysis in terms of an inability to speak or move the limbs, or to freely breathe. When the Quadracursor instead becomes akinetic within the Left-Chiral side of Layer 4, the individual experiences what are called hypnagogic or hypnopompic representations, whereby she/he may feel that "somebody is in the room" who is realistically not there, or feels the factitious application of a constant pressure pushing the body down. The fixism of a Cursor in the perceptive slant (left-chiral localization) is what creates this type of sensation. A few people have well reported feeling chilled or freezing during the experience. It only takes for someone else to touch or move the individual for the sensation to quickly dissipate as known. The interaction with someone else then simply forces the Cursor as a focus of attention and intent to drift away from the pensive partition it was held captive to. Again, only the natural transitioning dynamic that is part of the Quadratic Norm saves sufferers from full and persistent akinetic states of this Cursor and the negative consequences thereof. From that point of view, it is not a coincidence either that nature has chosen to entrust the Quadracursor with administration of the necessary biological cycling or fluctuation between entropic/metabolic activity and rest-oration in the prosecution of the thread of life.

It is interesting that Priyanka Vaidya, MD, a licensee in Behavioral Psychology, has described the representations in *Sleep Paralysis* of paranoid nature. Effectively, there is indeed an indisputable paranoid tone to the representations in Sleep Paralysis, which are clear in the doom aura that surrounds them: feeling that someone is lurking in the room, feeling that something is uncomfortably pushing you down as to cause harm, feeling of being dragged from the bed, even reportedly the sensation that one is going to die, and the very real difficulty to breathe. Therefore the term hypnopompic (during wake up process) and hypnagogic (during transitioning into sleep) to qualify those types of hallucinations are well justified in order to differentiate them in their intimate nature from the psychotic type of hallucinations.

There is a singular flurry of these types of hallucinations in the syndrome, of visual, olfactory, tactile and auditory nature, therefore at the PASSIVE-RESPONSIVE side of the nosology. We report them in the *Commented Bibliography* section. The two most important features of this experience is (1) they occur during transition in and/or out of sleep and (2) the aura of paranoid persecution that surrounds them, as profusely described in the clinical report quoted in the *Commented Bibliography*. In that regard, we expressly remind the reader that *Paranoia* is a Layer-4 Disorder, and that the form of tangential awareness that subsumes these representations is experienced by patients feeling they are both awake and in the cloudiness of sleep. Their inherent coherence makes them feel to the clinician a mix of realistic and unrealistic symptoms, leaving indeed no clear space to decisively settle the mark.

We nevertheless take serious issue with the characterization that the underlying mechanism of this Disorder involves a dysfunction in REM sleep, taxing it an unfounded hypothesis. We are far and away from pure sleep or deep sleep here, the individual being quite aware of what is happening in the environment while being in this paralysis or catatonic-like state, whether she/he is slowly waking up from sleep or transitioning into it from awakefulness. The level of awareness during sleep paralysis varies with sufferers. While some individuals insist they feel well awake and aware of their surroundings, others describe only a partial conscious awareness of their surroundings. This condition is totally incompatible with REM sleep, which only develops under the fullness of a Hypercursor in which awareness is absolutely unconscious.

Even though the ability to move the eyes is preserved in *Sleep Paralysis* as it is in REM sleep, constrastingly in REM sleep dreamers do not attempt to scream or call out for help as a result of a realization that their limbs are paralyzed during that state of sleep. They do not attempt to vocalize their fear and discomfort which only weakly come out as a whisper, a squeal, a grunt, or a groan due to paralysis of the muscles related to vocalization. The differences between one state of sleep and the other in our sense are major.

Furthermore, very infrequently, sufferers may report an out-of-body experience, whereby they bear the awareness of having been outside of their bodies, such as floating above the bed in a duplicate self and looking at themselves. This may be an interesting paranormal extension of the syndrome, which we are unable to eloquently discuss at this time in the lack of a larger metric framework presentation. It is all the more interesting that the catatonic feature of this Disorder, normally unidentified in psychiatry to this point, somehow relates to and brings back a psycho-paranormal element central to human ontology evoked at the very end of the study of *Catatonia*. The literature on trance phenomena[36] [37] in psychiatry i.e. does exist and is formally gathered under *Personality Dissociation* disorders for the most part. Under many latitudes of the globe the clinical

---

[36] **Culture, Trance and the Mind-Brain**, Richard Castillo, January 2008, Article in *Anthropology of Consciousness*, University of Hawaii, Division of Social Science

[37] **Electroencephalogram characteristics during possession trances in healthy individuals**, Norie Kawaia et al, NeuroReports, 2017, 28:949–955 – National center of Neurology and Psychiatry, Kodaira - Japan

presence of trance and related phenomena are to this day still a fact for psychiatric science to deal with. However despite the psychopathological and ethnographic aspect that frequently accompanies such phenomena, their verifiable presence with healthy individuals of all races begs for a deeper formal psychophysics approach to their understanding. Said approach is deemed to unravel the analytic elements capable of not only discerning between the normal and the abnormal, but furnishing adequate etiologic exegesis for the abnormal. We shall reserve presentation of a mature theoretical study of these questions in due course.

BEHAVIORAL FLIPS

Going from the feeling of complete limb paralysis and inability to move to sensations of a completely chilled or frozen body. Flips from the feeling of someone dragging you out of bed or pushing you down to the feeling that someone in a dark or ghostly figure up to no good is present in the room.

DERIVED DISABILITIES

Inability to sleep on certain physiognomic parts of the body, due to their triggering the Disorder. Most people with *Sleep Paralysis* report its occurence when sleeping on their backs. Some other people have however reported it occurring specifically when sleeping on their stomachs as well as their sides.

AWARENESS

Semi-Conscious (Neuro-psychotic Disorder)

CHARACTEROLOGICAL FILIATION

Hyperbolic

QG LAYER-PARTITIONS

4[(-4, -3, -2, -1) (+1, +2, +3, +4)]

MENTATION CURSOR

Quadracursor over accrued, in akinetic dynamics or slow motion.

STATISTICS

Estimated to occur in about 20% of otherwise healthy people.

Turbulent Sleep Disorder

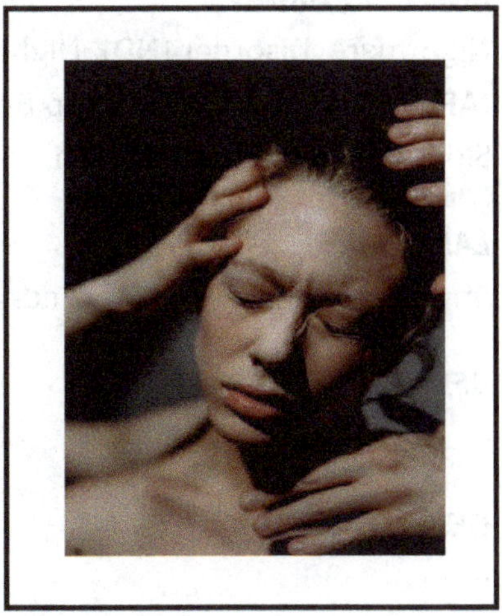

In the previous Chapter we have gathered under the new label *Turbulent Sleep Disorder* the forms of sleep eliciting clear disruptive behavior that is further deleterious to the individual and/or others. We have redimensioned the parasomnia label in a way that allows us to regroup a number of disruptive syndromes under *Turbulent Sleep Disorder*, while segregating other formerly related disorders such as Somnambulism and Confusional Arousal. We are now going to take a closer look at these variants, in particular their relationship with one another. We advance the corresponding etiological interpretation in the ***INSIGHTS*** block.

SYMPTOMS

Frequent nightmares projecting life-threatening or risky personal safety situations. Deeply disturbing and awaken the dreamer. Generally occur in the last third of the night *(Nightmare syndrome)*. Screaming while asleep and unresponsive to any other stimuli, with no memory of incident upon wake *(Night Terror syndrome)* - Sleep may become hyperactive, agitated, with the dreamer tossing and turning, doing too much at a time. Unusual word-like vocalizations, complex dream motor activity related to the dream content. May assault bed partner with fist hits and/or strangulation attempts or jump out of bed to fracture body parts. Patients wake up abruptly at the end of the episode *(Aggressive REM Sleep syndrome)*. Teeth grinding or clenching, which can be so strong that teeth may become fractured, chipped or loose *(Sleep-Related Bruxism syndrome)*. Urinating in bed *(Sleep-Related Enuresis syndrome)*. Tired or tight jaw muscles, jaw and face soreness. Sleep session disruptions. After wake, dull headache starting in the temples, poor concentration.

KNOWN VARIANTS

Nightmare Disorder (ND). Night Terrors (NT). Aggressive REM Sleep Disorder (ARSD) also called REM Sleep Behavior Disorder. Sleep-Related Bruxism (SRB). Sleep-Related Enuresis (SRE).

LANGUAGE

Strange word-like or distorded-word vocalizations.

BEHAVIORAL FLIPS

--

DERIVED DISABILITIES

--

AWARENESS

Unconscious (Psychotic Disorder)

CHARACTEROLOGICAL FILIATION

Paradoxical

QG LAYER-PARTITIONS

7[(-4, -3, -2, -1) (+1, +2, +3, +4)]

MENTATION CURSOR

Hypercursor over accrued.

STATISTICS

The Sleep Foundation states that *"studies have shown males and females [to be] equally susceptible to disorders of arousal, though age appears to play a role. Parasomnias have been reported in roughly 17% of children ages three to 13. For children and adults 15 and older, the prevalence rate falls between 2.9% and 4.2%."*

INSIGHTS

The most important character to all the symptom subsets that we reported in the nosology block is unquestionably their Layer-**7** sadomasochistic twist in phenomenology. Even *Sleep-Related Enuresis,* which seems to be the most inocuous among those profoundly disruptive syndromes, must be brought to a sadomasochistic account, given that even toddlers have learned to retreat in intimacy to satisfy the urge of urinating. They will further feel embarrassed to urinate on themselves and their clothing. Therefore, there is ample space to justifiably consider sleep occurring enuresis an act of self-depreciation. It is unnecessary to discuss the aggressive and disruptive character manifest in those sleep syndromes, given that they are so unmistakably observable, from terrors to self-harming teeth grinding to the point of fracture to loud audible screaming to violent assaults by strangulation, etc.

This account becomes very transparent and quite prevalent once we de-emphasize the REM/NREM distinction in those syndromes which has received so much attention. In other words, it might be more productive to look at these disorders from the viewpoint of a Layer-**7** storm within the psyche affecting REM sleep than the state of REM sleep causing or being concurrent to these syndromes. We know that just as late-night ingestion of indigestible or stomach-disrupting food may trigger nightmares within the night sleep cycle, an internalized psychosocial aura of intense stressors may trigger gastric disruption or ulcers possibly leading to frequent nightmares. Likewise we well know about the physiological underpinnings that accompany REM sleep, and they are many.

As discussed in the previous Chapter, many areas in the brain are very active during REM sleep and even more active then than during wakefulness. In REM sleep there is a loss of functional regulation, which is almost at par with the physiology of wakefulness, requiring even a reinforcement of the mechanisms that place the body in the state of atonia so that the dreamer does not materially enact her/his dreams. Quite notably, the body does not exercise thermic regulation during the REM phase of sleep, breathing and heart rate increase and become irregular. Atonia hence becomes an absolute necessity for normalcy in the development of REM sleep. Therefore the question is not to recognize that in the event of a breakdown in the regulatory mechanism atonia may be lost and dream enacting behavior will occur, but most tellingly to inquire about what causes the breakdown of this neuro-hormonal mechanism? Could there be instead of a breakdown a masking of the neuro-hormonal mechanism rather which is psychogenically triggered? To breakup the course of a developing REM sleep in a *Disruptive Sleep Disorder* sufferer is just as hard as it is in a dreamer developing any other kind of REM sleep, suggesting that the neural stimulus thresholds in the former and subsequent impulses through the afferent intra-brain pathways and circuits remain unaltered.

Our answer to these questions is one: an overaccrued intensity in a Hypercursor longitudinally sojourning over a paroxysmal Layer-7 of the Mental Foliate. Such levels of accretion (both Cursor and Partitions) create a conversion response directly inhibiting the atonia regulatory mechanism, just like an overload of internalized psychosocial stressors or a super intense stressor get to cause gastric ulcers through atonia of the gastric glands releasing hydrochloric acid constantly.

It may help to remind the reader that in organic medicine, atonia is a condition in which a muscle has lost its strength, this condition being frequently associated with so-called choreatic atonia or choreoathetosis, uterine atonia, and most interestingly gastrointestinal atonia as well, among others.

Addendum

Logorrhea

Logorrhea is a constant need to endlessly talk. It represents a single symptom. In its mild form, it is not a Disorder but a characterological attribute. Logorrhea becomes morbid however when it takes a certain intensity of speech or a certain magnitude among the diverse states or activities of daily living. An unmistakable sign of morbidity is when the flow of speech becomes rambling.

Morbid Logorrhea is frequently associated with tachyphemia characterized by rapid speech with erratic rhythm. The patient with Logorrhea talks for prolonged periods of time, with disjoint discourse and moving from one subject to another. Sometimes speech develops with leaked ideas.

Because Language is the realm par excellence for association, Logorrhea must be causally attributed to the Trinary Mental Normal, which embodies the typology of Association. When Logorrhea develops as a single but very intense symptom, the morbid behavior is rooted on the partitions of the Trinary Mental Layer.

When participating in a larger syndrome, Logorrhea must be understood to be a secondary symptom that does not belong to the causal root Layer of the syndrome, such as Schizophrenia or, more frequently, the manic phase of Bipolar Disorder. In that event, Logorrhea only occurs as a response to the overactive charge coming from the main root Layer responsible for the disease via orthoflows. Speech will then take a certain "color" informed by the main disease, i.e. echolalia in Bipolar Disorder.

Therefore, our pathological adscription for the dysfunction of Logorrhea is as follows:

AWARENESS
Conscious

CHARACTEROLOGICAL FILIATION

Intellectual

QG LAYER-PARTITIONS

3 [(-1, -2, -3, -4) (+1, +2, +3, +4)]

Copromania

Copromania is the obsession with one's own feces. In QG biophysics, human feces, both in its chemical nature and as a product of the Digestive System, which is a destructive system par excellence, respond to the the Paradoxical Norm (or the typological Norm of Destruction).

The following elements are unsurprisingly known to be concomitant with Copromania:

- Use of alcohol
- Use of narcotic drugs
- High stress level
- Chronic or permanent stress resulting from poverty, homelessness and/or family problems
- Sleep deprivation which may be caused by the same above predicaments
- Deleterious side effects of medication

They are for the most part expression of the Norm of Destruction in the biophysics context for themselves. Therefore the dysfunction of Copromania is to be rooted on the Paradoxical Mental Layer with the following adscription:

AWARENESS

Conscious

CHARACTEROLOGICAL FILIATION

Paradoxical

QG LAYER-PARTITIONS

7 [(-1, -2, -3, -4) (+1, +2, +3, +4)]

INSIGHTS

As a simple symptom, Copromania does not qualify as a Disorder. In that condition, it may just be part of the syndrome making up the main Disorder. In this context, Copromania becomes a secondary or consequential symptom that develops from orthoflow impulses rooted on the main Normal characterizing the Disease. Only when the intensity of the symptom reaches a certain magnitude can it be considered a Disorder in its own right, in which case it is deemed to be primarily rooted on the Paradoxical Normal of the Mental.

Taxonomic Index of Disorders

– Sector [Right-Chiral] –

Foliate Sector Localization: [Entire Right-chiral Sector] of Foliate
Principal
Narcissistic Personality Disorder
Alternative Labels: None
Partitions (facultative): 6 [(+1, +2, +3, +4)]
Allotropic Cause: Unknown
Psychophysics Etiology: Complete
IC-10-CM: F60.81
Page No: 502

Foliate Sector Localization: [Entire Right-Chiral Sector] of Foliate
Principal
Histrionic Personality Disorder
Alternative Labels: None
Partitions (facultative): 6 [(+1, +2, +3, +4)]
Allotropic Cause: Unknown
Psychophysics Etiology: Complete
IC-10-CM: F60.4
Page No: 499

Foliate Sector Localization: [Entire Right-Chiral Sector] of Foliate – Disparity between Biological and Mental Body sexuation
Principal
Gender Identity Disorder (Men)
Alternative Labels: Gender Dysphoria
Allotropic Cause: Biological, Unknown
Psychophysics Etiology: Complete
IC-10-CM: F64.9
Page No: 459

– Sector [Left-Chiral] –

Foliate Sector Localization: [Left-Chiral sector] of Foliate – Disparity between Biological and Mental Body sexuation
Principal
Dysthymia
Alternative Labels: None
Allotropic Cause: Unknown, Biological, Trauma
Psychophysics Etiology: Complete
IC-10-CM: F34.1
Page No: 372

Foliate Sector Localization: [Entire Left-Chiral Sector] of Foliate
Principal
Gender Identity Disorder (Women)
Alternative Labels: Gender Dysphoria
Allotropic Cause: Biological, Not well known
Psychophysics Etiology: Complete
IC-10-CM: F64.9
Page No: 459

Foliate Sector Localization: Entire Left-Chiral Sector (Depression) or Right-Chiral Sector (Agitation)
Class Disorder
Obsessive Disorders
Alternative Labels: Depression-Agitation Disorders
Psychophysics Etiology: Complete Foliate's Chiral Sector
Allotropic Cause: Unknown
Psychophysics Etiology: Complete
IC-10-CM: F42
Page No: 286

[2]
Principal
Voyeuristic Disorder
Alternative Labels: None
Foliate Sector Localization: Left-Chiral Sector Overaccrued
Partitions: 2 or 7 [(-4, -3, -2, -1) (+1, +2, +3, +4)]
Allotropic Cause: Unknown
Psychophysics Etiology: Complete
IC-10-CM: F65.3
Page No: 493

– Layers [1, 2, 3] –

[1, 2, 3]
PA to Insomnia
Insufficient Sleep Syndrome
Alternative Labels: Sleep deprivation
Foliate Sector Localization: Hypocursor over accrued - Layers 1, 2, 3 Overaccrued
Allotropic Cause: Unknown, Biological
Psychophysics Etiology: Complete
IC-10-CM: F51.12
Page No: 594

[1, 2, 3]
Principal
Insomnia
Alternative Labels: None
Foliate Sector Localization: Hypocursor over accrued
Layers 1,2,3 Overaccrued
Allotropic Cause: Unknown, Biological
Psychophysics Etiology: Complete
IC-10-CM: G47.00
Page No: 592

– Layer [1] –

[1]
PA to Burnout
Abulia
Alternative Labels: None
Foliate Sector Localization: Left+Right
Partitions: 1 [(-4, -3, -2, -1) (+1, +2, +3, +4)]
Allotropic Cause: Unknown
Psychophysics Etiology: Complete
IC-10-CM: R68.89
Page No: 360

[1]
Principal
Agressiveness
Alternative Labels: Intermittent Explosive Disorder
Foliate Sector Localization: Left+Right
Partitions: 1 [(-4, -3, -2, -1) (+1, +2, +3, +4)]
Allotropic Cause: Unknown
Psychophysics Etiology: Complete
IC-10-CM: R45.6
Page No: 378

[1]
PA to Burnout
Chronic/Persistent Vertigo
Alternative Labels: Dizziness
Foliate Sector Localization: Left-Chiral
Partitions: 1 [(-4, -3, -2, -1) (+1, +2, +3, +4)]
Allotropic Cause: Unknown,Biological
Psychophysics Etiology: Partial
IC-10-CM: R42.0
Page No: 359

[1]
PA to Social Anxiety Disorder
Selective Mutism
Alternative Labels: None
Foliate Sector Localization: Left-Chiral
Partitions: 1 [(-4, -3, -2, -1) (+1, +2, +3, +4)]
Allotropic Cause: Unknown
Psychophysics Etiology: Complete
IC-10-CM: F94.0
Page No: 380

[1]
PA to Social Anxiety ds
Avoidant Personality Disorder
Alternative Labels: None
Foliate Sector Localization: Left-Chiral
Partitions: 1 [(-4, -3, -2, -1) (+1, +2, +3, +4)]
Allotropic Cause: Unknown
Psychophysics Etiology: Complete
IC-10-CM: F60.6
Page No: 378

[1]
Principal
Burnout syndrome
Alternative Labels: Asthenia, Neurasthenia
Foliate Sector Localization: Left+Right
Partitions: 1 [(-4, -3, -2, -1) (+1, +2, +3, +4)]
Allotropic Cause: Unknown
Psychophysics Etiology: Complete
IC-10-CM: Z73.0
Page No: 357

[1]
Principal
Hoarding
Alternative Labels: None
Foliate Sector Localization: Left+Right
Partitions: 1 [(-4, -3, -2, -1) (+1, +2, +3, +4)]
Allotropic Cause: Unknown
Psychophysics Etiology: Complete
IC-10-CM: F42.3
Page No: 466

[1]
Principal
Social Anxiety Disorder
Alternative Labels: Timidity, Social phobia
Foliate Sector Localization: Left-Chiral
Partitions: 1 [(-4, -3, -2, -1) (+1, +2, +3, +4)]
Allotropic Cause: Unknown
Psychophysics Etiology: Complete
IC-10-CM: F40.10
Page No: 378

– Layer [2] –

[2]
PA to ADHD
Agitation Disorder
Alternative Labels: None
Foliate Sector Localization: Left+Right
Partitions: 2 [(-4, -3, -2, -1) (+1, +2, +3, +4)]
Allotropic Cause: Unknown
Psychophysics Etiology: Complete
IC-10-CM: R45.1
Page No: 269

[2]
Principal
Attention Deficit/Hyperactivity Disorder
Alternative Labels: None
Foliate Sector Localization: Left (inattentive)
Right (hyperactive), R+L (Combined type)
Combined 2 [(-4, -3, -2, -1) (+1, +2, +3, +4)]
Allotropic Cause: Biological, Substance use during pregnancy, Neurologic
Psychophysics Etiology: Complete
IC-10-CM: F90.0
Page No: 351

[2]
Principal
Authoritarianism
Alternative Labels: None
Foliate Sector Localization: Right-Chiral
Layer 1
Partitions: Hyper-Quantum Operator
Allotropic Cause: Unknown
Psychophysics Etiology: Complete
IC-10-CM: N/A
Page No: 541

[2]
Principal
Fetishism
Alternative Labels: Transvestic Fetishism is a putative PA to Fetishism
Foliate Sector Localization: Left-Chiral
Partitions: 2 [(-4, -3, -2, -1) (+1, +2, +3, +4)]
Allotropic Cause: Unknown
Psychophysics Etiology: Complete
IC-10-CM: F65.0
Page No: 392

– Layer [3] –

[3]
PA to Mental Confusion
Language Disorder
Alternative Labels: None
Foliate Sector Localization: Left-Chiral
Partitions: 3 [(-4, -3, -2, -1) (+1, +2, +3, +4)]
Allotropic Cause: Unknown
Psychophysics Etiology: Complete
IC-10-CM: F80
Page No: 267

[3]
Principal
Logorrhea
Alternative Labels: Excessive Talking
Foliate Sector Localization: Left+Right
Partitions: 3 [(-4, -3, -2, -1) (+1, +2, +3, +4)]
Allotropic Cause: Unknown
Biological

Psychophysics Etiology: Complete
IC-10-CM: R47.89
Page No: 631

[3]
PA to Inferiority Complex
Intellectual Disability
Alternative Labels: Mental Retardation
Foliate Sector Localization: Left+Right
Partitions: 3 [(-4, -3, -2, -1) (+1, +2, +3, +4)]
Allotropic Cause: Unknown
Psychophysics Etiology: Partial
F70-F79
Page No: 414

[3]
Principal
Approval Compulsion
Alternative Labels: None
Foliate Sector Localization: Left+Right
Partitions: 3 [(-4, -3, -2, -1) (+1, +2, +3, +4)]
Allotropic Cause: Unknown
Psychophysics Etiology: Complete
IC-10-CM: F42
Page No: 406

[3]
Principal
Developmental Coordination Disorder
Alternative Labels: None
Foliate Sector Localization: Left-Chiral Only
Partitions: 3 [(-4, -3, -2, -1)]
Allotropic Cause: Unknown
Psychophysics Etiology: Complete
IC-10-CM: F82
Page No: 585

[3]
Principal
Impostor Syndrome
Alternative Labels: Fraud syndrome, Neurosis of Failure
Foliate Sector Localization: Left+Right
Partitions: 3 [(-4, -3, -2, -1) (+1, +2, +3, +4)]
Allotropic Cause: Unknown
Psychophysics Etiology: Complete
IC-10-CM: N/A
Page No: 363

[3]
Principal
Inferiority complex
Alternative Labels: None
Foliate Sector Localization: Left+Right
Partitions: 3 [(-4, -3, -2,-1) (+1, +2, +3, +4)]
Allotropic Cause: Unknown
Psychophysics Etiology: Complete
IC-10-CM: N/A
Page No: 412

[3]
Principal
Mental Confusion
Alternative Labels: Delirium
Foliate Sector Localization: Left+Right
Partitions: 3 [(-4, -3, -2, -1) (+1, +2, +3, +4)]
Allotropic Cause: Little known, Biological, Neurological
Psychophysics Etiology: Partial
Page No: 265

[3]
Principal
Perfectionism
Alternative Labels: None
Foliate Sector Localization: Left+Right
Partitions: 3 [(-4, -3, -2, -1) (+1, +2, +3, +4)]
Allotropic Cause: Unknown
Psychophysics Etiology: Complete
IC-10-CM: R46.89
Page No: 400

[3]
Principal
Specific Learning Disorder
Alternative Labels: None
Foliate Sector Localization: Left+Right
Partitions: 3 [(-4, -3, -2, -1) (+1, +2, +3, +4)]
Allotropic Cause: Unknown, Biological
Psychophysics Etiology: Complete
IC-10-CM: F81.0
Page No: 418

– Layer [4] –

[4]
PA to Paranoia
Paranoid Personality Disorder
Alternative Labels: None
Foliate Sector Localization: Left+Right
Partitions: 4 [(-4, -3, -2, -1) (+1, +2, +3, +4)]
Allotropic Cause: Unknown
Psychophysics Etiology: Complete
IC-10-CM: F60.6
Page No: 439

[4]
PA to RLS
Periodic Limb Movement Disorder
Alternative Labels: None
Foliate Sector Localization: Left-Chiral, Quadracursor
Partitions: 4 [(-4, -3, -2, -1) (+1, +2, +3, +4)]
Allotropic Cause: Unknown, Biological
Psychophysics Etiology: Complete
IC-10-CM: G47.61
Page No:

[4]
PA to Sleep-Wake Disorders
Sleep Paralysis Disorder
Alternative Labels: None
Foliate Sector Localization: Left+Right
Partitions: 4 [(-4, -3, -2, -1) (+1, +2, +3, +4)]
Allotropic Cause: Unknown
Psychophysics Etiology: Complete
IC-10-CM: G47.53
Page No: 623

[4]
Principal
Guilt syndrome
Alternative Labels: None
Foliate Sector Localization: Left+Right
Partitions: 4 [(-4, -3, -2, -1) (+1, +2, +3, +4)]
Allotropic Cause: Unknown
Psychophysics Etiology: Complete
IC-10-CM: N/A
Page No: 422

[4]
Principal
Mythomania
Alternative Labels: Pseudologia Fantastica
Foliate Sector Localization: Left+Right
Partitions: 4 [(-4, -3, -2, -1) (+1, +2, +3, +4)]
Allotropic Cause: Unknown, low self-esteem
Psychophysics Etiology: Complete
IC-10-CM: N/ or F69
Page No: 385

[4]
Principal
Paranoia
Alternative Labels: Megalomania
Foliate Sector Localization: Left+Right
Partitions: 4 [(-4, -3, -2, -1) (+1, +2, +3, +4)]
Allotropic Cause: Unknown, Neurological, Biological
Psychophysics Etiology: Complete
IC-10-CM: F23
F60
Page No: 439

[4]
Principal
Restless Legs Syndrome
Alternative Labels: None
Foliate Sector Localization: Left-Chiral Quadracursor
Partitions: 4 [(-4, -3, -2, -1) (+1, +2, +3, +4)]
Allotropic Cause: Unknown, Biological
Psychophysics Etiology: Complete
IC-10-CM: G25.81
Page No: 602

[4]
Principal
Sleep-Wake Disorder
Alternative Labels: None
Foliate Sector Localization: Left+Right
Partitions: 4 [(-4, -3, -2, -1) (+1, +2, +3, +4)]
Allotropic Cause: Unknown, Biological
Psychophysics Etiology: Complete
IC-10-CM: G47.20
Page No: 619

[4]
Variant of Sleep-wake Disorder
Shift Work Sleep Disorder
Alternative Labels: None
Foliate Sector Localization: Left+Right
Partitions: 4 [(-4, -3, -2, -1) (+1, +2, +3, +4)]
Allotropic Cause: Unknown
Psychophysics Etiology: Complete
IC-10-CM: G47.26
Page No: 619

[4]
Variant of Turbulent Sleep Disorder
Non-Rapid Eye Movement Sleep Arousal Disorder
Alternative Labels: None
Foliate Sector Localization: Hypercursor over accrued
Partitions: 7 [(-4, -3, -2, -1) (+1, +2, +3, +4)]
Allotropic Cause: Unknown
Psychophysics Etiology: Complete
IC-10-CM: G47.5
Page No: 315

– Layer [5] –

[5]
PA to Hysteria
Somatic Symptom Disorder
Alternative Labels: None
Foliate Sector Localization: Left+Right
Partitions: 5 [(-4, -3, -2, -1) (+1, +2, +3, +4)]
Allotropic Cause: Unknown
Psychophysics Etiology: Complete
IC-10-CM: F45.9
Page No: 356

[5]
PA to Pseudocyesis
Couvade Syndrome
Alternative Labels: None
Foliate Sector Localization: Left+Right
Partitions: 7 [(+1, +2, +3, +4)]
Allotropic Cause: Unknown
Psychophysics Etiology: Complete
IC-10-CM: F44.89
Page No: 498

[5]
PA to Split PD
Dissociative Amnesia
Alternative Labels: None
Foliate Sector Localization: Left+Right
Partitions: 5 [(-4, -3, -2, -1) (+1, +2, +3, +4)
Allotropic Cause: Unknown, Biological, Trauma
Psychophysics Etiology: Complete
IC-10-CM: F44.0
Page No: 430

[5]
Principal
Compulsive Gambling Disorder
Alternative Labels: None
Foliate Sector Localization: Left+Right
Partitions: 5 [(-4, -3, -2, -1) (+1, +2, +3, +4)]
Allotropic Cause: Unknown
Psychophysics Etiology: Complete
IC-10-CM: F63.0
Page No: 432

[5]
Principal
Hypochondria
Alternative Labels: Illness Anxiety Disorder
Foliate Sector Localization: Left+Right
Partitions: 5 [(-4, -3, -2, -1) (+1, +2, +3, +4)]
Allotropic Cause: Unknown
Psychophysics Etiology: Complete
IC-10-CM: F45.21
Page No: 442

[5]
Principal
Hysteria
Alternative Labels: Conversion Disorder
Foliate Sector Localization: Left+Right
Partitions: 5 [(-4, -3, -2, -1) (+1, +2, +3, +4)]
Allotropic Cause: Unknown
Psychophysics Etiology: Complete
IC-10-CM: F44.4
Page No: 354

[5]
Principal
Pseudocyesis
Alternative Labels: False Pregnancy, Phantom Pregnancy
Foliate Sector Localization: Left+Right
Partitions: 5 [(-4, -3, -2, -1) (+1, +2, +3, +4)]
Allotropic Cause: Unknown
Psychophysics Etiology: Complete
IC-10-CM: F45.8
Page No: 496

[5]
Principal
Sleepwalking
Alternative Labels: Somnambulism
Foliate Sector Localization: Left+Right, Hypercursor
Partitions: 5 [(-4, -3, -2, -1) (+1, +2, +3, +4)]
Allotropic Cause: Unknown
Psychophysics Etiology: Complete
IC-10-CM: F51.3
Page No: 608

[5]
Principal
Split Personality Disorder
Alternative Labels: Dissociative Identity Disorder, Multiple PD
Foliate Sector Localization: Left+Right
Partitions: 5 [(-4, -3, -2, -1) (+1, +2, +3, +4)]
Allotropic Cause: Unknown, Trauma and Abuse
Psychophysics Etiology: Complete
IC-10-CM: F44.81
Page No: 428

– Layer [6] –

[6]
Principal
Catatonia
Alternative Labels: None
Foliate Sector Localization: Left+Right
Partitions: 6 [(-4, -3, -2, -1) (+1, +2, +3, +4)]
Allotropic Cause: Unknown
Psychophysics Etiology: Complete
IC-10-CM: F06.1
Page No: 611

[6]
Filiation: class Disorder
Depressive Disorders
Alternative Labels: Depression
Foliate Sector Localization: Left-Chiral Only
Partitions: 6 [(-4, -3, -2, -1)]
Allotropic Cause: Unknown, Biological
Psychophysics Etiology: Complete
IC-10-CM: F33.0
Page No: 269

[6]
PA to Bipolar Disorder
Adjustment Disorder
Alternative Labels: None
Foliate Sector Localization: Left+Right
Partitions: 6 [(-4, -3, -2, -1) (+1, +2, +3, +4)]
Allotropic Cause: Unknown
Psychophysics Etiology: Complete
IC-10-CM: F43.23
Page No: 366

[6]
PA to Bipolar Disorder
Melancholy
Alternative Labels: None
Foliate Sector Localization: Left+Right
Partitions: 6 [(-4, -3, -2, -1) (+1, +2, +3, +4)]
Allotropic Cause: Unknown
Psychophysics Etiology: Complete
IC-10-CM: F32.9
Page No: 366

[6]
PA to Bipolar Disorder
Borderline Personality Disorder
Alternative Labels: None
Foliate Sector Localization: Left+Right
Partitions: 6 [(-4, -3, -2, -1) (+1, +2, +3, +4)]
Allotropic Cause: Unknown
Psychophysics Etiology: Complete
IC-10-CM: F60.3
Page No: 366

[6]
PA to Bipolar Disorder
Cyclothymia
Alternative Labels: None
Foliate Sector Localization: Left+Right
Partitions: 6 [(-4, -3, -2, -1) (+1, +2, +3, +4)]
Allotropic Cause: Unknown
Psychophysics Etiology: Complete
IC-10-CM: F34.0
Page No: 366

[6]
PA to Bipolar Disorder
Disruptive Mood Dysregulation Disorder
Alternative Labels: None
Foliate Sector Localization: Left+Right
Partitions: 6 [(-4, -3, -2, -1) (+1, +2, +3, +4)]
Allotropic Cause: Unknown
Psychophysics Etiology: Complete
IC-10-CM: F34.81
Page No: 561

[6]
PA to Bipolar Disorder
Hypomania
Alternative Labels: Mania
Right-Chiral
Partitions: 6 [(-4, -3, -2, -1) (+1, +2, +3, +4)]
Allotropic Cause: Unknown, Biological
Psychophysics Etiology: Complete
IC-10-CM: F31.0
Page No: 366

[6]
PA to Bipolar Disorder
Narcomania
Alternative Labels: Drug addiction
Foliate Sector Localization: Left+Right
Partitions: 6 [(-4, -3, -2, -1) (+1, +2, +3, +4)]
Allotropic Cause: Unknown, Biological
Psychophysics Etiology: Complete
IC-10-CM: F19.10
Page No: 457

[6]
PA to Bipolar Disorder
Peripartum Dysphoria
Alternative Labels: None
Foliate Sector Localization: Left+Right
Partitions: 6 [(-4, -3, -2, -1) (+1, +2, +3, +4)]
Allotropic Cause: pregnancy
Psychophysics Etiology: Complete
IC-10-CM: F53.0
Page No: 371

[6]
PA to Bipolar Disorder
Postpartum Dysphoria
Alternative Labels: None
Foliate Sector Localization: Left+Right or either Right or Left-Chiral only
Partitions: 6 [(-4, -3, -2, -1) (+1, +2, +3, +4)]
Allotropic Cause: Hormonal
Psychophysics Etiology: Complete
IC-10-CM: F53.0
Page No: 371

[6]
PA to Bipolar Disorder
Postpartum Psychosis
Alternative Labels: None
Foliate Sector Localization: Left+Right or either Right or Left-Chiral only
Partitions: 6 [(-4, -3, -2, -1) (+1, +2, +3, +4)]
Allotropic Cause: Hormonal
Psychophysics Etiology: Complete
IC-10-CM: F53.1
Page No: 371

[6]
PA to Bipolar Disorder
Premenstrual Dysphoria
Alternative Labels: PMS, PMDD
Foliate Sector Localization: Left+Right
Partitions: 6 [(-4, -3, -2, -1) (+1, +2, +3, +4)]
Allotropic Cause: Hormonal
Psychophysics Etiology: Complete
IC-10-CM: F32.81
Page No: 370

[6]
PA to Bipolar Disorder
Seasonal Dysphoria
Alternative Labels: Winter blues

Foliate Sector Localization: Left+Right
Partitions: 6 [(-4, -3, -2, -1) (+1, +2, +3, +4)]
Allotropic Cause: Seasonal light alternation
Psychophysics Etiology: Complete
IC-10-CM: F39
Page No: 366

[6]
PA to Dependent Personality Disorder
Obsessive-Compulsive Personality Disorder
Alternative Labels: None
Foliate Sector Localization: Left+Right
Partitions: 6 [(-4, -3, -2, -1) (+1, +2, +3, +4)]
Allotropic Cause: Unknown
Psychophysics Etiology: Complete
IC-10-CM: F60.5
Page No: 286

[6]
PA to Grief Reaction
Passion Blues
Alternative Labels: Prolonged Grief
Foliate Sector Localization: Left-Chiral Only
Partitions: 6 [(-4, -3, -2, -1)]
Allotropic Cause: Unknown
Psychophysics Etiology: Complete
IC-10-CM: F43.0
Page No: 426

[6]
Principal
Separation Anxiety
Alternative Labels: None
Foliate Sector Localization: Left-Chiral
Partitions: 6 [(-4, -3, -2, -1) (+1, +2, +3, +4)]
Allotropic Cause: Unknown
Psychophysics Etiology: Complete
IC-10-CM: F93.0
Page No: 544

[6]
Principal
Bipolar Disorder
Alternative Labels: Manic Depression
Foliate Sector Localization: Left+Right or either Right or Left-Chiral only
Partitions: 6 [(-4, -3, -2, -1) (+1, +2, +3, +4)]
Unknown, Biological
Psychophysics Etiology: Complete
IC-10-CM: F31
Page No: 366

[6]
Principal
Body Dysmorphic Disorder
Alternative Labels: Dysmorphophobia
Foliate Sector Localization: Left+Right
Partitions: 6 [(-4, -3, -2, -1) (+1, +2, +3, +4)]
Allotropic Cause: Unknown
Psychophysics Etiology: Complete
IC-10-CM: F45.22
Page No: 535

[6]
Principal
Dependant Personality Disorder
Alternative Labels: None
Foliate Sector Localization: Left+Right
Partitions: 6 [(-4, -3, -2, -1)(+1, +2, +3, +4)]
Allotropic Cause: Unknown
Psychophysics Etiology: Complete
IC-10-CM: F60.7
Page No: 538

[6]
Principal
Disinhibited Social Engagement Disorder
Alternative Labels: None
Right-Chiral
Partitions: 6 [(-4, -3, -2, -1) (+1, +2, +3, +4)]
Allotropic Cause: Unknown
Psychophysics Etiology: Complete
IC-10-CM: F94.1
Page No: 585

[6]
Principal
Grief Reaction
Alternative Labels: Sadness
Foliate Sector Localization: Left-Chiral Only
Partitions: 6 [(-4, -3, -2, -1)]
Allotropic Cause: Unknown
Psychophysics Etiology: Complete
IC-10-CM: F43

Page No: 425

[6]
Principal
Infantile Neglect Disorder
Alternative Labels: None
Right-Chiral
Partitions: 6 [(-4, -3, -2, -1) (+1, +2, +3, +4)]
Allotropic Cause: Unknown
Psychophysics Etiology: Complete
IC-10-CM: T74.02
Page No: 547

[6]
Principal
Psychogenic Stuttering
Alternative Labels: Stammering
Foliate Sector Localization: Left+Right
Partitions: 6 [(-4, -3, -2, -1) (+1, +2, +3, +4)]
Allotropic Cause: Unknown, Neurological in Neurogenic form
Psychophysics Etiology: Complete
IC-10-CM: F80.81
Page No: 403

[6]
Principal
Reactive Attachment Disorder
Alternative Labels: None
Foliate Sector Localization: Left-Right
Partitions: 6 [(-4, -3, -2, -1) (+1, +2, +3, +4)]
Allotropic Cause: Unknown
Psychophysics Etiology: Complete
IC-10-CM: F94.1
Page No: 551

[6]
Filiation: Variant of Catatonia
Malignant Catatonia
Alternative Labels: None
Foliate Sector Localization: Left+Right
Partitions: 6 [(-4, -3, -2, -1) (+1, +2, +3, +4)]
Allotropic Cause: Unknown
Psychophysics Etiology: Partial
IC-10-CM: F06.1
Page No: 611

[6]
Filiation: Variant of Catatonia
Stupor
Alternative Labels: None
Foliate Sector Localization: Left+Right
Partitions: 6 [(-4, -3, -2, -1) (+1, +2, +3, +4)]
Allotropic Cause: Biological
Psychophysics Etiology: Complete
IC-10-CM: R40.1
Page No: 611

– Layer [7] –

[7]
PA to Body Dysmorphic Disorder
Avoidant/Restrictive Food Intake Disorder
Alternative Labels: None
Foliate Sector Localization: Left+Right
Partitions: 7 [(-4, -3, -2, -1)]
Allotropic Cause: Unknown
Psychophysics Etiology: Complete
IC-10-CM: F50.82
Page No: 569, 573

[7]
PA to Antisocial Personality Disorder
Pyromania
Alternative Labels: Fire setting
Foliate Sector Localization: Right-Chiral Only
Partitions: 7 [(+1, +2, +3, +4)]
Allotropic Cause: Unknown
Psychophysics Etiology: Complete
IC-10-CM: F63.1
Page No: 514

[7]
PA to BIDD
Factitious Disorder
Alternative Labels: None
Foliate Sector Localization: Left+right
Partitions: 7 [(-4, -3, -2, -1) (+1, +2, +3, +4)]
Allotropic Cause: Unknown
Psychophysics Etiology: Complete
IC-10-CM: F68.10
Page No: 264

[7]
PA to Bulimia/Anorexia Nervosa
Binge Eating Disorder
Alternative Labels: Clastomania
Foliate Sector Localization: Right-Chiral Only
Partitions: 7 [(+1, +2, +3, +4)]
Allotropic Cause: Unknown
Psychophysics Etiology: Complete
IC-10-CM: None
Page No: 568

[7]
PA to Bulimia
Rumination Disorder
Alternative Labels: None
Foliate Sector Localization: Left+Right
Partitions: 7 [(-4, -3, -2, -1) (+1, +2, +3, +4)]
Allotropic Cause: Unknown, Biological
Psychophysics Etiology: Complete
IC-10-CM: F98.21
Page No: 573

[7]
PA to Cotard
Depersonalization Disorder
Alternative Labels: None
Foliate Sector Localization: Left+Right
Partitions: 7 [(-4, -3, -2, -1) (+1, +2, +3, +4)]
Allotropic Cause: Unknown
Psychophysics Etiology: Complete
IC-10-CM: F48.1
Page No: 397

[7]
PA to Cotard
Derealization Disorder
Alternative Labels: None
Foliate Sector Localization: Left+Right
Partitions: 7 [(-4, -3, -2, -1) (+1, +2, +3, +4)]
Allotropic Cause: Unknown
Psychophysics Etiology: Complete
IC-10-CM: F48.1
Page No: 397

[7]
PA to Erectile Disorder
Delayed Ejaculation
Alternative Labels: Male Orgasmic Disorder
Foliate Sector Localization: Left-Chiral Side
Partitions: 7 [(-4, -3, -2, -1) (+1, +2, +3, +4)]
Allotropic Cause: Unknown
Psychophysics Etiology: Complete
IC-10-CM: N53.11
Page No: 484

[7]
PA to Erectile Disorder
Male Hypoactive Sexual Desire Disorder
Alternative Labels: None
Foliate Sector Localization: Left-Chiral Side
Partitions: 7 [(-4, -3, -2, -1) (+1, +2, +3, +4)]
Allotropic Cause: Unknown
Psychophysics Etiology: Complete
IC-10-CM: F52.0
Page No: 483

[7]
PA to Erectile Disorder
Premature Ejaculation
Alternative Labels: None
Foliate Sector Localization: Left-Chiral Side
Partitions: 7 [(-4, -3, -2, -1) (+1, +2, +3, +4)]
Allotropic Cause: Unknown
Psychophysics Etiology: Complete
IC-10-CM: F52.4
Page No: 484

[7]
PA to Exhibitionistic Disorder
Frotteuristic Disorder
Alternative Labels: None
Foliate Sector Localization: Left-Chiral Only
Partitions: 7 [(+1 ,+2, +3, +4)]
Allotropic Cause: Unknown
Psychophysics Etiology: Complete
IC-10-CM: F65.81
Page No: 453

[7]
PA to Female Sexual Interest-Arousal Dis-
order
Female Orgasmic Disorder
Alternative Labels: Frigidity
Foliate Sector Localization: Left-Chiral Side

Partitions: 7 [(-4, -3, -2, -1) (+1, +2, +3, +4)]
Allotropic Cause: Unknown
Psychophysics Etiology: Complete
IC-10-CM: F52.31
Page No: 478

[7]
PA to Obsessive-Convulsive Disorder
Tics Disorders
Alternative Labels: None
Foliate Sector Localization: Left+Right
Partitions: 7 [(-4, -3, -2, -1)(+1, +2, +3, +4)]
Allotropic Cause: Unknown
Psychophysics Etiology: Complete
IC-10-CM: F95.9
Page No: 289

[7]
PA to Separation Anxiety
Generalized Anxiety Disorder
Alternative Labels: None
Foliate Sector Localization: Left+Right
Partitions: 7 [(-4, -3, -2, -1) (+1, +2, +3, +4)]
Allotropic Cause: Unknown, Biological
Psychophysics Etiology: Complete
IC-10-CM: F41.10
Page No: 438

[7]
PA to PTSD
Anxiety Syndrome
Alternative Labels: None
Foliate Sector Localization: Left-Chiral
Partitions: 7 [(-4, -3, -2, -1) (+1, +2, +3, +4)]
Allotropic Cause: Unknown, Biological
Psychophysics Etiology: Complete
IC-10-CM: F41.9
Page No: 559

[7]
PA to PTSD
Panic Disorder
Alternative Labels: None
Foliate Sector Localization: Left-Chiral
Partitions: 7 [(-4, -3, -2, -1) (+1, +2, +3, +4)]
Allotropic Cause: Unknown, Biological
Psychophysics Etiology: Complete
IC-10-CM: F40.10
Page No: 559

[7]
PA to Transvestic Disorder
Transvestic Fetishism
Alternative Labels: None
Foliate Sector Localization: Left+Right
Partitions: 7 [(-4, -3, -2, -1) (+1, +2, +3, +4)]
Allotropic Cause: Unknown
Psychophysics Etiology: Complete
IC-10-CM: F65.1
Page No: 395

[7]
Principal
Body Integrity Identity disorder
Alternative Labels: Apotemnophilia
Foliate Sector Localization: Left+Right
Partitions: 7 [(-4, -3, -2, -1) (+1, +2, +3, +4)]
Allotropic Cause: Unknown
Psychophysics Etiology: Partial
N/A
Page No: 375

[7]
Principal
Bulimia-Anorexia Nervosa
Alternative Labels: BAN Syndrome
Foliate Sector Localization: Left+Right
Partitions: 7 [(-4, -3, -2, -1) (+1, +2, +3, +4)]
Allotropic Cause: Unknown
Psychophysics Etiology: Complete
IC-10-CM: F50.2
Page No: 568

[7]
Principal
Conduct Disorder
Alternative Labels: None
Foliate Sector Localization: Right-Chiral Only
Partitions: 7 [(+1, +2, +3, +4)]
Allotropic Cause: Unknown
Psychophysics Etiology: Complete
IC-10-CM: F91.9
Page No: 565

[7]
Principal
Cotard's Syndrome
Alternative Labels: Delire des Negations
Foliate Sector Localization: Left+Right
Partitions: 7 [(-4, -3, -2, -1) (+1, +2, +3, +4)]
Allotropic Cause: Unknown
Psychophysics Etiology: Complete
IC-10-CM: F22.0
Page No: 397

[7]
Principal
Dermatillomania
Alternative Labels: Excoriation
Skin picking
Right-Chiral
Partitions: 7 [(-4, -3, -2, -1) (+1, +2, +3, +4)]
Allotropic Cause: Unknown
Psychophysics Etiology: Complete
IC-10-CM: F42.4
Page No: 579

[7]
Principal
Erectile Disorder
Alternative Labels: Impotence
Foliate Sector Localization: Left-Chiral Side
Partitions: 7 [(-4, -3, -2, -1) (+1, +2, +3, +4)]
Allotropic Cause: Unknown
Psychophysics Etiology: Complete
IC-10-CM: N52.9
Page No: 480

[7]
Principal
Exhibitionistic Disorder
Alternative Labels: None
Foliate Sector Localization: Left-Chiral Only
Partitions: 7 [(+1, +2, +3, +4)]
Allotropic Cause: Unknown
Psychophysics Etiology: Complete
IC-10-CM: F65.2
Page No: 450

[7]
Principal
Female Sexual Interest-Arousal Disorder
Alternative Labels: Frigidity
Foliate Sector Localization: Left-Chiral Side
Partitions: 7 [(-4, -3, -2, -1) (+1, +2, +3, +4)]
Allotropic Cause: Unknown
Psychophysics Etiology: Complete
IC-10-CM: F52.22
Page No: 478

[7]
Principal
Homosexuality/Lesbianism (if causing distress)
Alternative Labels: None
Foliate Sector Localization: Left+Right
Partitions: 7 [(-4, -3, -2, -1) (+1, +2, +3, +4)]
Allotropic Cause: Unknown, Genetical
Psychophysics Etiology: Complete
IC-10-CM: N/A
Page No: 282

[7]
Principal
Intermittent Explosive Disorder
Alternative Labels: None
Foliate Sector Localization: Left+Right
Partitions: 7 [(-4, -3, -2, -1)(+1, +2, +3, +4)]
Allotropic Cause: Unknown
Psychophysics Etiology: Complete
IC-10-CM: F63.81
Page No: 382

[7]
Principal
Juvenile Delinquency
Alternative Labels: None
Foliate Sector Localization: Right-Chiral Only
Partitions: 7 [(+1, +2, +3, +4)]
Allotropic Cause: Unknown, Biological
Psychophysics Etiology: Complete
IC-10-CM: Z72.810
Page No: 565

[7]
Principal
Kleptomania
Alternative Labels: Pathological Stealing

Foliate Sector Localization: Left-Chiral Only
Partitions: 7 [(-4, -3, -2, -1)]
Allotropic Cause: Unknown
Uncontrollable impulse
Psychophysics Etiology: Complete
IC-10-CM: F63.2
Page No: 389

[7]
Principal
Neglect syndrome
Alternative Labels: Hemispatial Neglect, Unilateral Neglect, Hemi-inattention, Hemi-neglect
Foliate Sector Localization: Left+Right
Partitions: 7 [(-4, -3, -2, -1) (+1, +2, +3, +4)]
Neurological
Psychophysics Etiology: Partial
IC-10-CM: R41.4
Page No: 409

[7]
Principal
Nymphomania
Alternative Labels: Don Juanism, Satyriasis, Erotomania, Hypersexuality
Foliate Sector Localization: Left-Chiral in W and HomoMen
Right-Chiral in Men and lesbian f
Partitions: 7 [(-4, -3, -2, -1) **or** (+1, +2, +3, +4)]
Allotropic Cause: Unknown
Psychophysics Etiology: Complete
IC-10-CM: F52.8
Page No: 487

[7]
Principal
Oppositional Defiant Disorder
Alternative Labels: None
Right-Chiral
Partitions: 7 [(-4, -3, -2, -1) (+1, +2, +3, +4)]
Allotropic Cause: Unknown
Psychophysics Etiology: Complete
IC-10-CM: F91.3
Page No: 555

[7]
Principal
Turbulent Sleep Disorder
Alternative Labels: None
Foliate Sector Localization: Left+Right
Partitions: 7 [(-4, -3, -2, -1) (+1, +2, +3, +4)]
Hypercursor over accrued
Allotropic Cause: Unknown, Biological
Psychophysics Etiology: Complete
IC-10-CM: F47.50
Page No: 627

[7]
Principal
Pedophilic Disorder
Alternative Labels: None
Foliate Sector Localization: Left-Chiral Sector of Foliate
7[(-4, -3, -2, -1) (+1, +2, +3, +4)]
Allotropic Cause: Unknown
Psychophysics Etiology: Complete
IC-10-CM: F65.4
Page No: 470

[7]
Principal
Phobia
Alternative Labels: None
Foliate Sector Localization: Left-Chiral
Partitions: 7 [(-4, -3, -2, -2) (+1, +2, +3, +4)]
Allotropic Cause: Unknown
Psychophysics Etiology: Complete
IC-10-CM: F40.00
Page No: 435

[7]
Principal
Post traumatic stress disorder
Alternative Labels: None
Foliate Sector Localization: Left-Chiral
Partitions: 7 [(-4, -3, -2, -1) (+1, +2, +3 +4)]
Allotropic Cause: Unknown
Psychophysics Etiology: Complete
IC-10-CM: F43.10
Page No: 555

[7]
Principal
Sadistic (Antisocial) Personality Disorder
Alternative Labels: Psychopathy, Sociopathy
Foliate Sector Localization: Right-Chiral Only
Partitions: 7 [(+1, +2, +3, +4)]
Allotropic Cause: Unknown
Psychophysics Etiology: Complete
IC-10-CM: F60.2
Page No: 506

[7]
Principal
Sexual Masochistic Disorder
Alternative Labels: Masochism
Foliate Sector Localization: Left-Chiral Only
Partitions: 7 [(-4, -3, -2, -1)
Allotropic Cause: Unknown
Psychophysics Etiology: Complete
IC-10-CM: F65.51
Page No: 490

[7]
Principal
Sexual Sadism Disorder
Alternative Labels: Sexual Sadism
Foliate Sector Localization: Right-Chiral
Partitions: 7 [(+1, +2, +3, +4)]
Allotropic Cause: Unknown
Psychophysics Etiology: Complete
IC-10-CM: F65.52
Page No: 455

[7]
Principal
Suicidal Obsession
Alternative Labels: None
Foliate Sector Localization: Left-Chiral
Partitions: 7 [(-4,- 3, -2, -1) (+1, +2, +3, +4)]
Allotropic Cause: Unknown
Psychophysics Etiology: Complete
IC-10-CM: F42.0
Page No: 531

[7]
PA to Trichotilomania-Dermatilomania
Stereotypic Movement Disorder
Alternative Labels: None
Foliate Sector Localization: Left+Right
Partitions: 7 [(-4, -3, -2, -1) (+1, +2, +3, +4)]
Allotropic Cause: Unknown
Psychophysics Etiology: Complete
IC-10-CM: F98.4
Page No: 583

[7]
Principal
Transvestic Disorder
Alternative Labels: None
Foliate Sector Localization: Left+Right
Partitions: 7 [(-4, -3, -2, -1) (+1, +2, +3, +4)]
Allotropic Cause: Unknown
Psychophysics Etiology: Complete
IC-10-CM: F65.1
Page No: 462

[7]
Principal
Trichotillomania-Dermatillomania
Alternative Labels: None
Foliate Sector Localization: Left+Right
Partitions: 7 [(-4, -3, -2, -1) (+1, +2, +3, +4)]
Allotropic Cause: Unknown
Psychophysics Etiology: Complete
IC-10-CM: --
Page No: 575

[7]
Principal
Trichotillomania
Alternative Labels: Hair-Pulling
Foliate Sector Localization: Left-Chiral
Partitions: 7 [(-4, -3, -2, -1) (+1, +2, +3, +4)]
Allotropic Cause: Unknown
Psychophysics Etiology: Complete
IC-10-CM: F63.3
Page No: 575

[7]
Filiation: Variant of BAN
Anorexia Nervosa
Alternative Labels: BAN syndrome
Foliate Sector Localization: Left+Right
Partitions: 7 [(-4, -3, -2, -1) (+1, +2, +3, +4)]

Allotropic Cause: Unknown
Psychophysics Etiology: Complete
IC-10-CM: F50.0
Page No: 568

[7]
Filiation: Variant of Bulimia/Anorexia Nervosa
Bulimia
Alternative Labels: None
Foliate Sector Localization: Left+Right
Partitions: 7 [(-4, -3, -2, -1) (+1, +2, +3, +4)]
Allotropic Cause: Unknown
Psychophysics Etiology: Complete
IC-10-CM: F50.2
Page No: 568

[7]
Filiation: Variant of Bulimia/Anorexia Nervosa
Purging
Alternative Labels: None
Foliate Sector Localization: Left+Right
Partitions: 7 [(-4, -3, -2, -1) (+1, +2, +3, +4)]
Allotropic Cause: Unknown
Psychophysics Etiology: Complete
IC-10-CM: F50
Page No: 568

[7]
Filiation: Variant of Parasomnia
Enuresis
Alternative Labels: Bedwetting
Foliate Sector Localization: Left+Right
Partitions: 7 [(-4, -3, -2, -1) (+1, +2, +3, +4)]
Allotropic Cause: Unknown, Biological
Psychophysics Etiology: Partial
IC-10-CM : N39.44
Page No: 628

[7]
Filiation: Variant of Phobia
Acrophobia
Alternative Labels: Fear of heights
Foliate Sector Localization: Left-Chiral
Partitions: 7 [(-4, -3, -2, -2) (+1, +2, +3, +4)]
Allotropic Cause: Unknown
Psychophysics Etiology: Complete
IC-10-CM: F40.241
Page No: 436

[7]
Filiation: Variant of Phobia
Agoraphobia
Alternative Labels: Fear of open spaces
Foliate Sector Localization: Left-Chiral
Partitions: 7 [(-4, -3, -2, -2) (+1, +2, +3, +4)]
Allotropic Cause: Unknown
Psychophysics Etiology: Complete
IC-10-CM: F40.01
Page No: 436

[7]
Filiation: Variant of Phobia
Animal Phobia
Alternative Labels: None
Foliate Sector Localization: Left-Chiral
Partitions: 7 [(-4, -3, -2, -2) (+1, +2, +3, +4)]
Allotropic Cause: Unknown
Psychophysics Etiology: Complete
IC-10-CM: F40.218
Page No: 435

[7]
Filiation: Variant of Phobia
Blood-Injection-Injury Phobia
Alternative Labels: Hemophobia
Foliate Sector Localization: Left-Chiral
Partitions: 7 [(-4, -3, -2, -2) (+1, +2, +3, +4)]
Allotropic Cause: Unknown
Psychophysics Etiology: Complete
IC-10-CM: F40.23
Page No: 435

[7]
Filiation: Variant of Phobia
Claustrophobia
Alternative Labels: Fear of closed spaces
Foliate Sector Localization: Left-Chiral
Partitions: 7 [(-4, -3, -2, -2) (+1, +2, +3, +4)]
Allotropic Cause: Unknown
Psychophysics Etiology: Complete
IC-10-CM: F40.240
Page No: 436

[7]
Variant of Phobia
Natural Environment Phobia
Alternative Labels: None
Foliate Sector Localization: Left-Chiral
Partitions: 7 [(-4, -3, -2, -2) (+1, +2, +3, +4)]
Allotropic Cause: Unknown
Psychophysics Etiology: Complete
IC-10-CM: F40.228
Page No: 435

[7]
Variant of Phobia
Specific Phobia
Alternative Labels: None
Foliate Sector Localization: Left-Chiral
Partitions: 7 [(-4, -3, -2, -2) (+1, +2, +3, +4)]
Allotropic Cause: Unknown
Psychophysics Etiology: Complete
IC-10-CM: F40.2
Page No: 435

[7]
Filiation: Variant of PTSD
Acute Stress Reaction
Alternative Labels: Stress
Foliate Sector Localization: Left-Chiral
Partitions: 7 [(-4, -3, -2, -1) (+1, +2, +3, +4)]
Allotropic Cause: Unknown
Psychophysics Etiology: Complete
IC-10-CM: F43.0
Page No: 556

[7]
Filiation: Variant of Turbulent Sleep Disorder
Nightmare Disorder
Alternative Labels: Dream Anxiety Disorder
Foliate Sector Localization: Hypercursor over accrued
Partitions: 7 [(-4, -3, -2, -1) (+1, +2, +3, +4)]
Allotropic Cause: Unknown
Psychophysics Etiology: Complete
IC-10-CM: F51.5
Page No: 628

[7]
Variant of Transvestic Disorder
Autogynephilia
Alternative Labels: Eonism, Automonosexuality
Foliate Sector Localization: Left+Right
Partitions: 7 [(-4, -3, -2, -1) (+1, +2, +3, +4)]
Allotropic Cause: Unknown
Psychophysics Etiology: Complete
IC-10-CM: F65.1
Page No: 463

– Layer [8] –

[8]
PA to Schizophrenia
Autism
Alternative Labels: None
Foliate Sector Localization: Left+Right
Partitions: 8 [(-4, -3, -2, -1) (+1, +2, +3, +4)]
Allotropic Cause: Biological, Genetic
Psychophysics Etiology: Complete
IC-10-CM: F84.0
Page No: 446

[8]
PA to Schizophrenia
Schizoid Personality Disorder
Alternative Labels: None
Foliate Sector Localization: Left-Chiral
Partitions: 8 [(-4, -3, -2, -1) (+1, +2, +3, +4)]
Allotropic Cause: Unknown
Psychophysics Etiology: Complete
IC-10-CM: F60.1
Page No: 448

[8]
PA to Paranoia
Schizotypal Personality Disorder
Alternative Labels: None
Foliate Sector Localization: Left+Right
Partitions: 4 [(-4, -3, -2, -1) (+1, +2, +3, +4)]
Allotropic Cause: Unknown
Psychophysics Etiology: Complete
IC-10-CM: F21
Page No: 448

[8]
PA to Schizophrenia
Copromania
Alternative Labels: None
Foliate Sector Localization: Left+Right
Partitions: 8 [(-4, -3, -2, -1) (+1, +2, +3, +4)]
Allotropic Cause: Unknown
Psychophysics Etiology: Complete
IC-10-CM: N/A
Page No: 632

[8]
PA to Schizophrenia
Social Communication Disorder
Alternative Labels: None
Foliate Sector Localization: Left+Right
Partitions: 8 [(-4, -3, -2, -1) (+1, +2, +3, +4)]
Allotropic Cause: Unknown
Psychophysics Etiology: Complete
IC-10-CM: F80.82
Page No: 268

[8]
Principal
Schizophrenia
Alternative Labels: Dementia precox
Foliate Sector Localization: Left+Right
Partitions: 8 [(-4, -3, -2, -1) (+1, +2, +3, +4)]
Allotropic Cause: Biological, Trauma, Genetic
Psychophysics Etiology: Complete
IC-10-CM: F20.9
Page No: 445

[8]
Variant of Burnout Syndrome
Asthenia
Alternative Labels: Neurasthenia
Foliate Sector Localization: Left-Chiral
1[(-4, -3, -2, -1), (+1, +2, +3, + 4)]
Allotropic Cause: Unknown
Psychophysics Etiology: Complete
IC-10-CM: F48.8
Page No: 358

[8]
Variant of Turbulent Sleep Disorder
Rapid Eye Movement (REM) Sleep Behavior Disorder
Alternative Labels: None
Foliate Sector Localization: Hypercursor over accrued
Partitions: 7 [(-4, -3, -2, -1) (+1, +2, +3, +4)]
Allotropic Cause: Unknown
Psychophysics Etiology: Complete
IC-10-CM: G47.52
Page No: 315

– Layer [9] –

[9]
PA to Hypersomnia
Kleine-Levin Syndrome
Alternative Labels: Sleeping Beauty Syndrome
Foliate Sector Localization: Hypercursor over accrued
Layer 9 Overaccrued
Allotropic Cause: Biological
Psychophysics Etiology: Complete
IC-10-CM: G47.13
Page No: 598

[9]
PA to Hypersomnia
Narcolepsy Type 1 and 2
Alternative Labels: None
Foliate Sector Localization: Hypercursor over accrued
Layer 9 Overaccrued
Allotropic Cause: Unknown, Biological
Psychophysics Etiology: Complete
IC-10-CM: G47.419
Page No: 601

[9]
Principal
Alzheimer's Disease
Alternative Labels: Dementia
Foliate Sector Localization: Left+Right
Partitions: 9 [(-4, -3, -2, -1) (+1, +2, +3, +4)]
Allotropic Cause: Biological, Trauma, Vascular

Psychophysics Etiology: Partial
IC-10-CM: G30.9
Page No: 526

[9]
Principal
Epilepsy
Alternative Labels: Seizures
Foliate Sector Localization: Left+Right
Partitions: 9 [(-4, -3, -2, -1) (+1, +2, +3, +4)]
Allotropic Cause: Unknown, Biological, Trauma
Psychophysics Etiology: Partial
G40
Page No: 515

[9]
Principal
Hypersomnia
Alternative Labels: Hypersomnolence
Foliate Sector Localization: Hypercursor over accrued
Layer 9 overaccrued
Allotropic Cause: Unknown, Biological
Psychophysics Etiology: Complete
IC-10-CM: G47.10
Page No: 596

[9]
Symptom of Narcolepsy Type 1
Cataplexy
Alternative Labels: None
Foliate Sector Localization: Hypercursor over accrued
Layer 9 Overaccrued
Allotropic Cause: Unknown
Psychophysics Etiology: Complete
IC-10-CM: F47.411
IC-10-CM: F20.2
Page No: 601

Commented Bibliography

ATTENTION DEFICIT HYPERACTIVITY DISORDER (ADHD)

"ADHD symptoms can change over time as a person ages. In young children with ADHD, hyperactivity-impulsivity is the most predominant symptom. As a child reaches elementary school, the symptom of inattention may become more prominent and cause the child to struggle academically." -- https://www.nimh.nih.gov/health/topics/attention-deficit-hyperactivity-disorder-adhd/index.shtml

HYSTERIA

"Hysteria provokes convulsions, violent migraines and vomiting. To convulsions and vomiting, limb paralyses follow suit.(p.139)... Abundant flow of words, torrents of tears and laughter. Laments, at times in a yelling fashion. Insults." (p. 141) – ***Les Prodigieuses Victoires de la Psychologie, Pierre Daco, Les Nouvelles Editions Marabout, 1977.***

Tears and laughter are each behavioral expressions located at a different side of the distribution. As are laments and insults, laments being passive-responsive behavior and insults active-motivational behavior. These things are all happening in the moment and sometimes in phases. Now "Yelling laments" stands for another interesting hybrid bit of metamorphogenic behavior that is in fact a flashing dystonic shift between active and passive mode of the mood.

BURNOUT SYNDROME

Despite having been deprecated in DSM-5, the Burnout dysfunction has been restored to the status of a legitimate mental disorder by the World Health Organization in the International Classification of Diseases, catering to a large incidence of this illness among health professionals. In restoring this illness in official taxonomy, we heeded its essential aspect as a dysfunction, which is excessive mental fatigue or mental exhaustion. In that quality, Burnout Syndrome belongs to the former legitimate family of mental dysfunctions classified under the nomer of Asthenia.– *The American Journal of Medicine, https://www.amjmed.com/article/S0002-9343(19)30757-0/pdf -- https://www.doctissimo.fr/html/dossiers/depression/articles/9032-deprime-signes.htm*

"Asthenia is a lack of energy. It causes exhaustion from wake in early morning as well as a difficulty to work further. The difficulty to manifest "willpower" is there as well (abulia). Impossibility to focus one's attention, sensation of void in the head. Asthenia shares many of the symptoms of depression, with which it is often conflated." (p.250)

"Neurasthenia is a permanent Asthenia. It is a generalized depression of the nervous system, whose potential is severely diminished. The neurovegetative system goes out of order; depletion of

brain capacity is sometimes very significant... The person affected by Neurasthenia exhibits reactions that are quite unexpected, changing, sudden, paradoxical, illogical and out of proportion. ***He/she goes from merry excitation to the most profound dispiritedness in a completely unpredictable manner***[instance of Behavioral Flip].*"(p. 251)*

"Psychastenia is about the flow of ideas. Numerous disparate ideas cross the mind with the subject being unable to prevent them. It is indeed a psychic weakness, and not exactly a nervous asthenia akin to Neurasthenia. There is a drop of psychological tension; mental synthesis is difficult to realize. The Psychastenic patient is challenged to accomplish intellectual mentation, however his automatic reflexes are not affected..." ***(p.254) – Les Prodigieuses Victoires de la Psychologie, Pierre Daco, Les Nouvelles Editions Marabout, 1977.***

IMPOSTOR SYNDROME

It is noteworthy that this syndrome is known in francophone culture as *peur de l'échec, syndrome d'échec* ou *syndrome de l'imposteur.* While it is characterized by unjustified concerns around failure, it should not be confused with the dysfunction designated *Neurosis of Failure (Névrose d'Échec).* Neurosis of failure is a veritable need for failure, which does not see the mind deploy in discernment or perspicacious faculties at the active-latent side of Layer **3**, as it does in Impostor Syndrome, but restricted to the negative passive-latent partitions.

Note that in the Impostor Syndrome, which involves the entire partition set of Layer **3**, in general, the behavioral flips occur between intense feelings of fear of failure with sentiments of poor self-esteem, on one side, and, on the other side, positive deployment of intelligent intellect often leading even to overachievement. Over-achievement is a key artifact in the expression of the swing, since there would arguably be no visible, explicit reason for the extra push if it were not to be in reaction to an antithetic feeling. *"Many people who feel like impostors grew up in families that placed a big emphasis on achievement. In particular, parents who send mixed messages —* ***alternating between over-praise and criticism*** *— can increase the risk of future fraudulent feelings."* —says psychologist Suzanne Imes, one of the co-inventors of the designation, very interestingly.-- *https://www.apa.org/gradpsych/2013/11/fraud*

Admittedly psychoanalysis in its tendency to find mandatory unconscious drives to morbid behavior, commonly seeks to etiologically attribute unconscious motives to this disorder, such as putative non-conscious culpability in terms of self chastisement for inacceptable unconscious desires. For instance, one may read: *"Outre le trouble de l'estime de soi, l'auto-dénigrement du moi dominant, la culpabilité non-consciente (se punir de désirs inconscients) pourrait fournir une explication à ce comportement répétitif. Il pourrait s'agir d'un masochisme primaire qui renvoie à un trouble plus profond de la personnalité, éventuellement forgé dans l'enfance, qui peut être en relation avec la morbidité."*Note the conjectural tone of the interpretation. Ofentimes, the analyst seeks a connection with the Oedipus complex and the sentiments of culpability and urges of castration or masochism emerging from it. Nonetheless, straight observation shows at work here, in the specific case of Impostor Syndrome, the simple mechanism of compensation, involving a flip from sentiments of self-denigration and broad intelligent mentalization producing visible over-achievement, through a direct Transflow, in broad conscious daylight, so to speak. In the case of Neurosis of Failure, we face the simple case of Transflows involving such root thought partitions as *Aberration, Idiocy, Disorientation* and *Doubt* as the engine at work.

It may well be that the reason for deprecating this disorder, along with many others, in the pragmatic Anglo-American psychology is due to dubious or uncertain conjectural etiologies of the kind resulting from over-analysis in orthodox psychoanalysis.– *Les Prodigieuses Victoires de la Psychologie, Pierre Daco, Les Nouvelles Editions Marabout, 1977, p.467.*

The above remains valid even though the original designation for the illness was *"Imposter experience" (Expérience de l'imposture)* as proposed in 1978 by psychologists Pauline Rose Clance and Suzanne Imes, who did not quite think of it in terms of an illness but a psychological mechanism. However, given the details of its nosology and how widespread it turns out to be, and not restricted to just women as proposed by the original authors, we find it no less of a legitimate mental disorder than any other.

BIPOLAR DISORDER

"Bipolar I is defined by the appearance of at least one manic episode. You may experience hypomanic or major depressive episodes before and after the manic episode. This type of bipolar disorder affects men and women equally." - https://www.healthline.com/health/bipolar-disorder#types

*"The label 'mixed or rapid cycling' applies to the illness when four or more episodes of mania and depression in a year has been registered."*https://www.healthline.com/health/bipolar-disorder#facts – Unless they occur in polar alternation, this is not quite to be confounded with our so-called Behavioral Flips which involve phases of high mood subsequently followed or immediately preceded by a low mood phase in a rather short period of time. The latter duly corresponds to what has been designated "Mood Swings".

It is important to remain cognizant that what the established distinction between Bipolar I and Bipolar II seeks to highlight is matter-of-factly the prevalence over time of one polar phase (manic in Bipolar I or depressive in Bipolar II) in the course of the illness with respect to the other, as clinically observed. What constitutes the essence of the polarization is not at all well understood in current psychology, due to a veritable lack of clarity in the role of the entire spectrum of mind fits underlying the expression and development of the symptom set of the illness. This has led to a contentious classificatory taxon of Bipolar NOS (Non Otherwise Specified), a catch-all for bipolar-like symptoms that do not fit in their entirety Bipolar I or Bipolar II. Taxonomic controversy set aside, Bipolar NOS is at least commonly regarded as a precursor to either Bipolar I or bipolar II disorder. Nothing less than a recognition that there exists a full spectrum of mentation fits (moods) in their own rights underlying the illness of Manic Depression, which is the QG set of

Mentation Partitions of Layer 6 in our approach. Because analytic psychology has not ascertained thus far that bipolarization swings exist in all mental dysfunctions, it has been unable to formulate the question of why it seems to be so peculiar to and extreme in Manic Depression, why it seems to be dependent on seasons of the year, and why it seems to have such a negative impact on these patients' sleep cycle through the circadian rythmns than no other disorder and why they seem to be able to live over prolonged periods of time without energy recovery provided by night sleep. The simple answer to this question lies in the pineal gland.

Bipolar disorder is associated with high rate of chronicity and inter-episodic recovery. Women with bipolar disorder may also relapse more often. Hormonal changes related to menstruation, pregnancy or menopause seem to be responsible for these frequent relapses, which takes us right back to the pineal gland. Finally, mortality studies indicate that the rate of premature mortality is significantly elevated in bipolar disorder.

BODY INTEGRITY IDENTITY DISORDER (BIID)

"The studies we reviewed present individuals willing to amputate a limb, independent of the underlying etiology. However, two recent surveys highlight that the desire to modify the body might also present with non-amputation variants.Before these two studies, in 1997, Bruno noticed that individuals with ***apotemnophilia could present a peculiar desire to be paralyzed. He described in detail the case of a woman who was willing to be paralyzed and who pretended to be so, using a wheelchair.*** *However, Bruno did not include this desire within apotemnophilia. Rather, he proposed a psychological concept to explain not only a fascination for being with disabled persons, but also a desire to pretend to be disabled, and even to become disabled: "factitious disability disorders" (see First and Fisher for a discussion).*

Alternatively, two more recent reports suggest that the desire to be paralyzed is a variant of apotemnophilia/BIID. It should be noted that, in these cases, the adoption of the term xenomelia is not appropriate, as individuals who want to become paraplegic do not want to lose their limbs.

These surveys adopted questionnaires developed ad hoc to screen individuals about their desire, age at its onset, sexual compulsions, comorbid psychiatric pathologies, and other relevant clinical features.

Forty-four percent of the 54 individuals recruited by Blom et al reported a wish to be disabled, but not through amputation. Twenty-four of these individuals (seven females; 29% of the sample) desired to become paralyzed (about 44% of the entire sample) and indicated the exact location of the desired paralysis. The majority of individuals who desired paralysis were heterosexual, while seven individuals were homosexual and four were bisexual. Further, 11 individuals also presented with sexual arousal that was related to seeing persons with the desired disability. The same number of interviewed persons described a psychiatric comorbidity during their lifetime (eg, depression, anxiety, psychosis). The authors suggested that those individuals with the paralysis version of the desire did not differ in clinical features from those wanting an amputation. They concluded that this variant is a manifestation of the same desire. However, the authors did not provide a hypothesis to explain the existence of two variants of the same desire."

The results below clearly show that expectedly women are more affected by activity of the root partitions at the left side of the distribution on Layer 7, which are promoters of the Anima characterization define the female gender psychologically. There are significantly more women who report experiencing the desire of limb paralysis than there are men.

"In their study, Giumarra et al[4] enrolled 16 individuals with the paralysis variant and reached a conclusion in favor of a variability that can be attributed to gender differences. As for the clinical features (psychiatric comorbidities, sexual arousal), the rates are similar between the two studies, equally supporting the inadequacy of psychotic or mood disorders to explain the desire. Giumarra et al also reported that all participants who wanted a paralysis were able also to define a clear demarcation line for the desired spinal cord injury, as do subjects seeking amputation. Secondly, a higher proportion of women (37.5%) was found to have this desire variant. Thus, the authors hypothesized that the desire to be paralyzed is neurologically-based, as it is for amputation, and suggested that women are more inclined toward paralysis, as they have a less marked lateralization of the corpus callosum, which could lead to a "bilateral desire".

While this explanation seems appealing, it should be noted that the paralysis variant also manifests in men (though to a lesser degree than in woman, [15% versus 29%, respectively]). Thus, a different lateralization of the body representation, as a function of gender, does not fully account for all of the cases.—

... Further, they have been inspired mainly by First's observation that most of these individuals seek a limb amputation primarily "to feel complete" and not for a sexual reason.
https://www.ncbi.nlm.nih.gov/pmc/articles/PMC4094630/

'I have this limb that should not be' Mr. H, age 31, is a white male of Eastern European descent who was born, raised, and resides in a major metropolitan area in the western United States. -- ***Xenomelia: Profile of a man with intense desire to amputate a healthy limb,Current Psychiatry Vol. 17, No. 8***

SOCIAL ANXIETY DISORDER

"Heterogeneity of Social Anxiety. *At least some socially anxious people attempt to escape aversive states of self-awareness and unwanted anxious reactions by engaging in risk-taking behaviors such as substance abuse (e.g., Burke & Stephens, 1999). Socially anxious people with beliefs that alcohol can increase social assertiveness or alleviate anxiety symptoms exhibit the most problematic drinking patterns (e.g., Ham & Hope, 2005). However, only a few studies extended this line of inquiry to other risky behaviors such as aggression and unsafe sex (Erwin, Heimberg, Schneier, & Liebowitz, 2003; Kashdan et al., 2006).*

Three independent studies provide evidence for a subset of people suffering from social anxiety reporting disinhibited behavior tendencies. In one study, cluster analytic techniques were used to determine whether the interpersonal behavior dimensions of dominance-submissiveness and nurturance-cold-heartedness provide a framework for classifying people with SAD (Kachin et al., 2001). There was support for two groups with the first characterized by prototypical avoidant and submissive behaviors and the second by dominant and hostile behaviors. In a second unpublished study, cluster analytic techniques were used to determine whether people with social anxiety disorder (SAD) can be classified according to temperamental novelty-seeking (Kashdan & Hofmann, in press). Results supported the presence of two distinct subgroups with the first characterized by low novelty seeking and over-regulated and controlled behaviors and the second by high novelty seeking and exploratory tendencies in response to impulsive decision-making. In a third study, people with excessive social anxiety with positive expectancy beliefs for risky behaviors reported the greatest intentions to engage in aggressive acts and unsafe sexual practices over the next six months (even more than people with minimal social anxiety and positive expectancies; Kashdan et al., 2006).

These findings converge with work by Higgins and colleagues to suggest that attending to regulatory focus is not sufficient in the study of social anxiety. It may be overly broad to define people with excessive social anxiety as prevention focused and reliant on inhibited means to desired goals. People with excessive social anxiety are inclined toward behavioral inhibition but at least a subset of people engages in behavioral production strategies characterized as excitable, impulsive, quick-tempered, and unpredictable. Self-regulatory strength models provide additional insight into why social anxiety might be associated with behaviors such as excessive substance use and lack of sexual restraint. People with excessive social anxiety who strenuously resist their frequent anxious feelings and vigilant thought processes are likely to deplete limited self-regulatory resources that effectively prevent socially undesirable behaviors. This includes being aggressive, self-destructive, and hedonistic (e.g., Tice, Bratslavasky, & Baumeister, 2001; Vohs, Baumeister, & Ciarocco, 2005). People with excessive social anxiety vary in the amount of energy devoted to inhibiting and controlling their natural emotional reactions (Kashdan & Steger, 2006) and therefore, only a subset may regularly expend themselves to the point of being more impulsive, fickle, and quick-tempered than their more inhibited peers (Kashdan & Hofmann, in press). Since emotional well-being and self-regulation are significant contributors to success, being socially anxious and risk-prone is expected to characterize a particularly impaired subgroup of people.

Although the extant data are limited to date, existing theoretical models (Clark & Wells, 1995; Gilbert, 2001; Leary, 2001; Rapee & Heimberg, 1997) suggest conditions linking social anxiety to increased risk-prone activity. We present several speculations based on these theories. First, due to excessive self-presentation concerns, risk-taking may increase if these behaviors are associated with greater social status and power (e.g., people will perceive them as "cool" for consuming copious amounts of alcohol). Second, as a result of hypersensitivity to criticism, risk-taking behaviors such as aggression may increase if attacking others in social situations is viewed as an effective tactic to minimize critical evaluation and regain some semblance of power and control. Third, due to a preoccupation with unmet feelings of belonging, risk-taking behaviors such as unsafe sex with a prostitute may increase if it is believed that feelings of safety and security can be temporarily restored. Fourth, when socially anxious people believe they have a lot to offer other people in terms of physical attractiveness, intelligence, wit, or other qualities, they may engage in dominant risk-taking behaviors. Fifth, socially anxious people who experience high levels of curiosity, or ap-

praise certain events as having a high possibility to satisfy curiosity, may be more likely to engage in approach behavior amidst conflicting avoidance motivations. Exposure to novel and challenging situations such as risk-taking sports or meeting new people often evoke feelings of both anxiety and curiosity (Kashdan, 2004; Silvia, 2006; Spielberger & Starr, 1994). Although socially anxious people are defined by frequent, intense, enduring, and easily triggered anxious reactions, exploratory responses can derive from situations that evoke intense curiosity from potential incentives.

*Engaging in risky behaviors may serve the function of avoiding unwanted anxious thoughts, feelings, and sensations or temporarily restoring a sense of personal control over personal fears. Risky behaviors may also serve as a potential source of reward or strategy to appear more socially attractive to other people (even if it is illusory; Baumeister & Tice, 1990; Gilbert, 2001). Yet, frequent and impulsive risk-taking is unlikely to have a healthy influence on psychological and social well-being. In general, higher frequencies of unsafe sexual practices, aggression, and substance use are associated with psychological and physical health problems (e.g., Centers for Disease Control and Prevention, 2003; Wilson & Joffe, 1995). Coupled with the morbidity of social anxiety, being risk-prone is proposed to seriously compromise psychological, social, and physical well-being." --**Social anxiety and disinhibition: An analysis of curiosity and social rank appraisals, approach-avoidance conflicts, anddisruptive risk-taking behavior – Todd B Kashdan et al***

The elements of bipolar behavior between retreat and disinhibition have been clearly put in evidence by the above-mentioned studies. The fluctuation between one type of behavior and the other is further clearly spelled out from clinical evidence accumulated by Dr Pierre Daco, as reported below.

"The complex game of Timidity – *It is an infinitely complex game. Since the timid is never just a timid. Depending on the circumstances, he goes through all the phases involved in timidity. He will be shy now, then a perfectionist, and an aggressive tomorrow. We know that the wounds of timidity are: impotence, impossibility to "want", impossibility to adapt right away to a particular circumstance. In summary:*

- *Timidity and hyper-emotiveness are always linked to one another.*
- *With the timid there is always either an inner retreat or a violent projection outside of himself.*
- *He is always ruminating his failures.*
- *The timid's ambition (who is oftentimes quite clever) is always countervened by his timidity, from which pride ensues.*
- *Timidity always liberates protection reflexes (presumption, briskness and bluntness)*

(p.86) – Les Prodigieuses Victoires de la Psychologie, Pierre Daco, Les Nouvelles Editions Marabout, 1977."

INTERMITTENT EXPLOSIVE DISORDER

"Individuals with intermittent explosive disorder sometimes describe intense impulses to be aggressive prior to their aggressive acts. Explosive episodes may be associated with affective symptoms, such as irritability or rage, increased energy, racing thoughts during the aggressive impulses and acts, and the rapid onset of a depressed mood and fatigue after the acts. Some individuals may also report that their aggressive episodes are often preceded or accompanied by symptoms such as tingling, tremors, palpitations, chest tightness, head pressure, or hearing an echo." - https://www.psychologytoday.com/us/conditions/intermittent-explosive-disorder

PSEUDOLGIA FANTASTICA

*"In reviewing the case report literature on the subject, we identified a compensatory enhancing of self-esteem in the face of shame as a common qualitative theme among many of the stories. For example, Teaford et al. described a 14-year-old girl with pervasive developmental delay who began making up self-aggrandizing stories of academic success and intelligence when she became aware she was lagging behind her peers academically, while Snyder described a case of an 18-year-old man who told stories about being a well-connected drug dealer in response to feelings of inadequacy when compared to his brothers. From a psychodynamic perspective, pseudologic tales may be conceptualized as manifestations of a constellation of primitive defenses against painful affects that may be seen in a range of psychiatric disorders. Not only do pseudologues reject reality, but they also actively create a new reality that allows for wish fulfillment. Dissociation, temporary but drastic modification of one's personal identity to relieve distress, is also a hallmark defense of pseudologia fantastica. The pseudologue moves between conscious deceit and delusion, at times believing his tales while at others able to acknowledge their mendacity, thereby demonstrating a dissociative quality. As summarized by Deutsch, the psychic function of storytelling in pseudologia fantastica is not focused on achieving goal-directed external gain, but rather on the gratification inherently tied to the communication of the story itself. Communicating pseudologic daydreams as if they were reality serves the function of relieving the pseudologue of the obligations of real life.- **Case ReportPseudologia Fantastica in the Emergency Department:A Case Report and Review of the Literature,** HindawiCase Reports in PsychiatryVolume 2017, Article ID 8961256, 5 pages-ttps://www.ncbi.nlm.nih.gov/pmc/articles/PMC5442346/#B16*

*"**Personality Disorders** - Pathological lying is a possible symptom of certain personality disorders, including:*

- *Borderline personality disorder (BPD)*
- *Narcissistic personality disorder (NPD)*
- *Antisocial personality disorder (APD)*

*BPD is a condition that makes it difficult for a person to regulate their emotions. **People with BPD may experience severe mood swings, feel greater instability and insecurity,** and not have a stable sense of self.*

The hallmarks of NPD are fantasies of immense importance and the need for admiration and special treatment.

Researchers argue that while pathological lying may, in theory, occur in people with APD, those with this condition often lie for personal gain or pleasure.

A person with BPD or NPD may lie to distort reality into something that fits with the emotions that they are feeling, rather than the facts.

These personality disorders can lead to significant challenges with interpersonal relationships."

https://www.medicalnewstoday.com/articles/325982#causes

Fetishism
https://link.springer.com/chapter/10.1057%2F9780230601208_2

Stuttering
https://www.karger.com/Article/PDF/452215

Approval Compulsion
https://whywesuffer.com/the-futility-of-compulsive-approval-seeking/

COTARD'S SYNDROME

Le délire des negations – Psychopathologie du syndrome de Cotard – De la mélancolie anxieuse à la folie systématisée - dans la collection Le Discours psychanalytique

Editions de l'Association Freudienne Internationale , Le Discours psychanalytique, 1993. 1ere édition, 1993 Book ConditionAvant-propos et introduction - 1. Sémiologie, évolution, étiopathogénie : Séméiologie d'un délire hypocondriaque qui n'est ni exclusif, ni prodromique de la paralysie générale - Evolution d'un délire mélancolique qui n'est pas le délire de persécution - Etiopathogénie, de l'origine psycho-sensorielle à l'origine psycho-motrice du délire - D'un délire d'infinitude qui n'est pas non plus le délire de grandeur, le délire d'énormité - 2. Du délire des négations au syndrome de Cotard, le Congrès de Blois : L'historique du délire - Le débat et la place nosologique - 3. Approfondissement clinique, enjeu théorique : Approfondissement clinique - L'enjeu théorique, de la mélancolie à la paranoia, à propos des Leçons cliniques de Jules Seglas - Conclusions, notes et bibliographie.

Le syndrome de Cotard est une maladie rare se présentant sous la forme d'un syndrome délirant décrit en 1880 par le neurologue français Jules Cotard (1840-1889), observé au cours de syndromes dépressifs graves appelés syndromes mélancoliques. Ce syndrome ne figure pas spécifiquement (c'est-à-dire sous cette appellation) comme un trouble particulier dans le DSM-5. Cette affection mentale reste cependant inventoriée dans la Classification Internationale des Maladies,

10e révision (CIM-10) dans son chapitre consacré aux « Troubles délirants ». Ce syndrome est classé dans la « liste de codes CIM-9 » en tant que trouble de nature paranoïaque. - Le nom de ce syndrome est lié au Docteur Cotard, médecin, qui donna une description des délires de négation d'organes dans certaines formes d'hypochondrie. Les formes les plus extrêmes de ce délire seront dès lors ainsi baptisées d'après le nom de ce psychiatre français qui fut élève des professeurs Jean-Martin Charcot et Alfred Vulpian à la Salpêtrière à Paris, durant la dernière décennie du Second Empire. - Le malade, après avoir développé des préoccupations hypocondriaques et des troubles cénesthésiques graves, sent ses organes se putréfier et se détruire. Le syndrome associe anxiété intérieure effroyable, hallucinations visuelles, stupeur extrême, auto-accusation, auto-mutilation, voire suicide. Ce syndrome rare est rencontré au cours de certaines dépressions mélancoliques dont il constitue un indice de gravité. Les autres signes de dépression mélancolique sont également présents. Contrairement à ce qui se passe dans l'hypocondrie névrotique, le patient ne consulte pas pour ses problèmes corporels, et ne pense pas pouvoir être guéri (idées d'incurabilité). Ce tableau nécessite des soins urgents en milieu hospitalier car le risque suicidaire est maximal. (source : Wikipedia)"

STUTTERING

The Stuttering Foundation – *"After Willis came onto the radar screen in 1985 with his role as David Addison in the hot TV show Moonlighting, the actor would occasionally discuss his past struggles with stuttering in both print and television interviews.*

In the 1997 book, Bruce Willis: The Unauthorized Biography, by British author John Parker, Willis is quoted as saying, "I could hardly talk. It took me three minutes to complete a sentence. It was crushing for anyone who wanted to express themselves, who wanted to be heard and couldn't. It was frightening. Yet, when I became another character, in a play, I lost the stutter. It was phenomenal."

APPROVAL COMPULSIVE DISORDER

Approbativeness – *"It is a mental fit; the subject immediately approves his/her interlocutor's words, with mimics and stereotypical words. At times, he/she echoes the other person's words and copies that person's mimics.*

... the subject approves out of fear of contradicting or displeasing... Some cases of approbativeness show a lack of judgement and critical thinking. Found in mental retardation, manias, etc." ***– Les Prodigieuses Victoires de la Psychologie, Pierre Daco, Les Nouvelles Editions Marabout, 1977 (p. 456).***

NEGLECT SYNDROME

"In addition to these pen-and-paper tasks testing for neglect in peripersonal space, there are several tests that tap into the different types of neglect behaviour. For example, personal neglect can

be assessed through ecological tests where patients are asked to mime combing their hair or other grooming activities. Asking people to name items in the room around them tests for neglect in far extrapersonal space: patients with neglect often ignore objects on the left side. Patients can even be examined for representational neglect by asking them about landmarks in a familiar place (eg, the main square in their home town) and noting whether they omit items on the left side of a remembered scene or mental image.

Interestingly, an individual patient's degree of neglect can fluctuate strikingly,even within the same day. This depends upon factors such as overall arousal, which is known to be affected by right hemisphere stroke. In addition, although many people show neglect on more than one type of task, some groups of patients show dissociations, demonstrating a lateralised bias on only one test and normal performance on others; even these characteristics may vary over time. A battery of tests is therefore more sensitive to the presence of neglect than is one single task. This variability probably reflects the underlying heterogeneity of each individual's cognitive deficits. Although the core deficit in neglect clearly involves a spatial bias towards ipsilesional space and away from contralesional space, most patients also have several other deficits, some of which are not spatially lateralised but may still contribute to the clinical severity of the syndrome. This, in turn, reflects the underlying neuroanatomy, as discussed below."-- ***Spatial Neglect – Korina Li, Paresh A Malhotra -- Centre for RestorativeNeuroscience, Division of BrainSciences, Imperial College London, London, UK2 Department of Neurology, University Hospital Coventry, Coventry, West Midlands, UK***

INFERIORITY COMPLEX

"They experience the need to teach others, to direct and lead, they feel the need to counsel others...

They do not conceive of being "equal" to anyone. They either feel inferior or they believe they are superior. When a "compensating" neurotic patient feels inferior, he/she will do anything to astonish, to be admired for his knowledge, his intelligence, his elevated thoughts, his regards and courtesy towards others, his human warmth, etc... They are obviously thirsty of prestige." – ***Les Prodigieuses Victoires de la Psychologie, Pierre Daco, Les Nouvelles Editions Marabout, 1977 (p. 207).***

GRIEF REACTION

https://www.cancer.org/content/dam/CRC/PDF/Public/6036.00.pdf

COMPULSIVE GAMBLING

"Compulsive Gambling and Substance abuse have a number of similar characteristics that mimic each other; however, like other illnesses, there are distinct differences as well. The lists below will attempt to show both similar and differences, listed first are the similarities to Substance Abuse.

- *Inability to stop*

- *Denial*
- ***Severe depression and mood swings***
- *Progressive disease with phases and stages*
- *Chasing the first win/high*
- *First drink remembered, first win remembered*
- *Blackouts from drinking/using, Brownouts from gambling*
- *Activity used to escape from pain*
- *Preoccupation*
- *Low self-esteem and high ego*
- *Dysfunctional families*
- *High of gambling similar to rush or high of cocaine*
- *Use of rituals"*

Compulsive Gambling: An examination of compulsive gambling, including pathology, chemistry exchange, similarities to and differences from substance abuse, gambling phases, and assessment questionnaires. – Journal of Addictive Disorders, 2004, Breining Institute, Retrieved from http://www.breining.edu.

SCHIZOPHRENIA

"The schizophrenic patient withdraws onto himself in an absolute manner (autism). His mind is completely severed from reality. A fragmentation of psychic associations take place in the disorder... in the mind of the schizophrenic, a hallucinating world, comparable to the a "desocialized" dream is unfolding." – ***Les Prodigieuses Victoires de la Psychologie, Pierre Daco, Les Nouvelles Editions Marabout, 1977 (p. 274).***

SEXUAL SADISM DISORDER

"No clear lines divide sexual sadism and sexual masochism, and the predispositions are often interchangeable. The conditions may coexist in the same individual... This relationship is supported by the finding that those who entertain masochistic fantasies also engage in sadistic fantasies." *https://www.psychologistanywhereanytime.com/sexual_problems_pyschologist/psychologist_sadomasochism.htm*

FETISHISM

"The fetishist experiences the need to contemplate or imagine the object or body part in order to obtain an erection or sexual satisfaction... The fetishist tends to collect either the fetish objects of his interest or the images thereof.—p. 401

Mr. X was 50 years old, single, filled with shame, having a large collection of women shoes, having never had sexual intercourse with a woman, came to see me...-- p. 389 - ***Les Prodigieuses Victoires de la Psychologie, Pierre Daco, Les Nouvelles Editions Marabout, 1977***

GENDER IDENTITY DISORDER

Origin of the term

“Magnus Hirschfeld coined the word transvestite in 1910 (from Latin trans-, "across, over" and vestitus, "dressed") to refer to the sexual interest in cross-dressing.[9] He used it to describe persons who habitually and voluntarily wore clothes of the opposite sex. Hirschfeld's group of transvestites consisted of both males and females, with heterosexual, homosexual, bisexual, and asexual orientations.[10]

Hirschfeld himself was not happy with the term: He believed that clothing was only an outward symbol chosen on the basis of various internal psychological situations.[9] In fact, Hirschfeld helped people to achieve the very first name changes (legal given names were and are required to be gender-specific in Germany) and performed the first reported sexual reassignment surgery. Hirschfeld's transvestites therefore were, in today's terms, not only transvestites but a variety of people from the transgender spectrum.

Hirschfeld also noticed that sexual arousal was often associated with transvestism. In more recent terminology, this is sometimes called transvestic fetishism.[11] Hirschfeld also clearly distinguished between transvestism as an expression of a person's "contra-sexual" (transgender) feelings and fetishistic behavior, even if the latter involved wearing clothes of the other sex.

Cross-dressers

One of the fiercest activists to come out of the Stonewall Riots was Sylvia Rivera, who set up Street Transvestite Action Revolutionaries. In a 1971 essay, "Transvestites: Your Half Sisters and Half Brothers of the Revolution", Rivera wrote, "Transvestites are homosexual men and women who dress in clothes of the opposite sex."[12]

After all the changes that took place during the 1970’s,a large group was left without a word to describe themselves: heterosexual males who wear traditionally feminine clothing. This group was not particularly happy with the term "transvestism", and therefore took on the term "cross-dresser".[13] Cross-dressers are men who wear female clothing and often both admire and imitate women, but self-identify as different from both gay men and transsexuals, and generally deny having fetishistic intentions.”

“When cross-dressing occurs for erotic purposes over a period of at least six months and also causes significant distress or impairment, the behavior is considered a mental disorder in the Diagnos-

tic and Statistical Manual of Mental Disorders, and the psychiatric diagnosis "transvestic fetishism" is applied."" **Wikipedia - https://en.wikipedia.org/wiki/Transvestism**

TRANSVESTIC DISORDER

"A 17-year-old Indian male presented to the psychiatry outpatient department with the complaint of having recurrent desires to wear the clothes of his mother. The thought was very distressing to the patient and came to his mind again and again until he wore those clothes and masturbated in it. For this purpose, he stole a complete set of his mother's clothes. He has been wearing the clothes secretly for the past 2 years solely for the purpose of pleasure. Recently he was caught by the parents while wearing the clothes and masturbating and then beaten by the parents. On further enquiry he admitted that the thought is obsessive in nature, he tries to control it but is not able to do so. He added that he experiences restlessness until he wears the clothes and masturbates in order to overcome the anxiety. The thought caused significant impairment in his studies and other social functioning. He did not have any desire to be treated as female nor did he have any preoccupations regarding hormonal or surgical treatment for sex change therapy. There was a past history of ***homo-sexual activity*** *but upon presentation he denied having any sexual relationship. His general physical and neurological examinations were within normal limits. On investigations, contrast-enhanced CT scan of the brain and electroencephalograph were also found to be normal."* ***Treatment of Transvestic Fetishism With Fluoxetine: A Case Report-*** *https://www.ncbi.nlm.nih.gov/pmc/articles/PMC3940015/*

VOYEURISM AND FROTTEURISM

"A six-year-old boy was referred to the psychiatrist while accompanied by his mother and grandmother with the complaint of excessively rubbing his genitalia many times a day against his female family members' bodies, primarily their buttocks. Similar behaviors were first noticed by the child's mother at the age of 18 months during breastfeeding. His mother said that during breastfeeding, her baby usually rubbed his genitalia against her body. This behavior worsened at the age of four, when he started rubbing his genitalia many times a day against his grandmother's hand, foot, and back; the grandmother reported this behavior to the mother.

...His mother reported that her son exhibited voyeurism by experiencing sexual arousal while watching pornographic TV channels. However, because the patient is not currently attending school and is not a member of any social group, his sexual behavior in crowds cannot be evaluated. ***Atypical Frotteurism Associated with Voyeurism and Obsession in a Six-Year-Old Boy - https://sites.kowsarpub.com/thrita/articles/18258.html***

COURTSHIP DISORDERS: VOYEURISM, EXHIBITIONISM, & FROTTEURISM

In clinical settings which specialize in the treatment of Paraphilias, people with these disorders have an average of from three to four different Paraphilias – ***Mapping the Boundaries of Courtship Disorders.- The Journal of Sex Research – Freund Kurt, Robin Watson.***

Voyeurism, exhibitionism, and frotteurism may be different behavioral expressions of a single underlying courtship disorder. The overt behaviors differ, but can also be conceptualized as different stages on a continuum – different degrees of proximity to the victim. Voyeurism involves viewing the victim from a distance, exhibitionism involves approaching the victim, and frotteurism involves physically touching the victim. The preference for rape over consensual sexual activity (termed the preferential rape pattern) may represent the fourth phase in the courtship disorders (Freund et al., 1983). ***A common etiological factor has not been identified although evidence indicates that the courtship disorders are associated with a preference for eliciting an alarmed reaction from an unfamiliar target rather than any lack of interest in intercourse (Freund & Watson, 1990). A high degree of comorbidity exists between these disorders and even when no overt comorbid behavior is present, some evidence suggests that presence of one disorder predisposes to another such disorder (Freund et al., 1983).***

... Frotteurism involves "intense sexually arousing fantasies, sexual urges, or behaviors involving touching and rubbing against a nonconsenting person" (American Psychiatric Association, 1994). The majority of published articles on this disorder group frotteurism with other paraphilic disorders or report cases of men with multiple paraphilias, including frotteurism. ***Abel et al. (1987) examined 62 males diagnosed with frotteurism, as well as other paraphilic disorders, and found that, at the time of the interview, they had committed an average of 849 frottage acts. Rooth (1973) interviewed 561 nonincarcerated men with paraphilias and found that of those exhibiting frotteurism, 79% had other paraphilias, with an average of 4.8 paraphilias each.***

DELAYED EJACULATION

Men diagnosed with DE experience difficulties in ejaculating and reaching an adequate orgasm, both of which may occur during self-masturbation or manual, oral, vaginal, or anal stimulation by the partner. Problems with "difficulty" in ejaculating may range from varying delays in the latency-to-ejaculation interval to complete inability to ejaculate (anejaculation). Reductions in the volume, force, and sensation of ejaculation may occur as well. Although DE is commonly encountered, it can be confused with anejaculation (measured in time) and retrograde ejaculation (direction) by physicians and patients alike. Typically, the man has little or no difficulty achieving and maintaining an erection, but finds it extremely difficult, or impossible, to reach ejaculation and orgasm despite "adequate" sexual stimulation. The difficulty may occur in all situations (generalized) or be limited to only certain situations (situational). It may be primary (lifelong) or secondary (acquired). The most common clinical pattern of DE is a man who is unable to ejaculate in the presence of a partner (especially during intercourse) while he has little difficulty reaching orgasm and ejaculation during solo masturbation (5).

Perelman and Rowland identified three factors that disproportionately characterized patients with DE: (I) high frequency masturbation (age-dependent, with a mean of greater than 3×/week); (II) idiosyncratic masturbatory style; (III) disparity between the reality of sex with a partner and preferred sexual fantasy during masturbation. They defined an idiosyncratic masturbatory style as a technique not easily duplicated by the partner's hand, mouth, vagina, or anus. Furthermore, those authors noted that many men with DE engaged in a pattern of self-stimulation that was notable for its speed, pressure, intensity, duration, and specificity of focus on a particular "spot" of sensitivity in order to produce orgasm/ejaculation. In this way, they preconditioned themselves to possible difficulty in attaining orgasm with a partner and, as a result, experienced "acquired" DE (3).

There are many psychological and relational factors that have been traditionally implicated as predisposing and/or confounding factors in the etiology of DE, such as fear and/or ambivalence regarding pregnancy and fertility issues, hostility and anger, fear of loss of control, fears of abandonment/rejection, fears of intimacy and loss of autonomy, paraphilic inclinations/interests, and fears of hurting/defiling the partner (6). Although some of these factors may contribute to the etiologies of individual men with DE, no well controlled studies have provided comprehensive support for any of the various hypotheses.

However, Jern et al. and Bancroft et al. demonstrated that men with homosexual orientations had a significantly higher frequency of DE than heterosexual men (23,24). ***The Pathophysiology of Delayed Ejaculation – Translational Andrology and Urology doi: 10.21037/tau.2016.05.03, Juza Chen***

SADISTIC (ANTISOCIAL) PERSONALITY DISORDER

"Pyromaniacs. *Pyromaniacs are pathological firesetters. They seem to have no practical reasons for setting the fires and receive no material profit from them. Their only motive seems to be some sort of sensual satisfaction, and the classic "irresistible impulse" is often a factor. The behavior of pyromaniacs was best described during the early 1950s by Lewis and Yarnell in their well-known study* ***Pathological Firesetting****:*

The reasons for the fires are unknown; the act is so little their own that they feel no responsibility for the crime. . . . These offenders are able to give a classical description of the irresistible impulse. They describe the mounting tension; the restlessness; the urge for motion; the conversion symptoms such as headaches, palpitations, ringing in the ears, and the gradual merging of their identity into a state of unreality; then the fires are set. . . . Once they have started the fires, thrown the neighborhood into confusion, and are assured the fire engines are working, the tension subsides, and they can go home and drop into a peaceful sleep. The majority of pyromaniacs, incidentally, start fires in their own neighborhood. With some the impulse asserts itself episodically with extended periods of "normality" intervening; with others, it controls them night after night; in either instance they almost always have to set a fire when the impulse appears. Such offenders will continue, each fire being a facsimile of the first, until a more powerful force, usually embodied in the "arm of the law," steps in and commands them to stop. (p. 87)

These are the mysterious "firebugs" who terrorize neighborhoods by going on solitary fire-setting sprees, often nocturnal, during which they touch off trash fires in one building after another without regard to property or life. Many suffer from low-level mental deficiencies, are persons who derive sexual satisfaction from watching fires, or are chronic alcoholics, and they encompass the full range of ages.

Many pyromaniacs bring arrest upon themselves by making certain that the identity of the firebug will be easily found, by being conspicuously present watching all of the fires, by repeatedly contacting police or fire officials as to the whereabouts of fires or with information about the "identity" of local arsonists, or by going directly to the police and asking to be protected from their own "criminal desires." Once they are arrested the irresistible impulse ceases, and for some it never returns. The sprees of pyromaniacs last from a few days to a few months or even years, but discovery and arrest tend to put an end to each particular episode."

https://law.jrank.org/pages/529/Arson-Behavioral-Economic-Aspects-Offender-types.html

https://www.ncbi.nlm.nih.gov/pmc/articles/PMC4649950/pdf/nihms-704544.pdf

https://www.ncbi.nlm.nih.gov/books/NBK546673/

POST TRAUMATIC STRESS DISORDER

The following excerpt is meant to exemplify the serious comorbidity problem in Psychiatry. It reveals the exegetic death that the notion of comorbidity has brought to Pschiatric science when it comes to unequivocal diagnosis, let alone effective diagnosis that can lead to successful therapy.

"Epidemiologic samples have demonstrated that over 90% of people with PTSD have at least 1 lifetime comorbid mental disorder. Some of the most prevalent comorbid conditions with PTSD are major depressive disorder, alcohol abuse and (or) dependence, and another anxiety disorder. Self-medication of PTSD symptoms with alcohol and illicit drugs has been demonstrated to be associated with comorbid alcohol or drug use disorders. Among Axis II disorders, there has been increasing evidence that PTSD is associated with borderline personality disorder and antisocial personality disorder. It is possible that personality styles associated with impulsivity may put the person at risk of exposure to traumatic situations.

Suicidal behaviour and comorbid mental and physical disorders are associated with PTSD and traumatic events. It remains unknown whether it is the trauma or the PTSD symptoms that drive the associations with suicidal behaviour. For example, Wilcox et al demonstrated that suicidal behaviour was associated with PTSD, but not with exposure to traumatic events. However, other studies have demonstrated that childhood adversities and traumatic events are associated with suicidal behaviour. Similar issues have been considered in understanding the comorbidity of PTSD with substance use and physical illness. It seems that both stressful life events and PTSD are independently associated with comorbidity and with suicidal behaviour.

...

As PTSD is highly comorbid with other mental disorders, aside from trauma exposure, what differentiates PTSD from other disorders is the re-experiencing symptoms (for example, nightmares and flashbacks). Many of the other symptoms of PTSD, such as hyperarousal, avoidance, and numbing, overlap with other mental disorders, such as generalized anxiety disorder, panic disorder, and depression. Thus it is important to delineate whether the person is re-experiencing symptoms in relation to a traumatic event." - ***Posttraumatic Stress Disorder in Adults: Impact, Comorbidity,***

Risk Factors, and Treatment - www.LaRCP.ca460 W La Revue canadienne de psychiatrie, vol 59, no 9, septembre 2014 CanJPsychiatry 2014;59(9):460–467 - *Jitender Sareen, MD, FRCPC11 Professor of Psychiatry, Psychology, and Community Health Sciences, University of Manitoba, Winnipeg, Manitoba.*

SLEEP PARALYSIS DISORDER

The following excerpt is from a website writing of a clinician who has observed the many hallucinations elicited in Sleep Paralysis. Although the author has not underscored the sense of doom and dread evidenced in these symptoms as pertaining to Paranoia, it is clear that they are projecttions of a paranoid nature.

[HALLUCINATIONS IN SLEEP PARALYSIS]

"Vivid hallucinations may be part of this experience. In other words, you perceive an experience of something that is not there. It is like you are dreaming while awake. In a broad sense, the hallucinations associated with sleep paralysis can be divided into four categories: visual, auditory, olfactory, and tactile experiences.

Visual Hallucinations

The visual experience can be quite profound. Many people report seeing the presence of a human figure, often described as being a dark figure, shadow, or ghost. This figure may be standing at the bedside, just at the periphery of your vision. Some people report seeing multiple people in the room.

Others report that they see flashes, bright colors, or lights. Sometimes the visual hallucination can be quite elaborate. For example, some have reported seeing a disembodied hand, a gargoyle, bugs, or even a cat.

In other cases, the visions are vague, described as being blurry or shimmering or simply having a sense that things in the room are floating.

Auditory Hallucinations

Similarly, the experience of auditory hallucinations in sleep paralysis can range from the routine to the bizarre. Many people hear various noises. It is most common for people to hear voices. The language used might seem foreign. There may be the perception of whispering, screaming, and laughing.

Nearly as often, a loud buzzing or static noise is reported, much like the sound of a radio that is on but not tuned to a station. Some people hear breathing, footsteps, knocking, or a ringing sound.

Even unusual sounds like a horse carriage or growling may be perceived. Sometimes the sounds heard during sleep paralysis are nonspecific, difficult to characterize, or not well remembered.

Tactile Hallucinations

One of the most often reported phenomena of sleep paralysis is a tactile hallucination, the experience of being touched when you are not. Many people describe feeling a pressure or contact, often sensed as if something (or someone) is holding them down.

Some people with sleep paralysis describe tingling, numbness, or a vibrating sensation. Others describe a sense of floating, flying, or falling. A few people report feeling chilled or freezing.

Less frequently, there may even be a sense that you are being physically moved or dragged from your bed. Some people report sexual contact, including physical sensations involving the genitalia or even rape.

Other physical experiences have been reported as well, including a sense of being bitten, bugs crawling on the skin, breathing in the ear, or an uncontrolled feeling of smiling.

Olfactory Hallucinations

The least common hallucination in sleep paralysis is of an olfactory nature, relating to your sense of smell. As with the other types of hallucinations, you could imagine a range of possible imagined smells that you might experience." **What the Scary Symptoms and Hallucinations of Sleep Paralysis?** – Very Well Health, May 2020 - Brandon Peters, MD - *https://www.verywellhealth.com/symptoms-of-sleep-paralysis-3014781#:~:text=Some%20people%20with%20sleep%20paralysis%20describe%20tingling,%20numbness,,being%20physically%20moved%20or%20dragged%20from%20your%20bed.*

Chapter 6

PSYCHOMETRICS OF THE NORMAL AND ABNORMAL MENTAL FOLIATE

Our ambition throughout this study has been to provide an extensive and rigorous framework to evaluate the Human Mental in its totality, however the nature of the normal or abnormal conditions it presents. It is well known that about one half of all clinical psychological patients do not receive a clear diagnosis because their impairments do not fit the generic or neatly predefined criteria and categories in Psychiatry and Psychology of the day. In cases where the predefined criteria and categories seem to fit, undesirable misdiagnoses frequently occur. Further, a significant percentage of cases of CPP's[38] addressed by clinicians do not qualify as legitimate 'mental disorders' because they may be, per the current classifications, 'sub-threshold', or 'sub-clinical', or situation-specific (i.e. evidenced only in an occupational settings). In the Characterological area, practice is even merkier since there is no clear consensus on defined types, let alone demonstrable validity of types. To the aims of putting a final cure to these drawbacks, the many different metric elements of diagnosis that we have described in previous chapters we will now turn into broader and more stringent measurement methologies. Along that line, some may have found the Mental Foliate map, in both Layer and Thread categorizations, directly redolent of the Psychometric tests that currently exist in Psychotherapy. Effectively, the metric elements of measurement are innately built-in within our psychophysics frame-

[38] CPP in clinical psychology stands for Clinical Psychological Problem.

work. We shall therefore shortly present the Psychometric system naturally deriving from our psychophysics vision of the Human Mental as a differential geometry Foliate, which we hope will at the same time firmly contribute to significant amelioration in clinical diagnosis.

6.1 Language-Based Psychometrics

One of the questions often debated in cognitive science and philosophy concerns the preeminence of language over thought or vice versa, often with no conclusive outcome. Our layered psychophysics representation of the Mental seems to make the case for root partitions as pure pensive primitives devoid of linguistic potentiality, with language intervention principally at the representational level within surface sublayers. Be that as it may, in the human context of the living, language plays a seminal phenomenological role in the expression of the mentation experience. We next offer an analytic study of linguistic structures from the QG psychophysics standpoint and subsequently present language-based psychometric canvases as principal methods of measurement and gauging of mental activity.

6.2 Formed Words and their Association

Words are generally treated in linguistics and sciences of the mental as phenomenological entities with teleology primarily relating to orthography and syntax. The evocative association of words has been studied by J. Mem Lang and others through what this author called *index of semantic relatedness* of words. In his attempt to tie words structurally to psychology, he devised this index to measure "associative strength" at the basis of the lexicon developed by the Human mental. Effectively, J. Mem Lang writes:

"The index of semantic relatedness is associative strength and it has been shown repeatedly to be predictive of lexical processing and retrieval in adults (e.g., Nelson, Schreiber, & McEvoy, 1992; Steyvers, Shiffrin, & Nelson, 2005) and more recently, to also be predictive of the order of acquisition of nouns by young children (Hills et al., 2009a). Associative strength is itself an index derived from stu-

dies in which researchers provide word cues (e.g., dog) and participants give back the first word that comes to mind (e.g., cat). Associative strength is thus a property of large data sets of answers given back by the individual participants in an odd laboratory task. Presumably these association norms reflect in some aggregate way important regularities in language, language use, and the world (Deese, 1965). It would seem that they must in that adult association norms are strongly predictive of adult performance in many different kinds of language processing tasks (e.g., Nelson, Schreiber, & McEvoy, 1992). Still, adult association norms are best considered a statistical portmanteau—holistically useful but without a well-articulated link to the psychological mechanisms or the substructure of the language they carry. They may for example represent semantic relationships—the shared semantic context of "soap" and "bath"—and they may just as easily reflect compound words, where semantic relationships are less precise—like "bird" and "bath." This makes the fact that adult association norms also predict the order of acquisition of words by toddlers intriguing and potentially revealing."

The observation by J. Deese (1965) that presumably these association norms reflect in some aggregate way important regularities in language, language use, and the world represents an important insight in suggesting that language may be regulated by the same norms that regulate the natural world. We are going to further develop and solidly ground this prelude within our psychophysics framework to the aims of laying down the targeted psychometric methods.

6.3 Inner Teleology in Pronouns

The most towering linguistic entity concerning formed words in universal human language is the set of pronouns upon which fluent speech is built. In and of themselves, they stand for a class of words, arguably the primitives of locution. We grant them that elevation because speech or locution starts with a living entity that has assumed the Self, the qualities of the Self as well as the acknowledgement of kindred. Even if we should assume phenomenal qualities to words, as otherwise surmised in magic or myths of the ages, they must be primordially recognized as a faculty of Self. Therefore, the notions of self, same and other become primitives that transpire in the order of speech pronouns, a quality that the latter well preserves in structured language. In a human sense, indeed they are teleologically the first of all words since their semantics are innately tied to the actor of the action.

Common pronouns in the French language:

JE – TU – IL/ELLE – NOUS – VOUS – ILS/ELLES

In the English language:

I – YOU – HE/SHE/IT – WE – YOU – THEY

In the Spanish language:

YO – TU – EL/ELLA/ELLO/USTED – NOSOTROS – VOSOTROS/USTEDES – EL-LOS/ELLAS

In the Romanian language (a Romance language):

EU - TU - EL/EA - NOI - VOI – EI/ELE

As we can see, some languages advance more pronoun elements than others. The Romance languages, such as Spanish, French and Romanian, generally present a much richer set of pronouns than the Anglo-Saxon languages such as English and German.

PLURAL	SINGULAR
WE	I
YOU	YOU
THEY	HE-SHE-IT

Fig. 6.1 Binary order of pronouns in human languages

In particular, the second person pronoun (You) is rank- or seniority-sensitive and presents one version for informality (French: Tu) and another for formality (French: Vous). There is no unique plural form for He and She, in English, which are all rendered with They, unlike the Romance languages which present a plural form for each, i.e. in Spanish Ellos and Ellas. Almost universally, He and It share the same plural pronoun (English: They). The 3rd person in the Romance languages holds an alternative form, now in quasi obsolescence, to convey reverence, i.e. in French *Sa Majesté, Son Excellence*. This form is adulterated in English with *Your Majesty* (not His Majesty). It is meant to accord highest honor by amplifying the distance between oneself and the other person, Royalty or Presidency in this case. For people other than Royalty or representative of the highest echelon of power, in the Spanish language the form *Su Merced* is used in that case. It must be noted, however, that in Spanish as much as in English the 3rd person pronoun Ello (Spanish) or It (English) has no match in the French language. It is, in French, a neutral that blends with the pronoun for masculine: il.

From these particulars emerges a universal binary order of pronouns as depicted in Fig. 6.1, which we will further study in greater depth.

6.4 Structural Teleology of a Sentence

In most languages, the sentence appears to be the most irreducible element of speech that is semantically complete in itself. One does not expect anything else to be added to speech after the dictation of a sentence, except when context otherwise determines.

English grammar has it that: A sentence expresses a complete thought and consists of a subject and a predicate. It is interesting that linguists define a sentence to be an expression of a complete thought. In the light of all that we have studied about thoughts thus far, specifically the many different categories of abstractions that the Mind elicits, it is unclear what a thought would specifically mean in linguistics, let alone the boundaries that would define its completeness as claimed. Nevertheless, the statement makes it clear that verbal human language is a translation of and means to be the expression of thoughts or mental activity. Let us consider the following simple sentence:

The holiday sales | were nearly over. In this example "The holiday sales" is the subject and "were nearly over" is the predicate.

English grammar rules further pose that: The subject of a sentence is the person, object or idea being described. The predicate is an explanation of the action, condition or effect of the subject.

Subjects are nouns, pronouns or phrases used as nouns. Predicates are verbs and the words used to express the action or condition.

Hence, the predicate includes two critical components: a word category denoted a verb and a group of words that express the condition, attributes, effect or action either qualifying or undertaken by the subject. Hence, breaking down the sentence:

The holiday sales | were | nearly over.

As French grammatical analysis rightly has it, the part of the predicate that is not the verb qualifies as a complement. The complement qualifies the subject. In the English language it may be understood as the complementary part of the predicate, which altogether qualifies the subject. Linguists of the Spanish language have also distinguished a predicate portion (predicado) in the structure of a sentence. They acknowledged however that the verb constitutes the nucleus of the predicate, giving it thereby a stature of its own.

Therefore, a sentence consists of three separate generic components: Subject, Verb and Complement.

COMPOSITE	SIMPLE
PHRASE	SUBJECT
VERB	VERB
CLAUSE	COMPLEMENT

Fig. 6.2 Triplet structure of a sentence

In Fig. 6.2, we show the two different forms of the triplet structure in a sentence in universal analysis. Further down, we will analyze the composite form.

A phrase is a group of words that are closely related but have no subject or predicate. It is a mere juxtaposition of words.

Example: nearly over

It plays the role of a complement in the above sentence. A phrase in a sentence can either be a complement, a subject or even a verb.

The Christmas holiday is around the corner. In this case, both "The Christmas holiday "and "around the corner" are phrases.

The Christmas season could not have been more joyful this year. The group of words "could not have been" is a phrase in the role of a verb.

When the phrase class takes a complex expression, it becomes a clause. A clause, unlike the phrase, is a semi-independent group of words within the sentence which does have a subject and a predicate. A main clause makes for a sentence within a sentence; it might even stand alone as a primary 3-component sentence. Such sentences with clauses are, per our own qualification, complex or composite. An example of a complex sentence with a subject in the form of a clause is stated below:

These are the big Christmas season discounts that financial analysts have well predicted earlier in the year.

"These are the big Christmas season discounts" is a clause, specifically a main clause in regards to the rest of the sentence, per English grammar rule. The rule adds that a subordinate clause is incomplete and used with a main clause to express a related idea. An example of a subordinate clause in a complex sentence follows:

If the discounts are big enough, I will take advantage of the Christmas sales this year.

6.5 Anti-Symmetry Undergirding Pronouns

The entire linguistic developments beyond the two basic grammatical structures of pronouns and sentences concern their QG Quintessential Triplet instances. As a reminder, QG Quintessence consists of a hyper quantum operator or tier, a hyper space operator or tier and a hyper quadratic operator or tier. We have seen how the multiplicity of pronouns develops within each of their subclasses along the Triplet main vectors.

It is a transverse development over abstract transversal Layers. It is noteworthy that, in virtually none of the prominent Western languages, the 1st pronoun identifying the Self holds gender distinction. Both men and women say Yo, I, Je, etc. when referring to themselves individually. That artifact invalidates a construction for pronouns according each gender a longitudinal course, if ever considered, and validates longitudes or threads based on plural and singular forms instead. Such a construction would be very deficient for the Anglo-Saxon languages in particular, the 3rd person singular being the only conjugation person showing gender differentiation therein.

6.6 Longitudinal Undercurrents in a Sentence

Each of the three levels staged in a sentence counts with a significant population of distinct elements of their own. Subject can be plain nouns, common nouns and proper nouns, phrases or clauses. Verbs can be transitive, intransitive, and with a panoply of accessible tenses and different voices. Complementary elements of the sentence may be adjectives, adverbs, clauses, phrases, and in some languages so-called attributes, etc.

In most languages, the relationship between the three tiers of a sentence is a critical element that warrants cohesion and intelligibility of speech. Rules of many different orders norm this cohesion which is frequently viewed as concordance, harmonization or unity. This form of cohesion may be generalized with the notion of inheritance. Most common sentences in these many languages will exemplify at least partially these tier-to-tier connections and connections inside tiers. Let us thus examine the sentence below of the French language.

Marie et Juliette | s'étaient dédiées | tout entières à l'étude de la faune vivante répandue sur ces îles lointaines où elles avaient fini par établir leur résidence.

In this example for the circumstance, one can see how epithets accord with the nouns they qualify in gender and numeric form (faune vivante – îles lointaines), adjectives must accord with the subject they qualify (Marie et Juliette – entières), verb gender must accord with the subject (Marie et Juliette – dédiées), and the tense of verbs must be conserved throughout the sentence (s'étaient dédiées – avaient fini). In addition, the verb must agree with its subject not only in gender but in number as well. Accordingly, the plural subject "Marie et Juliette" demand the verb in plural form "s'étaient dédiées". Finally, the subject in the subordinate clause "elles" concords not only with the gender of the main subject "Marie et Juliette" as two females but with the plurality of the subject as well.

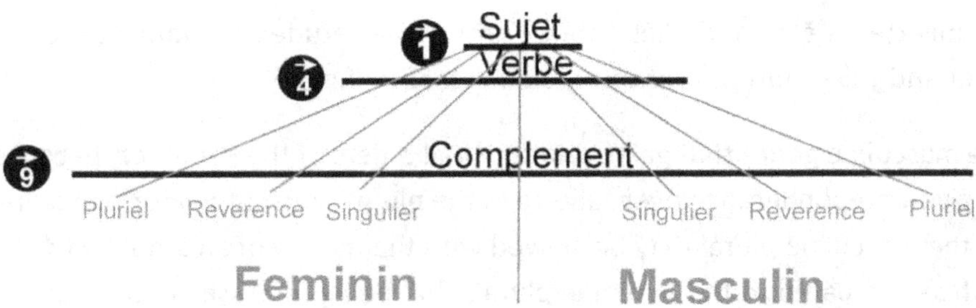

Fig. 6.3 Complete QG canvas of a sentence in universal language based on Quintessence

It is not difficult to see how both the gender in the subject of the sentence and the plurality of the subject propagate through the verb tier and the complement tier as distinct inheritance longitudes or threads throughout the entire sentence (Fig 6.3). Notably, the plurality feature takes the form of individual longitudes exhibiting (1) a simple singular line (for object or person), (2) a deferential singular for high-ranking personae, and (3) the normal plural form. The masculine and feminine gender forms appear instead as two chiral properties splitting the structure of the sentence longitudinally all across. They exist at all levels of the Triplet while all forms of plural, deferential singular and simple singular, can be either feminine or masculine. Those characteristics are given in Western languages that are structurally rich, the likes of Spanish or French.

Furthermore, even though we have aligned two sets of longitudes with the exact same nomenclature, it is of import to understand that there exist higher-level linguistic rules which make the two sets dissimilar from one another. In male-dominated societies, even though different epochs may have seen different rules, when a subject joins a male and a female person (i.e. Paul and Juliette), the plural form they represent preferentially takes after the masculine tenet for a masculine plural. This meta-level rule gives to the plural longitude on the masculine chiral side of the distribution a different tone than that of the plural longitude on the feminine chiral side. Accordingly, the verb inherits the masculine genre, and the complement alike. An example in the French language below:

Paul et Juliette | s'étaient dédiés | tout | entiers | à l'étude de la faune de la région quand | ils | durent presenter leurs thèses de fin d'études.

It is the masculine genre that gains priority at all 3 tiers of the sentence, because Paul is given preponderance over Juliette in the plural subject they form. Accordingly, the masculine plural may be viewed with the quality of an amplified strength as compared to the feminine plural. That being the case, it automatically means that the masculine singular longitude itself bears the same amplified strength over its feminine counterpart at the other chiral side of the distribution as well. The reader can understand the difficulty we face in finding the correct nomenclature for these nuances of language about language itself at the level of its very towering primitives! They shall forgive the repetition of same nomers at each chiral side, which should formally be dissimilar (their lexicon simply does not exist in current linguistics). Therefore, at the very least, we could add a positive sign to the thread nomers for the masculine genre to mean their amplified strength, and a negative sign to the thread nomers for the feminine genre to mean attenuation in the absolute or with respect to their counterparts. The ensuing representation is shown in Fig. 6.4.

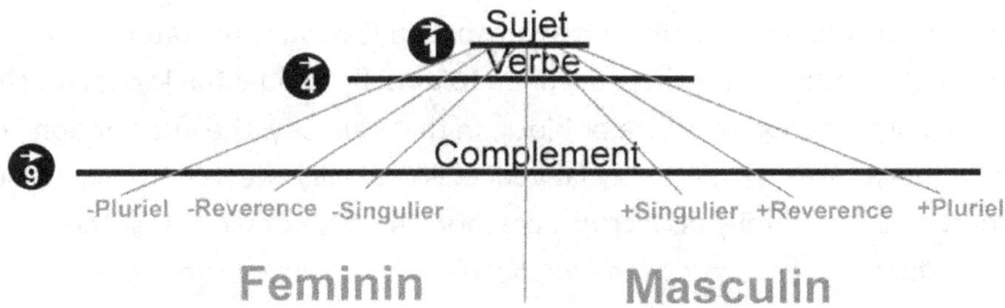

Fig. 6.4 The nature of longitudinal threads in the QG distribution subtending the structure of a sentence in universal language

It would be quite interesting to discuss for instance the plural genre of the subject "Julie et son chien" by stipulation of the French Language Academy[39]. Long time controversies of a different order indeed persist to this day regarding the rules for genre determination in the French language. Interesting though it might be, we will not however address this topic in our study.

6.6.1 Structures of Artificial Information Languages

Artificial Information Languages are devised to:

- Define artificial objects in modeling hardware systems and abstract computing systems.
- Exercise direct control over input-output logical systems.

As a collection of artificial objects, every information language, also denoted programming language, represents an unspoken lexicon destined to animate a hardware arrangement intended to function as a tool. The tool may be entrusted to produce a form of intelligence (computing gadget) or mediate the production of physical effects in the real world (hardware input-output system). Generally, this type of written authored work is qualified as object-oriented programming and designated a source code algorithm. A full algorithm is the equivalent of a literary book.

---

[39] https://www.leparisien.fr/societe/des-enseignants-refusent-que-le-masculin-l-emporte-sur-le-feminin-08-11-2017-7381113.php

A low level information language is an unspoken lexicon with statements arranged in strict sequential order destined to directly handle the logical mechanisms of a microprocessor device or block. In that capacity, the information language, otherwise called assembly language, is especially devised for a particular microprocessor or family of microprocessors. This type of written authored work exploits the resources of the applicable microprocessor to produce a universe of input-output controls or processes (Fig. 6.5). This sort of authored algorithm is said to be procedural, by contrast with the object-oriented attribute.

```
*dpx-4s.txt - Notepad
File  Edit  Format  View  Help

;Program Start

start               clrf        FSR             ;ensure FSR register bits 5,6 are reset
                                                ;for RAM page 0 to be selected

;implement delay before launching main program
                    pagesel     makeDelay       ;set page bits for out of page jump
                    goto        makeDelay       ;jump

; initialize all ports (inputs with high impedance and outputs with 0)

init_PORTS          movlw       0xFF            ;
                    tris        PORTA           ;set PORTA as an input port
                    movlw       0x0F            ;
                    tris        PORTB           ;set bits 0 to 3 of PORTB as inputs and 4 &
                    bcf         PORTB, 4        ;reset all doorstrike I/O's
                    bcf         PORTB, 5        ;       /
                    bcf         PORTB, 6        ;       /
                    bcf         PORTB, 7        ;       /
                    clrw                                ;set PORTC as an output port
                    tris        PORTC           ;       /
                    movwf       PORTC           ;reset all PORTC I/O's
                    movlw       B'00100000'     ;configure RC5  as an input
                    tris        PORTC           ;       /


;initialize voice page and music buffers

                    movlw       0x01            ;
                    movwf       RAM10           ;store initial value of 01 in music buffer R
                    clrw                        ;reset W
                    movwf       RAM9            ;clear voice page buffer RAM9
                    movwf       RAM14           ;clear distinctive chime buffer

                                    Ln 159, Col 2      100%   Windows (CRLF)   UTF-8
```

Fig. 6.5 Excerpt of a microprocessor program or firmware tasked to control a home automation system. Written in Assembly language (Author: Joseph J. Jean-Claude).

Of note is a third form of information language built to transform object-oriented source code or program to assembly language. The assembly language is the only language that the physical microprocessor system understands in its specificity and all source code programs must be translated into that language for the physical microprocessing block to execute it. This third form of language is denoted a compiling language and the machine which is able to understand and manipulate compiling language a compiler. There also exists a family of programming languages called scripting languages which represent a hybrid or mix between the object-oriented language and the procedural language.

Interestingly, here again we see the unintended sketch of the Triplet principle or Quintessence, to show that nothing humans do, as much as natural physical realizations, can escape the set of principles assembled within the Quanto-Geometric canon.

What we will retain from this exposé is that the advent of object-oriented algorithm had exploded the exploitation of the capabilities ascribed to hardware information systems by making it possible to utilize one device, system or machine, for the implementation of a universe of different tools or system realizations potentially. We believe that this tremendous potentiality, instrumental to the revolution of the information age as it was, is a direct result of the application of natural linguistic attributes in object-oriented information languages as well as a thorough emulation of the attributes of real world objects, even though their ultrastructural primitives had not been understood.

6.6.2 An Inner Look at Objects in Object-Oriented Information Languages

In programming languages of the object-oriented class, there is one universal signature for abstract information objects. Yet again, it is the Triplet structure of Quintessence joined to the transverse symmetry of longitudinal threads, as seen in natural languages. In a word, the signature is:

1. Identity
2. Attributes
3. Functions or Methods
4. Inheritance

The first three elements, Identity, Attributes and Functions (Methods), constitute the Quintessential Triplet while the fourth element, Inheritance, represents symmetric longitudinal threading. In other words, Identity, Attributes and Functions (or Methods) are a representation of the Triplet in QG Quintessence, while Inheritance translates into the set of orthogonal lines linking one level to the next.

An abstract object must belong to a class as a primal descriptor of its identity. The program must make an express enunciation of classes, along with their ascribed attributes and functions as one of its principal characteristics.

An object will have a declared name as its primary identity, but it shall be declared as a member of a particular class. From there, the object acquires its attributes and functions as class-derived properties. In that manner, an information object becomes an instantiation of a class, in object-oriented programming.

Attributes of class are data types or data structures offered by the class. Thus, they automatically become the attribute of member objects of the class.

Functions inherent to a class, also referred to as methods in some cases, represent the dynamic part of the class element and define the behavior or dynamic incline of member objects.

One can see that, in this form of encapsulation of objects through classes, inherit-ance is automatically built in, because all object properties at all three tiers are inherited from the class descriptors. What's more, encapsulation is a nomer very specifically used in object-oriented languages or programming to mean an instance when a behavior is joined to attributes, in a clear realization of what our framework denotes a longitude or thread.

We conclude this review with Larry O'Brien's iconic assessment:

"Programming is mirroring the world inside a computer."

We could add: through language.

6.7 Principle of Locutional Resonance

Our main objective in laying down these psychometric methods is to rate the predominance of a particular Mentation Layer within an individual's Mental Foliate through his/her sensitiveness to linguistic structures. Both the set of linguistic structures that we have identified and the Foliate consist of a universal QG Spectrum of 9 Normal Layers. We make the capital assumption that a direct parallel mapping exists between the two spectra, so that the typified linguistic structure the individual is most sensitive to, or resonates with, corresponds to the Layer of Mind that is predominant.

This assumption is based on the known important artifacts of catharsis and abreaction in Psychoanalytic Theory. They both ultimately consist in triggering psychological discharges, whether of emotional nature or otherwise, from the evocation of linguistic elements, words, phrases or sentences, that is. Naturally, the response expectedly occurs when the evoked word or linguistic element is particularly meaningful to the individual. It is however imperative to recognize that meaningfulness or teleology in our framework is not unspecific but essentially typed. We have shown how the most important analytic categories in Psychoanalytic Theory map to the QG psychophysics categories which broadly encompass them, owing to higher elevation. By virtue of this higher insight we are able to discern psychological meaning in locutional elements, beyond the level of representational teleology familiar to psychoanalists. In catharsis, it is the root sub-stratum of a Layer of Mind that becomes resonant and disburses "energy" under a particular linguistic trigger. Compare to the soldiers marching in step on the bridge (the bridge being the root Stratum), which will resonate and ultimately crumble should the vibrating steps (the steps being the evoked words or phrases) match the natural vibrating wavelength of the bridge.

Note further that the word cathartic has become part of common language ever since it has been coined by S. Freud in developing the psychoanalytic method. It is not rare at all to hear henceforth the common man express something the like "this talk has been cathartic" to qualify an exercise of locution or dialogue he or she found emotionally liberating.

Based on these premises, and for the purpose of these psychometric methods, we coin the following so-called principle of locutional resonance which stipulates that:

If an individual psychologically resonates with a speech mode as categorized in QG psychophysics, it denotes a natural or abnormal mirroring in the corresponding Foliate Layer, chiral side or cursor state in the Mental Body under examination.

We remind the reader that there is a total of 72 pensive partitions, 9 Layers, 9 Mood tones, 2 Animic chiral sides and 3 cursor states possibly subject to evaluation by the analyst.

Speech mode is any of the typified elements of speech above distinctly studied.

Scale:

The measurement scale that we uphold is modeled in quantity and quality after the symmetric set of longitudes or threads inherent to the Mental Manifold.

SCORE	MODE	MODEL
[-4]	Absolutely not	Dramatism
[-3]	Very unlikely	Pessimism
[-2]	Fairly unlikely	Negativity
[-1]	Maybe not	Disapprobation
[0]	Don't Know	Indecisive – Split
[+1]	Probably yes	Assent
[+2]	Fairly likely	Assurance
[+3]	Very likely	Optimism
[+4]	Absolutely yes	Excitement

Table 6.1 Parallel between the QG psychophysics scale (Model) and the conventional psychometric scales (Mode)

The Mode is the set of 9 choices which shall be given to the individual for the posed Speech element or Statement (Table 6.1). Eventually , the corresponding scoring numbers are to be algebraically computed. They altogether dictate the following forms of questions about the Statement, which are all equivalent to one another:

Which [Mode choice] for this Statement =▶

1. Do you resonate with?
2. Do you prefer?
3. Is appealing to you?
4. Do you identify with?
5. Are you agreeable to?

In devising this language-based psychometry, we must keep in mind the cultural nuances imbued in forms of speech under different latitudes. Some have been traditionally more utilized in certain cultures in literary works of different nature than others do, turning them into preferential figures for those nationals. This condition may skew the accuracy of the test, reason why we present multiple examples for every category for the professional's election. Should the therapist prefer to devise his or her own questionnaire based on our examples, special attention must be paid to this potential caveat.

The analytic literature on figures of speech is extremely prolific, with different proposed types of classification. We have made a selection which we normalized and mapped to the QG Mental Foliate distribution for the purpose of these psychometric methods. We do not recommend the use of those figures of speech which do not appear in this proposal.

For certain, all languages use figures of speech. Different languages, however, dictate different stylistic criteria. Arabic literature, with a wealth of similes and metaphors, proposes constructions that are very different from those familiar to the West, making even eventual translation much of a work of adaptation. This condition applies to both oral and written literature in Africa alike. Classical Greek and Roman traditions make for the basis of the stylistic developed in Western languages. Some figures in use in the Greco-Latin tradition may be entirely absent in others. Japanese poetry for its own appears to be heavily based on delicate structures of implication and an entire vocabulary of aesthetic values which many believe are quasi non-translatable to Western languages.

All in all, it is important to bear in mind that at this point we are not focusing on rating the predominance or paroxysm of Layers of the Foliate. Our focus is instead to determine which Layer is paroxysmal within the individual's Mental Manifold. Further down, we will rate the paroxysm by adjoining the metric elements proposed in Chapter 4 concerning the Disease Model. For every individual, there is only one single profile from the normalcy of Character or Temperament to the Manageable Abnormality of Neurosis to the Catastrophic Abnormality of Psychosis: essentially one Layer of the Foliate stepping to different successive levels of accrual.

6.8 Pre-Testing Character through the Quintessential Elements of Locution

This is a pretest to show where the individual's Character or Temperament is leaning. It is a test to show the tendency. We present 3 samples of locution as shown further down, from which the individual must select only one descriptive sentence of his or her preference.

In all 3 samples, the first description denotes an open-ended mind defined by the Hyper Space operator. The third sentence denotes a closed-loop mind defined by the Hyper Quantum operator. The second sentence invokes mid-level ambivalence marked by the Hyper Quadratic operator. The first choice signals a temperament leaning toward undergirding by Primitive Layers 1 to 3 or straightly the Hyper quantum operator. The third choice signals a temperament leaning toward undergirding by Primitive Layers 5 to 9 or straightly the Hyper space operator. The second choice signals undergirding by Primitive Layer 4 or straightly the Hyper Quadratic operator.

[Sample 1]

> □ None had succeeded in their effort to change the club statutory document as much as Joseph did.

□ He had been undertaking changes to the club statute.

□ Joe changed the club statute.

[Sample 2]

□ Hewlett Packard and its teams of professionals have built generations and generations of printing machines.

□ The Co Hewlett Packard has been building printers.

□ HP builds printers.

[Sample 3]

□ The oceans' spreads around the continents of the world extend in vast bodies of waters with different currents.

□ The oceans of the world are vastly spread and have undercurrents.

□ Oceans are vast and active.

A scoping test on the 3 samples further enhances the accuracy of the determination. The individual will be asked to determine the scope of the description as a whole in each sample. Sample 1 has a narrow scope because it essentially involves one person. Sample 3 has a broad scope because it involves the entire natural world on earth. Sample 2 has an intermediate-level scope because it involves a company with its people that is conceivably of a sizable geographic occupation.

The scale for the scoping test is:

1. Narrow
2. Broad
3. Fair

6.9 Diagnosing Sexual Identity Strength and Gender Disparity

Passive voice = Female. It is a *PASSIVE LATENT* property.

Active voice = Male. It is an *ACTIVE LATENT* property.

It is important in the proposed tests below that the individual perfectly understand it is not about choosing for best grammar or style, but selecting an option that matches the verbal language in which he/she would express himself/herself. It is not about how they would write these ideas, but how they would verbally express themselves conversationally.

Option A

Select one of the two statements that most resembles the way you would express yourself:

1. As he was given ample time and allowed to speak of his great qualities and successes, I was reminded when he was chased by the police for having fled the scene of an accident and left the injured person on the pavement.
2. His constant boasting talk about personal qualities and his successes in life only remind me of his predicament with the police when he fled the scene of an accident almost taking an old man's life he left lying on the pavement.

Option B

Select one of the two statements that most resembles the way you would express yourself:

1. After he was let in, Peter was served hot tea and given great deference by the agent. The firearm given him for his own protection by the officer was in appreciation for his services to city law enforcement.
2. The agent greeted Peter into the room with ample deference and served him hot tea. He also gave Peter a firearm for enhanced self-

protection in a show of appreciation for his services to the crime fighting unit.

Option C

Select one of these two statements that most resembles the way that you would express yourself:

1. The savannah is roamed by beautiful giraffes. Nowadays, their living area is protected by wild life preservation laws enated by National Congress. They were almost driven to extinction by avid and aggressive hunters not in the long gone past. But who is to say what a savannah tree would be left feeling, if it could, when its leaves are broiled by the giraffes' hungry teeth and its branches grazed by their long reaching necks.
2. Beautiful are the giraffes that roam the savannah. The National Congress has enacted wild life preservation laws to protect their living areas, ever since avid and aggressive hunters almost drove them to extinction in recent past. But one wonders, if a savannah tree could feel, what it would when the giraffes' hungry teeth broil its lushy leaves and their long-reaching necks graze its many branches.

Option D

Select one of these two statements that most resembles the way that you would express yourself:

1. Anita was driven to the theater by her aunt Carla. She was sent by her mother to visit her sister Carla for a few days. But Carla was never advised by her sister that that her niece would be visiting during the weekend. Plans were made with her husband for a getaway that weekend, which they had to cancel so her niece could be attended to.
2. Anita's aunt, Carla, drove her to the theater. She was on a visit with her aunt for a few days. Anita's mother never advised her sister Carla, however, that Anita was going to spend the weekend with her. She and her

husband had made plans for a getaway, which they had to cancel in order to attend to Anita.

Three or more passive voice choices lead to an indication of an Anima-dominant Foliate. Three or more active voice choices lead to an indication of an Animus-dominant Foliate. Two passive voice choices and two active voice choices lead to an indication of a possible asexual Foliate. Additionally, in the case of indication of a sexuate Foliate, the contrasting with the observable biological gender will determine whether there is a gender identity disparity or not.

6.10 Diagnosing the Predominant Layer of the Mental Foliate

We make extensive use of figures of style in locution for this test. It is based on the principle that the vast majority of linguistic figures of style are QG typed. We recommend the inclusion of at least 12 sentences for each set in order to increase the accuracy level of the test.

The scale to be used is the main scale proposed in Section 3.

6.10.1 Determination of Layer 1 Predominance through Metonymy

Metonymy is all about summary or summarizing. It is a dense or condensed form of figure of style – it is conciseness literally. This kind of figure of style implodes a representation into a condensed form. For instance, "Nixon bombed Hanoi" means: The Nixon administration with the use of US Armed Forces bombed Hanoi.

The question to ask is: How much do these statements resonate with you? It is not about whether the individual agrees with the statement or not, but whether not he or she would express himself/herself in that way.

Sentences based on metonymy:

1. I have never read Auburn.
2. I've got new wheels.

3. Nixon bombed Hanoi.
4. Acrylic is now prevailing in art.
5. The White House announced plans against the avian flu epidemic.
6. Money talks.
7. One pen is mightier than a thousand swords.
8. New blood is now a must in this organization.
9. Pull them back in the box.

Test whether conciseness is appealing to the individual by making him/her identify the condensed part(s) of the sentence that may be exploded for greater clarity. This is to further extol the monolithic typology tendency being tested. At the same time, this particular questionnaire seeks to counteract a stylistic sense that the individual might have acquired by education, which might have somewhat skewed his/her answers to the first questionnaire.

The question to ask: How likely are you to express your thoughts in the way expressed in the sentences below?

Use the main Scale as is for this Test.

1. I have never read any book written by Auburn.
2. I bought myself a brand new car.
3. The Nixon Administration through the use of the US Armed forces bombed Hanoi.
4. Paintings in acrylic have taken over the art world.
5. The president and his cabinet announced a preparedness plan for the avian flu.
6. The influence of money is everywhere.
7. Countering an enemy with ideas has proven more effective than wars.
8. We need to bring into this organization new capable personnel.
9. Can you tell them to consider approaching this problem in a more conservative way?

6.10.2 Determination of Layer 2 Predominance Through Puns

Puns are equivocal or ambivalent statements. The marked tendency to use them signals an Ambivalent Layer 2 predominance.

The question to ask is: How much do these statements resonate with you?

1. I once heard a joke about amnesia, but I forgot how it goes.
2. Reading while sun bathing makes you well red (to be asked to fair skin individuals).
3. Never lie to an x-ray technician. They can see right through you.
4. His theory on inertia never seemed to gain momentum.
5. To the guy who invented Zero: Thanks for nothing!
6. His fear of moving stairs is escalating.
7. I used to have a fear of hurdles, but I got over it.
8. Two antennas got married last Saturday. The reception was fantastic.
9. Writing with a dull pencil is pointless.
10. I meant to look for my missing watch, but I could never find the time.

6.10.3 Determination of Layer 3 Predominance Through Rethoric

Rethoric may be defined as phrasing, or even talking for talking. In Rethorical locution, the individual is mainly associating words with one another, with the actual circumstance being a pretense for talking. In this form of locution, clichés are often amply used.

The question to ask is: How much do these statements resonate with you?

1. Marriage is a wonderful institution, but who would want to live in an institution? And freedom is one of those transcendent values one should never renounce to, even in marriage.
2. How can I express my thanks to you? You have done so much to make my stay feel so very pleasurable. Your hospitality has no par that I know.

3. First and foremost, as an invited guest he showed an unexpected utterly arrogant attitude. Little did she know she was going to be the first prey to his arrogance.
4. The big moment came when she, slowly but surely in the 5-minute conversation, started to unveil her true feelings toward him. Curiouser and curiouser.
5. The ability to think outside the box conditions success in any enterprise. Some people however are too extreme in their views and ambitions. Bringing them back into the box is often an uphill battle you lose before even starting.
6. Life is about seizing opportunities and to live every moment at the fullest. To be or not to be. But as true as this is, I shall acknowledge it is easier said than done.
7. In that section of the bookstore with displays of philosophy and psychology books, George was like a kid in a candy store. It is so difficult to play your cards right sometimes. It is true, never judge a book by its cover.
8. Putting all your eggs in one basket is, of course, always a bad idea. No question about it. Just as always going for the low-hanging fruits without thinking it twice is a recipe for disaster. Caution is advisable always.
9. "With experience comes wisdom, and with wisdom comes experience" is not true for everyone's life. How can one shoe ever be a good fit for all? In my experience, you can never satisfy everyone and your father at the same time.
10. "It's better to have loved and lost, than to have never loved at all." Love is a universal experience that everyone should have at least once. But if you've ever had a lost love, I know exactly how you feel.

6.10.4 Determination of Layer 4 Predominance through Hyperbole and Antimetabole

Hyperbole in speech is grandiloquence, exaggerated statements about facts, objects or events. Antimetabole is a form of twinning presenting ambivalent realities. They are both Quadratic figures of speech in QG analysis.

The question to ask is: How much do these statements resonate with you?

Hyperboles:

1. Pete was so mad he could chew nails.
2. I know in your younger years you could run faster than the wind.
3. As you must know, your bag feels weighing like a ton.
4. Your cousin looks as tall as a house.
5. Your shopping costed me a million dollars and more.
6. My dad will kill me if he sees you messing with his bike.
7. The skin of your cousin Jane feels softer than silk.
8. You were then trying to become skinny as a toothpick.
9. She was so happy that you could see in her a mile-wide smile.
10. I'm so hungry I could eat a horse.
11. Next Sunday is never going to arrive.
12. I know you love this book, you must have read it a hundred times.
13. My hand hurts so much it's going to drop off.
14. Your elder brother is stronger than iron.
15. You, my dear, are my guardian angel.

6.10.5 Determination of Layer 5 Predominance through Metaphors – Personification & Simile

These figures of speech amount to comparative statements based on evocations or splits in relation to facts, objects or events. They stand for transformational figures of speech in QG analysis.

The question to ask is: How much do these statements resonate with you?

1. Wary of the coming winter, trees in the fall shed their leaves to rocky breezes that make them dance like a hover waltz over ground.
2. The clouds look like cotton balls and the fields underneath an endless sea of greenery.
3. The dish ran away with the spoon. (Blake)
4. Little sorrows sit and weep. (Boccaccio)
5. She was in the sunset of her days. She has now fallen asleep.

6. Compassionate like an angel, she was the shining star of her family.
7. The childhood of the world; the anger of the tempest; the deceit-fulness of the riches: wine is a mocker.
8. The edge of this snow shovel is sharp like a knife. It's not like every snowfall dreams of turning icy.
9. He had this Je ne sais quoi that gave him this air of an angel.
10. His out-of-this-world mastery of both the cello and the piano made him a musician extraordinaire.
11. Although it meant walking on eggshells, her boyfriend decided not to wait for the other shoe to drop and brought up the subject to her.
12. Boy, when she wakes up on the wrong side of the bed, it is war zone around her all day!

6.10.6 Determination of Layer 6 Predominance through Alliteration & Assonance

These figures of speech essentially present repetition of the same sound akin to rhythms or chorus of a song.

The question to ask is: How much do these statements resonate with you?

1. She sells sea shells by the sea shore.
2. Peter Piper picked a peck of pickled peppers.
3. "The rain in Spain stays mainly on the plain."
4. “I saw a saw that could outsaw any other saw I ever saw.”
5. Sheep should seek to sleep in a shed.
6. Black bug bit a big black bear bearing back white spots.
7. A good cook should cook cookies like goodies crooks will never re-ward.
8. Finn fell for Phoebe in Phenix before his fate befell to felony in Fresno.
9. Easy come, easy go, like teasing a busy bee to get on its knee in the honey.
10. On the dock, she was locked on a face that would stop a clock on a 6:00 o'clock look.

11. To fight fire with fire in the night is fighting the good fight.
12. A persistent fly in flight around his fluffy mouth flies in the face of debate etiquette.
13. They say Jacque is a Jack-of-all-trades who dislikes facts, lacks focus and likes putting black jack paint on everything but sacks.

6.10.7 Determination of Layer 7 Predominance through Antithesis – Paradox & Oxymoron

To the above mentioned figures of speech, one might also add combination of words that contradict each other or make up irony or sarcasm.

The question to ask is: How much do these statements resonate with you?

1. Hatred stirs up strife; but loves covers all sins.
2. He is not that smart and will never ever be. A peapod is bigger than his brain.
3. Being born in a stable does not make a horse out of a pig.
4. Dumb as he is, he will only succeed if failure leads to success.
5. The only certainty in this life is the perenniality of uncertainty.
6. Rarely have I seen someone so derailed and clueless. Worse than a lost ball in the weeds.
7. A bad penny always turns up unexpectedly. Like a slap in the face.
8. I got these superb vintage shoes at a price you will never believe. It was a steal.
9. A deafening silence, a muted cry, a stubborn abandonment, will a pinch wake up inanity?
10. Is she oddly normal if she reacts abnormally to an abnormal situation or if she does not?
11. Unfaithful faith kept him falsely true.
12. Why, then, O brawling love! O loving hate!
13. Artfulness is long, Time is fleeting.
14. Many are called but so very few are chosen.
15. The fire station ragingly burned down to ashes.
16. The well-known marriage counselor Peter Arnett files for divorce.

17. One of the impounded cars in the police station's parking lot got robbed last night.
18. Among the many Facebook posts are a few complaining how useless Facebook is.
19. Because of unpaid parking tickets, this town's traffic cop gets his license suspended.
20. This airline pilot who had one of the best flight records always had a fear of heights and blindness.
21. You and your buddy are telling us fairy tales. Liar, liar, pants on fire.
22. "When truth is replaced by silence, the silence is a blatant lie."
23. How I know you are lying is simple: we both speak and understand the English language.
24. With so much dedication to community service, it was for her a slap in the face to have not been mentioned as a contributor in the celebratory gathering. Ugly as sin.
25. George meant to describe the huge overnight storm, when he said: "Looks like it rained a bit last night!"

6.10.8 Determination of Layer 8 Predominance through Apostrophe & Exclamations

These elements of speech invoke reverence, the artifact of belief and a form of self-detachment characteristic of Layer 8 ontology.

The question to ask is: How much do these statements resonate with you?

1. How big a deal it would be if our pool of tickets hit the Power Ball! A very big deal!
2. Oh God! His standup shows are killers. We go to his shows knowing we are going to die laughing.
3. Twinkle, twinkle, little star, O wonderful night of the birth of a new star!
4. Oh George! Once bitten, twice shy, Eh? It is quiet and sleepy now. No danger!
5. What an odd duck this boy is! No friends! No toys! No hobbies!

6. Holy night! ...
7. O, pardon me, thou bleeding piece of earth, when will be the next eruption?
8. Roll on, thou deep and dark blue Ocean – roll! O thrill of high surf!
9. Welcome, O life! I have been for months on fours. Take me off the ground, please!
10. "O, happy dagger! This is thy sheath. Thus let me rust and die."

6.10.9 Determination of Layer 9 Predominance through Silence

Speech that invokes silence or the preeminence of silence characterizes Layer 9 mentation.

The question to ask is: How much do these statements resonate with you?

1. Timeless truth: Never miss a good chance to keep silent.
2. Complete silence is so overwhelmingly loud!
3. Time for them never passes and what a meaningless thing to be racing against time all the time.
4. God is silent. Now, if only man would shut up, would it not be grace?
5. "Does not everything depend on our interpretation of the silence around us?"
6. "Silence is an unending source of Great Strength."
7. Entrepreneurship is all about deferred gratification.

6.10.10 Determination of Hyper-Ego Predominance through the Use of Imperatives

The question to ask is: How much do these statements resonate with you?

1. Get me the best exemplars available!
2. Tell me at once who won that race!
3. Don't insult my intelligence!
4. Start the engine immediately!
5. Expedite the shipping of this item!

6. Hurry up, the plane is leaving!
7. Dare say the truth for once!
8. Countdown zero, blast off!
9. Leave me alone!
10. Don't you give a damn about it!

6.10.11 Determination of Hyper-Hyperbolic Predominance through the Use of Antimetaboles

The question to ask is: How much do these statements resonate with you?

1. Eat to live, not live to eat. Love some food but if food gets to love you, it will be forever at your mouth!
2. Fair is foul and if foul is fair too, then fairness lives together with foolishness.
3. If you fail to plan, you have planned to fail.
4. You do what you like and you like what you do. – Andrew W.K., "Party Hard"
5. To be found innocent and yet have to pay a big fine is no better than to be found guilty and yet not receive any sanction.
6. Pyrrhic victories which give a taste of bitter sweet are yet preferable over straight loss to sour losers. (or straight win over sour losers).
7. Bargain without quality are raw deals for the foul.

6.10.12 Determination of Hyper-Asymptotic Predominance through the Use of Extrapolations

We understand extrapolation to be the act of arriving at conclusions or results by hypothesizing or projecting from known facts or observations. We alternatively understand the concept to be an inference, estimation or speculation by extending or projecting known information. In those conditions, extrapolation is an artifact of the expansiveness propensity characterizing Layer 9 mentation.

The question to ask is: How much do these statements resonate with you?

1. When it rains it pours and pours. That seems to make some people feel like a million, but others not!

2. Nathanael is a person of few words. He is at a loss of words though when his siblings tell him that he is always chasing rainbows!
3. Life without liberty is like a body without spirit.
4. Qué será será. What will be will be.

6.11 Probing Layer Paroxysm from Visual Cues

This test may be performed in two different ways. One approach is to have the patient put a face on a partition. The test probes the individual's ability to image a face or body expression that represents a pensive partition of the Foliate. The clinician shows an image to the individual for him or her to mimic. The image must accuse the pensive mental fit at its best. An ease of execution and a perfect mimic by the individual evidence propensity to or habit of experiencing this thought or mental fit, which amounts to a personal attribute from a paroxysmal condition. We only expect a palette of partitions at the same Layer or the same chiral side of a Layer to jointly produce this overtone. Otherwise, the test must be evaluated to have failed calling for a do-over or settle for the alternate test explained below. The caveat to avoid in this test is the selection of imageries which might at the end put in evidence only a thread quality, i.e. distress, instead of an authentic Layer pensive partition. The pilot imageries must unequivocally portray a specific partition of the Mentation Foliate, else accuracy in determining the paroxysm will suffer.

One other way to conduct this test is to name a thought partition and ask the subject to express it facially or with the body. It is obviously most appropriate for blind individuals for whom replicating presented imageries with facial expression would be unfitting. Here, also an ease of execution and a perfect mimic would evidence propensity to or habit of experiencing this thought or mental fit.

The scale for this test for every partition is:

1. [-4] Poor
2. [±] or [0] Average
3. [+4] Excellent

There are 72 partitions to probe. A successful test must have identified at a minimum 7 out of the 8 partitions of one particular Layer and they must all have the the Excellent ranking. **This result is to be matched with the paroxysmal level that determines Character.**

This test gives the clinician a deeper level of prospection of the patient's Mental Body. Unlike the previous tests, it probes the Foliate at the granular partition level, not just a Layer level.

6.12 Processing Foliate Chiral Sector Paroxysm

If what emerges from the granular partition test is a random pattern of partitions throughout the entire Foliate, then we advise to repeat the test as previously indicated. However, if the picture that emerges from the granular partition test is instead a prevalence of a group of partitions cross Layer, the practitioner must then further examine the possibility of a sketch of Foliate Chiral Sector paroxysm.

Should there be a clear prevalence of partitions matching an entire chiral sector of the Foliate (Anima or Animus Sector) for the most part, this result must be compared to that of the gender identity test. In that event, the two results should be in line with one another to establish the strength of the individual's self-conscious gender identity or whether there is gender disparity between the psychogenic gender identity and the biologically determined gender.

6.13 To Determine the Representations on the Predominant Layer

To determine the representations on the predominant Layer is an important prospection task in the diagnosis of mental pathology. This is done by eliciting them through meta-representations, that is to say the representation of our percepts and incepts performed by the very Unconscious Cognos for the most part. They are a result of intense activity between the root Layer and what we have called the representational sublayer superimposed on the latter. The meta-representations resulting from this interaction feed back into the representational sublayer to become essentially part of Memory. It is by virtue of this indelible retention that the Unconscious Cognos is able to conduct an unbroken thread of life through the day-to-day or night-to-night cycle of dreams which delivers the bulk of this activity.

It is important to distinguish here two different trends in the meta-representational activity in human mentation: one that is geared by continuity and the other by repetition. The patterns that we have studied in the establishment and development of NREM and REM phases of night sleep are only the beginning of the meta-representational orchestration of the Mind, keeping in mind that dreams do fully develop during NREM sleep as well. In conscious life, social organization is what dictates both the continuity and repetitiveness in an individual's life thread as an external constraint tended by the Conscious Cognos. During the nocturnal phase of life, the methology of continuity and repetitiveness in both keeping and developing the thread of life does not disappear in the absence of social organization and interaction. This methology remains whole in the execution of the meta-representational activity tended by the Unconconscious Cognos. The continuity methology is clearly evident is some forms of sleep disorders and states of provoked sleep, on one hand, and on the other, most normal people know that many of their nightly dreams are repetitive over long periods of their lives, sometimes in slightly different imageries and other times in the exact same ones. To fully comprehend this, one ought to remember the cases of split personality disorder whereby the Unconscious Self-Awareness may even switch back and forth across decades between different forms of personality expressions that are unequivocally different from one another. Understand the distinct personalities as very active clusters of Layer partitions / representational sublayer almost with a life of their own within the Normal Layer, in this case Mentation Layer 5. When the splits occur, awareness of the newly explicit personality connects back to what it was before, put in a different way, to where its thread of life was left before.

Each Layer of the Mind projects in a different manner and according to its inherent Norm. Of all the objects present in the natural world and internalized as percepts, as much as the elements of the subject's psychosocial experience, each Layer selectively and primarily retains in the representational and Memory strata those that are compatible with the Layer's Norm and ensuing primitive phenomenology. The subtending root stratum of the Layer projects from this content to give rise to the meta-representational activity occurring globally on the Layer. *Therefore, it is perfectly possible to identify the mark or stamp of a Layer on a particular meta-representational product, such as the distinct imageries or scenarios making up the content of nightly dreams.*

Beyond ethnic, cultural and psychosocial differences in the human conglomerate, there exists commonalities in the meta-representations of the human mind under different latitudes, a fact known ever since the early psychoanalytic studies, which technically termed them symbols. What makes this commonality possible, however, is because of the very subtending Mentation Layers that spur these meta-representations, which are absolutely universal in their primitive tenure across not only humans but all forms of the living.

In actual fact, the fullness of the many different mentation categories that make up the Mental Foliate as extensively studied throughout, not just the Normal Layers, transpire through the root-layer/meta-representational activity occurring every night in the thread of life.

6.14 Importance of Dream Recurrence

In light of the above discussion, the recurrence or frequency of a particular dream (or type thereof) is a particularly meaningful psychophysics diagnostic element in that it signals an accrual of a Mentation Layer, partition, partition set, or Chiral Sector of the Foliate. Most people are aware of those dreams that they keep making year after year and may readily supply them to the analyst. Keep in mind, in this context, that an accrual is not necessarily of a negative tone but may be positive when the involved meta-representations are felt as such by the subject.

In therapy, the conditions for determination of the frequency of these dreams should be expressly established such as keeping a diary of nightly dreams. Narcosis for the purpose of remembering frequently projected dreams is another appropriate means to that end. At very least, a clue as to the frequency of a certain type of dreams is a clue to specific Layer prevalence in a particular Mentation Foliate, once one is able to identify Layers behind meta-representations. Further, this clue may help narrow and even expedite the psychophysics diagnostic prospection by judiciously helping zero in on a particular mentation element of the Mental Foliate.

Lastly, a few sporadic dreams gathered across a few nights, while useful to establish the subject's psychological climate in general, may not provide the needed elements for pathological diagnosis. So it is even though they may be emotionally intense such as nightmares, or those other dreams which finalize with sudden wake of the dreamer, mainly for reasons of possible exogenous triggers.

6.15 Diagnosis Confirmation with QG Foliate Signatures from Dreams

For diagnosis confirmation, we present a glossary of meta-representations at the end of the Chapter, which the reader should now take the time to visit. It is based on real-life nightly dreams drawn from clinical practice, many of which from psychoanalyst Pierre Daco's[40]. It would be a vast enterprise to compile an exhaustive list of different types of dreams with their particular psychological interpretation. We have restrained the glossary to about 100 different keys common to dreams by Westerners which can hopefully serve as a universal guide to therapists under all latitudes. While we support the psychoanalytic interpretation for the most part, which is dicated by syllogistic inference and effected through transposition, we present key novel elements of interpretation concordant with the QG psychophyics hitherto developed. The main goal of the glossary is two-fold:

1. to aid in the psychological interpretation of the meta-representations displayed in those dreams, and

---

[40] **L'interpretation des Rêves**, Pierre Daco, Les Nouvelles Edition Marabout, Verviers, 1979

2. to present a systematic method to relate dream imageries to QG Psychophysics elements of the dreamer's Mental Foliate.

What we have in mind with the second objective as firstly indicated is to present a conclusive probing element of the pathological diagnosis that previous tests have elicited consistent with the conventional psychometric prescription. This test speaks to the reliability of the entire diagnostic method in that it comes from a totally different mentation resource than the ones previously utilized. If the results of both are concordant, then the diagnosis is firmly confirmed.

6.16 Utilizing the Glossary of Meta-Representations

It is important to acknowledge that Meta-Representations may symbolize different things to different people in general, even though a universal representational common core may well exist. Therefore, one should not expect a unijective relationship between a meta-representation and its symbolic value. There may be several symbolic values to one same meta-representation as displayed in a number of keys of the glossary.

Some dreams are simple and others more elaborate. As discussed throughout this study, there are two coordinates to the mental fits encapsulated in the mentation partitions: there is the Layer coordinate and the anti-symmetric thread coordinate. These two coordinates determine the nature and layout of the meta-representation that emerge from the interaction betwen the partition root and the super-imposed representational stratum. We denote this projection[41] product an *Abstraction Vector*. For every meta-representation, which are the keys or main labels of the glossary, there may be several *abstraction vectors*.

In simple terms, what is the kind of imagery that the partition of terror i.e. will project in the context of the meta-representational activity of a dream? It is important to always determine the main theme of a dream, whether it is a snippet

[41] The term projection here is not being used in its usual psychoanalytic meaning of seeing or unleashing one's own defects onto someone else, but in its straightforward meaning of a spur.

or a more elaborate piece. Three important questions ought to be asked at the outset in relation to the overall theme:

- Does the dream develop like a forceful outward mobilization or deployment of things (as in an explosion)?
- Does the dream develop like a forceful inward constriction of things (as in an implosion)?
- Does the dream develop like a somewhat static state of equilibrium or balance between the several parts of the content?

If the answer to question 1 is yes, then the abstraction vector is on the [+4] thread. If the answer to question 2 is yes, then the abstraction vector in on the [-4] thread. If the answer to question 3 is yes, then the abstraction vector is on the [±/0] or Hybrid thread.

The other 6 threads are the next ones to probe for. To probe for the [-3] and [+3] threads one ought to examine how the dream answers the question: is the glass half-empty or half-full in terms of the scope or perspective the dreamer seems to bear on the situation? If the dream presents a lack of something, then the perspective is that of a lack and the abstraction vector is very likely to be on the pessimism thread ([-3]) for the vertical component. If the dream instead presents a gain or an addition of something in its imagery, then the perspective is that of a gain and the abstraction vector is very likely to be on the optimism thread ([+3]) for the vertical component.

The other 4 threads are next to be probed for. To probe for the [-2] and [+2] threads, one examines the question of whether there is a measure of a positive or a negative tone setting in the narrative. And finally to probe for the [-1] and [+1] thread, one looks for any form of permission giving, an affirmative slant of some sort, or else an invalidation of tenets of any kind. Note that the steps for probing the 8 threads are not at all mutually exclusive. Following the indicated order will make it generally easier to conduct the analysis. All threads must be probed for.

When it comes to the Layer identity for the meta-representation, there is always a relatively clear element in the dream narrative that points to the identity of the Layer the meta-representation is being profiled from.

We are going to show an example of how to conduct this sort of meta-representational analysis by debunking the *Adventurer* key in the glossary. *'Black man adventurer dancing with the woman dreamer like a forest vine*[42]*'* is the main theme. She is seeking harmony with her natural resources of free mobilization, which are no other than the [Animus Sector]. 'She' as a woman means her prevalent [Anima Sector]. She may well be a Matrixial character (Layer 6) as well because of the artistic dexterity of her [Animus Sector] which moves like a forest vine (flamenco dance) and her engaging in a dance with 'him'. The dream expresses a balance problem between the two sectors, which is an over prevalence of the [Anima Sector] over the [Animus Sector]. The repulsion that she feels for 'him' extols the discordance there exists between the two sectors in her Mental Foliate. The pleasure that she feels reflects the search or desire to gain that measured equilibrium.

The first 3 questions are to be answered in the negative: nothing extreme and no balance. The next two questions ought to be answered in the positive: there is a gain (thread [+3]), which is the pleasure that she felt, and a positive tone setting (thread [+2]) which is the dancing together with sure and agile steps. But there is also a negative tone (thread [-2]) introduced by the repulsion that she felt for the black adventurer.

The dance element is an important phenoma that pertains to the Layer characterization, extolling it as a prevalent Layer 6 within the Manifold. It is important because the abstraction vector – *which is the representation of a female dancing with an unknown free spirit* – is all about dancing, not a walk with a visitor or a simple company.

Note that we have not filled up the *Abstraction Vector* field in the rest of the glossary, due to the fact that some complex keys bear more than one vector.

---

[42] **L'interpretation des Rêves**, Pierre Daco, Les Nouvelles Edition Marabout, Verviers, 1979, p.189

We have purposely left that field empty for uniformity. There is no doubt however that the *Abstraction Vec*tor is an important entity in the mechanism of thought formation within the human Mentation Manifold at the level of the Unconscious Cognos. It is also part of the mechanism of thought formation within the Conscious Cognos to the extent that projection is inherent to that mechanism as well.

Furthermore, there is an element of impairment or dysfunction in this meta-representation spelled out in the quasi impossible constraint of being enchanted and repugnated at the same time. It is the mark of what conventional psychoanalysis would call a conflict or conflictive drive. In fact, from our perspective, it is the result of a disproponately hyperactive [Anima Sector] of a Caucasian woman compared to the Animus Sector of her Foliate which she perceives as an inferior and repulsive side of self. This interpretation is supported by the fact that in the matter of mobilization, in the global culture, motional and speed attributes are eponymously conferred to the "primitive" blacks associated with "forest vines". Therefore, the nature of the dysfunction is not a conflict per se but an overdrive that creates a steep unbalance between an over accrued Passive-Responsive Sector of a female Mental Foliate and its conjugate Active-Reactive Sector. Interestingly, one can see in this case how culture can contribute to dysfunction in a predisposed Mental Foliate.

6.17 QG Color Space

The metric in color psychology may be taken by the analyst either as one more psychometric category in the diagnostic process or a probing element to confirm the results cast by the previous diagnosis regime which we have outlined and studied to this point. What confers this virtue to color psychometric in this context is its complete independence from the previous diagnosis exegetic elements. The metric at work in color psychology, otherwise denoted human behavioral and neurobiological response to color, pertains to the very physics of nature, namely particle physics, and responds to the material wavelength metric in the *space momentum* dimension.

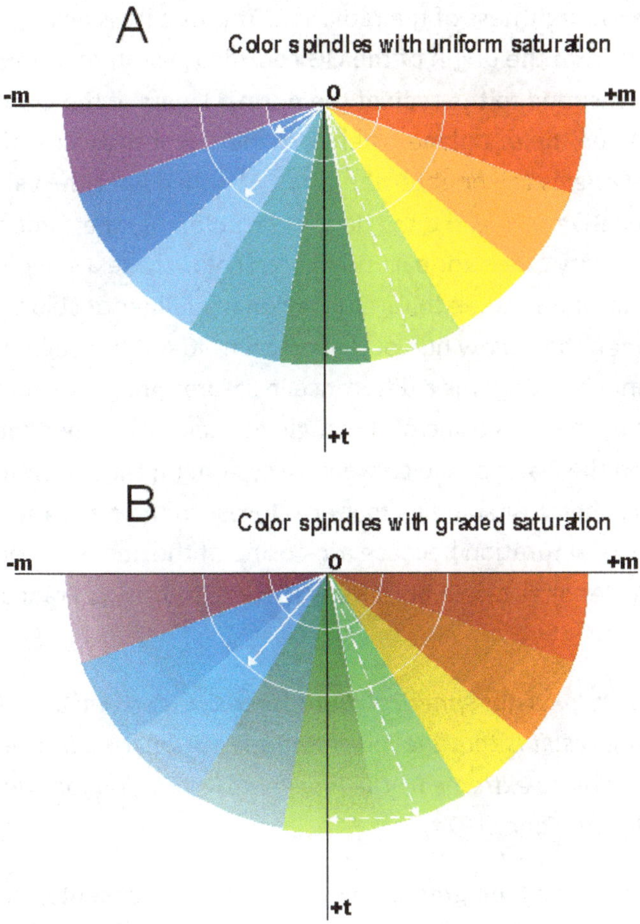

Fig. 6.6 Color space emanating from the QG physical framework

In the QG physics relating to single photon theory, there is both a zenithal and azimutal dimension to the real-valued space that gives rise to elementary particles. In the case of photon particles in the color space inherent to their material configuration, there are three foundational constructs that support the three primary qualities known to color as observed in electromagnetic radiation. The first qualifier of color is hue or tint, which is modeled by the QG *m*-axis evolving from a *-m* side to a *+m* side. This axis ascribes to radiation the 8 observable primary colors or hues (Fig. 6.6). We discuss later how the progression from *-m* to *+m* is reflected in the primary palette of colors. The second qualifier of color is the luminance or brightness of the radiation. This quality is given by radial longitudes that start from the origin of the QG coordinate system or the color space. These lines correspond to the radii of the normal layers of the QG Manifold when projected on the *m-t* plane. Therefore the larger the value of these radii on the positive *m*-axis the brighter the color, and the lesser the value of these radii on the negative *m*-axis the the darker the color. By the same token, this makes the geometry of a color partition in our color space a spindle. Lastly, saturation or colorfulness is the third foundational qualifier of color. The difference i.e. between the yellow hue of the lemon fruit and the yellow hue of mustard which is much stronger is a difference in saturation. In our color space saturation is given by the arc-cosine of the angle formed by the median line of the hue spindle and the *t*-axis of the coordinate system (in trigonometry the cosine axis). Therefore the color spindles that are closest to the *t*-axis must exhibit the minimum level of saturation because arc-cosine of the angle is around its minimum value. As Jennifer Marie Binzak Fugate and Courtny L. Franco well acknowledge:

"... the space of color is not spherical, but rather lopsided and a partially flattened globe. The result is that the maximum saturation for a hue near "bluish-green" is not nearly as extreme as the maximum saturation for hues near "red" (see D'Andrade and Egan, 1974)."

As we shall shortly see blue-green does occupy an almost center position with respect to the cosine axis in our color space, giving it a minimum saturation delta or gradation.

6.18 Metric of Color Psychology

Color psychology has long been studied, to no firm conclusive determinants to this day however[43], despite the enormous interest in the subject both by academia and industry.

---

[43] **Color and Psychological Functioning: a Review of Theoretical and Empirical Work**, Andrew J Elliot, Frontiers in Psychology, 2015, doi: 10.3389/fpsyg.2015.00368

Dra-matism *[-4]*	*Pessim-ism* *[-3]*	*Nega-tivity* *[-2]*	*Disap-proval* *[-1]*	*Neutral [±]* *[0]*	*Assent* *[+1]*	*Assur-ance* *[+2]*	*Optim-ism* *[+3]*	*Excite-ment* *[+4]*
Implo-sion or inward constrict-ion of things	Perspec-tive of Subtrac-tion or Lack: glass half-empty	Nega-tive tone setting	Invalida-tion of tenets	Equili-brium between 2 or more binary tenets	Affirma-tive slant on things or per-mission giving	Positive tone setting	Perspec-tive of Addition or Gain: glass half full	Explo-sion: forceful outward mobiliz-ation
Violet	Indigo	Blue	Blue-Green	Green	Lime	Yellow	Orange	Red
400 nm	*437nm*	*475 nm*	*513 nm*	*550 nm*	*587 nm*	*625 nm*	*663 nm*	*700 nm*
1[-4]	1[-3]	1[-2]	1[-1]	1[±/0]	1[+1]	1[+2]	1[+3]	1[+4]
2[-4]	2[-3]	2[-2]	2[-1]	2[±/0]	2[+1]	2[+2]	2[+3]	2[+4]
3[-4]	3[-3]	3[-2]	3[-1]	3[±/0]	3[+1]	3[+2]	3[+3]	3[+4]
4[-4]	4[-3]	4[-2]	4[-1]	4[±/0]	4[+1]	4[+2]	4[+3]	4[+4]
5[-4]	5[-3]	5[-2]	5[-1]	5[±/0]	5[+1]	5[+2]	5[+3]	5[+4]
6[-4]	6[-3]	6[-2]	6[-1]	6[±/0]	6[+1]	6[+2]	6[+3]	6[+4]
7[-4]	7[-3]	7 [-2]	7[-1]	7[±/0]	7[+1]	7[+2]	7[+3]	7[+4]
8[-4]	8[-3]	8[-2]	8[-1]	8[±/0]	8[+1]	8[+2]	8[+3]	8[+4]
9[-4]	9[-3]	9[-2]	9[-1]	9[±/0]	9[+1]	9[+2]	9[+3]	9 [+4]
→1[-4]	→1[-3]	→1[-2]	→1[-1]	→1[±/0]	→1[+1]	→1[+2]	→1[+3]	→1[+4]
→4[-4]	→4[-3]	→4[-2]	→4[-1]	→4[±/0]	→4[+1]	→4[+2]	→4[+3]	→4[+4]
→9[-4]	→9[-3]	→9[-2]	→9[-1]	→9[±/0]	→9[+1]	→9[+2]	→9[+3]	→9[+4]

Table 6.2 Mapping QG color space to the Mentation Foliate Manifold. QG color space is embodied in the longitudinal threads of the Manifold.

The conclusion that researcher Andrew J Elliot drafted in the following lines in his 2015 review of the subject is still current as of this writing today:

"First, the focus of theoretical work in this area is either extremely specific or extremely general. A precise conceptual proposition such as red signals dominance and leads to competitive advantage in sports (Hill and Barton, 2005) is val-

uable in that it can be directly translated into a clear, testable hypothesis; however, it is not clear how this specific hypothesis connects to a broader understanding of color–performance relations in achievement settings more generally. On the other end of the spectrum, a general conceptualization such as color-in-context theory (Elliot and Maier, 2012) is valuable in that it offers several widely applicable premises; however, these premises are only vaguely suggestive of precise hypotheses in specific contexts. What is needed are mid-level theoretical frameworks that comprehensively, yet precisely explain and predict links between color and psychological functioning in specific contexts."

As he further points out:

"All color effects undoubtedly depend on certain conditions – culture, gender, age, type of task, variant of color, etc. – and acquiring an understanding of these conditions will represent an important marker of maturity for this [research]."

Color symbolism has changed over time both in particular cultures and cross-culture. There is a general disagreement over whether reactions to color and their symbolism stem from cultural conditioning or instinct. Several studies have concluded that color partakes of the social learning process owing to the significant symbolic value it is accorded in all cultures. What we believe is that reaction to color exists instinctually at a basis state, that is to say, that which would be found in a Foliate at birth. The basis response to color is modeled according to azimuthal symmetry or anti-symmetric threading parity. In Table 6.2 we show the palette of color primitives and their wavelengths in the radiation format. We so propose that every human temper, type regardless, would react to color in the same way in terms of the psychological and neurobiological quality inherent to the longitudinal anti-symmetric threads.

As previously dicussed, the main color quality is hue or tint, an attribute by which color is discernible by red, green, blue, etc. This attribute is dependent on wavelength and independent of intensity or brightness. Quite well known are a few facts about color, both cast by formal research results and cultural traditions, which support the fullness of our characterization. Let us analyze psychological color response and color metaphors by hue. Note that most colors of the palette have only received a modicum of attention in research, which is also the case in human culture for some other important colors in metaphoric attributions.

It is important to underscore the notable fact that, in the ignorance of the true nature of primal qualifiers behind color primitives, research studies have confused these qualifiers with mental states or fits that stand instead for partitions pertaining to normal Layers of the Mentation Manifold. Consequently, our analysis will take into account this important caveat and provide the necessary redress.

6.18.1 Red Longitude

Red is a color that is well acknowledged to cause *excitation* in behavior. It fittingly sits on the thread of *excitement* in the Foliate map. It is not at all a coincidence that admittedly it represents thus far the most studied of all colors, a clear indication of the excitement it elicits in everyone's mind including researchers'.

Elliot has found in his review that *"Research focused on color and aggressiveness/dominance evaluation has shown that viewing red on self or other increases appraisals of aggressiveness and dominance (see Krenn, 2014, for a review)... In research on color and attraction, viewing red on or near a female has been shown to enhance attraction in heterosexual males (see Pazda and Greitemeyer, in press, for a review)."*

As previously noted, we can see in this case that the attribution of the chromatic effect has gone to the partition of *fury*, perhaps *cupidity* as well, in the *"aggressiveness/dominance"* wording for theme of the research. Translation of the latter to *fury/cupidity (greed)* is not at all far fetched. Furthermore, Eliott also reports that *"in research on color and attraction, viewing red on or near a female has been shown to enhance attraction in heterosexual males."* In this case red equates *passion*, which is a Layer 6 partition lining up along the same *excitement* thread. In addition, research has understandingly demonstratred that red stimuli or perception of red commands observers' attention. Research has also demonstrated that wearing red tends to enhance both actual performance and perceived performance in sport competitions and tasks.

6.18.2 Magenta Longitude

Magenta or violet is the color of penitence or constriction for both the Anglican and the Catholic Church. In traditional Chinese symbolism it is the color of immortality, ascribed to the immortal Gods. Considering that the mental fit of inanition, which is synonym to the constriction of hibernation, is on the same [-4] or dramatism thread, it is fair to conclude a reasonable amount of conformity to our psychophysics visualization in the religious adjucation.

6.18.3 Green Longitude

Green is a color that is well acknowledged to contribute to appeasement and tranquility. It neither excites nor constricts: it fittingly sits on the Neutral thread of the Foliate map. The progression in two opposite directions from the green color is consequently clear (from green to red and from green to purple) and authorizes us at a stroke to establish an equal gradation scale at both sides of the *Neutral* green color.

This partitioning gives us two wings of colors, one that is of bright or brighter colors at the right-chiral side of the palette (lime to red) and the other being of darker colors at the left-chiral side of the palette (blue-green to magenta). This attribute is also called *luminance*.

6.18.4 Orange Longitude

Orange is acknowledged to be a warm and welcoming color in the culture of the West. We shall take these attributes to make it a color of *optimism*, in conformity with the [+3] thread.

6.18.5 Yellow Longitude

Next is the royal yellow, often associated with sunshine. Children, with their natural spontaneity and genuine joy, knowingly tend to be fond of the bright yellow color generally. Does this not factually make it a color of *positive tone setting*?

6.18.6 Lime Green Longitude

Lime Green is a bright green color which is close to that of the citrus fruit. This color is said to depict *"nature, confidence, abundance and yield"*. Does that not make it the color of *Assent* or *permission giving* as described for the [+1] thread?

6.18.7 Indigo Longitude

At the anti-symmetric position to orange on the color palette is the indigo color. Our review of the literature at large gathers a lot of spirituality associated with indigo, much of it of a new age taint. We will retain none of it however, since they appeared to be adscriptions by the culture and clearly do not stringently or sufficiently describe human behavioral or emotional response to the color.

A research study review by Jennifer Marie Binzak Fugate and Courtny L. Franco[44] found more reliable results for the indigo color from application of formal methods and reported the following:

"Indigo" was indicated among the top three colors for only one emotion, sadness, *making it potentially specific. The intensity of "indigo" was moderate for* sadness, *and the agreement among raters was low-medium, Kendall's* W = *0.243. Using bootstrapping, we found that the probability of selecting a sample in which the intensity of "indigo" given to* sadness *exceeded the intensity of "indigo" to another emotion was always < 62%. Therefore, it is unlikely that "blue" is specific to* sadness, *even though participants never picked "indigo" as one of the top three colors for any other emotion."*

The distinctive association with sadness puts the color on the [-3] or *pessimism* thread of the Foliate, as predicted.

6.18.8 Blue Longitude

Next color in that chiral wing is blue. Eliott's review of research about color psychology has found related researches with the common conclusion that *"Partic-*

---

[44] **What color is your anger? Assessing color emotion pairings in English speakers,** Frontiers in Psychology, 2019, Jennifer Marie Binzak Fugate and Courtny L. Franco, doi: 10.3389/fpsyg.2019.00206

ipants exposed to blue (relative to yellow) illumination reported greater mental alertness" and that *"Blue light has [contributed] to increase subjective alertness and performance on attention-based tasks."* Translate the latter to be a moderate form of perception that equates *devoted attention to elements of reality,* which we had ascribed to the *superficiality* fit on Layer 2 and which lines up with the matching [-3] thread of the Foliate.

When it comes to adscription by human cultural traditions, several sources indicate that in most human cultures blue can also mean sadness. Psychologist Pierre Daco goes so far as to wonder *"if the deep-seated melancholy of the many Mediterranean peoples do not stem from immateriality of this blue in which body and spirits are immersed..."* Effectively, melancholy or *sorrow* is one of the mental fits on the [-3] or negativity thread which corresponds to the blue longitude, thereby justifying the attribution.

6.18.9 Blue-Green Longitude

Lastly, the blue-green color comes into consideration. This color is also called cyan, of which turquoise and teal are some of the varied tones or tint. Our review of the literature addressing color influence on behavior found squint references of its putative psychological impact. The most prominent reference we have found dwells in pre-Columbian and colonial religious traditions in the Americas. The color was known in pre-Columbian cultures under the name of Maya blue. On manuscripts, the blue color was sometimes diluted to take the express and close appearance of turquoise. The blue-green color became prominent in the colonial era with the iconography associated with the Virgin of Guadalupe of Mexico often representated wearing a blue-green robe. As a religious figure she came to play a prominent role in the formation of Mexico as a nation. If any symbolic value must be drawn from the display of this color under the Mexican Marian tradition, it is definitely that of disapproval or invalidation of the colonial trend pursued both by the conquistadores and the Catholic Church itself. Effectively, the Virgin of Guadalupe is first of all a virgin of 'color' or a black virgin. With this manifest ontology, she was thereby clearly siding with the indigenous side of the colonial enterprise. First, she chose to appear to Juan Diego Cuauhtlatoatzin, a young local Amerindian. There is of course the conquista-driven interpretation that her brown complexion expressly makes her relatable to people in Latin America in a bid for more Catholic converts. Inarguably, her avowed intention was to make Diego speak to the Catholic pontiffs and request them to honor her by building her, the black virgin, a temple. Bishop Zumárraga was skeptical of the apparition and requested evidence to Juan Diego, which was severally supplied by the virgin again through Juan Diego and which the bishop denied time and time again. So much for insistence, disapproval and invalidation on both sides. As an interesting side note, after almost 500 years the turquoise color of what became the sacred mantle remains inexplicably bright, and no one is yet apparently able to credibly explain why.

After much searching, we have yet to find a formal study that specifically addresses the blue-green color.

6.19 Metaphoric Value of Color

Researchers have found it possible that *"biologically-derived color-emotion associations might be modified, reinforced or conventionalized as a result of frequently-paired associations. That is, initial tendencies can be exaggerated by the constant associations of color-emotion within a culture. From a very young age, people are constantly exposed to explicit and implicit pairings, and once these pairings are learned they can be associated with knowledge and behaviors outside the realm of consciousness (Bargh, 1990; Elliot et al., 2007). They can also serve as unconscious primes to automatically influence cognitive processing. Put into practice, "red" and its association with danger, is reinforced in our culture by the "red" of stoplights and stop signs, the "red" of fire alarms, the "red" of pens used to correct papers, etc. (Elliot et al., 2007).*

Other theories of emotion, however, do not treat emotions as biological entities, but rather explanatory constructs that a person evokes to explain the primitive changes in his or her own internal sensations or such similar changes within another person (Russell, 1980; Barrett, 2006a,b)... Consequently, specific color-emotion associations should be based on a person's beliefs as experienced in their culture and through their language, rather than on evolutionary honest signals."

We do not find these two theoretical viewpoints to be mutually exclusive, although we strongly disagree with the definition of emotions as explanatory constructs of any kind. It is obvious that color metaphors or color-emotion pairings promoted by the culture are internalized within the individual's Mentation Foliate, specifically within the mnemonic substratum. This does not preclude the instinctual response to color that is germane to antisymmetric orthoflow dynamics of the Foliate.

Psychological response to color can be studied in its various facettes in the meta-representational language of dreams, instead of response to stimuli while the subject is in the conscious awake state. In the meta-representational language, color primarily responds to its foundational azimuthal antisymmetric quality formalized in the mathematics of trigonometry, as drafted in previous discussion. Note well that it is only because of this quality, which is accountable by vector algebra, that color shows mixing properties exhibited in the existence of the conventional color spaces and mixing within these spaces, which all derive from the fundamental real-valued QG color space.

Below is a dream from psychoanalyst Pierre Daco's clinical record to help us undertake this analysis[45].

I was walking down a narrow trail. To my left, vast blooming fields of tropical crops. To my right was flowing a river filled with red hot waters. There was an end-of-war atmosphere all around. The river was slowly flowing, and at a certain point in the remote distance changed into a sort of lake, that one of a dark red color, and as if contained by a levee. I knew the war was over.

This dream clearly outlines a broad depiction of the dreamer's Foliate while in therapy. The dreamer has a presence that is flanked by two different settings, one at his left (left-chiral side) and the other at his right (right-chiral side). Further, what is laying at the left takes the passiveness or staticity of a tropical plantation – translate the PASSIVE-RESPONSIVE side of his Mental Foliate. And what is laying at the right takes the mobility of a flowing river – translate the

---

[45] **L'interpretation des Rêves**, Pierre Daco, Les Nouvelles Edition Marabout, Verviers, 1979, p.200

ACTIVE-REACTIVE side of his Mental Foliate. Of notable interest to us is the color of the river, which is initially bright red. Transposition onto the Foliate gives us action occurring on the [+4] thread of *excitement*, with this red 'longitudinal' river. The bright red river here is a meta-representation of a Right-Chiral Sector broadly overaccrued and in particular in the excitement thread. An ultrastructural interpretation may come to visualize the 'bright red longitudinal river' to be in and of itself a meta-representation of the entire Right-Chiral Sector of the Foliate geared by what bright red generally represents in human culture, as argued by Eliott. It would signal in this case an over accretion experienced by all the threads in that Sector. In this event we are dealing with a representation of a meta-representation, in simple terms a meta-symbol.

In the next projected scenery in the dream, the flow of the river disappears into what is a stagnant lake formation that is contained by dikes, in other words a sort of dam. Therefore, what was a strident morbid accretion of an overbearing Animus Sector has now been tapered down to something like a dam – translate a de-emphasis of the overbearing accretion. This mobilization drawdown is further stamped by the metaphor of the bright red intensity of the river changing to dark red, a higher level of saturation, which in the culture means less excitement or agitation, or perhaps more wisdom or ponderation. The term ponderation here is not at all far-fetched, it is clearly associated with the combative introspection the dreamer was undertaking in analysis, since she pointedly mentioned that a whole atmosphere of war was emanating from the developing scenery of the dream and, once the river had turned into a dark red dam, it became an after-the-war atmosphere. Introspection is obviously and unequivocally about self-debunking and taking down one's own internal bunkers.

As to the tropical fields at the left side of the scenery, the dreamer could not ascertain their true colors in the dream. We only know that they were blooming crops, an indication of an appropriately balanced PASSIVE-RESPONSIVE Foliate Sector. The meta-representation of the dream was definitely mostly concerned with the state of the Animus Sector.

In conclusion, when all the qualifiers and attributes of color are taken into consideration, the universal psychological metaphoric or symbolic values of color are not mutually exclusive with instinctually driven response to color. The latter stems from the very physics of color as it emanates from photonic radiation. Further elaboration and research in that direction are well granted in order to further evolve Color Theory and broaden the systematic basis of human color response, starting from the QG color space in its zenithal and azimuthal dimensions. It is worth stressing that we do not see any contradiction or inconsistency between conscious color response and unconsciously-driven color response because these properties stem from top-down cross Foliate longitudinal threading, independent of Cognos realm delimitation. However, color projection in metarepresentations may be at the outset the best cast for color-mood pairing which is the primitive for emotional evocation elicited by color.

6.20 Color-Driven Diagnosis Confirmation

What we have shown is that there is no color-emotion pairing per se, a terminology in use in many studies, but color-mood pairing, mood being viewed as previously defined in our psychophysics analysis. As such a color is a pointer to many different emotions localized on the same threading longitude of the Mentation Manifold. Only moods and pensive longitudes can be matched with one another.

Hence response to color can only elicit disorders that are marked by the chirality of the Manifold. It can be used to determine left-chiral or right-chiral over accretion as well as gender disparity and gender balance (a-sexuation). It cannot directly probe Layer-prevalent neuroses or psychoses, but only when there is a prevalent chiral side of the normal Layer within the morbid Foliate. Note that it can specifically be used in the case of psychoses, either as an aid in confirming a diagnosis or a partial means to establish one, since it is not subject to the patient's views about or own perception of his/her impairment or the elements thereof.

6.21 Diagnosing the Specificities of a Particular Disorder

Once the QG psychophysics signature of a disorder has been determined by virtue of the application of the diagnosis regime above offered, it is not difficult to zero in on particular nosological cadre to finally put a label on the patient's dysfunctional behavior. The *Taxonomic Index of Disorders* in which they are arranged by Layer groupings is a first-order resource in pinpointing a particularly applicable disorder. It is not our objective in this treatise to present 150 different disorder tests for clinical diagnosis of mental disorders. At this stage, we will leave it to the clinician to modify existing tests to suit their practice based on the QG psychophysics principles that we have so extensively presented in this Treatise.

We will however make a critique of one commonly used diagnostic test as an example of how to adapt a test to suitability, namely the Young Mania Rating Scale (YMRS). We do not believe that when self-awareness is impaired as in the case of the psychosis of Bipolar Disorder a mentally ill person can properly self-administer any test. Any effort to make available to the public testing samples for self-assessment, as good intentioned as their authors may be, is probably futile.

There are 11 groups of statements or key areas in the YMRS questionnaire. The first serious problem with the questionnaire is that the 11 areas of testing are not normalized since we do not know what standard they respond to other than what appears to be semiological criteria.

The YMRS is reported below.

1. Elevated Mood

1. Absent
2. Mildly or possibly increased
3. Definite subjective elevation; optimistic, self-confident; cheerful; appropriate to content
4. Elevated, inappropriate to content; humorous
5. Euphoric, inappropriate laughter, singing

2. Increased Motor Activity or Energy

1. Absent
2. Subjectively increased
3. Animated; gestures increased
4. Excessive energy; hyperactive at times; restless (can be calmed)
5. Motor excitement; continuous hyperactivity (cannot be calmed)

3. Sexual Interest

1. Normal; not increased
2. Mildly or possibly increased
3. Definite subjective increase
4. Spontaneous sexual content; elaborates on sexual matters; hypersexual
5. Overt sexual acts

4. Sleep

1. No decrease in sleep
2. Sleeping less than normal amount by up to one hour
3. Sleeping less than normal by more than one hour
4. Decreased need for sleep
5. No need for sleep at all

5. Irritability

1. Absent
2. Subjectively increased
3. Irritable at times; recent episodes of anger or annoyance
4. Frequently irritable; short, curt
5. Hostile, uncooperative

6. Speech: Rate & Amount

1. No increase
2. Feel talkative
3. Increased rate or amount at times, verbose at times

4. Push; consistently increased rate and amount;
5. Pressured; uninterruptedly, continuous speech

7. Language: Thought Disorder

1. Absent
2. Circumstantial; mild distractibility; quick thoughts
3. Distractible; loses goal of thought; change topics frequently; racing thoughts
4. Flight of ideas; tangentially; difficult to follow; rhyming, echolalia
5. Incoherent; communication impossible

8. Content

1. Normal
2. Questionable plans, new interests
3. Special project(s); hyper religious
4. Grandiose or paranoid ideas; ideas of reference
5. Delusions; hallucinations

9. Disruptive or Aggressive Behavior

1. Absent
2. Sarcastic; loud at times, guarded
3. Demanding; threats
4. Threats, shouting
5. Assaultive; destructive

10. Appearance

1. Appropriate dress and grooming
2. Minimally unkempt
3. Poorly groomed; moderately disheveled; overdressed
4. Disheveled; partly clothed; garish make-up
5. Completely unkempt; decorated; bizarre garb

11. Insight

1. Present; admits illness; agrees with need for treatment
2. Possibly ill
3. Admits behavior change, but denies illness
4. Admits possible change in behavior, but denies illness
5. Denies any behavior change

Appearance and Sexual Interest are partition qualities. *Increased Motor Activity and Energy are threading qualities. Irritability* is a Layer quality (Layer 7 – Wickedness and Fury partitions). *Insight* is a self-awareness quality. *Disruptive or Aggressive Behavior* is a Foliate Sector property. *Content* is a normal Layer quality. *Language and Speech* are Layer qualities as they reflect pensive partitions. *Sleep* is only a semiologic quality (lack of sleep is present with many disorders). *Elevated Mood* is a threading quality.

Elements that bear Layer quality have priority over all others. Join them together into one section of the Test and accord that section the highest proportion or percentage of the scale grade. Elements that bear a chiral sector quality are second in the priority level. Determine whether pensive chirality prevalence applies to that Layer or the entire chiral Sector. Join those elements together under a single section of the Test. As to elements that bear partition quality, join them with the Layer elements. This effort would renormalize the test according to our psychophysics diagnostic drivers.

In regards to speech and language, we have already made copious and sufficient speech and language analytics in this chapter, in showing how they are both put to work in the construction of this psychometrics regime. What proceeds here is a semiologic approach geared at drawing on the typical language elements reported in the Language key of the canvasses, in this case the Bipolar Disorder canvas. Rhyming and echolalia are to a large extent typical of manic morbidity.

One important remark about Mood. *Euphoria* is not a mood element, it is a pensive partition in its full right. Likewise *cheerful* is not a mood attribute per se either, instead it relates to the *Euphoria* partition as an explicit expression of the same. Note that *Admiration* may also lead to an explicit expression of cheerfulness (i.e. clapping).

6.22 Young Mania Rating Scale (YMRS) Redesigned

Following is an example of rework of the YMRS by applying the above criteria. The clinician administers the evaluation and looks for genuine and truthful answers to the fullest extent possible. Each question or evaluative element of the test is marked with the assigned score points. They each call for a yes or no answer and receive either the full score or a 0 score as indicated.

The numeric scale itself is built in for a total of 100 points. A total of 70 to 100 points is required for a qualifying diagnosis of Mania. A total that lies between inclusive 50 to 69 points qualifies a diagnosis of Hypomania. Any accumulated total that is below 50 points disqualifies the diagnosis of Mania or Hypomania. Note as well that the diagnosis of Hypomania additionally requires at least two of the group of items 6, 7 and 8 to be positive.

It is also clear that what is being evaluated here is Mania alone as a single instance Disorder. It is not a test of Mania in the context of the cluster of Bipolar Disorder syndromes. Therefore a negative result here may still leave the possibility of Manic dysfunction as the Manic phase of Bipolar Disorder, particularly when the final score is in the high 40's or the majority of the questions rated at 1.36 points receive a positive answer. In that event, the clinician may quickly test for the Bipolar context by probing the existence of behavioral swings among the patient's symptoms. This probe equates a differential diagnosis assessment destined to widen the diagnostic scope to a broader dysfunctional context. Should the swing probe be positive, the clinician could then execute a thorough evaluation for Depression as known in the Depressive phase of Bipolar Disorder.

The reworked YMRS follows:

1. Noticeable decrease in sleep - (1.25) / (0)
2. Sleeping less than normal amount by two hours or more - (1.25) / (0)

3. Only sleeps for one hour or two through the night - (1.25) / (0)
4. Decreased need for sleep - (1.25) / (0)
5. No need for sleep at all - (1.25) / (0)
6. Admits important behavior changes - (1.25) / (0)
7. Admits illness or being impaired - (1.25) / (0)
8. Acknowledges need for treatment - (1.25) / (0)
9. Defiant when told no to anything - (1.0) / (0)
10. Intractable in desire and behavior - (1.0) / (0)
11. Recent episodes of anger or annoyance - (1.0) / (0)
12. Imposes her presence and breaks into anyone's space - (1.0) / (0)
13. Frequently irritable and curt - (1.0) / (0)
14. Lots of agitation and disquiet - (1.0) / (0)
15. Uncooperative - (1.0) / (0)
16. Imposes her/his talk on anyone - (1.0) / (0)
17. Sarcastic attitude - (1.0) / (0)
18. Demanding; threats ; hostile behavior - (1.0) / (0)
19. Shouting - (1.0) / (0)
20. Assaultive; destructive - (1.0) / (0)
21. Disparages or denigrates loved ones - (1.0) / (0)
22. Apt at unearthing other people's weaknesses or defects - (1.0) / (0)
23. Alcohol use – Drug use - (1.0) / (0)
24. Definite subjective elevation; - (1.0) / (0)
25. Increased speech rate or amount at times - (1.0) / (0)
26. Push - Pressured speech - (1.0) / (0)
27. Uninterrupted - continuous speech - (1.0) / (0)
28. Elevated Mood - (1.0) / (0)
29. Increased excitement - (1.0) / (0)
30. Definite subjective elevation; - (1.0) / (0)
31. Optimistic, self-confident - (1.0) / (0)
32. Cheerful - (1.0) / (0)
33. Elevation in mood that is inappropriate to content; humorous - (1.0) / (0)
34. Increased Motor Activity or Energy - (1.0) / (0)
35. Pacing or frequently moves from one location to another - (1.0) / (0)
36. Animated; gestures increased - (1.0) / (0)
37. Excessive energy; hyperactive at times; restless - (1.0) / (0)
38. Motor excitement; continuous hyperactivity that cannot be calmed - (1.0) / (0)
39. Erratic motor behavior, ie reckless driving - (1.0) / (0)

40. Euphoric, inappropriate laughter (laughters for no reason) - (1.36) / (0)
41. Frequent singing - (1.36) / (0)
42. Playing and listening to music all day and overnight - (1.36) / (0)
43. On spur of moments feels driven to play musical instruments the person never played before - (1.36) / (0)
44. Definite subjective increase of sexual interest - seeks to revive old loves - (1.36) / (0)
45. Spontaneous sexual content - (1.36) / (0)
46. Elaborates on sexual matters - (1.36) / (0)
47. Hypersexual (sexual advances or persistent seduction) - (1.36) / (0)
48. Overt sexual acts - (1.36) / (0)
49. Feeling excessive need for admiration - (1.36) / (0)
50. Distractible, loses goal of thought - (1.36) / (0)
51. Changes topics frequently - (1.36) / (0)
52. Racing through thoughts - Flight of ideas - tangential ideation - (1.36) / (0)
53. Difficult to follow; rhyming, echolalia - (1.36) / (0)
54. Incoherent; communication impossible - (1.36) / (0)
55. Undertakes endless simultaneous tasks without completing them - (1.36) / (0)
56. Questionable plans of travel - (1.36) / (0)
57. Questionable plans for or effecting untimely tourism, visits to remote natural parks or entertainment park - (1.36) / (0)
58. Ex-abrupto and impulsive travel without adequate planning, accomodation and discussion with family members, which may lead to disruptive consequences. - (1.36) / (0)
59. Desire for reckless adventures - (1.36) / (0)
60. Sudden new inordinary or unusual interests - (1.36) / (0)
61. Gives away significant amount of money to friends or charity indiscriminatingly - (1.36) / (0)
62. Makes unsound investment(s) - (1.36) / (0)
63. Spends money incontrolably in anything and everything - (1.36) / (0)
64. Shows little interest in work or to make money from work - (1.36) / (0)
65. Blatant downplay of or irresponsibility with financial obligations - (1.36) / (0)
66. Hearing or seeing God, the Devil or Angels - (1.36) / (0)
67. Hearing or seeing or talking to deceased relatives - (1.36) / (0)
68. Singing religious songs even at the wee hours - (1.36) / (0)

69. Ideas of reference: incessant, frantic and solemn talk about national history, political/historic figures in one-way impenetrable conversations or monologues - (1.36) / (0)
70. Expresses baseless determination to lead the nation, become president or first lady - (1.36) / (0)
71. Expresses determination to change the Constitution - (1.36) / (0)
72. Garb with extremely bright eye-catching colors - (1.36) / (0)
73. Overdressed - (1.36) / (0)
74. Garish make-up - (1.36) / (0)
75. Bizarre garb - (1.36) / (0)
76. Sexually provocative vestimentation - (1.36) / (0)
77. Obsession with order, lush and light - (1.36) / (0)
78. Turns virtually ALL home lights ON, day and night and/or adds more lights to windows and outlets - (1.36) / (0)
79. Decorates and/or cleans the home constinually, day and night and over-decorates - (1.36) / (0)
80. Fixation with shiny and colorful objects - rings decorative bells - (1.36) / (0)
81. Prepares lavish meals and drinks - (1.36) / (0)
82. Prepares large amounts of stocked food - Endless cooking - (1.36) / (0)
83. Serves dinner with full china to no invite and never discharges the table - (1.36) / (0)

6.23 Conclusion

This psychometrics regime altogether is a theoretical product resulting from the analytic psychophysics perspective central to this treatise. It has been guided by the authors' critical personal life experience and clinical practice as relates to observation in particular. As is, it does not pretend to be valid, accurate or reliable to any particular degree, as we understand that only in the foundry of broad empirical experimentation undertaken in research labs and across clinical settings it may garner adequate performance ratings and subsequent applicable corrections. Initial and adopted use of these prescriptions should therefore be considered at this stage experimental and the clinician should be prepared to tweak them as necessary toward exacting and perfecting them to fitness for proficient practice. The authors make no representation of any other claims thereof.

Glossary of Meta-Representations

Abyss

***Abstraction Vector:* --**

Symbolic Value: mother's matrix - **QG Foliate Signature: [Layer 6]**

Symbolic Value: Unconscious Cognos - **QG Foliate Signature: [Layers 5 through 9]**

Symbolic Value: menacing unknown - QG Foliate Signature: [Layer 7]

Meta-Representation Exemplification: *I find myself at the top edge of a canyon. I look down and I felt very afraid of falling down into this giant rift.*

Adventurer

Abstraction Vector: *female dancing with an unknown free spirit*

Symbolic Value: inner creativity - **QG Foliate Signature: [Layer 5]**

Symbolic Value: deployment and mobilization abilities.

QG Foliate Signature: [Animus Sector]

Meta-Representation Exemplification: *A Caucasian woman dreams that she had met an adventurer who was a black man. He took her in hers arms and they started dancing. She felt pleasure and repulsion at the same time. He was dancing like a forest vine as she felt.*

Amputation

***Abstraction Vector:* -- --**

Symbolic Value: a physical disruption (fear of impotence and castration) - **QG Foliate Signature: [Layer 7]**

Symbolic Value: a harsh punishment (feelings of shame or guilt) - **QG Foliate Signature: [Layer 4]**

Meta-Representation Exemplification: dreaming of losing a leg, foot or tooth: *I was in my office. I realized that my right arm was amputated and I was terrified. I said to my boss: please do not lay me off, find me work I can do with my left arm!*

Angel

***Abstraction Vector:* --**

Symbolic Value: Androgyny

QG Foliate Signature: [Anima or Animus Sector]

Meta-Representation Exemplification: *I saw an all whitish winged angel standing on the ground and he was smiling.*

Army

***Abstraction Vector:* --**

Symbolic Value: Aggressive instincts

Symbolic Value: a blind pugnacious force (fear of rape or violation in women)

QG Foliate Signature: [Layer 7]

Meta-Representation Exemplification: *A marching army on its way*

Ascension (Flight)

***Abstraction Vector:* --**

Symbolic Value: a transition from low to high (desire for self-perfecting or sublimation)

QG Foliate Signature: [Layer 9]

Meta-Representation Exemplification: *I frequently dream I am flying quite high and going through the tree foliages and over roofs. I could keep the height for a long stretch, though worried about keeping myself afloat. Most of the time*

I end up disappointedly landing on the ground unable to stay in flight.

Attic

Abstraction Vector: --

Symbolic Value: past, childhood - QG Foliate Signature: [Unconscious Cognos]

Symbolic Value: Elevation

QG Foliate Signature: [Layer 9]

Meta-Representation Exemplification: *I climb up to the attic to discover a nice mess of things thrown away here and there, although in real life I keep my attic well ordered.*

Automobile

Abstraction Vector: --

Symbolic Value: means of or path to freedom

QG Foliate Signature: [Layer 5]

Meta-Representation Exemplification: *I was at the steering wheel of a running car which did not belong to me.*

Baptism

Abstraction Vector: --

Symbolic Value: internal purification, washing the soul

QG Foliate Signature: [Layer 6] or [Layer 8]

Meta-Representation Exemplification: *see Water*

Bath (see Baptism)

Abstraction Vector: --

Bicycle

Abstraction Vector: --

Symbolic Value: means of independence and freedom, the mobilizing self.

QG Foliate Signature: [Animus Sector]

Meta-Representation Exemplification: *The dreamer is on a bike pedaling hard to get up the hill. The bike becomes squeaky and moves very little forward.*

Bird (see Ascension)

Blood

Abstraction Vector: --

Symbolic Value: energy, vital force (relates to fire)

QG Foliate Signature: [Layer 1]

QG Foliate Signature: [Layer 6]

Meta-Representation Exemplification: *The dreamer is enraged against a white lily plant. He takes a knife and plunges it in. Red blood comes out of the lily. He feels sexually aroused.*

Box

Abstraction Vector: --

Symbolic Value: a mystery or secret of a feminine tenure

QG Foliate Signature: [Layer 6]

Meta-Representation Exemplification: *a female sees herself receiving a beautiful box with an enticing design; she opens it up but became fearful of its content.*

Canoe

Abstraction Vector: --

Symbolic Value: inner voyage of self-discovery, bold introspection

QG Foliate Signature: [Layer 4]

Meta-Representation Exemplification: *attempting to jump off a boat or missing a boat that just took off.*

Castle

Abstraction Vector: --

Symbolic Value: noble action in a difficult enterprise
QG Foliate Signature: [Layer 4]
Meta-Representation Exemplification: *I am heading to a castle built on top of a rocky hill, stones are rolling under my feet. I intend to save someone in danger, somebody young, a woman perhaps. I had to fight against the guards to make my way in. They let me in and then I found myself in pitch darkness.*

Catastrophe
Abstraction Vector: --
Symbolic Value: anxiety, internal turmoil (fear of incapacitation)
QG Foliate Signature: [Layer 7]
Meta-Representation Exemplification: *all forms of nightmarish dreams familiar to most and which generally see the dreamer waking up in emotional turmoil.*

Child
Abstraction Vector: --
Symbolic Value (positive): an essential element of personality sprouting - QG Foliate Signature: [Layer 5].
Symbolic Value (negative): an essential element of personality being lost - QG Foliate Signature: [Layer 7]
Meta-Representation Exemplification: *the dreamer loses a child in a big crowd of people.*

Church
Abstraction Vector: --
Symbolic Value: mother figure, affectiveness, deeper unconscious or spirituality.
QG Foliate Signature: [Layer 9]
Meta-Representation Exemplification: *to get into a church (initiate a spiritual renovation).*
to get out of a church (undertake the rite of initiation toward a higher plane in life).

Cliff (see Abyss)
Abstraction Vector: --

Colors (see p. 707-719)

Cow
Abstraction Vector: --
Symbolic Value: Mother figure
QG Foliate Signature: [Layer 6]
Meta-Representation Exemplification: *The dreamer walks on a green pasture and finds himself in the middle of a herd of cows. Hunger gets the best of him as he attempts to milk a cow.*

Cradle
Abstraction Vector: --
Symbolic Value: safety, maternal safety (in that it is an extension of the mother's safe arms)
QG Foliate Signature: [Layer 6]
Meta-Representation Exemplification: *The dreamer sees a small boat on the water in which there is a child. The boat is moving along with the water that was flowing in quiet. He wakes up feeling happy.*

Crowd
Abstraction Vector: --
Symbolic Value: blind extant force
QG Foliate Signature: [Layer 7]
Alternatively:
if naked within a crowd, feeling of inferiority and guilt - QG Foliate Signature: [Layer 4].

if fusing within the crowd, desire to return to mother's care and attention - QG Foliate Signature: [Layer 6]
Meta-Representation Exemplification:

Dance
Abstraction Vector: --
Symbolic Value: birth or rebirth of internal harmony
QG Foliate Signature: [Layer 6]
Meta-Representation Exemplification: *the dreamer attends to a tribal dance while of a Safari trip.*

Dead Leaves
Abstraction Vector: --
Symbolic Value: end of life (sadness and melancholy, remote past) - QG Foliate Signature: [Layer 6]
Symbolic Value: feeling of anxiety, horror - QG Foliate Signature: [Layer 7]
Meta-Representation Exemplification: *the dreamer finds himself/herself buried to the neck into a stack of dead leaves.*

Decapitation
Abstraction Vector: --
Symbolic Value: death of sane mental life
QG Foliate Signature: [Layer 7]
Meta-Representation Exemplification: *to dream of being beheaded by brutal rebels.*

Departure
Abstraction Vector: --
Symbolic Value: abandonment (angst or fear of abandonment)
QG Foliate Signature: [Layer 6]
Meta-Representation Exemplification: *to dream that someone familiar to the dreamer is leaving or moving away.*

Fire
Abstraction Vector: --
Symbolic Value (positive): Father figure, constructive energy or light that guides toward internal truths
QG Foliate Signature: **[Animus Sector of Foliate] influenced by positive Father figure**
Symbolic Value (negative): Father figure, destructive energy
QG Foliate Signature: [Animus Sector of Foliate] influenced by negative Father figure + [Layer 7]
Meta-Representation Exemplification: *a dream vision of one setting a camp on fire without use of matches.*

Fish
Abstraction Vector: --
Symbolic Value: inner harmony
QG Foliate Signature: [Layer 6]
Meta-Representation Exemplification: dream of a large number of fish of every color swimming in clear water.

Flag
Abstraction Vector: --
Symbolic Value: union between male and female (totality)
QG Foliate Signature: [Right + Left Chiral Sectors]
Symbolic Value for a flag at half staff: internal pain or distress
QG Foliate Signature: [Layer 6 Left-chiral]
Meta-Representation Exemplification: *to erect or plant a flag into the ground*

Flowers
Abstraction Vector: --
Symbolic Value: contentment of heart

QG Foliate Signature: [Layer 6 Right-Chiral]
Meta-Representation Exemplification: *to dream of picking daffodils down the valley and making a necklace of them.*

Flying Saucer
Abstraction Vector: --
Symbolic Value (positive): hope of a better world - QG Foliate Signature: [Layer 8]
Symbolic Value (negative): psychological apocalypsis - QG Foliate Signature: [Layer 7]
Meta-Representation Exemplification: *Bright and silent, an unidentified craft flies at low altitude. Then it stops and lands on the ground. A kind man comes out, he is getting ready to speak. The dreamer wakes up.*

Fog
Abstraction Vector: --
Symbolic Value: a state of indifferentiation furnishing a potential ground to change, a change underway.
QG Foliate Signature: [Layer 5]
Meta-Representation Exemplification: *a vision of being lost on a foggy beach and unable to find one's way to safety.*

Forest
Abstraction Vector: --
Symbolic Value: a vast natural (non men-made or self-made) asset.
QG Foliate Signature: [Unconscious Cognos]
Meta-Representation Exemplification: *The dreamer steps into a vast forest or the dreamer comes out of the forest.*

Fountain
Abstraction Vector: --
Symbolic Value: accumulating fluid of an elemental source (like a spring) - **QG Foliate Signature:** [Anima Sector]
Symbolic Value: an active flow or jet of elemental fluid (like a geyser) - **QG Foliate Signature: [Animus Sector]**
Symbolic Value: rejuvenation - **QG Foliate Signature: [Layer 5]**
Symbolic Value: a dry fountain has value of scarcity of the elemental resource, for a stamp of self-devalorization or incapacitation - **QG Foliate Signature: [Layer 3 Left-chiral]**
Meta-Representation Exemplification: *I am in a giant forest that feels like a jungle. I took a slim way to a secret location deep inside of it where a treasure has been waiting for me.*

Hero
Abstraction Vector: --
Symbolic Value: aspiration to social significance
QG Foliate Signature: [Layer 4]
Meta-Representation Exemplification: *I was going around on my Harley-Davidson. My moves were fantastic and attracted hundreds of looks. Other motorists joined me while the crowd pushed back. I believe we were up to a bank robbery when I suddenly woke up.*

Hippie
Abstraction Vector: --
Symbolic Value: a shadowy character (another shadowy side of self)
QG Foliate Signature: [Layer 5]
Meta-Representation Exemplification: *Somebody knocked at my door. When I opened the door, I saw a rough man in black, messy hair, unshaven with a very puffy beard. He said: love running after the seasons.*

Horse
Abstraction Vector: --
Symbolic Value: fitness with humans to support human locomotion
QG Foliate Signature: [Layer 8]
Meta-Representation Exemplification: *The dreamer sees himself on a white horse that was slowly moving with classy steps toward a forest. He wakes up amidst a sensation of wonder.*

Hospital
Abstraction Vector: --
Symbolic Value: place to be taken care of (desire of a regression toward the fostering of childhood)
QG Foliate Signature: [Layer 6]
Meta-Representation Exemplification: *the dreamer wakes up in a hospital and cannot get out of bed.*

Hospital Operation Room
Abstraction Vector: --
Symbolic Value: removal of parts of the body in operation rooms (fear of mutilation and castration of one's personality)
QG Foliate Signature: [Layer 7 Left-Chiral]
Meta-Representation Exemplification: *a vision of being in an operation room and hoping for the doctor not to induce you.*

Hotel
Abstraction Vector: --
Generic Symbolic Value: Associativity in fact of one concierge kiosk controlling access to and exit out of all rooms, and all rooms only able to call or interact with concierge.
QG Foliate Signature: [Layer 3]
(1) Symbolic Value: interim care
QG Foliate Signature: [Layer 3 Left-chiral]
Meta-Representation Exemplifications: *To be in a shoddy hotel but felt comfortable enough to not want to leave.*
(2) Symbolic Value: one's own status or worth (miserabilism, feeling of inferiority)

House
Abstraction Vector: --
Generic Symbolic Value: entire self in social life
QG Foliate Signature: [Layers 1 through 9]
Meta-Representation Exemplification: *Touring all the rooms of a simple but beautiful home. Many roads are tied to the house as in a mandala.*

Shutters
Abstraction Vector: --
Symbolic Value: a mask shielding the real inner self.
QG Foliate Signature: [Layer 6]
(2) Door and doorstep
Symbolic Value: passage toward the inner self
QG Foliate Signature: [Layer 4]
(3) Windows
Meta-Representation Exemplification: *a vision of window shutters in one's home while trying to isolate oneself.*

Hunt
Abstraction Vector: --
Symbolic Value: prosecution (repressed sadism in men or male lesbian tendencies in women)
Symbolic Value: victimization urges (repressed masochism)

QG Foliate Signature: [Layer 7 Right-Chiral or Left-chiral]
Meta-Representation Exemplification: *a vision of going hunting in the woods with friends and continually missing targets.*

Island
Abstraction Vector: --
Symbolic Value: paradise (sun-star), autonomy in isolation
QG Foliate Signature: [Layer 1]
Meta-Representation Exemplification: *I was on an island. I ignore how I got there. I was alone. It is a radiant and nurturing island. Looking at the horizon, I thought for myself the earth is so round.*

Jewel
Abstraction Vector: --
Symbolic Value: stellar balance of the personality
QG Foliate Signature: natural balance (within disparity) between the two Chiral Sectors of Foliate
Meta-Representation Exemplification: *I invested my entire fortune in a large diamond stone. Then I saved it in a small box and buried it in the back yard garden.*

King / Queen
Abstraction Vector: --
Symbolic Value: father and mother
QG Foliate Signature: Anima and Animus Sectors
Meta-Representation Exemplification: -

Locomotive
Abstraction Vector: --
Symbolic Value: inner projective power, creative affectiveness
QG Foliate Signature: [Animus Sector]
Meta-Representation Exemplification: *I was in a luxury train, first class. But this train was not moving. I leaned through the window and saw a deficient locomotive, driven by an unskilled engineer.*

Marriage
Abstraction Vector: --
Symbolic Value: union of inner aspects of the personality or between self and the natural world - harmonization between Anima and Animus
QG Foliate Signature: [Anima Sector] + [Animus Sector]
Meta-Representation Exemplification: vision of *getting married with an unknown man or woman.*

Moon
Abstraction Vector: --
Symbolic Value: freedom of romantic expression
QG Foliate Signature: [Layer 6]
Meta-Representation Exemplification: *the dreamer flies in a rocket by the moon and touches it with his palm.*

Mud
Abstraction Vector: --
Symbolic Value: being obnoxiously stuck or incapacitated
QG Foliate Signature: [Layer 7]
Meta-Representation Exemplification: vision of *being stuck in a mud field - getting drown in a mud field.*

Music
Abstraction Vector: --
Symbolic Value: personal expressiveness
QG Foliate Signature: [Layer 6]

Meta-Representation Exemplification: *I a dream vision of hearing discordant musical notes on the piano while laying in bed.*

Notebook

Abstraction Vector: --
Symbolic Value: anxiety of being tested or submitted to stressing work, feelings of abandonment by mother to the stress work of school during childhood. - Same as Separation Anxiety
QG Foliate Signature: [Layers 6-7]
Meta-Representation Exemplification: *I was on the bus going to work. In my pits, my workbooks along with a small mysterious package. While still on my way, I opened the package: my true primary school notebooks were in there. I became anxious and wanted to leave the bus.*

Nudity

Abstraction Vector: --
Symbolic Value: freedom from "social rules and customs"
QG Foliate Signature: [Layer 4]
Meta-Representation Exemplification: *I was heading to my mother's house. There was a crowd on the street. Suddenly my zipper opened and my pant belt gave way. I became bottom naked in the middle of the street and was in complete embarrassment.*

Ocean (see Water)

Numbers (see p.55-58)

Party

Abstraction Vector: --
Symbolic Value: celebration of a participatory transformation
QG Foliate Signature: [Layer 8]
Meta-Representation Exemplification: *I was singing a religious air. It was blissfull. All the women came out to sing with me. The tree tops were going up and down in accord with with the tone of the music that seemed like a Gregorian. A majestuous tune. I was surprised at myself who normally does not sing, and so were the women who were happy to sing with me.*

Plane positive

Abstraction Vector: --
Symbolic Value: to be in a plane is a quest for spirituality
QG Foliate Signature: [Layer 9]
Meta-Representation Exemplification: *the dreamer is aboard a plane which he is piloting himself.*

Plane negative

Abstraction Vector: --
Symbolic Value: a plane crash is an imminent crash of inner structures
QG Foliate Signature: [Layer 7]
Meta-Representation Exemplification: *Passenger in a plane where the pilot turned to a nose dive, impervious to the dreamer's screams of terror.*

Prince and Princess

Abstraction Vector: --
Symbolic Value: if dual, bipolar Sexual expression of the personality - if single, unipolar sexual expression as male or female
QG Foliate Signature: [Anima Sector] and/or [Animus Sector]
Meta-Representation Exemplification: a male dreams that he is in the company of the most beautiful princess. All of her attention was put on him.

Prostitute
***Abstraction Vector:* --**
Symbolic Value: the bad mother
QG Foliate Signature: hyperactive or over accrued [Anima Sector]
Meta-Representation Exemplification:
a dream vision by a female that she is a prostitute and feels eager to meet with another prostitute in the new brothel.

Rainbow
***Abstraction Vector:* --**
Symbolic Value: a celestial bridge (one that unifies the personality) or a higher alliance
QG Foliate Signature: [Layer 9]
Meta-Representation Exemplification:
to dream that one is flying on a rainbow.

Ring
***Abstraction Vector:* --**
Symbolic Value: union of opposite poles or alliance of matching parts
QG Foliate Signature: [Layer 6]
Meta-Representation Exemplification:
the dreamer wears a ring that is too tight. It has to be adjusted.

River (see Valley)

Rose
***Abstraction Vector:* --**
Symbolic Value positive: woman, female bloom, blooming feminity
QG Foliate Signature: [Layer 6 Right-Chiral]
Meta-Representation Exemplification:
to dream that one receives beautiful roses of several different color tones.
Symbolic Value negative: sentimental deception
QG Foliate Signature: [Layer 7 Left-Chiral]
Meta-Representation Exemplification:
to dream that one receives fake roses of different color hues.

School Test (see School Notebooks)

Sea
***Abstraction Vector:* --**
Symbolic Value: untamed immensity
QG Foliate Signature: [Layer 6 Left-Chiral]
Meta-Representation Exemplification:
the dreamer finds herself lost at sea in a small canoe. Then a cruise ship approaches the canoe to rescue her.

Secret
***Abstraction Vector:* --**
Symbolic Value (positive): a hidden treasure
QG Foliate Signature: [Layer 6 Right-Chiral]
Meta-Representation Exemplification:
the dreamer takes to a long journey around the world. Along the way she meets with a secret admirer.

Ship
***Abstraction Vector:* --**
Symbolic Value: Mother figure
QG Foliate Signature: [Layer 6]
Meta-Representation Exemplification: *I was aboard a ship headed to the Bermuda Triangle. In the middle of high seas I realized that there was no captain. The crew men were running up and down with no direction and the boat started speeding up. I woke up (female dream).*

Shoe

Abstraction Vector: --
Symbolic Value: vagina in sexual intercourse
QG Foliate Signature: [Layer 6]
Meta-Representation Exemplification: *A male dreams he is busily putting his foot into a white shoe or a white sock tendered to him by the mother of his spouse.*

Sibling

Abstraction Vector: --
Symbolic Value: duality and ambivalence
QG Foliate Signature: [Layer 2]
Meta-Representation Exemplification: *A male dreams he is taking a walk with his brother who resembles him like a twin. He is happy and apprehensive at the same time. He told his brother: I was born in 1922 (in reality he was born in 1927).*

Socks

Abstraction Vector: --
Symbolic Value: when putting socks onto one's feet, sexual intercourse
QG Foliate Signature: [Layer 6]
Meta-Representation Exemplification: *A male dreamer sees himself busily putting his foot into a white sock tendered to him by the mother of his spouse. He wakes up aroused.*

Sky

Abstraction Vector: --
Symbolic Value: open ended vastness above (Hyper-asymptotic personality center)
QG Foliate Signature: [Hypercursor] dynamics
Meta-Representation Exemplification: *The dreamer insistently scrutinizes and stares at the blue sky and realizes it is limitless.*

Snake

Abstraction Vector: --
Symbolic Value: dangerous biting snake
Symbolic Value: Erect Cobra: Mankind, human phylogenesis
QG Foliate Signature: [Layer 8]
Meta-Representation Exemplification: *a female dreamer sees herself following a blue snake. They arrive at the edge of a large river. The snake sneaks into the river and crosses through. She follows the snake swimming after her.*

Spider

Abstraction Vector: --
Symbolic Value: mutation, personality transformation
QG Foliate Signature: [Layer 5]
Meta-Representation Exemplification: *a female dreamer sees a big white spider somewhere she cannot tell. It was soft like velvet. (She is normally afraid of spiders!). The web was detached and filled up with iridescent water droplets.*

Stable positive

Abstraction Vector: --
Symbolic Value: desire for inner changes for the better (cleaning up a stable)
QG Foliate Signature: [Layer 8]
Meta-Representation Exemplification: *to clean up the stable for the next derby in one's dream and hoping to win a trifecta.*

Stable negative

Abstraction Vector: --

Symbolic Value: feeling of disquiet or threat of destruction of one's inner world (i.e. stable destroyed).

QG Foliate Signature: [Layer 7]

Meta-Representation Exemplification: *The dreamer arrives at an old animal barn, wants to get in but a log blocks its door.*

Staff (same as Tree trunk)

Stairs

Abstraction Vector: --

Symbolic Value: work and effort to ascend to a higher level or the degradation of descending to a lower level

QG Foliate Signature [Hybrid Thread]

Meta-Representation Exemplification: *the dreamer stands in front of a long stairway. He then takes to climb the stairs one after another. When he reached the top, he started feeling dizzy.*

Stool

Abstraction Vector: --

Symbolic Value (positive): vital forces, personal freedom of expression.

Abstraction Vector: --

QG Foliate Signature: [Right-chiral Foliate Sector]

Meta-Representation Exemplification:--

Symbolic Value (negative): indication of personality retention

Abstraction Vector: --

QG Foliate Signature: [Left-chiral Foliate Sector]

Meta-Representation Exemplification:--

Sun

Abstraction Vector: --

Symbolic Value: enlightenment, fortitude, power.

QG Foliate Signature: [Right-chiral Foliate Sector]

Meta-Representation Exemplification: *to dream of seeing the sun coming out in the middle of the night.*

Torn Clothing

Abstraction Vector: --

Symbolic Value: feelings of anxiety and impotence

QG Foliate Signature: [Left-chiral Layer 7]

Meta-Representation Exemplification: *the dreamer sees himself dressed up in torn clothing.*

Trains

Abstraction Vector: --

Symbolic Value: social life

Symbolic Value: to miss the train is parting with the rest of society (reflects feelings of inadequation or inferiority in comparison to others)

QG Foliate Signature: [Layer 4]

Meta-Representation Exemplification: *frequently dreamer misses the train schedule and commits errors in navigation, i.e seizing the wrong operator control device or being in the wrong compartment per the fare paid for, etc.*

Tree

Abstraction Vector: --

Symbolic Value: virility, Father.

Symbolic Value (If with lots of foliage): safety, refuge, Mother

Roots of the Tree

Symbolic Value: Foundation

QG Foliate Signature: [Unconscious Cognos]
Trunk of the Tree
Symbolic Value: Personal level of empowerment or projective capacity
QG Foliate Signature: [Right-Chiral Sector of Foliate]
Meta-Representation Exemplification (for Trunk): *the dreamer finds himself in a forest of dead tree trunks and waits for the rain to bring them back to life.*

Triangle
Abstraction Vector: --
Symbolic Value: Social life of dreamer
QG Foliate Signature: [Conscious Cognos]
Meta-Representation Exemplification: *the dreamer finds himself motionless on a horizontal plane. Two obliquous paths start from this plane, without ever intersecting however.*

Valley
Symbolic Value: fertility, rich inner life
QG Foliate Signature: [Layer 8 right-chiral]
Meta-Representation Exemplification:

War
Abstraction Vector: --
Symbolic Value: affective and/or moral conflicts
QG Foliate Signature: [Layer 7]
Meta-Representation Exemplification:

Wardrobe
Abstraction Vector: --
Symbolic Value: psychosocial norms of the dreamer
QG Foliate Signature: [Layer 4]
Meta-Representation Exemplification: a vision that the dreamer's wardrobe is outdated and no longer fits in the closet.

Water
Abstraction Vector: --
Symbolic Value (positive): flexibility, softness, fluidity - QG Foliate Signature: [Layer 8]
Symbolic Value (negative): black water, agitated waters - **QG Foliate Signature: [Layer 7] or [Depressive Left-Chiral Sector of Foliate]**
Meta-Representation Exemplification: *I was in the midst of a vast ocean with menacing waters. Was trying to get out and resisting getting drowned.*

Window
Abstraction Vector: --
Symbolic Value: level of openness to the world in consideration of the future from present
QG Foliate Signature: [Layer 4]
Meta-Representation Exemplification: *dreamer is looking through the window (See House)*

Woods
Abstraction Vector: --
Symbolic Value: one's internal world (quest for spirituality)
QG Foliate Signature: [Unconscious Cognos]
Meta-Representation Exemplification: *heading the way of a secret place inside the woods or forest where a hidden treasure is awaiting.*

Bibliography

(n.d.). Retrieved from Stanford University's Plato Encyclopedia: https://plato.stanford.edu/entries/plato/

(2000). "Chapter 16: Personality Disorders". In *DSM-IV-TR Diagnostic and Statistical Manual of Mental Disorders.* American Psychiatric Publishing.

Abramowitz, J. S. (2002). A Contemporary Conceptual Model of Hypochondriasis. *Mayo Clin Proc , 77,* 1323-1330.

Adibhatla, R. M. (2007). Role of Lipids in Brain Injury and Diseases. *Future Lipidol. , 2* (4), 403-422.

Adorno, T. W. (1950). *The authoritarian personality.* New York: Harper.

Al-Zaben, F. N. (2012). Suicidal Obsessions in a Patient with Obsessive Compulsive Disorder: A Case Report. *JKAU: Med Sci , 19* (4), 121-127.

Alzheimer's Disease Facts and Figures. (2021). *Alzheimers Dement , 17* (3).

American Medical Association. (2020). *ICD-10-CM 2021: The Complete Official Codebook with Guidelines (ICD-10-CM the Complete Official Codebook)* (First ed.). USA: AAPC.

American Psychiatric Association. (2013). *Diagnostic and statistical manual of mental disorders: DSM-5* (Fifth ed.). Washington, D. C.: American Psychiatric Association.

American Psychiatric Association. (2013). *Diagnostic and Statistical manual of mental disorders: DSM-5* (Fifth ed.). Washington, D. C.: American Psychiatric Association.

American Psychiatric Association. (1994). *DSM IV: Diagnostic and Statistical Manual of Mental Disorders* (Fourth ed.). Washington, D. C.: American Psychiatric Association.

Amy L. Price, G. R.-N. (2012). Bipolar Disorders: A Review. *American Family Physician , 85* (5), 483-493.

Antúnez, L. (1979). *Anatomía Funcional del Sistema Nervioso.* Editorial Limusa.

Araji, S. F. (1985). Explanations of pedophilia: Review of empirical research. *Bull Am Acad Psychiatry Law , 13* (1), 17-37.

Arda, E. C. (2016). Primary Nocturnal Enuresis: A Review. *Nephrourol Mon , 8* (4).

Ardila, A. (1979). *Psicofisiología de los Procesos Complejos.* Editorial Trillas.

Arseni, C. a. (1977). Logorrhea syndrome with hyperkinesia. *Eur Neurol , 15* (4), 183-187.

Arvaniti, A. L. (2018). Measuring authoritarianism in a Greek health care setting. *Psychiatriki , 29* (3), 240-248.

Arvaniti, A., Livaditis, M., Kalamara, E., Vorvolakos, T., Serdari, A., & Samakouri, M. (2018). Measuring authoritarianism in a Greek health care setting. *Psychiatriki , 29* (3), 240-248.

Baggiani, G. A. (2018). Psychotropic Medication of Acute Episodes of Mood Disorders: Current Prescription Attitude in Two Psychiatric Wards in Cagliari, Italy. *Clin Pract Epidemiol Ment Health , 14*, 236-249.

Bakker, G. M. (2019). A new conception and subsequent taxonomy of clinical psychological problems. *BMC Psychology , 7* (46).

Barnet, S. a. (1975). *Barnet and Stubbs's Practical Guide to Writing.* Little Brown and Company.

Bauer, M. P. (2005). Epidemiology of Bipolar Disorders. *Epilepsia , 46* (Suppl.4), 8-13.

Benazzi, F. (2006). Various forms of depression. *Dialogues Clin Neurosci , 8* (2), 151-161.

Bereczkei, T. G. (2004). Sexual imprinting in human mate choice. *Proc Biol Sci , 271* (1544), 1129–1134.

Biederman, J. P. (2008). The long-Term Longitudinal Course of Oppositional Defiant Disorder and Conduct Disorder in ADHD boys: findings from a controlled 10-year longitudinal follow-up study. *Psychol Med , 38* (7), 1027-1036.

Binzak Fugate, J. M. (2019). What Color Is Your Anger? Assessing Color-Emotion Pairings in English Speakers. *Front Psychol , 10*, 206.

Blum, K. B. (2015). Retracted: Hypersexuality Addiction and Withdrawal: Phenomenology, Neurogenetics and Epigenetics. *Neurogenetics and Epigenetics , 7* (7).

Bravata, D. M. (2019). Prevalence, Predictors, and Treatment of Impostor Syndrome: a Systematic review. *J Gen Intern Med* , 1-24.

Cantor, J. M. (2005). Handedness in Pedophilia and Hebephilia. *Arch Sex Behav , 34* (4), 447-459.

Cantor, J. M. (2004). Intelligence, Memory and Handedness in Pedophilia. *Neuropsychology , 18* (1), 3-14.

Capra, G. A. (2014). Current Scientific Research on Paedophilia: A Review. *Journal of Psychopathology , 20*, 17-26.

Castillo, R. J. (2008). Culture, Trance, and the Mind-Brain. *Anthropology of Consciousness , 6* (1), 17-34.

Castillo, R. J. (2008). Culture, Trance, and the Mind-Brain. *Anthropology of Consciousness , 6* (1), 17-34.

Claiborn, J. P. (2002). *The BDD Workbook.* Oakland, California: New Harbinger Publications.

Collins, G. (1985, December 2). Women and Masochism: Debate Continues. (Section B), p. 12.

Cortiella, C. H. (2014). The State of Learning Disabilities: Facts, Trends and Emerging Issues. New York, NY, USA.

Daco, P. (1979). *L'Interpretation des Rêves, Editions Marabout.* Editions Marabout.

Daco, P. (1977). *Les Prodigieuses Victoires De La Psychologie.* Les Nouvelles Editions Marabout.

Daco, P. (1977). *Les Triomphes de la Psychanalyse.* Marabout: Editions Gérard et Co 1965.

Daley, M. D. (1946). Pseudocyesis. *Post-Graduate Medical Journal*, 395-399.

Daley, M. D. (1946). Pseudocyesis. *Post Med J*, 395-399.

Daley, M. D. (1946). Pseudocyesis. *Post-Graduate Medical Journal*, 395-399.

Das, J. M. (2020). *Abulia.* Treasure Island: StatPearls Publishing.

Dawson, G. (2015). Measuring Brain Lipids. *Biochim Biophys Acta.*, *1851* (8), 1026–1039.

Dawson, G. (2015). Measuring Brain Lipids. *Biochim Biophys Acta.*, *1851* (8), 1026–1039.

Day, M. (2014). Guilt. In T. R. Levine, *Encyclopedia of deception* (pp. 427-429). Thousand Oaks, California: Sage Publications.

De Leon, J. (2013). Is Psychiatry Scientific? A letter to a 21st Century Psychiatry Resident. *Psychiatry Investig*, *10* (3), 205-217.

De Neef, N. C. (2019). Bondage-Discipline, Dominance-Submission and Sadomasochism (BDSM) From an Integrative Biopsychosocial Perspective: A Systematic Review. *Sex Med*, *7* (2), 129-144.

Dena M. Bravata, S. A. (2019). Prevalence, Predictors, and Treatment of Impostor Syndrome: a Systematic review. *J Gen Intern Med*, 1-24.

Derbyshire, K. L. (2015). Compulsive Sexual Behavior: A Review of the Literature. *J Behav Addict*, *4* (2), 37-43.

Dodson, E. R. (2010). Therapeutics for Circadian Rhythm Sleep Disorders. *Sleep Med Clin*, *5* (4), 701-715.

Drouin, E. P. (2017). Demonic possession by Jean Lhermitte. *L'Encephale , 43,* 394-398.

Drouin, E., Péréon, T., & Péréon, Y. (2017). Demonic possession by Jean Lhermitte. *L'Encephale , 43,* 394-398.

Eaton, W. W. (2018). Specific Phobias. *Lancet Psychiatry , 5* (8), 678–686.

Edwards, B. (1994). *Larson, R., and Hostetler, R. Calculus of a single variable.* D.C. Heath and Company.

Ehrenreich, J. T. (2008). Separation Anxiety Disorder in Youth: Phenomenology, Assessment, and Treatment. *Psicol Conductual , 16* (3), 389–412.

Elliot, A. J. (2015). Color and psychological functioning: a review of theoretical and empirical work. *Front. Psychol , 6,* 368.

Ellis, A. A. (2009). *Personality Theories: Critical Perspectives.* Thousand Oaks, CA: Sage Publications.

Embley, D. W. (1992). *Object-Oriented System Analysis, A Model-Driven Approach.* Prentice Hall P T R.

Fedoroff, J. P. (2008). Sadism, Sadomasochism, Sex, and Violence. *Can J Psychiatry , 53* (10), 637-646.

First, M. B. (2014). DSM-5 and Paraphilic Disorders. *Journal of the American Academy of Psychiatry and the Law , 42* (2), 191-201.

Frances, A. W. (2012). Sexual Sadism: Avoiding Its Misuse in Sexually Violent Predator Evaluations. *J Am Acad Psychiatry Law , 40,* 409-416.

Frick, P. J. (2012). Current Issues in the Diagnosis of Attention Deficit Hyperactivity Disorder, Oppositional Defiant Disorder, and Conduct Disorder. *Annu Rev Clin Psychol , 8,* 77-107.

Furman, Y. W. (1997). Shakespeare and sleep disorder. *Neurology , 49* (4), 1171-1172.

Goldstein, I. (2000). Female sexual arousal disorder: new insights. *International Journal of Impotence Research , 12* (4), S152-S157.

Grant, J. E. (2016). Trichotillomania. *Treatment in Psychiatry , 173* (9), 868-874.

Grant, J. E. (2009). Update on pathological skin picking. *Current Psychiatry Reports , 11*, 283–288.

Hales, E. a. (2003). *The American Psychiatric Press Textbook of Psychiatry.* Washington DC: American Psychiatric Publishing, Inc.

Halliday, D. R. (1997). *Fundamentals of Physics* (Fifth ed.). USA: John Wiley & Sons, Inc.

Histrionic Personality Disorder. (Archived from the original on 2018-03-16). *Courses Lumen* .

Holt, R. R. (2015). On Freud's Authoritarianism. *The Psychoanalytic Review , 102* (3).

https://www.leparisien.fr/societe/des-enseignants-refusent-que-le-masculin-l-emporte-sur-le-feminin-08-11-2017-7381113.php. (2017, 11 8). Retrieved from LeParisien: https://www.leparisien.fr/societe/des-enseignants-refusent-que-le-masculin-l-emporte-sur-le-feminin-08-11-2017-7381113.php

Jagot, P.-C. (1975). *Méthode Pratique de Magnétisme, Hypnotisme et Suggestion.* Editions Dangles.

Jean-Claude, J. J. (1995). *La Quanto-Géométrie* (Vol. Tome I). Quantometrix, Inc.

Jean-Claude, J. J. (2015). *Quanto-Geometry, Overture of Cosmic Consciousness and Universal Knowledge for All* (Vol. I & II). Quantometrix, Inc.

Jean-Claude, J. J. (2015). *The Human Mind Inside.* Quantometrix, Inc.

Kaga, J. a. (1968). *Psychology An Introduction.* Hartcourt, Brace & World, Inc.

Kaufman, C. (2007, January 24). *Three-dimensional Villains: Finding Your Character's Shadow*. Retrieved from Ezinearticles:

https://ezinearticles.com/?Three-Dimensional-Villains---Finding-Your-Characters-Shadow&id=428279

Kaur, J. (2014). Bondage/Discipline, Dominance/Submission, Sadism/Masochism – The Emerging Subculture. *UC Merced Undergraduate Research Journal, 7* (2), 68-73.

Kawaia, N. e. (2017). Electroencephalogram characteristics during possession trances in healthy individuals. *Neuroreports, 28* (15), 949-955.

Kaylor, L. J. (2016). Examining the Impact of Technology on Exhibitionistic Behavior. *Deviant Behavior, 37* (10), 1152-1162.

Kelleher, I. C. (2014). Whither the psychosis-neurosis borderline. *Schizophr Bull, 40* (2), 266-268.

Kessing, B. F. (2014). Current diagnosis and management of the rumination syndrome. *J Clin Gastroenterol., 48* (6), 478-483.

Kessler, R. C. (2005). Prevalence, severity, and comorbidity of 12-month DSM-IV disorders in the National Comorbidity Survey Replication. *Arch Gen Psychiatry, 62* (6), 617-627.

Kessler, R. C. (2006). The prevalence and correlates of DSM-IV intermittent explosive disorder in the National Comorbidity Survey Replication. *Arch Gen Psychiatry, 63* (6), 669-678.

Kimberly B. Werner, L. R. (2015). Epidemiology, Comorbidity, and Behavioral Genetics of Antisocial Personality Disorder and Psychopathy. *Psychiatr Ann., 45* (4), 195-199.

Korolev, I. O. (2014). Alzheimer's Disease: A Clinical and Basic Science Review. *MSRJ, 4* (Fall), 024-033.

Kovacick, G. L. (1999). *High Technology Crime Investigator's HandbooK* (Second ed.). Butterworth-Heinemann.

L.in, T. (1997). *INFERIORITY COMPLEX. Prevention in Children and Relief from It in Adults.* Biblical Studies Ministries International, Inc.

Leonhardt, M. B. (2017). All Impostors Aren't Alike – Differentiating the Impostor Phenomenon. *Front. Psychol.*

Lessin, D. S. (2017). The impact of perfectionism on anxiety and depression. *Journal of Psychology and Cognition*, *2* (1).

Lung, D. W. (2018). Voyeuristic Disorder and Internet Pornography Addiction: A Case Report. *Mal J Med Health Sci*, *14* (3), 54-56.

Mackenzie, K. (2018). Stereotypic Movement Disorders. *Semin Pediatr Neurol*, *25*, 19-24.

Maldonado, J. R. (2008). Delirium in the acute care setting: characteristics, diagnosis and treatment. *Crit Care Clin*, *24* (4), 657-722.

Marrus, N. H. (2017). Intellectual Disability and Language Disorder. *Child Adolesc Psychiatr Clin N Am.*, *26* (3), 539–554.

Martens, W. H. (2010). Schizoid personality disorder linked to unbearable and inescapable loneliness. *Eur. J. Psychiat.*, *24* (1), 38-45.

Martens, W. H. (2010). Schizoid personality disorder linked to unbearable and inescapable loneliness. *Eur. J. Psychiat.*, *24* (1), 38-45.

Martin, J. L. (2001). The authoritarian personality, 50 years later: What questions are there for political psychology? *Political psychology*, *22* (1), 1-26.

McIntyre, R. S. (n.d.). *Pharmacological Treatment of Bipolar Disorder:2017-2018 Update Summary*, 12-23.

McIntyre, R. S. (n.d.). *Pharmacological Treatment of Bipolar Disorder:2017-2018 Update Summary*, 12-23.

McShane, L. (2013, October 15). Man who jumped into Bronx Zoo tiger den gets year in mental health facility . *New York Daily News* .

Mehler, P. S. (2015). Bulimia Nervosa – medical complications. *Journal of Eating Disorders*, *3*, 12-16.

Messias, E. C.-Y. (2007). Epidemiology of Schizophrenia: Review of Findings and Myths. *Psychiatr Clin North Am , 30* (3), 323-338.

Michael Bauer, A. P. (2005). Epidemiology of Bipolar Disorders. *Epilepsia , 46* (Suppl.4), 8-13.

Mimura, M. (2001). Comorbidity of Depression and Other Diseases. *JMAJ , 44* (5), 225-229.

Mohammed Taouis, I. T.-A. (2019). Editorial: Insulin and The Brain. *Frontiers in Endocrinology , 10*, 1-2.

Moran, P. (1999). The epidemiology of antisocial personality disorder. *Soc Psychiatry Psychiatr Epidemiol , 34* (5), 231-242.

Morein-Zamir, S. P. (2014). The profile of executive function in OCD hoarders and hoarding disorder. *Psychiatry Research. , 215* (3), 659-667.

Neumann, C. S. (2008). Psychopathic traits in a large community sample: links to violence, alcohol use, and intelligence. *J Consult Clin Psychol , 76* (5), 893-899.

Nicoletti, A. L. (2013). Obsessive compulsive personality disorder and Parkinson's disease. *PLoS One , 8* (1).

Noppen, B. V. (2010). Retrieved from International OCD Foundation: http://www.ocfoundation.org

Noppen, B. V. (2010). Retrieved from International OCD Foundation: http://www.ocfoundation.org

O'Sullivan, R. L. (1997). Trichotillomania : Behavioural Symptom or. *Am J Psychiatry , 154* (10), 1442-1449.

Oakes, L. a. (2002, 2007). *Ancient Egypt, An Illustrated to the Myths, Religions, Pyramids and Temples of the Land of the Pharaohs.* Anness Publishing.

Ono, A. (2010). Viruses and Lipids. *Viruses , 2*, 1236-1238.

Ono, A. (2010). Viruses and Lipids. *Viruses , 2*, 1236-1238.

Oosthuizen, P. C. (1998). Dysmorphic Concern: Prevalence and Associations with Clinical Variables. *Australian and New Zealand Journal of Psychiatry , 32*, 129-132.

Papadopoulos, V. a. (2007). The rumination syndrome in adults: A review of the pathophysiology, diagnosis, and treatment. *Journal of Postgraduate Medicine , 53* (3), 203-206.

Patel, K. R. (2009). Schizophrenia: Overview and Treatment Options. *P&T , 39* (9), 638-645.

Phillips, K. A. (1997). *Learning to Live With Body Dysmorphic Disorder.* Connecticut, USA: Obsessive-Compulsive Foundation.

Picchioni, M. M. (2007). Schizophrenia. *BMJ , 303*, 91-95.

Pincus, A. L. (2010). Pathological narcissism and narcissistic personality disorder. *Annual Review of Clinical Psychology , 6*, 421-446.

Pine, D. S. (1999). Pathophysiology of childhood anxiety disorders. *Biological Psychiatry , 46* (11), 1555-1566.

Pineiro, V. (2009, February 14). *A Kiss Is a Mechanism For Mate Assessment.* Retrieved from Popten: http://www.popten.net/2009/02/a-kiss-is-a-mechanism-for-mate-assessment/

Price, A. M.-N. (2012). Bipolar Disorders: A Review. *American Family Physician , 85* (5), 483-493.

Raihani, N. J. (2019). An evolutionary perspective on paranoia. *Nat Hum Behav , 3* (2), 114-121.

Rao Muralikrishna Adibhatla, J. F. (2007). Role of Lipids in Brain Injury and Diseases. *Future Lipidol. , 2* (4), 403-422.

Rew, K. T. (2016). Erectile Dysfunction. *American Family Physician , 94* (10), 820-828.

Ribeiro, V. F., Valenti, V. E., Ferreira, M., Abreu, L. C., Carvalho, T. D., Xavie, V., et al. (2014). Prevalence of burnout syndrome in clinical nurses at a hospital of excellence. *International Archives of Medicine , 7*, 22.

Ribeiro, V. F., Valenti, V. E., Ferreira, M., Abreu, L. C., Carvalho, T. D., Xavie, V., et al. (2014). Prevalence of burnout syndrome in clinical nurses at a hospital of excellence. *Int Arch Med , 7*, 22.

Ronningstam, E. (2010). Narcissistic personality disorder: A current review. *Current Psychiatry Report , 12* (1), 68-75.

Ronson, J. (2012). *The Psychopath Test: A Journey Through the Madness Industry.* Pengiun Publishing Group.

Rumbaugh, J. B. (1991). *Object-Oriented Modeling and Design.* Prentice Hall.

Rushing, J. M. (2003). Bulimia Nervosa: A Primary Care Review. *Prim Care Companion J Clin Psychiatry , 5* (5), 217-224.

Sareen, J. (2014). Posttraumatic Stress Disorder in Adults: Impact, Comorbidity, Risk Factors, and Treatment. *Can J Psychiatry , 59* (9), 46-467.

Scherer, T. O.-A. (2011). Brain Insulin Controls Adipose Tissue Lipolysis and Lipogenesis. *Cell Metabolism , 13*, 183-194.

Schredl, M. (2009). Dreams in patients with sleep disorders. *Sleep Med Rev , 13* (3), 215-21.

Scriptures, N. W. (1971). *Song of Solomon.* New York: Watch Tower Bible and Track Society of New York.

Seay, S. J. (n.d.). *Suicide Obsessions: Fear of Killing/Harming Yourself.* Retrieved from http://www.psychologyandbehavior.com/suicide-obsessions-fear-killing-yourself/

Sementovski-Kurilo, N. (1985). *Astrología: Tratado completo teórico y práctico.* Editorial Planeta.

Seto, M. C. (2018). *Pedophilia and Sexual Offending Against Children, Theory, Assessment, and Intervention* (2nd ed.). American Psychological Association.

Sharma, R. P. (2007). Vol. 10 No.1 APRIL 2007 Pseudologia Fantastica. *Delhi Psychiatry Journal , 10* (1), 77-80.

Shea, S. E. (2012). Intellectual Disability (Mental retardation). *Pediatr Rev , 33* (3), 110-21.

Shertzer, M. (1986). *The Elements of Grammar.* Collier Books McMillan Publishing Company.

Shipman, K. T. (2009). Mental health treatment of child abuse and neglect: the promise of evidence-based practice. *Pediatr Clin North Am , 56* (2), 417-428.

Small, G. W. (1986). Pseudocyesis: an overview. *Can J Psychiatry , 31*, 452.

Solmi, M. e. (2018). Prevalence of Catatonia and Its Moderators in Clinical Samples: Results from a Meta-analysis and Meta-regression Analysis. *Schizophrenia Bulletin , 44* (5), 1133–1150.

Staniloiu A., M. H. (2014). Dissociative amnesia. *The Lancet Psychiatry , 1* (3), 226-241.

Stefani, A. a. (2021). Nightmare Disorder and Isolated Sleep Paralysis. *Neurotherapeutics. , 18* (1), 100-106.

Stein, D. J. (2019). Obsessive–compulsive disorder. *Nat Rev Dis Primers , 5* (1), 52.

Świtaj, P. A. (2012). Disability and schizophrenia: a systematic review of experienced psychosocial difficulties. *BMC Psychiatry , 12*, 193-204.

Taouis, M. T.-A. (2019). Editorial: Insulin and The Brain. *Frontiers in Endocrinology , 10*, 1-2.

Thippaiah, S. M. (2018). A Case of Concomitant Pseudocyesis and Couvade Syndrome Variant. *Psychopharmacol Bull , 48* (3), 29-32.

Thomas Scherer, J. O.-A. (2011). Brain Insulin Controls Adipose Tissue Lipolysis and Lipogenesis. *Cell Metabolism , 13*, 183-194.

Thomas, R. a. (1994). *The Analysis and Design of Linear Circuits,*. Prentice-Hall, Inc.

Thomas, R. M. (2016). Speech and language deficits in separation anxiety disorder. *Advances in Pediatric Research* .

Vivian F Ribeiro, C. F., Valenti, V. E., Ferreira, M., Abreu, L. C., Carvalho, T. D., Xavie, V., et al. (2014). Prevalence of burnout syndrome in clinical nurses at a hospital of excellence. *International Archives of Medicine , 7*, 22.

Werner, K. B. (2015). Epidemiology, Comorbidity, and Behavioral Genetics of Antisocial Personality Disorder and Psychopathy. *Psychiatr Ann. , 45* (4), 195–199.

Werner, K. B. (2015). Epidemiology, Comorbidity, and Behavioral Genetics of Antisocial Personality Disorder and Psychopathy. *Psychiatr Ann. , 45* (4), 195-199.

Wetzler, A. J. (2007). Suicidal ideation versus suicidal obsession: a case report. *CNS Spectr , 12* (7), 553-556.

Wilcox, J. A. (2015). The Syndrome of Catatonia. *Behav Sci , 5* (4), 576-588.

Wright, J. J. (2015). Female Sexual Dysfunction. *Med Clin N Am , 99*, 607-628.

Zwicker, J. G. (2012). Developmental coordination disorder: a review and update. *Eur J Paediatr Neurol , 16* (6), 573-581.

Index

A

B

C

D

E

F

G

H

I

N

O

P

Q

R

S

T

U

V

W

X

The authors may be reached via email sent to:

jjc@qgmindarchitects.com *(Joseph J. Jean-Claude)*

cso@qgmindarchitects.com *(Caroline Stamu-O'Brien)*

Book website:

https://www.qgmindarchitects.com

CPSIA information can be obtained
at www.ICGtesting.com
Printed in the USA
LVHW080726050822
724594LV00003B/8/J

9 781668 541623